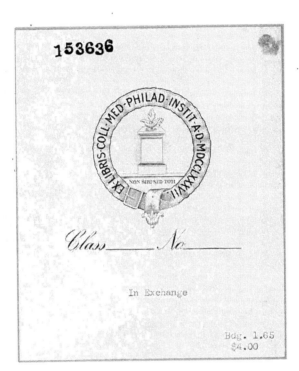

THE JOURNAL
OF THE
OKLAHOMA STATE MEDICAL ASSOCIATION

VOLUME XXXII   McALESTER, OKLAHOMA, JANUARY, 1939   Number 1

Published Monthly at McAlester, Oklahoma, under direction of the Council.

INDEX TO CONTENTS

Vol. XXXII   JANUARY   Number 1

EDITORIAL

INDEX TO ADVERTISERS ON
PAGE XIX

BALYEAT~BOWEN
HAY FEVER and ASTHMA CLINIC

OSLER BUILDING · · · · · OKLAHOMA CITY, OKLAHOMA

Devoted EXCLUSIVELY to the DIAGNOSIS and TREATMENT of ALLERGIC DISEASES

MEDICAL STAFF

Ray M. Balyeat, M.A., M.D., F.A.C.P.
Director

Ralph Bowen. B.A., M.D., F.A.A.P.
Pediatrics

George J. Seibold, B.S., M.D.
Gastroenterology

Carl L. Brundage, M.Sc., M.D.
Consultant in Dermatology

O. Alton Watson, B.S., M.D., F.A.C.S.
Consultant in Otolaryngology

GOLDFAIN RHEUMATISM-ARTHRITIS RESEARCH LABORATORY

MEDICAL ARTS BUILDING
OKLAHOMA CITY, OKLAHOMA

DEVOTED TO THE DIAGNOSIS AND TREATMENT OF RHEUMATIC DISEASES

X-RAY AND CLINICAL LABORATORY SURVEY OF EACH PATIENT

Special Attention:
Bacteriology of focal infections.
Serologic tests necessary to determine type of systemic invasion.
Preparation of vaccines.

E. GOLDFAIN, M.D.
Director

INDEX TO CONTENTS

INDEX TO ADVERTISERS ON
PAGE XIX

INDEX TO CONTENTS

Vol. XXXII   APRIL   Number 4

INDEX TO ADVERTISERS ON
PAGE VI

INDEX TO CONTENTS

Vol. XXXII   MAY   Number 5

INDEX TO ADVERTISERS ON
PAGE VI

INDEX TO CONTENTS

Vol. XXXII   JUNE   Number 6

INDEX TO CONTENTS

Vol. XXXII   JULY   Number 7

BALYEAT
Hay Fever and Asthma
Clinic

OSLER BUILDING · · · · OKLAHOMA CITY, OKLAHOMA

Devoted EXCLUSIVELY to the DIAGNOSIS and TREATMENT of ALLERGIC DISEASES

MEDICAL STAFF

Ray M. Balyeat, M.A., M.D., F.A.C.P.
Director

George R. Felts, B.S., M.D.
Pediatrics

Carl L. Brundage, M.Sc., M.D.
Consultant in Dermatology

Wayne M. Hull, M.S., M.D., F.S.C.P.
Gastroenterology

Onis Geo. Hazel, D.S., M.D.
Consultant in Dermatology

O. Alton Watson, B.S., M.D., F.A.C.S.
Consultant in Otolarynology

GOLDFAIN RHEUMATISM-ARTHRITIS RESEARCH LABORATORY

MEDICAL ARTS BUILDING
OKLAHOMA CITY, OKLAHOMA

DEVOTED TO THE DIAGNOSIS AND TREATMENT OF RHEUMATIC DISEASES

X-RAY AND CLINICAL LABORATORY SURVEY OF EACH PATIENT

Special Attention:
Bacteriology of focal infections.
Serologic tests necessary to determine type of systemic invasion.
Preparation of vaccines.

E. GOLDFAIN, M.D.
Director

INDEX TO CONTENTS

Vol. XXXII   AUGUST   Number 8

EDITORIAL

INDEX TO CONTENTS

Vol. XXXII   SEPTEMBER   Number 9

EDITORIAL

INDEX TO CONTENTS

Vol. XXXII   NOVEMBER   Number 11

INDEX TO CONTENTS

Vol. XXXII   DECEMBER   Number 12

EDITORIAL

solid union clinically and by X-ray in 17, 20 and 20½ weeks respectively. Two of the end-results could not be determined, but evidence of callous in the fourth was present by X-ray five weeks post-operatively. The patient obtaining solid union in 20 weeks to date has a normal extremity with the exception of slight posterior bowing resulting in one inch of shortening. In the sixth case, an inlay graft was successful, union being present clinically and by X-ray in 12 weeks, but the inlay graft used in another (No. 7) was a failure. Definite X-ray evidence of bony union of the fracture in which the osteoperiosteal split graft (No. 8) was employed a p p e a r e d in 20 weeks. To date this patient has a normal extremity. Solid bony union following the intramedullary graft (No. 9) was obtained clinically and by X-ray in 13 weeks. Clinical solid bony union was present in 10 weeks with the massive onlay graft (No. 10).

Humerus—Five p a t i e n t s were in this group, their ages ranging from 23 to 45 years. One was a compound fracture. All five resulted from automobile accidents. The site of the fractures were: (1) in the middle third, and (2) at the junction of the middle and distal thirds of the femur. The interval between the time of accident and operation v a r i e d from eight to 22 weeks.

Massive onlay grafts were used in all five patients. Autogenous pegs and chromic catgut were used to obtain fixation of the grafts in the first four cases, and beef bone screws were used in the fifth one.

Three of the patients developed a radial palsy following surgery. Two of these patients recovered, one a few weeks later, the other 13 months after operation. The period of immobilization varied from 14 to 40 weeks. Solid union of the first two fractures was present clinically and by X-ray in 18½ and 30 w e e k s respectively. Firm clinical union was present in one (No. 3) in 56 weeks and in another, (No. 4) in 14 weeks. The end-result of the fifth case could not be determined but beginning callous formation by X-ray was present 20 weeks post-operatively.

Femur—This group is comprised of three cases. The ages of the patients were 19, 45 and 46 years. All were simple fractures and all obtained union. The time interval

between accident and operation was nine, 16 and 24 weeks respectively.

Two of the fractures occurred as the result of violence. The youngest patient was in a motorcycle accident on June 15, 1934, sustaining a fracture which subsequently united in poor position. An osteotomy was later done, and skeletal traction applied correcting three inches of overriding plus anterolateral bowing.

Two fractures were in the middle third and one involved the distal third of the femur. An intramedullary graft was used in each case and osteoperiosteal g r a f t s were also placed about the fracture site in the middle aged patients (Nos. 2 and 3).

The average period of immobilization was about 18 weeks. Slight drainage from one operative wound occurred. Satisfactory u n i o n s were obtained in all three cases.

Ulna—E.M.S., white, male, age 39, was in a car accident August 15, 1935, receiving a compound fracture of both bones of the left forearm. The radius alone united. The fracture of the upper third of the ulna was bone-grafted 19 weeks after the accident using an intramedullary graft. In addition, two osteoperiosteal grafts were laid a c r o s s the fracture site and fixed with chromic catgut. Immobilization was continued for 20 weeks, at the end of which time no union was present, clinically or by X-ray. Any further record is unavailable.

Radius—This group consisted of two patients whose ages were eight and 24 years. In both patients the radius and ulna were fractured. The eight - year - old boy had fractured both bones of the forearm several times previously, suggesting a localized nutritional disturbance. The site of the fractures were: in the boy's case middle third of the radius, and in the adult's case the junction of the middle and distal thirds. The interval between the time of accident and operation for the boy was 10½ weeks, and for the adult 16 weeks.

An osteoperiosteal graft was used in the youngster and fixed with chromic catgut. The p e r i o d of immobilization was eight weeks after which solid c l i n i c a l union occurred. There was definite X-ray evidence of bony union six weeks post-operatively. In the second case a massive onlay graft was employed using autogenous pegs plus chromic catgut for fixation. Almost solid u n i o n was present by X-ray in 27 weeks and this patient now has a perfectly normal extremity.

Clavicle—One case, B.D., a white male, age 37, fell and obtained a simple fracture of the outer third of the clavicle on February 13, 1935. Ten weeks later a massive onlay graft was applied and fixation obtained by autogenous pegs plus chromic catgut. Shoulder immobilized for eight weeks after which there was solid union clinically and by X-ray.

2—NON-UNION

Tibia — Nine patients c o m p r i s e this group, seven of whom are males. Their ages range from nine to 52 years. Both bones were fractured in seven cases and three were compound. The causes of the fractures w e r e variable. Four resulted from car accidents, three were due to falls, one was due to d i r e c t violence and the cause was not stated in the record of one case. The site of the fractures were: (2) distal third, (2) middle third, (4) junction of middle and distal thirds, (1) junction of middle and proximal thirds. The time interval between time of accident and operation ranged from 35 to 163 weeks. In this series there were four sliding Albee inlay grafts, three tibial inlay grafts, one osteoperiosteal "split" graft, and one osteoperiosteal inlay graft. F i x a t i o n of the grafts consisted of chromic catgut in nine cases and autogenous pegs were the means of fixation with the osteoperiosteal "split" graft.

Eight cases were immobilized for eight, 11, 13, 20, 29, 31, 31, 33, and 48 weeks respectively. The record is incomplete in one case. Osteomyelitis of the t i b i a subsequently developed in each of the three compound fracture cases (Nos. 1, 7 and 8). An exacerbation of the infectious process occurred in two of these patients following surgery and necessitated the removal of a small sequestra in one (No. 7), and an incision and drainage of an abscess in the other (No. 8).

Satisfactory unions were obtained in all cases. The results of the sliding Albee inlay grafts were as follows: the first patient obtained solid union clinically and by X-ray in 18 weeks. The second, solid union clinically and by X-ray in 16 weeks and to date this patient has good function of the extremity although there is ¾ inch

shortening and s l i g h t posterior bowing. Another (No. 3) disclosed solid bony union by X-ray in 65 weeks. The fourth case, a 17-year-old boy, operated on a few months ago has at present good union clinically and by X-ray. The length and contour of his extremity is normal. The three patients (Nos. 5, 6 and 7), in whom inlay tibial grafts were used, obtained solid union clinically and by X-ray in 24, 29 and 48 weeks respectively. The patient immobilizd for 48 weeks had a compound fracture. In the last two cases (Nos. 8 and 9) solid union occurred clinically and by X-ray in 50 weeks using an osteoperiosteal "split" graft and in eight weeks with an osteoperiosteal graft.

Humerus—There were seven patients in this group, six were white males, one a negro male. Their ages were from 17 to 51 years. Three were compound fractures resulting f r o m gun-shot injuries and one compound fracture was comminuted. Two patients (Nos. 1 and 3) had open reductions and Lane plates were applied but one plate had to be removed five weeks later because of a soft tissue infection.

The time intervals between the accident and the operation were 28½, 36, 40, 47, 56, 72 and 75 weeks. The sites of the fractures were: (3) in the distal third, (1) at the junction of the distal and middle thirds, and (2) in the middle third. The period of immobilization varied from 14 to 44 weeks in six of the cases. The type of grafts applied were massive· onlay (5), osteoperi-osteal (1), intramedullary combined with osteoperiosteal (2), onlay intramedullary (1). In the non-unions resulting f r o m gun-shot injuries, a massive o n l a y was used in one patient (No. 4) and intramedullary grafts were employed in the other two cases (Nos. 5 and 6). The latter was supplemented by osteoperiosteal grafts.

One patient developed a radial palsy following surgery. In the first two patients autogenous pegs were used to secure fixation of the massive onlay grafts and in the third case they were used in both the first and second grafts. In the fourth case the first graft was fixed with beef bone screws and the second with chromic catgut. In c a s e s Nos. 5, 6 and 7, fixation was with chromic catgut.

It is not known if union was obtained in the first case as the record is incomplete, but fair u n i o n by X-ray was present 10 months post-operatively in the second case. Massive o n l a y grafts were used in the above two patients. The onlay graft employed in the fracture of the upper third of the humerus, case No. 3, was a failure and an onlay intramedullary graft used in a subsequent operation also proved unsuccessful. The fourth case, in whom a massive onlay graft had been unsuccessful, has to date, fair union by X-ray nine weeks after application of a second massive onlay graft. The fifth and sixth cases, in whom combined intramedullary a n d osteoperiosteal grafts were used obtained good bony union clinically and by X-ray in 16 and 37½ weeks respectively. An osteoperiosteal graft used in the last case, No. 7, resulted in abundant callous formation in 14 weeks.

Femur—This group is composed of two cases, a white male, age 53, and a white female, age 17. The male had a simple fracture of the middle third of the femur and the female a compound fracture in the same location. Osteomyelitis developed in the compound fracture which had been reduced by open operation one month after injury. The interval between the automobile accidents and operation was 41 months for the male and 42½ months for the female.

A massive cortical intramedullary graft and an osteoperiosteal graft were used in the compound fracture case. The simple fracture was treated with a massive onlay graft and f i x e d with autogenous pegs. Post-operative X-rays s h o w e d that the bone pegs had pulled loose from the shaft of the femur.

Solid clinical union occurred in 29 weeks in the 17-year-old patient and a re-check revealed solid union and good alignment one year and 11 months later.

The massive onlay graft was a failure and to date there is typical pseudo-arthrosis at the fracture site with three inches of shortening.

Ulna—Five patients comprise this group. The ages range from two to 37 years. The cause of injury varied from falls to fistic encounters. Three were compound fracture cases. One non-union, case No. 2, was the result of a two-inch subperiosteal resection of the shaft for an osteomyelitic infection. The fracture sites were as follows:

(1) the middle third, (2) the junction of the proximal and middle thirds, (2) the proximal thirds. The time intervals between the a c c i d e n t and operation were from seven to 45 months. The types of grafts used were massive onlay (3), "split" inlay (1), onlay intramedullary (1). The latter was used in the fracture at the junction of the upper and middle thirds (No. 5). Fixation of the massive onlay grafts were by means of autogenous pegs in three of the cases (Nos. 1, 2 and 3), and chromic catgut in the remaining two cases.

Two of the patients (Nos. 4 and 5) had previously had bone graft operations for delayed union. The fourth patient whose fracture had been a compound one developed osteomyelitis.

The period of immobilization averaged 14.6 weeks. Fracture of one massive onlay graft occurred. All grafts were successful with the exception of the s l i d i n g inlay graft (No. 4), which was employed in one of the two fractures occurring at the junction of the m i d d l e and proximal thirds. This patient had previously had a massive onlay graft applied to the fracture site 10 weeks following injury. To date he has a typical pseudo-arthrosis at t h e fracture site with limitation of supination and pronation of the forearm.

The result of the massive onlay grafts employed in the first three patients were as follows: *First case:* union present clinically and by X-ray in 24 weeks; solid clinically in 33½ weeks. To date this is not entirely satisfactory, but the result was complicated by a resection of the head of the radius for an anterior dislocation 14½ months after the original injury. There is a s l i g h t increase in the carrying angle, supination is one-quarter normal, pronation is completely absent, relationship of radius to ulna at wrist joint is altered and in addition he complains of pain along the radial side of the forearm on voluntary motion. *Second case:* clinically solid five months post-operatively w i t h moderate callous on X-ray. *Third case:* solid clinical union seven weeks post-operatively. This last patient to date has solid union clinically and by X-ray. The contour of the arm is normal, but function of the forearm as yet is not perfect due to slight limitation of pronation and supination.

The massive onlay intramedullary graft

TABLE OF DELAYED UNIONS
TIBIA

Case No.	Type of Graft	Result	Complications	Interval Between Inj. & Op.	Period of Immobilization
1.	Sliding Albee Graft	Good union clin. & by X-ray in 17 wks.	None	20½ wks.	18½ wks.
2.	Sliding Albee Graft	Union clin. & by X-ray in 20 wks.	None	16 wks.	9 wks.
3.	Sliding Albee Graft	Union clin. & by X-ray in 21½ wks.	None	20 wks.	15 wks.
4.	Sliding Albee Graft	X-ray evidence of callous in 5 wks.	None	21½ wks.	Incomplete
5.	Sliding Albee Graft	Incomplete	None	13 wks	Incomplete
6.	Inlay Tibial Graft	Firm clin. union in 9 wks. & solid bony union by X-ray in 12 wks.	None	15½ wks.	9 wks.
7.	Inlay Tibial and Osteoperiosteal	Failure	None	14 wks.	16 wks.
8.	Osteoperiosteal "Split" Graft	Definite X-ray evidence of union in 4 mos. To date solid union.	None	13 wks.	?
9.	Intramedullary Graft	Solid bony union clin. & by X-ray in 13 wks.	None	27½ wks.	9 wks.
10.	Massive Onlay	Solid bony union clin. in 10 wks.	None	20 wks.	24 wks.

HUMERUS

Case No.	Type of Graft	Result	Complications	Interval Between Inj. & Op.	Period of Immobilization
1.	Massive Onlay	Solid union clin. & by X-ray in 18½ wks.	Radial palsy with comp. recovery in 13 mos.	8 wks.	14 wks.
2.	Massive Onlay	Solid union clin. & by X-ray in 39 wks.	None	8 wks.	30 wks.
3.	Massive Onlay	Fairly firm clin. union & beg. callous formation by X-ray in 32 wks. Solid clin. union in 56 wks.	Radial palsy. It is not known if recovery occurred	21 wks.	40 wks.
4.	Massive Onlay	Solid bony union clin. in 14 wks. To date has solid union clin. & by X-ray	Radial palsy with comp. recovery in a few wks.	21½ wks.	14 wks.
5.	Massive Onlay	Beginning callous formation by X-ray in 20 wks.	Incomplete	22 wks.	Incomplete

FEMUR

Case No.	Type of Graft	Result	Complications	Interval Between Inj. & Op.	Period of Immobilization
1.	Intramedullary Plus Osteoperiosteal	Solid union by X-ray in 23 wks.	None	24 wks.	20½ wks.
2.	Intramedullary Plus Osteoperiosteal	Solid union clin. & by X-ray in 24 wks.	Slight drainage from wound subsided in 24 wks.	16 wks.	18 wks.
3.	Intramedullary	Solid clin. union in 18 wks.; solid union by X-ray in 23 wks.	None	9 wks.	18 wks.

RADIUS

Case No.	Type of Graft	Result	Complications	Interval Between Inj. & Op.	Period of Immobilization
1.	Osteoperiosteal Onlay	Definite X-ray evidence of union in 6 wks. & of solid clin. union in 8 wks.	None	19½ wks.	8 wks.
2.	Massive Onlay	Almost solid union by X-ray in 27 wks.	None	16 wks.	Incomplete

CLAVICLE

Case No.	Type of Graft	Result	Complications	Interval Between Inj. & Op.	Period of Immobilization
1.	Massive Onlay	Union present clin. & by X-ray in 8 wks.	None	10 wks.	8 wks.

TABLE OF NON-UNIONS

TIBIA

Case No.	Type of Graft	Result	Complications	Interval Between Inj. & Op.	Period of Immobilization
1.	Albee Sliding Inlay	Solid bony union clin. & by X-ray in 18 wks.	None	48 wks.	18 wks.
2.	Albee Sliding Inlay	Good bony union clin. & by X-ray in 16 wks.	None	48 wks.	11 wks.
3.	Albee Sliding Inlay and Osteoperiosteal	Solid union by X-ray in 65 wks.	None	25 wks.	31 wks.
4.	Albee Sliding Inlay	To date has good union by X-ray	None	56 wks.	29 wks.
5.	Tibial Inlay	Solid bony union clin. & by X-ray in 24 wks.	None	51½ wks.	8 wks.
6.	Tibial Inlay	Solid union clin. & by X-ray in 29 wks.	None	163 wks.	29 wks.
7.	Tibial Inlay	Solid bony union clin. & by X-ray in 48 wks.	Exacerbation of osteomyelitic infection	76 wks.	16 wks.
8.	Osteoperiosteal "Split" Graft	Solid bony union clin. & by X-ray in 50 wks.	Exacerbation of osteomyelitic infection	76 wks.	33 wks.
9.	Osteoperiosteal Onlay	Good bony union by X-ray in 8 wks.; solid bony union clin. in 15 wks.	None	25 wks.	13 wks.

HUMERUS

Case No.	Type of Graft	Result	Complications	Interval Between Inj. & Op.	Period of Immobilization
1.	Massive Onlay	Incomplete	Radial palsy; it is not known if recovery occurred	47 mos.	Incomplete
2.	Massive Onlay	Fair union by X-ray in 10 mos.	None	28½ wks.	Incomplete
3.	Massive Onlay 1st Operation	Failure	Autogenous pegs pulled loose from graft	49 wks.	28 wks.
	Onlay Intramedullary 2nd Operation	Failure	Graft fractured	78 wks.	24 wks.
4.	Massive Onlay 1st Operation	Failure	None	22½ wks.	44 wks.
	Massive Onlay 2nd Operation	Moderate callous by X-ray 9 wks. P.O.	None	72 wks.	In plaster to date
5.	Intramedullary Plus Osteoperiosteal	Solid union by X-ray in 16 wks.	None	36 wks.	16 wks.
6.	Intramedullary Plus Osteoperiosteal	Firm clin. union & moderate callous by X-ray in 37½ wks.	Serosanguineous drainage from wound for ½ wk.	56 wks.	37½ wks.
7.	Osteoperiosteal Onlay	Good new callous formation by X-ray 14 wks. P.O.	None	40 wks.	14 wks.

FEMUR

Case No.	Type of Graft	Result	Complications	Interval Between Inj. & Op.	Period of Immobilization
1.	Massive Onlay	Failure	Autogenous pegs pulled loose	42½ mos.	?
2.	Intramedullary Plus Osteoperiosteal	Solid union clin. & by X-ray in 29 wks.	None	41 mos.	22 wks.

ULNA

Case No.	Type of Graft	Result	Complications	Interval Between Inj. & Op.	Period of Immobilization
1.	Massive Onlay	Solid clin. union in 7 wks.; to date has solid union by X-ray	None	28 wks.	11 wks.
2.	Massive Onlay	Clin. solid in 5 mos. Moderate callous by X-ray	None	20 mos.	20 wks.
3.	Massive Onlay	16 wks.—slight callous by X-ray; solid clin. union in 33½ wks.	Fracture of graft	45 mos.	26 wks.
4.	Sliding Inlay	Failure		14½ mos.	22 wks.
5.	Onlay Intramedullary	Solid union clin. & by X-ray in 46 wks.	None	24 mos.	8 wks.

(No. 5) was employed in the non-union occurring at the junction of the middle and proximal third, resulting from a gun-shot injury. Clinical union was present in six weeks, but it was 46 weeks before bony union was solid. To date this patient has a s l i g h t increase in the carrying angle. Moderate medial bowing of the forearm is present, but the function is excellent. The bone is clinically solid, but the last X-ray fails to reveal solid bony union.

SUMMARY OF DELAYED UNIONS

Tibia—Seven patients are known to have obtained union. The onlay t i b i a l graft combined with an osteoperiosteal graft was a failure and the result could not be determined in two cases.

Humerus—Four massive o n l a y grafts were successful. The fifth record is incomplete.

Femur—Union was obtained in all three f r a c t u r e s. Intramedullary grafts were u s e d and supplemented with osteoperiosteal grafts in two cases. One patient developed a soft tissue infection.

Radius and Ulna—The delayed unions of the radius were successfully treated with onlay grafts. Osteoperiosteal grafts across the fracture site of the ulna combined with an intramedullary graft proved unsuccessful.

Clavicle—Union of the clavicle was obtained with a massive onlay graft.

SUMMARY OF NON-UNIONS

Tibia—There are no failures in this series.

Humerus—Three cases o b t a i n e d solid union and one other case fair union in 10 months. Moderate callous was present in nine weeks following a second operation in the fourth case. There was one failure and one record was incomplete.

Femur—One case obtained s o l i d union. The massive onlay graft was a failure.

Ulna—Four cases obtained u n i o n. One sliding inlay graft failed to stimulate osteogenesis.

---------------o---------------

Hyperthermic Epidermal Destruction

PATRICK S. NAGLE, M.D.
OKLAHOMA CITY, OKLAHOMA

Foreword: The following paper represents a frank experiment in Form. The intent of this form is that a long paper may be read through from beginning to end rapidly and without loss of continuity by reading only the text of the "thesis." Following this form a reader might pick up any particular point in the development of an author's thesis and follow through with him to its antithesis and cited data.

For example, one point that this paper wishes to bring out is cited in the first thesis. If the reader finds the generality unconvincing, he may accept the tendered elaboration of this point under the heading of "development." If the particular point sufficiently interests him, he may pursue it further through the "argument" and still further under "data" which might cite original or experimental work, anatomy, related chemistry, or a bibliography of the literature. With due apology for imposing this unconventional form upon the reader, the author hopes that negative critical comment may be responsibly presented by letter if serious.

* * * *

THESIS

This designation is employed because it denotes a situation that must be recognized and kept in mind if it is to be treated rationally. Hyperthermic epidermal skin loss exactly describes what occurs in 90 per cent of s e c o n d degree "burns and scalds."

The integument consists of non-vascular horny, protective epidermis and a thick, highly vascular d e r m i s. In superficial burns and scalds the so-called non-scarring, or second degree burns, the non-vascular epidermis is rendered avital by the heat of the offending a g e n t, but the protected, underlying, thicker, highly vascular derma rarely suffers full thickness devitilization.

DEVELOPMENT

Hyperthermic agents such as hot water, steam and the ignited gases of an explosion cool down so rapidly that full thickness "cooking" of the entire skin rarely occurs. Even in the skin damage incident to burning oils and burning clothes and other agents that do not "flash in the pan," but exert an effect over a considerable period of time, the victim will, unless unconscious, divest himself of his clothes or smother the flames and escape further and continued exposure to the burning agent. Here too, we r a r e l y see full thickness "cooking" burns of the skin. It is usually present in those who are restrained and cannot escape and thus remain in an environment of burning material over long.

ARGUMENT

This title obviously excludes such conditions as electric burns, acid and caustic burns and those cases in which full thickness "cooking" destruction of the skin does occur. These immediately a b o v e mentioned situations present additional problems not covered in this paper.

DATA

The integument may be considered under four headings:

1. The corneum.
2. The malpighian layer.
3. The derma.
4. The hypo-dermis.

The four divisions are generally present but in quite variable relationships. For the purpose of this paper we will stress the relative thickness of the derma regionally.

* * * *

THESIS

Characteristics of the derma to be signalled out are:

1. Highly vascular.
2. Contains the s e n s o r y end organs, pain, p r e s s u r e, temperature, and touch.
3. Glandular structures . . . sebaceous and sudoriferous glands.
4. Hair follicles.

5. White connective tissue fibers and an abundance of elastic fibers. (This is the crux of the situation. The preservation of these white and elastic connective tissue fibers is essential to the escape from contracting scars.)
6. Lymphatics.

It is apparent from the above mentioned constituents of the derma that it is the important, truly functional layer of the skin and must be preserved. Its loss or non-loss is a differential point in the prevention of scar contracture.

DEVELOPMENT

The corneum consists of the desicated dead, desquamating cells from the superficial layers of the Rete malpighii and its purpose is solely protective. Necessarily it is found in greatest thickness over those areas of the body which are constantly traumatized, i.e., the soles of the feet, and the palms of the hand, whereas it is very thin to absent in the more protected areas, i.e., the inter-a s p e c t s of the arms and thighs, and the abdomen.

The second division, the Rete malpighii, consists of four classical layers from without inward: the stratum lucidium, stratum granulosum, stratum spinosum, and stratum cylindricum. The report of Thuringer, who has studied the Rete malpighii relative to the percentage occurrence of mitotic figures in these four layers, indicates that mitosis is responsive to stimulation of the area, and that the percentage of occurrence for each stratum varies for different regions of the body, but the one and generally important finding shown by his work is that all cell reproduction does not occur in the stratum cylindricum and stratum spinosum, but that a goodly number of mitotic figures are discoverable in the stratum lucidium.

The basement membrane underlying the stratum cylindricum delimits the epidermis from the dermis. Note also that the epidermis from the basement membrane outward is non-vascular, and contains none of the truly functional tissues of the integument. Its sole purpose is to protect the delicate underlying functional derma from trauma (heat, pressure, and infection).

The f o u r t h division, the hypo-dermis consists of areolar tissue. It is the panniculus adiposus underlying the derma and overlying the fasciae. It is not important in this paper.

ARGUMENT

It is the observation of the writer, as indicated in the opening remarks, that a large percentage of skin area involved in the majority of the u s u a l run of "burn cases" suffers only devitalization of the epidermis. It is possible that some of the true dermis is involved, but we shall now attempt to show that the great thickness of the derma contraverts the probability of full thickness devitalization. The relationship of the thickness of the epidermis to the thickness of the dermis of the skin of the general body surface varies from one-twelfth to one-twentieth of the total thickness of the epidermis and the dermis, while in specialized tissue such as the soles of the feet and p a l m s of the hand, the thickness of the epidermis is much greater, reaching a maximum of about one-fifth of the entire thickness. The derma in general body surface is many times the thickness of the epidermis. It is the writer's belief that this great t h i c k n e s s of the derma, the protection of the epidermis, the great vascularity of the derma, prevent permanent full thickness devitalization of the derma.

As permanent devitalization is rare, it is quite likely that temporary anaphylactic disfunction of the derma frequently immediately supervenes. This anaphylaxis to the p h y s i c a l agent heat is admittedly a loose hypothesis but is the only concept that in any way clarifies the aphysiological process presenting itself immediately after the burn. The hypothesis of a "heat anaphylaxis" explains the initial shock, the disfunction of the undestroyed derma and the marked and rapidly developing, immediately subcutaneous edema, which is in relation to loss of blood plasma from the capillaries, and is hence in relation to the blood stream concentration described by Underhill. This extraordinary blood plasma loss from the capillaries into the tissues underlying the burn is the critical problem confronting us in our thinking about the pathologic physiology and the management of severe hyperthermic epidermal destruction.

* * * *

THESIS

Proper management of "burns" demands that surgeons regard them not as entities, b u t as dynamic unphysiological process. Phases in this process are set out below under the following headings:

1. Stage of shock.
2. Stage of blood stream concentration.
3. Stage of maximum peripheral sensory stimulation.
4. Stage of infection.
5. Stage of repair.

The stage of shock begins immediately after the burn and progresses more or less rapidly to a peak within an hour to three hours and then may blend symptomatically into the picture of the second stage. This shock is probably the same situation we see in surgical shock and it is attended by a drop of blood pressure, increase in heart rate, and diminution of the volume of the circulating blood.

DEVELOPMENT

Its immediate treatment is that of surgical shock and is of the same primary importance as surgical shock. Shock is the first thing to treat in the acute burn if it exists in an alarming degree. Its treatment is that of surgical shock, that is morphine, intravenous f l u i d s, transfusions, stimulation, and cortin.

ARGUMENT

It is very important that the treatment of shock not be sacrificed to the institution of r o u t i n e therapeutic measures which may be postponed until shock is controlled. It is true that in the average case shock is not a critical factor but it must be remembered that patients do die in the first few hours of s h o c k. Fortunately, the treatment of shock is consistent with and blends into the treatment of the second stage of burns; that is the stage of blood concentration.

More recently the writer has become reoriented to the problem that the shock in burns is not surgical shock but is a manifestation of an anaphylaxis. The tenableness of this hypothesis is enhanced because it fits in with and increases our insight into the extraordinary loss of blood plasma from the capillaries into the tissues underlying the b u r n e d area. The importance and significance of plasma loss was originally little appreciated and next was evaluated because of the importance of the related blood stream concentration. Replacement therapy with isotonic saline and glucose soon defined the critical importance of this plasma transudation edema, for we have now repeatedly o b s e r v e d that although the blood concentration is corrected, the edema, the loss of blood electrolytes, the development of pulmonary and cerebral e d e m a, and the emergency of right heart failure r e m a i n e d as major hazards to be overcome by direct attack upon the primary fault in the physiology of the burned victim.

It is quite clear now that the primary fault is the loss of blood plasma from the capillaries into the tissues. Recognizing this, it is the present practice of the writer not to employ isotonic intravenous solutions at all, but to employ hypertonic, intravenous solutions from the outset, and consistent with the hypothesis that "heat anaphylaxis" is responsible for the initial shock, the immediately supervening blood p l a s m a transudation, and subcutaneous e d e m a, ephedrine, adrenalin and large doses of adrenal cortical hormone are employed. Morphine is eschewed because it contributes to cerebral anoxemia. (Long continued cerebral anoxemia and cerebral edema are the f a c t o r s responsible for the subsequent appearance of the "burned brain.") The stage of blood stream concentration is second.

DEVELOPMENT

The stage of blood concentration is a phenomenon first observed (Underhill) in the 21 victims of the New Haven theater fire in 1923. This o b s e r v e r noted the marked increase in the hemoglobin of all the b u r n e d cases. This increase varied from 117 per cent to 209 per cent. Osterburg of the Mayo Clinic has reported consistent findings. The chart made of Underhill's reported case No. 13, is typical of this perversion of the normal physiology. The initial readings show hemoglobin 200, intake 3,000, urine zero on the first day. At the end of the second day the hemoglobin has dropped to 180, the intake is elevated to 5,000, and the output is elevated to 1,000. At the end of the third day the hemoglobin has dropped to 130, the i n t a k e has increased to 7,000, and the output has in-

creased to 3,000 cubic centimeters. By the end of the fifth day, adequate physiological balance has been recovered.

ARGUMENT

The concentration of the b l o o d is dependent upon the loss of the blood plasma into the t i s s u e s about the area burned. Everyone has noticed the striking edema developing on the second and third days. This loss of fluid from the blood stream is out of all proportion to the average normal fluid intake, and necessarily results in a marked diminution in the volume of the circulating blood with the attending kidney disfunction and accumulation of the nitrogenous waste in the blood s t r e a m. This edema is probably due to increased permeability of the capillaries about the burned areas, and according to Osterburg this loss may be as high as 70 per cent of the total blood volume. Such an uncompensated l o s s is obviously incompatible with life and the second stage of burns is frequently fatal. Fluids should be forced by mouth, by hypodermoclysis and intravenously until a total intake of some four to six thousand cubic centimeters per day is maintained. The efficacy of this may be checked by observation of the hemoglobin concentration. It is very probable that the importance of the extent of the burn is not so m u c h the interference with skin function as an excretory organ and the resultant increased load forced upon the kidneys, but rather that the greater the skin area involved, the g r e a t e r the area of edema, and the greater and more acute the diminution of blood volume.

*   *   *

THESIS

The stage of maximum peripheral sensory stimulation runs through the first two stages and is placed third in sequence since its treatment and management is third in importance.

DEVELOPMENT

It is not meant that these stages should be accepted as sharply defined. One or more may overlap. This designation is made to cover the management of the local lesion, that is the area of denuded dermis. Obviously the pain and temperature fibers are very superficial and are insulted by the lightest stimulation. Simple exposure to air of the d e n u d e d dermis in the early course of the burn may c a u s e sufficient pain to contribute to the initial shock.

The most practical management is an early and complete removal of devitalized epidermis and the application of four per cent tannic acid as a spray at intervals of 15 minutes until a suitable crust is secured. This treatment originally brought out by Davidson was originally suggested by Mason and was purposed to precipitate the split protein of the secretions of the burned areas, which were believed to be absorbed and to be the source of the toxemia.

ARGUMENT

This conception of absorption of the toxic material from the burned surface as being of primary importance in fatality of burns, has not been entirely substantiated, but the efficacy of t a n n i c acid in the early treatment of burns has been amply substantiated, being in general use since it was first brought out by Davidson.

* * * *

THESIS

The original factor in the stage of infection is the local infection of the burned area which is characteristically due to the growth of the beta streptococcus hemolyticus. This development is almost inevitable in all large burns and is a very important consideration in the intelligent c a r e of burns. This is the source of the general sepsis next discussed.

DEVELOPMENT

The frequency of the development of infection under the tannic acid crusts necessitating the removal of these crusts, is one of the disappointments in its use. Recently Aldrich has suggested the use of Gentian violet in lieu of tannic acid, and he states that it has the added advantage of having an inhibiting effect on the beta-hemolytic and gamma streptococcus, which he found to be the invading organisms in all extensive burns. It is probable that either of these agencies are satisfactory as an initial measure in the treatment of the local lesion. Tannic acid has proved to be very effective and valuable in covering over the burned area in such a manner that the burn, itself, may be dismissed from consideration for a period of a few days during which time measures are carried out to combat shock,

increased b l o o d concentration, fractures, and other complicating situations requiring immediate attention.

Position of the patient at this time should be one of c o m f o r t. It is impractical to make any effort to prevent contracture at this time. In as much as p o s s i b l e the burned surfaces should be exposed to the air, not subjected to dependent pressure, the pressure of h e a v y dressings or bed clothes. A light cradle should be employed to prevent contact of the bed clothes with the burned area and to m a i n t a i n body temperature. Caution w h e n first instituted as to the n u m b e r of lights and amount of heat should be observed in relation to the patient's temperature, since overheating of a dehydrated patient may contribute to a syndrome similar to sunstroke and cause death. Simple exposure of smaller areas to the air without dressing or medication, and protected by a l i g h t cradle from contacting bed clothes, may prove to be adequate treatment.

Aldrich has s h o w n that typically the beta-hemolytic and the gamma streptococcus is the invading organism in all extensive b u r n e d surfaces and that in those cases manifesting prolonged sepsis, blood cultures frequently revealed the same organisms. The w r i t e r has observed that large burned areas which are apparently uniformly burned and treated with tannic spray, would vary in their healing. Those areas in which the tannic acid crust would remain firm and adherent to the underlying skin w o u l d heal without event and without contracting scarring; w h e r e a s those areas in which the tannic acid crusts were f l o a t e d off by the underlying pus w o u l d inevitably granulate and necessitate ultimate skin grafting. It was apparent that infection was inhibiting epithelization and it later became apparent that it was causing a lysis of the skin which originally did not appear to be devitalized. The explanation of this was not clear but was originally assumed to be the lysis of the tissue by pus under any pressure. It was observed that as the infected crusts were removed early and the underlying area c l e a n e d repeatedly, that healing would take place with a m i n i m u m of scarring. In all tissue cells, particularly in the phagocytes of the blood stream there are proteolytic and a u t o l y t i c enzymes which are freed upon the death of the cell and which are active in an acid environment.

ARGUMENT

It is the writer's present belief that in these burns the full thickness of the derma was not devitalized but was subsequently destroyed by the action of the proteolytic enzymes of the dead phagocytes; that is, the pus cells in those areas in which pus was impounded under crusts of tannic acid or other debris. It is our contention that this inevitable phase of infection should be kept in mind in the very beginning of the management of burns and e v e r y effort made to preserve the delicate, exposed derma. It has been our observation that following the early removal of tannic acid crusts and the cleaning of the surface of the derma of pus, that prompt epithelization would result if no dependent pressure was permitted to effect the derma, but that in all areas in which it was inevitable that pressure should exert itself, we observed the effect to be that of destruction of the derma and ultimate healing by scarring. (The bath, a Kirschner wire suspension are of help here.)

* * * *

THESIS

The second i m p o r t a n t factor in the stage of infection is the g e n e r a l sepsis which inevitably manifests itself in those cases in which large infected non-epithelizing, granulating areas are not corrected.

DEVELOPMENT

In this situation whether the blood culture be positive or not (it is impractical to await a blood culture since a positive report on a streptococcus bacteremia may not be made under three or four week's time) intravenous 5/10 per cent Gentian violet has given in some cases dramatic results. The usual septic temperature of a duration of several weeks has been seen to disappear after a single administration of 15 cc. of one-half per cent Gentian violet. Other measures important in the management of this stage are wet saline packs removed at least once daily preferably left in place over night and removed during the day time. Their application and removal carried away the surface debris of crusts and pus, and their intermittent withdrawal for a period of 12 hours p e r m i t s marginal epithialization.

Certainly an essential item of treatment of this stage is frequent small blood transfusions. Few p a t i e n t s can be carried through the tedious weeks of the stage of infection except through the agency of multiple transfusions. Not to be overlooked is diet.

* * * *

THESIS

The stage of repair begins when, incident to the c e s s a t i o n of the marginal epithelization of the granulation areas, it becomes necessary to r e p l a c e the lost derma, and epidermis.

DEVELOPMENT

This replacement may be accomplished by any of the n u m e r o u s types of skin grafts. It is desirable. to so d i r e c t and manage the earlier phases in the progress of the case that this stage will begin as early as possible and before the patient is debilitated. If due to complications or inability to control and shorten the stage of infection, the patient bcomes wasted, anemic, and septic, much difficulty will be experienced in the securing of the deep split skin from the donor site. The limbs and torso will be so emaciated, the hypodermis will be so diminished and infirm that great difficulty will be encountered in splitting the skin from the donor site. In addition to this the viability of the graft after it is secured and placed in p o s i t i o n will be jeopardized by the inferior general constitutional condition.

The technic of the deep split graft is that of B l a i r and Brown. The implantation graft of Wangensteen, the small full thickness graft, the small Ollier-Thiersch graft, and other grafts consisting of transportation of small islands of epithelium to the granulating areas which stimulate epithelization and ultimately accomplish an epithelial surfacing of these areas, but are in no degree comparable in durability to the deep split graft. They should be only employed when the non-healing areas are so extensive as to leave no donor site available for split skin. Whenever donor sites are available the deep split grafts should be employed. The reason for this is apparent. Those areas repaired by the deep split graft have an underlying derma and ultimately function as full thickness skin, whereas the other types have no underlying derma and c o n s i s t only of a thin, non-resistant, epithelial s u r f a c i n g over scar tissue, which of course, c o n t r a c t s. (Carcinomous degeneration.)

T h e impracticability o f heterogenous and homogenous skin grafts has been so amply demonstrated, that it is only necessary to mention it. It has been our practice to place our deep split grafts not upon the granulating s u r f a c e s, but to excise such granulating surfaces with care so as to contaminate the site of removal as little as possible and place the g r a f t directly upon the hypodermis. Thus the true relationships of the n o r m a l skin are re-established. Experience has shown that these grafts are viable on this underlying areolar tissue. However in repair of areas which will ultimately demand full thickness graft, the deep split graft may be placed as a dressing and subsequently be replaced with full thickness skin.

* * * *

DISCUSSION

F. L. Flack, M.D., Tulsa.—A knowledge of anatomy and physiology is essential in the treatment of any condition, whether disease or injury. Certainly it is important to know that the derma contains essential elements including sensory nerve filaments, white and yellow elastic connective tissue, and a good blood supply. This must be borne in mind and carefully considered in order to obtain a good functional result and avoid disabling scars.

I have so many times seen patients die from shock following extensive burns that I consider the treatment of shock to be of primary importance. The sheet anchor in the treatment is adequate doses of morphine. It may require half a grain of morphine by hypodermic. I have r e c e n t l y been using morphine by vein and the results have been such as to recommend its further use. One hundred cc. of 50 per cent · glucose has, in my experience, been the best treatment for shock in addition to morphine. · This can be used immediately and before blood transfusions can be arranged. The treatment of shock should be started immediately. The use of concentrated glucose solution has a definite effect to counteract pulmonary and cerebral o e d e m a. I appreciate and am familiar with the fact that morphine is a medullary depressant but its v a l u e outweights the contra-indications.

There is a tremendous drop in b l o o d chlorides in severely b u r n e d cases and these must be replaced by the introduction of sodium chloride. Make repeated tests to determine the blood chlorides.

There is some question about the absorption of toxins from a burned area. One of the ideas in the use of tannic acid was the prevention of absorption of toxins from b u r n e d proteins. It has probably been shown that a burned area does not absorb toxins and that alkaloids such as strichnine are not absorbed from a burned area. The use of five per cent t a n n i c acid, in my hands, has been of definite v a l u e in the first aid treatment of burns, probably because it forms a protective coating over the peripheral sensory nerves which are exposed and c a r r y a constant bombardment of stimuli to the cerebral cortex. The use of tannic acid has been so extensive and has been used in so many thousands of cases that its value has been established by competent and careful observers.

As to the treatment of infection, no one method has been so valuable in my hands as the proper application and continued use of warm moist saline dressings. I use such treatment at some stage in practically every burned case of any extent that comes under my care. The best way to remove crusts and clear up infection is by this method.

Certainly the use of the new chemical "Prontylin," is of value in some infections, and is of particular value in the infections which occur in burns. ·

Frequent small blood transfusions every third or fourth day have a definite value in the treatment of these patients.

Sufficient fluids must be given in order to take care of the marked blood concentration which occurs in these cases.

In regard to the use of skin grafts, it is to be remembered that the grafting of skin is the healing of epidermis or dermis taken from one place and applied to another. Of course, autogenous g r a f t s are the only ones to be considered. Skin grafting is purely an experiment in wound healing. The point to be attained is to remove the graft to its bed before the serum has time to coagulate. The practice used years ago of floating a graft in saline solution was the worst practice possible because this tended to remove the serum whose coagulation produced a t t a c h m e n t. Fresh wounds heal themselves because they are presumably free from infection. Granulated surfaces must be accepted in many cases. If the granulations are young, excoriation with a piece of gauze is sufficient to produce e x u d a t e competent to take grafts. In order for grafts to grow, it is necessary for f i b r i n formation to take place. When the granulations have reached a certain age, in general three or four weeks, the v e s s e l s of the granular area u n d e r g o endovascular changes which make it impossible to secure a suitable serum in which to imbed grafts. In such cases these granulating surfaces must be removed by means of a knife or curet in order to secure a suitable surface. It is advisable, of course, for the bed to be smooth so that all grafts can lie evenly and have absorption and touch the grafted areas at all points. Split grafts are ideal and may be applied to muscle or fascia.

We know that the conjoined t e n d o n does heal to Poupart's ligament. Those of us who have had to re-operate h e r n i a s have found this out. Muscle fibers themselves do not heal. Healing occurs by virtue of the connective tissue of the muscle. In instances where this is not sufficient, one must so operate as to create fibrous tissue. We know that by sewing tightly the conjoined t e n d o n to Poupart's ligament, we p r o d u c e a fibrosing myositis. The newly produced fibrous tissue forms a real fibrous union. The kind of suture is of little importance. Sutures obtained from the patient's own fascia, either in the immediate site of the wound or elsewhere, as from fascia lata, has nothing to commend it aside from saving the price of a tube of catgut. The fibrosing myositis is the essential thing. The agent used is immaterial.

Between 65,000 and 75,000 lives are lost in the United States each year as a result of burns and of these about 45 per cent are children. The extent of a burn is more important than the depth. The majority of victims of severe burns s u f f e r from some degree of s u r g i c a l shock. When manifest, shock should be treated before attention is given to the wound. This is best done by the m e t h o d s described. Grease in any form, a h o m e remedy of long standing, should not be used; when applied to extensive burns it has to be removed before the injured surface can be properly treated and this may require an anaesthetic. The frequency of reactions following the use of picric acid in the form of severe dermatitis constitutes a valid objection to this agent.

Recently, Aldridge, following bacteriologic studies on a series of burned patients concluded that most of the fatalities following burns are due to secondary infection of the traumatized tissues and that the representative organism is the gram positive beta hemolytic strep. The most recent contribution to burn therapy is a compound of crystal violet, neutral acriflavine, and brilliant green which is reported to possess all the virtues of gentian violet plus the important additional advantage of exerting bactericidal influence on the gram negative organism. I have had no experience with this.

John F. Burton, M.D., Oklahoma City— I think the significant thing in Dr. Nagle's paper is that burns are a process and not an entity, and if we will keep that in mind in the rationale of treatment, it will be an advantage. There is one method of treatment that might be brought out here, and that is four per cent tannic acid with the immediate application of 10 per cent silver nitrate.

I enjoyed the paper.

————————o————————

Infant Mortality in Germany

In Germany, which has had sickness insurance longer than any other nation in the world, the infant mortality rate is higher than in any state in the United States that is in any way comparable with Germany as to climate and racial uniformity, The Journal of the American Medical association for Dec. 17 reports.

In the Deutsches Aerzteblatt, of Oct. 1, 1938, Hans Klepp reports on "The Struggle Against Infant Mortality," and gives a table showing the course of infant mortality during the present century. Although showing a fairly consistent decrease in the death rate per thousand live births, the 1935 rate in Germany was 69. In eleven northern states that have been in the registration area since 1920, the range of the infant death rate per thousand in 1935 was between 41.2 for Oregon and 53.9 for New Hampshire, according to a summary issued by the Bureau of the Census of the United States Department of Commerce.

Gastrointestinal Allergy*

GEO. J. SEIBOLD, M.D.
OKLAHOMA CITY, OKLAHOMA

Each day the a v e r a g e practitioner of medicine is confronted with a gastrointestinal problem that taxes his diagnostic and therapeutic acumen. Presumably s i n c e the beginning of mankind there have been gastrointestinal complaints. The B i b l e records no evidence of food idiosyncrasies, but Lucretius, an early Roman (96-55 B.C.) actually wrote, "One man's food may be highly poisonous to another." This statement has been revised with time to read, "One man's meat is another man's poison."

Salter, in 1860, published his work on a s t h m a, demonstrating that there was definite relationship between f o o d and asthma. In 1868, Salter[1] published a case report of gastrointestinal reaction in an asthmatic who was s e n s i t i v e to milk. Smith[2], in 1909, recorded symptoms referable to the gastrointestinal t r a c t f r o m buckwheat sensitization. The year 1914, saw the publication of the excellent work of Laroche, Richet, and Saint Girons[3] on "Gastrointestinal or Alimentary Anaphylaxis." Duke, Gay, Eyermann, Alexander, Vaughan and Rowe, have recorded and discussed many instances of this phenomenon in recent years.

The term "gastrointestinal allergy" will be u s e d throughout this discussion, and should not be confused with food sensitivity which might include all the allergic manifestations due to food, namely; respiratory, gastrointestinal, cutaneous, neurologic, and others. These remarks will be confined to the alimentary tract.

The incidence of these manifestations is not accurately known. Rackemann believes it to be extremely uncommon, while Rowe, on the other hand, doubts that its frequency is properly appreciated. Chaney[4] points out the frequency of abdominal reactions, and Graham, Cole, Copher and Moore[5] have long considered food sensitivity in the differential diagnosis of gall bladder disease,

*Read Before the Forty-sixth Annual Session of the Oklahoma State Medical Association at Muskogee, May 11, 1938.

placing it as high as third in importance. Ochsner[6] points to the allergic manifestations in the diagnosis of abdominal conditions as a very important pitfall and insists it must not be overlooked.

Females are most often affected, the proportion being about two to one (Rowe[7]). Positive personal and family histories are obtained in proportion to occurrence of other allergic manifestations.

ETIOLOGY

Heredity is evident in the majority of cases, and in some patients there is a tendency to inherit a sensitivity to a specific food. This has been demonstrated wherein several generations of one family react to the same allergen, as egg or milk. On the other hand, histories may be wanting in inherited manifestations and these apparently fall into a classification of an acquired type.

The ingestion of food and drugs is the common etiological f a c t o r in producing symptoms of gastrointestinal allergy. Its a c t i o n, as a rule, is a local one resulting from direct action of the allergen on the locally sensitized cells. Duke[8] has reported abdominal symptoms which apparently were due to pollen allergy. Eyermann and Freeman have recorded reactions after pollen injection and ingestion.

It is generally believed that the abdominal symptoms associated with migraine are cortical in origin rather than local from an offending food.[1-11] The mechanism is theoretically the same as for urticaria, and has been called intestinal hives.

SYMPTOMATOLOGY

Gastrointestinal symptoms begin at birth and are of great concern to the pediatricians, especially in the form of colic. The bottle-fed infant whose formula has to be altered repeatedly must be considered potentially allergic. Clinical manifestations and symptomatology are n u m e r o u s as shown in the following table, listed in order of frequency:

GASTROINTESTINAL

1. Nausea.
2. Distention.
3. Constipation.
4. Vomiting.
5. Epigastric heaviness.
6. Belching.
7. Intestinal cramping.
8. Canker sores.
9. Pain and soreness in epigastrium.
10. Pain in lower abdomen.
11. Sour stomach.
12. Coated tongue.
13. Pain in midabdomen.
14. Pain in right upper quadrant.
15. Mucous colitis.
16. Heavy breath.
17. Burning, pyrosis.
18. Diarrhea.
19. Ulcer type of pain.
20. Pruritis ani.
21. Proctitis.

GENERAL SYMPTOMS

1. Fatigue.
2. Weakness.
3. Mental dullness and confusion.
4. Nervousness.
5. Irritability.
6. General aching.
7. Fever.

Multitudes of apparent e n t i t i e s have been found to be produced by food sensitivity in a l l e r g i c individuals, namely; colic, pylorospasm, nausea, vomiting, cyclic vomiting, abdominal p a i n, diarrhea, and mucous stools in infants and children, and colic, distention, eructations, acidity, cholecystitis, appendicitis, mucous colitis, peptic u l c e r, nausea, vomiting, fatigue and weakness in adults. Erhlich[9] has reported two cases of prolapse of the rectum in children caused by food.

Two principal types can be distinguished in relation to symptomatology: Gastrointestinal disturbances o c c u r r i n g in patients with other clinical manifestations of allergy, and those occurring in patients in whom no other a l l e r g i c manifestation exists. The symptoms in both types may be acute and multiple in character, involving different portions of the gastrointestinal tract, as well as other tissues of the b o d y. Thus, the ingestion of even the

smallest amount of egg by a sensitive patient may produce swelling of the mouth, nausea, vomiting, and diarrhea in addition to sneezing and asthma. In o t h e r s all symptoms may tend to be chronic and localized to the alimentary tract.

In this discussion an a t t e m p t will be made to include the more important reactions occurring in the gastrointestinal tract, starting first with the buccal and pharyngeal symptoms.

(1) *Buccal and Pharyngeal:* Contact of the lips and buccal mucous membranes by even minute particles or weak dilutions of certain substances may cause immediate and intense swelling of the tissues in patients with a marked sensitivity. Reactions that may occur other than swelling are burning, itching, or puckering of the mucosa. Canker sores are common and the general consensus is that chocolate and nuts are the most frequent etiological factors. Heavy breath and c o a t e d tongue have been listed as other b u c c a l and pharyngeal manifestations. Swelling of the esophagus offers an explanation of globus hystericus.

(2) *Gastric:* Nausea, vomiting, anorexia, distention, epigastric discomfort, belching, heartburn and eructations a r e common gastric symptoms. T h e s e symptoms, so common to organic disease, would lead one to be suspicious of this type of pathology, and it is only through exclusion of organic pathology, plus allergic investigation, that gastrointestinal allergy can be listed as the final diagnosis and proper treatment instituted. Clinical trial will aid in diagnosis by elimination, and then reingestion of causative foods should produce recurrence of symptoms.

Nausea and vomiting are frequent symptoms of gastrointestinal allergy, but are also commonly associated with asthma and migraine.[3-11] In asthma the symptoms may be due to local contact with the offending allergen. In migraine the vomiting and nausea are cerebral in origin. Contrary to this, Rowe believes it to be an allergic reaction on the part of the liver.

Ulcer-like syndromes have been reported in patients due to sensitivity, with no evidence of organic lesion[1]. Gay[10] has reported a large group of ulcer cases (organic lesions demonstrable) in which milk and other foods were found to be causative factors by the leukopenic method of testing, and upon elimination of these allergens, immediate satisfactory results were produced. The similarity of this type of lesion and canker sores tend to lead Rowe to believe Gay's work will be reproduced by other clinicians.

(3) *Colonic Symptoms*: Diarrhea is the most common symptom of both the acute and chronic form of allergic reaction of the colon, particularly in association with mucous c o l i t i s. Constipation is frequently present and alternating with diarrhea is not uncommon. Cramping occurs in the presence of constipation.

The English describe the allergic colon as "irritable" because no true inflammation exists in the presence of symptoms of mucous colitis. Sigmoidscopic examination demonstrates excessive mucus secretion and oft-times presence of blood. There is unusual smooth muscle spasm accompanying this reaction.

Many gastro-enterologists believe t h i s "irritable" type of colon to be functional and psychogenic in origin, and that allergy plays little, if any, part.

Pruritis ani has been demonstrated by a number of authors to be due to food sensitivity.

(4) *Miscellaneous*: One of the most important symptoms of gastrointestinal allergy is grouped under this heading. It is abdominal pain, which may be localized to any quadrant of the abdomen and be associated with organic pathology of the underlying viscera. These pains may be associated with chronic appendicitis, but upon removal of the appendix, a benign, non-inflamed specimen is found, however, the caecum should be carefully noted to detect swelling, edema and possible induration.

Hepatic and biliary allergy f r o m food and probably bacteria accounts for many symptoms in these tissues.[13] Hepatic allergy is associated with edema, swelling of the liver, resulting in pain, soreness, jaundice, and d i g e s t i v e dysfunction. Pseudo-cholecystitis as discussed by Alvarez[12] has been demonstrated to be allergic in origin, and symptoms quite often return after operation for removal of the gall bladder. The foods that frequently disagree with h e a l t h y people, have been shown to be pathognomonic with biliary disease, and are not allergic in their reaction. Onion is the most frequent offender in this group.

Pain is sometimes acute and an acute abdominal catastrophe s e e m s imminent. This is produced by the allergic reaction and is termed acute abdominal angioneurotic edema, and has been demonstrated at laparotomy to be a large hive-like reaction in the intestinal mucosa. Intestinal obstruction, appendicitis, ruptured viscus, and other abdominal crises, are quite often imitated by gastrointestinal allergy and at times are needlessly operated.

Bleeding often simulates the findings in organic disease and the relationship between Henoch's purpura and allergy has been clearly demonstrated. It is fortunate that these acute crises are infrequent and it takes but little time and few procedures to rule out allergic manifestations in the presence of a bona-fide surgical abdomen.

The systemic, or general, reactions are quite variable. They include fatigue, weakness, drowsiness and mental confusion, and bodily aching.

The following reports of cases demonstrate the stormy course so frequently encountered by the allergic individual:

REPORT OF CASES

Case 1—C.E., a physician's wife, aged 47, came with a complaint of abdominal distress for 20 years, periodic sick headaches, and perennial itching of the nose and eyes, with occasionally m a r k e d symptoms of hay fever.

Appendectomy 12 years ago, but patient failed to obtain relief from abdominal distress. The diagnosis was chronic appendicitis. Eight years ago, cholecystectomy brought some improvement in her condition. In the interval between the two operations, the chronic abdominal disturbance was diagnosed as a peptic ulcer.

On questioning the patient, one is unable to obtain a history of an acute attack of appendicitis preceding the symptoms of the chronic appendix. No relief was derived from eating, the taking of soda, emesis, and use of cathartics, heat, or rest. The abdominal symptoms increased with the ingestion of milk. At times there would be mucus in the stool.

The patient was found very sensitive to milk and to a number of other foods. These were removed, with the r e s u l t that the abdominal s y m pt o m s disappeared. It was found by trial, that a teaspoonful of milk was sufficient to reproduce abdominal s y m p t o m s and headaches. Patient can tolerate daily as much as six ounces of superheated milk. If more is used, however, a congested nose, fullness in the upper abdomen, or headaches will occur.

This report demonstrates how frequently patients are subjected to polysurgery before the allergic diagnosis is made.

Case 2—W.E., a 34-year-old housewife, entered the clinic complaining of diarrhea of eight year's duration. Mild attacks of frequent loose stools have been experienced since childhood, but during the past eight years symptoms were considerably worse, consisting of four to six loose movements a day, occurring for the most part at night. Very little mucus, no red blood, and very little cramping accompanied bowel action. Nausea and loss of w e i g h t and strength also accompanied condition. Systemic symptoms consisted of malaise, insomnia, and nervousness.

Other history was essentially negative except for typhoid fever at age of 15, and appendectomy with unilateral oophorectomy and salpingectomy.

Physical examination and laboratory procedures, including X-ray, were essentially within normal limits.

Allergic investigation revealed a number of etiological factors in the form of foods. With elimination of these foods, definite clinical response was noted, and patient made g r a d u a l improvement. However, upon reingestion of one or several of the foods to which she was quite sensitive, there would be a recurrence of symptoms.

This case illustrates food sensitivity in the absence of other allergic manifestations.

Case 3—J.H., aged three years, was first seen at three w e e k s of age, suffering from colicky pains and persistent vomiting, by a pediatrician. Careful observation for a week lead the physician to believe the child was suffering from hy-

pertrophic pyloric stenosis. A surgical consultant concurred in the diagnosis. At four weeks of age, the abdominal cavity was explored. No evidence of pyloric stenosis or any other abnormality of the abdomen could be detected. After the operation, the child continued to vomit and cry with colic as before, but he retained a sufficient amount of food to sustain life and gain weight slowly.

Most of the time the patient suffered from constipation, but often would have loose bowel movements with a great deal of mucus. The abdominal symptoms interfered so seriously with his comfort and growth that the parents demanded something be d o n e. The pediatrician who first saw the child and the surgeon who operated upon him had an opportunity to observe him carefully over a period of three years, and they finally concluded that either the original diagnosis of hypertrophic p y l o r i c stenosis was correct and that in the exploratory operation the pathological condition had been overlooked, or adhesions had formed, which might have contributed to the present symptoms. The abdomen was again opened. S o m e adhesions were found, but they w e r e not causing obstruction. The p y l o r u s and stomach were both normal. After the second operation the symptoms continued as before.

Three weeks after the second operation this patient was brought to the clinic for study from the standpoint of food sensitization as a possible cause of the symptoms for which he had been twice operated. A careful history revealed the fact that besides the vomiting and collicky pains, from which he had suffered since three weeks of age, the patient had had from time to time eczema of a rather severe form, having been suffering from it at the time the pediatrician first saw him.

The patient's mother had migraine and e c z e m a; one maternal aunt had hayfever and asthma; the maternal grandmother had asthma; the maternal grandfather had eczema and migraine; the maternal great-grandmother had eczema.

The child had suffered from practically no disease except the gastrointestinal symptoms and the eczema.

At 14 months of age, eggs had been added to the diet, which caused violent attacks of vomiting. The parents had learned that foods which contained egg always increased vomiting, so eggs had been left out of the diet. They thought they had been excluding all foods which contained egg, but it was found that almost daily the child had been taking egg.

At the time of the first operation, the child's diet consisted entirely of breast milk. The mother reported that during this time, on account of the child's doing poorly, she was advised to have plenty of eggs and milk in her diet. About a week after the first operation, he was placed on lactic acid milk, and for the next three years his diet was modified from time to time with the addition of practically everything the child could be persuaded to eat.

Testing for protein sensitivity gave positive reactions to oats, egg, cow's milk, Irish potato, tomato, orange, and grapefruit, the greatest reaction being that produced by the egg.

Removal of the foods found positive on testing, alleviated all abdominal symptoms in 24 hours, and resulted in the disappearance of all skin lesions in one week. By clinical trial the following foods were added, one at a time: grapefruit, orange, tomato, Irish potato, oats, and then cow's milk, with the result that apparently the patient was able to tolerate all of these foods well with the exception of cow's milk. Because of his emaciated condition, milk was not entirely excluded from the diet. Then egg was tried in very small amounts. It caused a return of abdominal symptoms even when the smallest quantity was used. Frequently there has been a recurrence of severe colicky pains, and it was found that the child's parents or nurse had unknowingly given him egg-containing foods. During one attack, which was severe, adrenalin was given in six-minim doses, with relief of symptoms.

This case demonstrates the fact that a patient may clinically be extremely sensitive to two or more foods, developing a complete or partial tolerance to some of them, but retaining a marked sensitization to one. It also shows that a patient may be skin sensitive to many foods, but clinically sensitive to only one or two.

LABORATORY AND X-RAY FINDINGS

It is a well known fact that laboratory methods and roentgenological examinations are for the most part used to rule out organic pathology. Roentgenological studies of the gastrointestinal tract shows no typical picture for sensitivity, the important factor being exclusion of other existing lesions. Cases have been shown wherein there is hypotonicity of the caecal region and hypertonicity of the transverse and pelvic portions of the colon.

Examination of the stools for eosinophils is not a valuable procedure, as shown by many writers, and the presence of these cells in pathological numbers in the white cell differential is not diagnostic. Fecal examinations should be carried out to rule out parasites or other existing lesions.

Contrary to the work of Loveless[14] we have frequently found a state of subnormal free hydrochloric acid and oft-times achlorhydria existing in patients with gastrointestinal allergy. We have been impressed with the importance of maintaining normal acidity by the clinical response, when proper acid therapy is instituted, plus the allergic outline of each case. Gastric analysis should be a routine in the investigation of these cases.

DIAGNOSIS

In patients with history of hay fever, asthma, urticaria or other allergic conditions, the occurrence of gastrointestinal or abdominal symptoms should at once arouse suspicion that they may be due to food or drug allergy. In these cases it is not difficult to arrive at the correct diagnosis through history, skin tests and therapeutic trial.

Considerable difficulty may be encountered in determining, in the absence of any associated allergic manifestations, that the gastrointestinal complaints of the patient are the result of food sensitivity. It is in these cases that organic pathology must be carefully ruled out. After one is satisfied the condition existing cannot be demonstrated as organic, he is justified in trying to solve the problem from an allergic approach.

Listed according to importance as steps toward diagnosis are the following:

1. History.
2. Skin tests.
3. Elimination diets.
4. Clinical trial.
5. Leukopenic index.
6. Food diary.

Anomnesis is by far the most important item in the above list in the approach to diagnosis. One will be well rewarded by careful and well-planned routine of history taking.

Skin tests are of considerable aid but are by no means infallible. Sixty per cent has been an average figure of their accuracy. This report is by allergists, while gastro-enterologists feel they are p r a c t i c a l l y worthless.

Elimination diets and their clinical trial and observations of this trial by an accurately kept food diary are very important in both diagnosis and treatment.

The leukopenic index is still a disputed procedure as to its relative merits. There are many factors that enter into the test that may produce false readings, such as washing the hands, s m o k i n g, knitting, laughter, and many similar disturbances. In acute abdominal crises, adrenalin may be used. The e f f i c a c y of adrenalin in gastro-intestinal a l l e r g y is variable but warrants therapeutic trial, and the results are quite often diagnostic.

The patient should be carefully advised as to possible difficulties encountered in drugs that produce gastrointestinal symptoms, such as phenolphthalein, castor oil, and aspirin. It is as important to educate the patient against the use of certain medications as it is to remove certain foods from the diet.

TREATMENT

Elimination of the causative food or drug is necessary if results are to be obtained. Hyposensitization by the oral route is a tedious, difficult procedure and the percentage of satisfactory r e s u l t s by this method is very low. Many of the foods that produced weak skin reactions, can often be added gradually to the diet. If it is felt that they p r o d u c e recurrence of symptoms, they s h o u l d immediately be withdrawn.

Rowe has published excellent elimination diets based chiefly on egg, wheat, and milk exclusion. One must be careful of vitamin and mineral balance and adequate caloric intake while prescribing this type of diet. Hypodermic desensitization is occasionally employed and the plan of treatment is similar to pollen hyposensitization. This procedure is not without dangers and very severe reactions have been demonstrated. The work of Richet and Urbach, employing the oral administration of propetans, has not been clinically verified, and has been generally discarded.

Symptomatic therapy has to be carefully carried out in all cases, and all manifestations of coexistig organic pathology properly handled.

Particular i n t e r e s t to scientific food classification should be observed in prescribing diets, for example, a patient with marked sensitivity to peanuts should also avoid peas and lentils. When a patient is advised not to eat wheat he should be supplied with information concerning substitutes in the cereal group, and it should be called to his attention that wheat is contained in many foods among which are rye bread, wieners, gravy, and some commercial ice creams.

Hydrochloric acid in adequate dosage is very important to those patients with decreased or absence of the normal acidity figures.

Adrenalin should be given, especially in abnormal crisis, both for therapeutic purposes and as a means of differentiation, since, if symptoms are relieved, one feels the condition to be allergic.

SUMMARY

Gastrointestinal allergy refers to those clinical manifestations of allergy which are limited to the gastrointestinal tract and result from sensitization, either inherited or acquired, of the living cells of part or all of the mucosa. Although foods are usually responsible for the production of symptoms, in gastrointestinal allergy, food allergy may cause other sensitivity manifestations without gastrointestinal symptoms; hence, the two terms should not be used synonymously. Of the various foods which can produce symptoms, eggs, milk, wheat, and chocolate are probably the most frequent offenders. The symptomatology which can be produced is an extremely varied one, and can m i m i c almost any lesion of the gastrointestinal tract. When these symptoms occur in a patient who has some other allergic manifestation, it can u s u a l l y be assumed that they are most likely the result of gastrointestinal allergy. The diagnosis in these instances is accomplished in the same manner as in other allergic diseases, and treatment is similar.

REFERENCES

1. Tuft, Louis: Clinical Allergy, W. B. Saunders, Philadelphia, 1937.

2. Smith, H. C.: Buckwheat Poisoning, Archives of Internal Medicine 3:350, 1909.

3. Laroche, Richet and Saint Girons: Gastrointestinal or Alimentary Anaphylaxis, Paris, 1919.

4. Chaney, W. C.: Southern Medical Journal, 30:12; 1185, 1937.

5. Graham, E. S., Cole, W. H., Copher, G. H., and Moore, S.: Diseases of the Gall Bladder and Bile Ducts. Lea & Febiger, Philadelphia, 1928.

6. Ochsner, Alton: Pitfall in Diagnosis of Abdominal Conditions. Personal communication.

7. Rowe, A. H.: Clinical Allergy, Lea & Febiger, Philadelphia, 1937.

8. Duke, W. W.: Archives of Internal Medicine, 28:151, 1921.

9. Ehrlich, M. A.: J.M.A. Gergia 26:5, January, 1937.

10. Gay, L. P.: G. I. Allergy. Exhibit in St. Louis, Interstate P. G. Medical Assembly, 1937.

11. Balyeat, Ray M.: Allergic Diseases, F. H. Davis & Co., Philadelphia, 1936.

·12. Alvarez, W. C.: J.A.M.A., 104:2053, 1938.

13. Hoge, Albert H.: Gastrointestinal Allergy, West Virginia Medical Journal, 3:296, July, 1937.

14. Loveless, Mary: Gastric Acidity and Acid Therapy in Allergy, Journal Allergy 7:203, March, 1936.

---o---

Insulin Treatment of Schizophrenia*
in the Western Oklahoma Hospital

JOHN L. DAY, M.D.
H. L. JOHNSON, M.D.
SUPPLY, OKLAHOMA

INTRODUCTORY

Dr. Manfred Sakel of V i e n n a read a paper November 14, 1933, describing a new treatment for schizophrenia. He had been using insulin for the amelioration of withdrawal symptoms in morphine addiction. Certain adventitious results prompted him to try large doses in the t r e a t m e n t of schizophrenia. Repeated d o s e s not only controlled excitement but produced definite mental improvement. He then proceeded to work out a plan of treatment, the alleged results of which have astonished the world. Psychiatrists began flocking to him to witness the work and then to return home and try it in their own hospitals. Beginning December 8, 1936, he gave a six-week's course of instruction in New York. Since then the treatment has been instituted in a considerable number of hospitals and several interesting reports have been published. The bibliography appended herewith is v e r y incomplete. Daily newspapers have carried sensational

*Condensed from a Paper Read at a Meeting of the Woodward County Medical Society, Supply, Oklahoma, December 14, 1937.

descriptions of the treatment and results and relatives of patients with mental disorders are appealing to psychiatrists for the treatment. Insulin had been used previously in the treatment of psychoses with malnutrition due to refusal of f o o d. In 1928, Dr. Julius Schuster of Budapest advocated the use of insulin in the treatment of schizophrenia and in that year reported its use in more than 60 cases. These earlier procedures, however, are not to be confused with the hypoglycemic shocks described by Sakel.

In order to promote therapeutic effort and research in Oklahoma Hospitals, the State Board of Public Affairs authorized a visit to the Mayo Clinic for the purpose of studying the insulin treatment. Accordingly, one of us, Johnson, spent some time there in August. The work was being done in the Rochester State Hospital under the direction of Dr. F. P. Moersch and Dr. E. F. Rosenberg and had been going on since the first of January, 1937. Upon return to Supply, we selected six female patients for treatment and on the first day of September work was actually begun. Later, a group of 12 male patients was started and this group is still receiving intensive treatment. The indications were restricted to schizophrenia. Hypoglycemic shocks may be of value in the treatment of other psychoses; that is a problem for f u t u r e research. Some work has already been done on the psychoneuroses. Some of the cases classified as schizophrenia or dementia praecox may have been incorrectly diagnosed. We have separated the types of schizophrenia b e c a u s e different results with them have been reported. Some investigators have obtained best results with the paranoid types, others with the catatonics.

TECHNIQUE

The technique of the treatment is based on that described by Sakel. It is strenuous but can be learned easily and requires no unusual manual skill. Because of the physical dangers it should be administered only in a hospital and because of the mental considerations it should be under the direction of a psychiatrist.

By c a r e f u l experiment the minimum dose of insulin necessary to produce coma is determined and this is given once a day, five or six days a week, for a p e r i o d of about eight weeks. Each day the coma is interrupted by the exhibition of a sugar solution, usually by gavage but occasionally intravenously.

The transition from somnolence to coma being g r a d u a l, any line of demarcation must of necessity be arbitrary. The onset of coma may be defined as that instant the patient becomes unable to drink. Instead of sinking into a stuporous coma, some patients go into a coma-vigil. Their eyes may remain open and they may carry on somnambulistic conversations and actions. There are so m a n y varieties of reaction that it is unsafe to define the general rule. Any one patient may react differently on different days.

Systematic routine, attention to details, team work, and the absence of outside distraction are important. The hypoglycemic attack is beset with dangers and the intelligent observer will maintain a continual watch over the patients in order to recognize trouble as soon as it develops. The

(FOOTNOTE)—Grateful acknowledgment is made to Eli Lilly & Company of Indianapolis, Indiana, for the insulin used.

danger to life is real and may be due directly to the treatment or indirectly to secondary complications. The mortality rate is not high. Including patient No. 11 of our series we have collected reliable information of nine deaths. In our opinion, an occasional death will occur even in the most expertly managed clinic. But considering the malignant n a t u r e of schizophrenia, there is ample justification for any procedure, regardless of its dangers, that may hold out a reasonable hope for cure.

The awakening from coma is sometimes spectacular. The mental transformation may appear to be miraculous. There is n e a r l y always euphoria. Patients who have for long periods been in a catatonic stupor, who have had to be tube-fed, and who have persistently maintained a state of apathetic mutism may ask for food, manifest an interest in what is going on, and talk readily and relevantly. The first utterances, however, may be silly and the patient may become amused at his own silliness. Logoclonia, echolalia, and echopraxia are common. Infantile t a l k and conduct suggest a psychological palingenesia. Laughter becomes contagious and the whole room may take on the aspect of a wild party. It is this that breaks the monotony and that may explain some of the enthusiasm of the experimenters. It is well for the workers to become imbued with cheerfulness but not to the degree of lowering their dignity.

Psychotherapy of the practical variety begins here. An attempt is made to restore and maintain the patient's cheerful interest in his surroundings. In order to avoid introversion, his prospects and the conditions of the other patients should not become conspicuous topics for conversation. Even if psychoanalysis were not impracticable, it is my opinion that it is contraindicated. Inhibitions being removed, there might be a temptation to try it but it seems that that would be taking an unfair advantage. The consent for psychoanalysis should be as nearly normally voluntary as possible. In cases receiving insulin treatment it is better to leave the unpleasant past buried in amnesic oblivion. Psychosynthesis, recreation, occupational therapy, industriousness, attention to personal appearance, and general hygiene are essential adjuncts in the treatment. All this extra individual attention may be responsible for much of the good results obtained.

The number of visitors in the treatment room should be kept at a minimum and should be restricted to persons with proper professional and official credentials. Relatives should not be admitted to the treatment room, but as soon as the patient is able to appreciate it, they may visit in the afternoon, the object being to encourage the patient's return to contact with reality.

The workers themselves should set good examples in language and conduct. They should be enthusiastic and optimistic without being fanatical. We undertook the work with as open minds as we could command. We tried to avoid prejudice. But we did not go so far as to discard notions and precepts previously handed down by authority and confirmed by observation. To our present satisfaction, we find those notions even more firmly established.

RECORDS

Until some general agreement has been r e a c h e d regarding the efficacy of this treatment, it is obligatory that the clinical records go into considerable detail. When a very large number of such records from a large number of sources can be assembled, it is hoped that some wise compiler will tell us where we are going. Then perhaps the records can be simplified. Important as records may be, their compilation must not interfere with a vigilant supervision of the patients. Comparatively few of the clinical phenomena resulting from glycopenia have been found to be generally true, and most of them have exceptions. The blood-sugar may descend to the level of 18 mg. per 100 cc or even lower. An occasional early morning glycosuria may be observed. General physical improvement, a healthier skin, and a gain of 15 to 23 pounds has been noted with our patients. The temperature usually falls during hypoglycemia; a minimum of 92 rectal has been observed. The surface temperature of the exposed extremities in ordinary room conditions has been observed as low as 80. The pulse and blood pressure curves are found to be fairly consistent in showing increases during hypoglycemia.

THEORIES

The physiology and the biochemistry of hyperinsulinism and hypoglycemia in the laboratory animal and in man are being studied by scientists. The changes in the sugar and m i n e r a l metabolism during treatment have been described and an effort has been made to discover some consistent relationship between the laboratory and clinical observations. The exact mechanism by which the glycopenia produces its effects on the nervous system remains a mystery. Sakel is quite modest in the presentation of his theory. He reminds one of the hostess who makes profuse apologies for a very excellent entertainment. He assumes that the abnormal activity in the nervous system of the psychotic individual consists of reactions to stimuli deserting their e a r l i e r pathways to flow through new and inappropriate channels. The glycopenia blockades these more recent channels first, thereby favoring the reestablishment of the older routes. This explains, too, the greater value of the treatment in the more recent cases. If an inappropriate pathway has been used long enough to have become as firmly established as its conventional predecessor, the glycopenic attack can only blockade them alike.

RESULTS

Excluding the insulin treatment, most of the recoveries from schizophrenia may be attributed to superior institutional care. Some are ascribed to empirical chemotherapy, some are spontaneous, and a few appear to be the result of shock. This use of the term "shock" is not to be confused with that in connection with the insulin treatment. An instantaneous r e m i s s i o n has been seen to follow an accident, a severe illness, a surgical operation, or a catastrophe. To go further than to mention those treatments and results is beyond the scope of this paper.

The Western Oklahoma Hospital had a total resident population on December 31, 1933, of 1,205. Of this number 455 or 38 per cent were diagnosed as having dementia praecox. During the calendar years, 1934, '35, and '36, there were admitted 195 additional cases of dementia praecox and during the same period 135 cases of dementia praecox were discharged, 15 as recovered, 111 as improved, and nine as unimproved. Expressed in percentages of the number of schizophrenics admitted e i g h t per cent were recovered, 56 per cent improved, and five per cent unimproved. The remaining 60 were not discharged and statistics as to their condition have not yet been completed. The foregoing data were compiled from records made before this study had been contemplated and show that the pre-insulin outlook for schizophrenia was not altogether hopeless. But in treating 300 cases with i n s u l i n Sakel reports 70 per cent recovered and an additional 10 per cent improved of those who had been psychotic less than six months and 40 per cent recovered of the chronic cases. Although the percentages are computed from different bases, such a score for insulin cannot be ignored.

In examining statistics on psychiatric observations the personalities and viewpoints of the different investigators must be taken into account. We believe that the average American state hospital psychiatrist is inclined to be conservative in reporting recoveries and liberal in reporting improvements. We should remove the beams from our own eyes before searching for motes in the psychological optics of our Viennese brethren. Dussik of Vienna considers that more than 70 per cent of all patients in hospitals for mental disease are schizophrenic. When we compare that with our 38 per cent we are handicapped at the very beginning of the statistical race.

We have not had a sufficient number of patients under treatment nor have we observed them over a long enough period of time to speak with much authority. We should be neither surprised nor perturbed if some of our conclusions were found to be erroneous. This report is preliminary and incomplete and no attempt is made to interpret the results in percentages.

CASE HISTORIES

Case 1, E. H., female, age 17 years. This patient had had one p r e v i o u s attack, spent three months and 23 days in the hospital and was discharged as recovered. The insulin treatment was terminated reasonably early in her case as her improvement appeared to have attained its maximum. She was p a r o l e d nine days after treatment was discontinued and a recent letter from her father states that she is in excellent physical health, still gaining in w e i g h t, and he makes only one complaint about her; she is disobedient and saucy at times. Some of

this may be due to improper training but there is a possibility that it is a sequel to the psychosis.

Case 2, R. E. B., female, age 35 years. This patient's physical appearance and health was much improved, her behavior was g o o d throughout the treatment but a nodding mannerism and her rather uncouth habit of belching persists. Her attitude toward her husband remains uncertain and when asked for an explanation of her conduct she evades the answer.

Case 3, F. B., female, age 28 years. This p a t i e n t required feeding and dressing throughout her entire hospital residence. Just immediately upon awakening she would talk freely, would feed herself, and showed signs of recovery. In a few hours she would relapse into her former negativistic attitude. Her husband took her home one month after treatment was discontinued. A recent letter from him justifies the conclusion that she is still gradually improving. He says that she talks freely, that she dresses herself and makes her bed but that she still refuses to eat unless someone carries the food to her mouth for her.

Case 4, L. R., female, age 19 years. This patient required careful watching during the treatment. She had a few grand mal convulsions. B e f o r e beginning treatment she had been incorrigible at times, saucy and indolent. Improvement at the end of treatment was very little. Her father took her home 18 days after treatment was discontinued. A recent letter of inquiry to him has not been answered.

Case 5, G. R. K., female, age 21 years. This patient is said to have had one previous attack. She spent nine months and 24 days in the hospital and was discharged as improved. She was rather irritable and would fight with very little provocation at the beginning of the treatment. There was some improvement in every way at the end of the treatment, but now six weeks later there has been some recession. An aggravated case of acne has almost completely disappeared.

Case 6, M. E., female, age 35 years. Before beginning treatment this patient had to be kept in a side room because of exhibitionism. During the treatments she seemed to be completely cured of this misconduct and remained so for s o m e time afterwards. Six weeks later she manifests an occasional sign of relapse.

Case 7, J. B., male, age 16 years. This patient had one previous attack from which he appeared to completely recover. On readmission he was very badly excited. By the time treatment was begun, he had a l r e a d y begun to improve. At the t i m e treatment was discontinued his mental condition seemed to be normal. Treatment was terminated a little early in his case because of the onset of pneumonia, due probably to aspiration of fluid from feeding and vomiting. Ten days after o n s e t of pneumonia thoracentesis was performed and 750 cc of mucopurulent f l u i d was withdrawn from the right chest. He is still in bed and is not yet out of danger.

Case 8, L. H., male, age 17 years. Because of the long duration of this patient's illness and the apparent mental deterioration the prognosis was unfavorable. His physical h e a l t h is improved. He has gained considerable weight but his ·reactions have been troublesome. He has had a few convulsions and there have been times when danger was threatened. During the treatment, which he is still receiving, he has talked a little, using an infantile vocabulary with logoclonia and echolalia. The prognosis remains unfavorable.

Case 9, L. M. P., male, age 23 years. Treatment was shortened because of an attack of tachycardia. His reactions during the treatment and since that time have b e e n satisfactory and his parole may be recommended.

Case 10, A. G., male, age 25 years. This patient has made much improvement in general appearance. Before beginning treatment he had b e e n combative at times. He has' given no trouble lately but he does not reply to q u e s t i o n s promptly and his mental condition remains unsatisfactory. He is still taking treatment.

Case 11, G. W. O., male, age 18 years. When this patient entered' the hospital he was practically maniacal. He was destructive. His clothes could not be kept on him and for a few days his general con-

dition was unsatisfactory. When treatment was begun he had already made some improvement. He reacted v e r y well until the eighth treatment at which time he received 80 units of insulin and went into what appeared to be a usual coma. When the time came to terminate the hypoglycemia s u g a r was administered but he did not wake up. Ceaseless efforts were then begun by using adrenalin, intravenous injections of glucose, and so forth in an attempt to arouse him, all without avail. He remained in this coma 12 days at the end of which time he died. He did not develop pneumonia nor did there appear to be any complication other than the persistent coma.

During the first few days of coma he would have occasional attacks of extreme opisthotonos and lordosis. Such attacks always yielded promptly to the intravenous i n j e c t i o n of glucose. During these 12 days all nourishment had to be given with a stomach tube and a number of special procedures were resorted to when necessary to combat transient symptoms.

Case 12, H. F., male, age 33 years. The patient's improved p h y s i c a l appearance constitutes the chief change due to his treatment. W h e n his parents visited him the other day he did a number of erratic things, for example, he sat in the automobile and talked to his father but refused to talk to the mother unless he were assured that he could go home. The prognosis remains unfavorable.· Treatment was discontinued a few days ago because of fever and an attack of tachycardia.

Case 13, A. P., male, age 21 years. Treatment has been without incident. He is still receiving treatment and it may be that he has made some mental improvement.

Case 14, C. C., male, age 22 years. This very q u i e t p a t i e n t has been quiet throughout the treatment and he too may have shown a little mental improvement. He is still receiving treatment.

Case 15, D. D., male, age 39 years. Treatment has been without incident. He is still receiving treatment and it may be that he has made some mental improvement.

Case 16, J. F. P., male, age 37 years. Treatment has been without incident. He is still receiving treatment and it may be that he has made some mental improvement.

Case 17, R. D., male, age 24 years. This patient was taken off treatment yesterday as his improvement seemed to have reached its maximum. His psychosis has been one a little difficult to describe. His symptoms have been somewhat elusive. He appears to be very much improved. The Examiner's prognosis is favorable but g u a r d e d. Considerable difficulty was had in f e e d i n g him with a tube. More than half the time the feeding tube would go into the trachea rather than the esophagus d u r i n g the insertion of the tube. He would struggle violently making it very difficult to feed him. He required the largest dose of any that we have used, sometimes as much as 120 units at a time.

Case 18, B. C. B., male, age 30 years. This patient is still receiving treatment. His behavior is satisfactory but he has not been tested recently regarding his paranoid delusions. No prediction is being made at this time regarding the outcome.

CONCLUSIONS

1. Induced insulin hypoglycemia is a positive contribution to the t h e r a p y of schizophrenia.

2. The percentage of favorable results in the Western Oklahoma Hospital has not been as high as that reported in much of the literature.

3. The treatment may hasten a remission already in progress.

4. The sooner treatment is begun after onset of the disorder, the better the prognosis.

5. Best results have been observed in cases of the catatonic type.

6. The concommitant psychotherapy and special attention is responsible for much of the good results.

7. Used indiscriminately some cases will be r e s t o r e d, some improved, some unchanged, and some made worse.

8. The permanency of these results cannot be evaluated for some time.

9. A gain in weight and a general improvement in physical health almost always takes place but occasionally a death will occur during treatment. Undesirable sequelae may develop late.

10. Unless the individual shall have acquired an immunity in addition to his remission, relapse will occur when he is returned to the offending situation.

11. The immediate problems are the perfection of the technique of treatment and the determining in advance more specifically the indications a n d contraindications.

12. The State Hospital should not be expected to pursue this treatment without additional financial support.

BIBLIOGRAPHY

Sakel, M.: A New Method of Treating Schizophrenia with Insulin, Wien. med. Wchnschrl, 84:1211, 1934.

Wilson, Isabel G. H.: A Study of Hypoglycemic Shock Treatment in Schizophrenia, Report to Board of Control of England and Wales, 1936.

Glueck, Bernard: The Hypoglycemic State in the Treatment of Schizophrenia, J.A.M.A., 107:1029 (September 26), 1936.

Steinfeld, Julius: Insulin Shock Therapy in Schizophrenia, J.A.M.A., 108:91 (January 9), 1937.

Sakel, M.: Translation, American Journal of Psychiatry, 93:829, 1933.

James, G. W. B. et al: Insulin Shock Treatment of Schizophrenia, The Lancet, Vol. 1, 1937, p. 1101.

Rosenberg, E. F. et al: Treatment of Schizophrenia, Mayo Clinic Proceedings, 12, 273.

Smith, H. Mason, Hypoglycemic Therapy, J.A.M.A., 108, 1959 (June 5) 1937.

Cameron, D. Ewen, and Haskins, R. G.: Insulin-Hypoglycemia Treatment of Schizophrenia, J.A.M.A., 109, 1246 (October 16) 1937.

Rymer, Charles A., et al.: Hypoglycemic Treatment of Schizophrenia, J.A.M.A., 109, 1249, (October 16) 1937.

Symposium on Therapy including Hypoglycemia: American Journal of Psychiatry, 94, 89, (July) 1937.

Importance of Instant Attention to Trivial Injuries

Instant attention to trivial injuries greatly reduces the incidence of felons, E. A. Devenish, M.D., London, England, points out in an article in The Archives of Surgery, an abstract of which appears in The Journal of the American Medical Association for Dec. 17.

Immediate treatment should include cleansing of the wound, its protection against contamination and a warning to patient to report to his physician immediately if the finger or hand becomes painful. A matter of a few hours' delay can bring about a condition that will require surgery or even amputation, whereas with earlier attention simple medical measures would have sufficed.

Swelling and congestion of the inflamed area should be reduced to a minimum by elevating the injured extremity. If splinting is used circulation must not be interfered with.

Although bone conduction seems to be the active cause of ear degeneration, air conduction likewise has been found to be responsible for deafness and deterioration of the auditory apparatus.—Hygeia.

Surgical Treatment of Maxillary Antrum Infections*

CLINTON GALLAHER, M.D.
SHAWNEE, OKLAHOMA

I should like to limit this paper to a discussion of the treatment of the pyogenic infections of the maxillary antrum. For the purpose of our discussion I would like to define such a condition as an abscess of and within the maxillary antrum. This would exclude from the discussion such subjects as the maxillary antrum with infection wherein the natural otsei afford adequate drainage. It would also exclude all conditions that are neoplastic in origin, tubercular or luetic. We wish to discuss the pus producing infections which invade the maxillary antrum and produce therein a reaction which has resulted in a partial or complete filling of the antrum with pus u n d e r pressure, and less than adequate drainage, if any.

It seems l i k e l y that every surgeon is aware of the principles involved in the treatment of an abscess. These principles are fairly well d e f i n e d and have been taught in the surgical departments of medical schools for many years. Briefly they are:

1. Attempt to secure adequate drainage.
2. Attempt to sterilize the cavity.
3. Attempt to obliterate the cavity.
4. Attempt to restore the tissues to normal functional integrity.

The p r o b l e m then is one of adapting these principles to the treatment of the maxillary antrum.

In attempting to secure drainage it will appear necessary to establish an opening sufficiently l a r g e to reduce the pressure within the antrum and to permit the continuous escape of the pus. This opening should be sufficiently large if possible to assure continuous drainage so long as it is needed. The determination of the time when such drainage should be instituted must rest with the judgment of the surgeon as with the treatment of any other

*Presented to the Pottawatomie County Medical Society in regular meeting of April 16, 1938, by Clinton Gallaher, M.D.

abscess. Practically we find that a large number of these cases come to our attention in a condition where there is some reason to doubt the necessity of the establishing of drainage by surgical means. We are justified therefore in attempting by medical treatment to establish adequate drainage. We conceive that it is also important to remember t h a t, whereas the patient will appreciate treatment without surgery, they will always condemn a protracted illness or a chronic infection which may result by delayed drainage.

Sufficient drainage in the acute pyogenic infection may be s e c u r e d through the natural osteum by needling. But the very fact that this condition is present usually constitutes good evidence that natural or accessory osteum d r a i n a g e has already proved inadequate and needling is a very poor assistant to drainage. It is therefore necessary in most of these cases to establish drainage through a large opening. We prefer to make this opening in the most dependent portion of the sinus available, and routinely use that point in the lateral wall which is inferior to the lower turbinate and two or three cm. posterior to the anterior tip. For some years we have preferred a drill for this purpose. We believe that this is particularly advantageous because of the fact that it is possible to obtain adequate drainage with less trauma to the tissues involved. We are especially anxious to produce as little damage as possible to the adjacent tissues. In keeping with the idea of securing adequate drainage, this opening is u s u a l l y made about one-fourth i n c h in diameter or slightly less. The desire to attempt to restore to normal function cautions us to make this opening at once sufficiently small so that we may expect it to close by the time the abscess has been sufficiently drained.

All manner of attempts to sterilize the cavity of the antrum have been proposed. Every antiseptic under Heaven, so far as we know, has been squirted into the antrum with the idea of combating the infection. We believe that as a principle the idea of sterilizing the cavity of the antrum is of considerable benefit. Our particular reason for objecting to attempts of sterilization lies in the fact that it appears to be impossible and anything which will produce a sterility as of micro-organisms, will undoubtedly produce a devitalizing or necrosing effect upon the ciliated epithelium which lines the cavity. Hence it would appear impossible to sterilize the cavity and at once maintain the hope of ultimately restoring the normal function of the tissues which line the c a v i t y. In view of these considerations we are at once convinced that normal saline washing is the method of choice, with or without 1/4 of 1 per cent ephedrin sulphate. One other detail we feel is important. Proetz has demonstrated beyond a d o u b t that ciliated epithelium is destroyed by temperatures of 42 degrees C. and above. He also states that temperatures below 37.5 degrees C. have a tendency to sharply retard the action of the cilia. But unless the temperature is actually freezing there is no harm done. It is therefore important to regard the temperature of the solution. It may be that we will sometime find a solution which will effectively produce a condition of sterility in the cavity without injury to the tissues. But until we are certain that the solution will produce this happy result I feel sure that we will repeatedly be disappointed in the results of treatment which includes attempts to sterilize the cavity.

When we consider this subject in relation to attempting to obliterate the cavity, our analogy begins to disintegrate. The only way in which an attempt is ever made to obliterate the cavity is in effect an attempt to exteriorize the cavity. It is true that p o l y p s and neoplasms occasionally obliterate the c a v i t y, but only through pathological processes is t h i s condition ever brought about. There is an advanced state of infection of the maxillary antrum wherein, in a relatively very small number of cases it appears impossible to re-establish a normally functioning antrum. The classical Caldwell-Luc operation has been suggested for this purpose. It generally consists of a l a r g e incision through the alveolar process and a large opening under

the inferior turbinate producing a through drainage. Extensive curretage is usually associated with this operation also. We see relatively few of those p e o p l e who have had this operation, but in our limited observation it seems that the results are often far from satisfactory. I doubt very much if I will ever do a Caldwell-Luc. I prefer rather the technique which is extensively employed, of simply making a large window under the inferior turbinate. Packing the cavity with gauze and removing a small portion each day apparently has a tendency to produce benefit. It is true that these cases will continue in many instances to e x h i b i t manifestations of chronic infection. But it is equally true that many of them will become entirely comfortable and heal to the extent that a very small amount of serous drainage is the only persisting sign. Under no circumstances will such an antrum ordinarily become acutely inflamed and if this should occur the signs and symptoms incident to the presence of pus under pressure and absorption are but moderate.

In relation to attempting to establish the normal function of the antrum, all of the procedures discussed apply. The original drainage is made large enough to be adequate but there is a definite attempt to keep it sufficiently small to assure ultimate c l o s u r e and re-establishment of drainage through the natural osteum. We believe that it is only in this manner that we may hope to re-establish the function of warming and moistening and aiding in the filtration of inspired air. We believe that it is especially important in this connection to improve such methods and technique as may be expected to produce the least possible damage to every tissue involved. I do not believe that it is possible to overstress the importance of this care and technique. It is reasonable to assume that an infection treated early, adequately and carefully, in a large majority will be healed within a few days and with a very few repeated washings.

In concluding I wish to again stress the following points. Let us attempt to secure adequate drainage as soon as the indication becomes definite. Let our attempts to sterilize the cavity be limited to washing with normal saline and to rely upon the natural physiological processes to produce that happy result. In cases where the effect of obliterating the cavity seems necessary let us use the most conservative means which may be expected to produce results and keep our operative proceedures relative simple and not extensive. In all advice and treatment e i t h e r medical or surgical, let us remember the delicate na-ture of the tissues involved, the physiological properties and the necessity of restoring to normal function in so far as possible. We believe that it is only with these factors in mind that we may work to the best interest of our patient and secure for them the most satisfactory and early results.

---o---

State Prenatal and Premarital Examination Laws

Chas. M. Pearce, M.D.
Commissioner, Oklahoma Health Department
David V. Hudson, M.D.
Consultant Genitoinfectious Diseases
Oklahoma State Health Department
OKLAHOMA CITY, OKLAHOMA

Public interest has been aroused to the importance of syphilis as a public health problem and one manifestation of this interest has been the attention paid to the passing of more effective laws for the control of syphilis. Two phases of syphilis control are commanding interest because of their importance. These are prenatal and p r e m a r i t a l examinations. Three states, New York, New Jersey, and Rhode Island have prenatal examination l a w s while 26 states have premarital examination laws. The Oklahoma laws do not require a physician's certificate from an applicant for a marriage license, nor is there any provision for serodiagnostic tests in pregnancy.

The H e a l t h Department is preparing P r e n a t a l and Premarital Examination Laws based upon the suggested forms reprinted below from the Journal of Social Hygiene. Space does not permit discussion of the reasons for the form of the following laws and the reader is referred to the November, 1938, issue of the Journal of Social Hygiene for the background and details.

It is important that physicians be familiar with these laws in o r d e r to answer questions from interested persons. They will become the subject of much discussion and it is imperative that the public have correct information regarding the contents and purposes of these laws.

"A Suggested Form of a State Prenatal Examination Law"

Section I—Serological b l o o d test for syphilis of pregnant women. Every physician attending a pregnant w o m a n in (name of state) during gestation shall, in the case of each woman so attended, take or cause to be taken a sample of blood of such woman at the time of first examination, and submit s u c h sample to an approved laboratory for a standard serological test for syphilis. Every other person permitted by law to attend upon pregnant women in the state but not permitted by law to take blood tests, shall cause a sample of the blood of such pregnant woman to be taken by a duly licensed physician and submitted to an approved laboratory for a standard serological test for syphilis. The term "approved laboratory" means a laboratory approved for this purpose by the state department of health. A standard serological test for syphilis is one recognized as such by the state department of health. Such laboratory tests as are required by this act shall be made on request without charge by the state department of health.

Section II—In reporting every birth and stillbirth, physicians and others permitted to attend pregnancy cases and required to report births and stillbirths, shall state on the b i r t h certificate or stillbirth certificate, as the case may be, whether a blood test for syphilis has been made during such pregnancy upon a specimen of blood taken from the woman who bore the child for which a birth or stillbirth certificate is filed and, if made, the date when such test was made, and, if not made, the reason why such test was not made. In no event shall the birth certificate state the result of the test.

Section III—The sum of ....dollars ($..............), or so much thereof as may be necessary, is hereby appropriated out of any moneys in the state treasury to the state department of health to cover additional clerical, p r i n t i n g, laboratory and other expenses in carrying out the provisions of this act.

Section IV—This act shall take e f f e c t immediately.

"A Suggested Form of a State Premarital Examination Law"

Section I—It shall be necessary for all persons intending to be married to obtain a marriage license from the (here insert the name of the person or persons authorized under the law of the state in question to issue such licenses) and to deliver said license, within sixty days from the date of issue, to the clergyman or other qualified person who is to officiate before the marriage can be performed.

Section II—Before any person, authorized by law to issue marriage licenses, shall accept an application for any such license each applicant therefor shall file with him a certificate from a duly licensed physician stating that such applicant has been given such examination, i n c l u d i n g a standard serological test, as may be necessary for the discovery of syphilis, made not more than thirty days p r i o r to the date of such application, and that,. in the opinion of the physician, the person therein named either is not infected with syphilis or, if so infected, is not in a stage of that disease which is or may become communicable to the marital partner.

Section III—Because of an emergency or other cause shown by affidavit or other proof, a j u d g e of the (name of proper) court, if satisfied by medical and/or other testimony that neither the health of the individuals nor the public health and welfare will be injuriously affected thereby, may make an order, on joint application of both of the parties desiring the marriage l i c e n s e, dispensing with those requirements of Sections II and IV which relate to the filing with the licensing authority by either or both of the parties of the physicians' certificates a n d t h e laboratory statements or, the s a i d certificates and statements having b e e n filed, extending the thirty day period following the examination and test to not later than ninety days after such examination and test. The order s h a l l be accompanied by a memorandum in writing from the judge, reciting his reasons for granting the order. Application for such extension may be made before, on or after the expiration of such thirty day period. The order and the accompanying memorandum shall be filed with the licensing authority and the latter shall thereupon accept the application for the marriage license without the production or filing of the physicians' certificates a n d the laboratory statements dispensed with by the order, or shall accept the application within any such extended period, as the case may be. The licensing authority and his clerks and employees shall hold such memorandum of the judge in absolute confidence.

Section IV—Each physicians' statement shall be acompanied by a statement from the person in c h a r g e of the laboratory making the test, or from some other person authorized to make such a statement, setting forth the name of the test, the date it was completed and the name and address of the person whose blood was tested, but not stating the result of the test. The physicians statement and the laboratory statement s h a l l be on the same form sheet. Upon a separate form a detailed report of the laboratory test, showing the result of the test, shall be transmitted by the laboratory to the physician who, after examining it and if he deems it desirable, discussing it with either or both the proposed marital partners, s h a l l file it with the state (or local) health officer, where it shall be held in absolute confidence and shall not be open to public inspection; provided that it shall be produced for evidence at a trial or proceeding in a court of competent jurisdiction, involving i s s u e s in which it may be material and relevant, on an order of a justice or a judge of such court requiring its production.

Section V—A standard serological test shall be a laboratory test for syphilis approved by the state commissioner of health and shall be performed by the state department of health, on request, f r e e of charge or at a laboratory approved for this purpose by the state department of health.

Section VI—Nothing in this act s h a l l impair or affect existing laws, rules, regulations or codes made by authority of law, relative to the reporting by physicians and others of cases of syphilis discovered by them.

Section VII—Marriage licenses shall be issued to all applicants who have complied with the provisions of this act and who are otherwise e n t i t l e d under the laws of (name of the state) to apply therefor and to contract matrimony.

Every such license, when issued, shall have endorsed thereon or annexed thereto at the end thereof, a statement, subscribed by the person issuing the license that the application for the l i c e n s e was accompanied by papers complying with the applicable requirements of Sections II and IV of this act relative to examination and health of the parties or, if such compliance was dispensed with, wholly or partly, by order of a judge, a statement to that effect.

The license issued, including the above statement and the certificate duly signed by the person who shall have solemnized the marriage therein authorized, shall be returned by him to the licensing authority who issued the same within five days succeeding the date of the solemnizing of the marriage therein authorized, and any person or persons who shall wilfully neglect to make such return within the time above required shall be deemed guilty of a misdemeanor and upon conviction t h e r e o f shall be punished by a fine of not less than .... dollars or more than .... dollars for each and every offense.

Section VIII—Any applicant for a marriage license, any physician or any representative of a laboratory who s h a l l misrepresent any of the facts called for by the physicians statement and the laboratory report or statement, or any licensing officer who shall accept an application for a license without the accompanying physicians statement and laboratory report, as required in Sections II and IV hereof, unless the same shall have been dispensed with by judicial order as provided in Section III, or who shall have reason to believe that any of the f a c t s contained in said statement or report h a v e been misrepresented and shall nevertheless issue a marriage license, or any health officer or his employee who shall not hold the laboratory record confidential, except as provided in Section IV hereof with respect to its production for evidence on order of a judge, or any officer, clerk or employee of the office issuing the license who shall not hold in strictest confidence the statement filed with him as to the reasons for granting a judicial o r d e r, as provided under Section III hereof, shall be guilty of a misdemeanor and punishable accordingly.

Section IX—The sum of ....dollars ($.................), or so much thereof as may be necessary, is hereby appropriated out of any moneys in the state treasury to the state department of health, to cover additional clerical, p r i n t i n g, laboratory and other expenses in carrying out the provisions of this act.

Section X—This act shall take effect on (a day specified at least three months after its passage).

REFERENCES

Johnson, Bascom: Premarital and Prenatal Examination Laws. Journal of Social Hygiene, Vol. 24, No. 8, November, 1938, p. 477.

———————o———————

Nicotinic Acid Reactions

The unpleasant reactions that often follow treatment with nicotinic acid may be due to the rate at which the drug is absorbed into the system, W. H. Sebrell, M.D., and R. E. Butler, M.D., Washington, D. C., report in The Journal of the American Medical Association for December 17.

Nicotinic acid is used in the treatment of pellagra (weakness and scaliness), which is due to a deficiency of certain vitamins.

The reactions are harmless to the individual and should not interfere with the use of the acid in treatment. They include tingling, dizziness, itching, rash, flushing of the skin and nausea.

———————o———————

The body requires mineral elements for growth, repair and regulation of body processes.—Hygeia.

———————o———————

Coronary thrombosis is that rather common accident in which a clot has shut off the blood supply to the heart.—Hygeia.

THE JOURNAL
OF THE
Oklahoma State Medical Association
Issued Monthly at McAlester, Oklahoma, under direction of the Council.
Copyright, 1938, by Oklahoma State Medical Association, McAlester, Oklahoma.

Vol. XXXII	JANUARY	Number 1

DR. L. S. WILLOUR..Editor-in-Chief
McAlester, Oklahoma

DR. T. H. McCARLEY..Associate Editor
McAlester, Oklahoma

Entered at the Post Office at McAlester, Oklahoma, as second-class matter under the act of March 3rd, 1879.

This is the official Journal of the Oklahoma State Medical Association. All communications should be addressed to The Journal of the Oklahoma State Medical Association, McAlester Clinic, McAlester, Oklahoma. $4.00 per year; 40c per copy.

The editorial department is not responsible for the opinions expressed in the original articles of contributors.

Reprints of original articles will be supplied at actual cost provided request for them is attached to manuscripts or made in sufficient time before publication.

Articles sent this Journal for publication and all those read at the annual meetings of the State Association are the sole property of this Journal. The Journal relies on each individual contributor's strict adherence to this well-known rule of medical journalism. In the event an article sent this Journal for publication is published before appearance in The Journal the manuscript will be returned to the writer.

Failure to receive The Journal should call for immediate notification of the Editor, McAlester Clinic, McAlester, Oklahoma.

Local news of possible interest to the medical profession, notes on removals, changes of addresses, births, deaths and weddings will be gratefully received.

Advertising of articles, drugs or compounds unapproved by the Council on Pharmacy of the A. M. A., will not be accepted.

Advertising rates will be supplied on application.

It is suggested that wherever possible members of the State Association should patronize our advertisers in preference to others as a matter of fair reciprocity.

Printed by News-Capital Company, McAlester.

EDITORIAL

OUR EXECUTIVE SECRETARY

Since the meeting of the House of Delegates at Muskogee, last May, when this body requested the Council to employ a full time Executive Secretary, the Council has had the matter under consideration. A Committee to consider applicants was appointed by the President composed of the following: Doctors J. D. Osborn, Jr., Frederick, James Stevenson, Tulsa, and P. M. McNeill, Oklahoma City, who immediately proceeded to their task of investigating and interviewing many applicants. The Council felt that the financial condition of the Association was such that an Executive Secretary could not be immediately employed, so the matter was put off from time to time until a called meeting of the Council at Oklahoma City, December 11th, 1938, when several applicants were presented by the Committee, and Mr. R. H. Graham of Peabody, Kansas, was employed, his services to begin January 1, 1939.

Mr. Graham is a young man, very enthusiastic about his proposed work. He is a graduate of Peabody High School and attended Kansas University. He is a young man of excellent presence and has many ideas relative to his work which the Council believe will improve the service of the State Association to its members as well as the service of Organized Medicine to the public.

The Council immediately voted sufficient funds for Mr. Graham to make a tour of inspection to some of the States where full - time, lay Executive Secretaries are employed and also to visit the headquarters of the American Medical Association in Chicago, and familiarize himself with the different departments. His office will be with the Secretary-Treasurer-Editor in McAlester, Oklahoma. However, it will be necessary for him to spend considerable time on the road visiting the various County Medical Societies and representing our interests wherever he may be most needed.

It is our opinion that this addition to the Staff of the Headquarters office of the State Association will be of great benefit and it is asked that the membership, in every way, give him complete co-operation and feel free to call for him for any assistance that he may be able to render.

---o---

INSURANCE MEDICAL DIRECTORIES*

The attention of all members is called to the following resolution adopted by the Society at the Hot Springs meeting April 29th:

"WHEREAS, certain commercial interests are publishing medical directories, listing physicians by specialty and otherwise, as available for insurance and compensation work, and other professional services, and

"WHEREAS, participation by listing in these lay publications merely serves for the profit of the promoters, and is

*Copied from Journal, Arkansas Medical Society.

furthermore technically indirect solicitation of patients.

"THEREFORE, BE IT RESOLVED, That the Arkansas Medical S o c i e t y condemns these practices as unethical and forbids its members to continue listing their names in such directories, and .

"BE IT F U R T H E R RESOLVED, That the Arkansas Medical S o c i e t y requests the House of Delegates of the American Medical Association to take similar action."

The resolution was p r e s e n t e d to the House of Delegates of the American Medical Association and referred to the Judicial Council for study. The Judicial Council approved the resolution a n d recommended its adoption, which the House of Delegates did at the session of May 14th, 1936.

The attention of our members has been previously called to the activities of these directory publishers. As is often the case, individual physicians felt that they might incur a loss if they removed their names from such directories while other members retained their listing. With this thought in m i n d, the above resolution has been adopted. The practice of so listing is declared unethical; no individual m e m b e r may now feel that should he remove his name that another physician will accept that listing. The benefit is direct to these physicians in the fees saved; the loss is entirely the promoters.

Some idea of the financial gains involved in the publication of these directories may be understood when we state that one directory now on our desk c o n t a i n s the names of approximately 5,000 physicians. Ninety-two Arkansas physicians are listed in the three directories available to The Journal. The fee charged for listing in this one directory is $15.00 per annum. A liberal estimate of the cost of publication and distribution is $15,000. The balance, $60,-000, is presumably divided between the promoter and his solicitors. Verily, a most altruistic motive prompts the publication.

Editorial Notes—Personal and General

DR. R. M. ANDERSON, Shawnee, has been appointed a member of the Council of the Southern Medical Association from Oklahoma for a regular Council term of five years, the appointment having been announced recently by the President, Dr. Walter E. Vest, of Huntington, West Virginia. Dr. Anderson succeeds Dr. W. K. West, Oklahoma City, who, having served the constitutional limit, was not eligible for reappointment.

DR. MORRIS FISHBEIN, Editor Journal American Medical Association, Chicago, will be the guest of Pottawatomie County Medical Society, March 14, 1939, at Shawnee.

DR. EDW. D. McKAY, formerly with the Miami Clinic at Miami, is now with the Wesley Clinic, Oklahoma City.

DR. W. JACKSON SAYLES, announces his association with the Miami Clinic, Miami.

DR. and MRS. ONIS HAZEL, Oklahoma City, have returned from a trip to Texas and Mexico. Dr. Hazel read a paper before the meeting of the North Texas Medical Society.

DR. E. S. KILPATRICK, formerly of Elk City, now of Erick, is reported recovering from an operation for a gall bladder condition.

DR. ELIZABETH CHAMBERLAIN, Bartlesville, is reported recovering from injuries received in an automobile accident some weeks ago.

DR. HENRY H. TURNER, Oklahoma City, was guest speaker before the regular December Staff meeting of the McAlester Clinic.

DR. GEO. S. KILPATRICK, McAlester, has returned from a visit to the Pacific Coast.

DR. EARL D. McBRIDE, Oklahoma City, had as guest of honor at a dinner given by him at his new Clinic Building, December 27, 1938, Dr. Edward L. Compere of the University of Chicago, who addressed the guests on some important orthopedic problems.

DR. HENRY H. TURNER, Oklahoma City, was guest speaker before the regular Staff Meeting of the McAlester Clinic, in December.

DR. M. B. GLISMANN, Okmulgee, will spend the next few months in New Orleans where he will do post graduate work at Tulane University.

———o———

News of the County Medical Societies

OKLAHOMA County Medical Society have the following officers for 1939:

President, Dr. Carroll M. Pounders; Vice-President, Dr. Tom Lowry; Secretary-Treasurer, Dr. Geo. H. Garrison; Board of Directors, Doctors Rex Bolend, John F. Burton, C. J. Fishman, Geo. H. Garrison, John E. Heatley, P. M. McNeill, Tom Lowry, Carroll M. Pounders, W. W. Rucks, Jr.; Board of Censors, Doctors Lea A. Riely, Walker Morledge, Dan R. Sewell; Delegates, Doctors, W. F. Keller, Walker Morledge, John F. Burton, C. R. Rountree, Geo. H. Garrison, Ben H. Nicholson, D. H. O'Donoghue, L. J. Moorman, W. W. Rucks, Jr., Allen G. Gibbs, Ralph Bowen and Wann Langston; Alternates, Doctors O. A. Watson, C. P. Bondurant, John E. Heatley, L. Chester McHenry, Lloyd C. Boatright, H. Dale Collins, J. C. Macdonald, L. J. Starry, C. M. Pounders, Hugh Jeter, Henry H. Turner, and E. S. Ferguson.

BLAINE County Medical Society elected the following officers for 1939 at their meeting December 15th: President, Dr. A. K. Cox, Watonga; Vice-President, Dr. Wm. F. Boheman, Watonga; Secretary, Dr. W. F. Griffin, Watonga.

PITTSBURG County Medical Society held their regular annual election in December and elected the following officers: President, Dr. Geo. S. Kilpatrick; Vice-President, Dr. C. O. Williams; Secretary, Dr. Edw. D. Greenberger, all of McAlester. Dr. T. H. McCarley held over as Delegate and Dr. E. H. Shuller was the newly elected delegate, for two years.

WAGONER County Medical Society elected the following officers for 1939 at their recent meeting: President, Dr. H. K. Riddle, Coweta; Vice-President, Dr. J. H. Plunkett, Wagoner; Secretary-Treasurer, Dr. Francis S. Crane, Wagoner.

LINCOLN County Medical Society met in December and elected the following officers to serve for 1939: President, Dr. Carl H. Bailey, Stroud; Vice-President, Dr. C. W. Robertson, Chandler; Secretary-Treasurer, Dr. E. F. Hurlbut, Meeker; Delegate, Dr. Ned Burleson, Prague; Alternate, Dr. W. B. Jenkins, Tryon.

WASHINGTON County Medical Society met December 14th and elected the following officers for 1939: President, Dr. L. D. Hudson, Dewey; Vice-President, Dr. William LeBlanc, Ochelata; Secretary, Dr. J. V. Athey, Bartlesville; Treasurer, Dr. O. I. Green, Bartlesville; Delegate, Dr. J. E. Crawford, Bartlesville; Alternate, Dr. E. E. Beechwood, Bartlesville.

JEFFERSON County Medical Society met December 12th electing the following officers for 1939: President, Dr. L. L. Wade, Ryan; Vice-President, Dr. W. M. Browning, Waurika; Secretary, Dr. J. I. Derr, Waurika; D e l e g a t e, Dr. C. M. Maupin, Waurika.

GRANT County Medical Society met November 23rd and elected the following officers for 1939: President, Dr. I. V. Hardy, Medford; Vice-President, Dr. S. A. Lively, Wakita; Secretary-Treasurer, Dr. E. E. Lawson, Medford.

CHOCTAW County Medical Society elected the following officers at their meeting in December: President, Dr. Robt. L. Gee, Hugo; Secretary, Dr. Floyd L. Waters, Hugo.

GARVIN County Medical Society elected the following officers for 1939 at their meeting in December: President, Dr. Edw. T. Shirley, Pauls Valley; Vice-President, Dr. Hugh Monroe, Lindsay; Secretary-Treasurer, Dr. John R. Callaway, Pauls Valley; Censor 1939 to 1941, Dr. Hugh Monroe; Delegate, Dr. Hugh Monroe; Alternate, Dr. Robt. M. Alexander, Paoli.

WOODWARD County Medical Society met December 13th for their annual election of officers. Dinner at 6:30 was followed by business meetings of both the Auxiliary and the Doctors. Their scientific program was as follows: Dr. H. L. Johnson, member of the Staff of the Western Hospital,

gave a report on the results of the insulin treatment in this hospital during the past year. Dr. Coyne H. Campbell, Oklahoma City, guest speaker, gave an interesting talk, and Dr. H. K. Speed, Sayre, President of the State Association, gave a very interesting talk.

The following officers were elected following the meeting: President, Dr. C. E. Williams, Woodward; Vice-President, Dr. Floyd Newman, Shattuck; Secretary, Dr. C. W. Tedrowe, Woodward.

POTTAWATOMIE County Medical Society elected the following officers at their meeting December 17th: President, Dr. E. Eugene Rice (re-elected), Shawnee; Vice-President, Dr. C. C. Young, Shawnee; Secretary-Treasurer, Dr. Clinton Gallaher (re-elected), Shawnee; Trustee, Dr. J. M. Byrum, Shawnee; (President and Secretary also Trustees); Board of Censors, Dr. Horton E. Hughes, Shawnee (elected for three years); other Censors, Drs. R. C. Kaylor, McLoud; M. A. Baker, Shawnee.

ROGERS County Medical Society elected Dr. Earle E. Bigler, Claremore, President, and Dr. P. A. Anderson, Claremore, Secretary, for 1939.

MURRAY County Medical Society met December 19th and elected the following officers for 1939: Dr. Warren E. Parker, President, Davis; Dr. Arthur Fowler, Vice-President, Sulphur; Dr. Richard M. Burke, Secretary-Treasurer, Sulphur; Dr. Ernest Rose, Delegate, Sulphur; Dr. P. V. Annadown, Alternate, Sulphur; Dr. Geo. W. Slover, Dr. F. E. Sadler, Dr. Ernest Rose, Councillors, all of Sulphur.

---o---

New Books

THE HEART IN PREGNANCY, by Julius Jensen, Ph.D. (In Medicine), University of Minnesota, M.R.C.S., (England), L.R.C.P. (London) Assistant Professor of Clinical Medicine, Washington University School of Medicine; Assistant Physician to Barnes Hospital; Physician to St. Louis Maternity Hospital and St. Louis City Hospital. Price $5.50. The C. V. Mosby Company, St. Louis, 1938.

This is a very timely book on a very important subject. There is a wide divergence of opinion among competent observers regarding the ability of the cardiac patient to bear children. This most complete volume on that subject should clarify some of these debated questions.

This book is divided into three parts: (1) The Effect of Pregnancy on the Normal Heart; (2) Abnormal Cardiac Impulse Formation During Childbearing, and (3) Organic Heart Disease and Pregnancy.

It should be of much use to any physician that comes in contact with obstetrical patients.

THE COMPLETE PEDIATRICIAN, Second, Completely Rewritten 1938 Edition, For the Use of Medical Students, Internes, General Practitioners, and Pediatricians, by Wilburt C. Davidson, M.A., D.Sc., M.D. Professor of Pediatrics, Duke University School of Medicine, and Pediatrician, Duke Hospital, Formerly Acting Head of Department of Pediatrics, The Johns Hopkins University School of Medicine, and Acting Pediatrician in Charge, The Johns Hopkins Hospital, Fellow American Academy of Pediatrics and American College of Physicians. Member White House Conference, American Pediatric S o c i e t y and American Board of Pediatrics. Durham, N. C., Printed by Seeman Printery for Duke University Press, 1938. (Adaption of the Title Page of The Compleat Angler by Izaak Walton, 1653).

This is a very unique book on Pediatrics. At

first glance it would appear that it is poorly connected, but if one will read the instructions at the beginning of the book it will be very easily understood. It combines in one volume the information usually found in several volumes. Of course if the reader desires a more complete description of a condition it would be necessary to consult more complete volumes.

The book is divided into groups of diseases: (1) Respiratory; (2) Gastro-Intestinal; (3) Skin and Contagious; (4) Neuro-psychiatric; (5) Circulatory Metabolic and Glandular; (6) Urological; (7) Orthopedic and (8) Unclassified.

This volume should be very useful to any physician who has anything to do with children. It should be especially useful to a very busy general practitioner.

CLINICAL LABORATORY METHODS AND DIAGNOSIS, A Textbook on Laboratory Procedures With Their Interpretation, by R. B. H. Gradwohl, M.D. Director of the Gradwohl Laboratories and Gradwohl School of Laboratory Technique; Formerly Director of Laboratories, St. Louis County Hospital; Pathologist to Christian Hospital; Director, Research Laboratory St. Louis Metropolitan Police Department, St. Louis, Mo.; Commander, Medical Corps, Fleet, United States Naval Reserve. With 492 Illustrations in the Text and 44 Color Plates. Second Edition, The C. V. Mosby Company, St. Louis, 1938.

The first edition of this text was received with considerable enthusiasm by both the laboratory specialists and technicians. The clinician as well has received much valuable information from this edition. It seems that all laboratory subjects were completely covered, however, in this new edition we find additional illustrations in black and white and 24 full page color plates; illustrations on the estimation of kidney function; description of newer concepts on nephrosis and nephritis; more recent data on origin and development of cells; more than 100 additional pages on hematology; new illustrations and text on parasitology and tropical medicine; information concerning the Black Widow Spider, and detection of crime by laboratory methods, and many other important facts in laboratory technique.

This is indeed a complete work and will be acceptable by everybody interested in laboratory technique, or the application of laboratory findings to clinical procedures.

ABSTRACTS : REVIEWS : COMMENTS
and CORRESPONDENCE

SURGERY AND GYNECOLOGY
Abstracts, Reviews and Comments from
LeRoy Long Clinic
714 Medical Arts Building, Oklahoma City

Fertility and Sterility after Extra-uterine Pregnancy by Mayo and Strassmann; Surgery, Gynecology and Obstetrics, July, 1938; Vol. 67, No. 1; page 46.

This is a report on 142 patients with ectopic pregnancies seen at the Mayo Clinic in the ten-year period, 1926 to 1935.

Of these, there was only one who died and she was admitted in shock and died before any surgical procedure was attempted. The remainder were operated upon without mortality.

One hundred of the 142 patients had the possibility of further pregnancy. Eighty-four of these 100 were traced and 31 became pregnant later. Of these 28 had intra-uterine pregnancies and three (3.6 per cent) had recurrent extra-uterine pregnancies. The 28 patients had 47 intra-uterine pregnancies with 32 full-time deliveries and the others resulting in miscarriage or premature delivery.

These authors have made a review of the literature, finding that recurrent ectopic pregnancies occur in about 3.9 per cent of the cases of ectopic pregnancy. Their figures of recurrence were in keeping with this one.

"Since the probability of intra-uterine pregnancy after one ectopic pregnancy is about 10 times larger than the probability of another ectopic pregnancy, conservative surgery is advisable in order to preserve fertility. Only if the other tube is severely diseased should it be removed. In this connection it should be kept in mind that the non-pregnant tube undergoes certain acute changes in more than 50 per cent of tubal pregnancies, such as swelling, redness, and peritoneal friction produced by hematomas. These changes, however, more or less disappear and do not interfere with subsequent fertility."

COMMENT: This is an interesting study and the last quoted paragraph is of great importance because of the soundness of judgment and experience drawn in these conclusions.

While it is to be expected that a group of patients seen at the Mayo Clinic would not represent those instances of tubal rupture with severe shock necessitating immediate emergency treatment, these figures as to the recurrence of ectopic pregnancy and as to the possibility of subsequent intra-uterine pregnancies are in keeping with series from other localities and hospitals.

Conservative surgical approach is certainly to be recommended in the care of this pelvic pathology as in all pelvic surgery.

Wendell Long.

The Persistence of Gonococcal Infection in the Adnexa by Studdiford, Casper, and Scadron; Surgery, Gynecology and Obstetrics; August, 1938, Vol. 67, No. 2, page 176.

This is a report of the bacteriological study of 24 patients which was undertaken "to determine, if possible, whenever the gonococcus is persistent in cases that are clinically and pathologically recognized as chronic salpingitis."

"Of this number 66.6 per cent were found to harbor gonococci in spite of the fact that none of them was in the acute stage of the disease." These findings are at variance with the older observations about the presence of gonococci in chronic inflammation of the uterine adnexa. . These authors reviewed the literature and particularly call attention to the work of Curtis in 1921 in which 192 cases were studied and gonococci were not demonstrated in any case that did not at the same time reveal evidence of recent inflammation. Curtis, therefore, felt that the organisms were rapidly killed and that they were rarely recoverable in culture later than two weeks after the disappearance of fever and leucocytosis. Studdiford and his co-authors point out the fact that no competent bacteriological investigation has been carried on since that of Curtis in 1921 and the present investigation is in direct variance with the findings of Curtis and others.

In one of Studdiford's cases it was most likely that the most recent infection took place at least 10 years before study. In another, fever therapy had apparently cured the local cervical infection, but the culture from the tube was positive. It was also significant that the gonococcus complement fixation tests were found to be frequently at variance with the results of culture.

The conclusions of the authors are quoted below since they are concise and to the point.

1. "Contrary to previous reports, the fallopian tubes may remain as active foci of gonococcal infection for long periods of time.

2. "Many cases regarded as acute exacerbations of chronic salpingitis may be due to recrudescences of residual infections rather than to reinfections.

3. "Gonococci may survive in the tube in the presence of turpentine and mineral oil.

4. "Gonococci may survive in the tube despite apparent cure of local cervical infection by hyperpyrexia."

COMMENT: This is an extremely practical subject and since the authors' results vary so greatly from that of the most recent investigation by Dr. Curtis in 1921, this report is deserving of critical study.

The present series is far too small for any comprehensive conclusions and it is to be hoped that these authors will extend their investigation over a large enough series of patients so that they can draw conclusions with more assurance.

However, the work of Curtis in 1921 has been used as a basis for the therapeutic management of gonococcal infection in the uterine adnexa and it is entirely possible that a review of the bacteriology of chronic inflammatory disease of the uterine adnexa will influence to no small degree the treatment of this annoying but common condition.

It must be added that these findings do not justify any but conservative treatment in the initial attacks of gonorrheal infection in women. This applies equally to the subacute stages of inflammation due to gonorrheal infection.

Wendell Long.

Glomus Tumor. Report of a Case. By Charles P. Larson, C. M. and R. J. Bennett, Fort Steilacoom, Washington. Western Journal of Surgery, Obstetrics and Gynecology, November, 1938.

This is an interesting article about a rare tumor, benign in character, which has received definite study only within recent years.

The authors credit Masson, pathologist for the Western State Hospital, Fort Steilacoom, Washington, with a description of the true origin of the tumor, he having described the detailed histology in 1924.

The authors say, "the neuromyo-arterial glomus is a normal vascular anastamosis which is distinctive in that it is arteriovenous with no intervening capillaries and that it has a peculiar architecture which includes smooth muscle and nerve fibers." It appears that the glomus tumors are usually located on the extremities, particularly under the nails (subungual position). They are sometimes found in the skin of the extremities, and other parts of the body. The authors report a case in a man 49 years of age, an inmate of a hospital for the treatment of mental diseases, where the tumor was located "on the flexor surface of the right wrist just above the ends of the radius and ulna." It had been present for about 12 years and was noticed because of excruciating pain, particularly on stimulation. It was a pale blue nodule about 2 cm. in diameter. "On the medial side of the nodule there was a darker colored, bluish-purple elevation, pinhead in size which was the 'trigger point' of the tumor." When this point was irritated, it produced great pain.

In the case of this particular patient, the true character of the tumor had been overlooked for a long time because it was supposed that the complaint of the patient was probably of a psychotic character.

The tumor was removed by surgical operation. The following is the microscopic report: "The tumor was surrounded by a thick layer of connective tissue, but this did not completely encapsulate the nodule as newly formed vessels surrounded by glomus cells were found lying free on the outer edge. A large nerve trunk was seen entering one side of the tumor. The body of the glomangioma was made up of distorted blood vessels having large lumens of irregular sizes and shapes. These vessels were lined internally by endothelium and some of them possessed a smooth muscle wall while others showed only a mantle of glomus cells. Elastic laminae were entirely lacking in the arterial walls. The glomus cells were found arranged in four different ways: (1) closely packed together in the walls of the vessels intermingled with smooth muscle cells; (2) forming a mantle around an endothelial-lined sinus; (3) clumped together into large masses without a vascular lumen; (4) loosely arranged and separated from each other by a homogeneous eosinophilic material containing an occasional collagen fiber. The cells were polygonal to round in shape, having a deeply basophilic nucleus and a clear eosinophilic cytoplasm. Mitoses were absent but in areas where new canals were being formed the glomus cells were much larger and more embryonic in appearance. With Mallory's phosphotungstic acid hemotaxylin stain numerous nerve bundles and fibers were demonstrated both in the cavernous portions of the tumor and between the individual glomus cells. Normal appearing arteries having a smooth muscle wall and elastic laminae were also present." The authors report that all symptoms were relieved after the excision of the tumor, but it had been only about two weeks before the article was written, so that it is uncertain about the final result.

The authors comment as follows:

"1. The tumor possessed a 'trigger point' of nervous excitation.

"2. The patient, being psychotic, caused the symptom of pain in the tumor to be regarded by the attending physicians as psychoneurotic in origin.

"3. On stimulation the tumor enlarged to twice its normal size and became darker in color. As this coincided with the onset of the pain, we may assume that the dilatation of the glomic vessels was the factor which stimulated the nerve endings.

"4. The nonencapsulation of the tumor suggests that it grew not merely by pushing aside the surrounding connective t i s s u e in a centrifugal manner, but by active infiltration and proliferation. This observation makes the possibility of recurrence a likely event in this particular case."

The authors report that only about 70 authentic cases have appeared in the literature.

LeRoy Long.

Acute Cholecystitis. The Results of Operation Within Forty-Eight Hours of the Onset of Symptoms; Henry F. Graham, and Milton E. Hoefle; Annals of Surgery; November, 1938; Vol. 108, No. 5; page 874.

During the past 10 years increasing interest has been shown in early operation for acute cholecystitis. However, the term "early operation," judging from various articles read, is used loosely by the various authors and seems to mean anything from early in the disease to soon after admission to the hospital, although the patient may have been previously ill at home for some days. These authors, in an effort to more definitely evaluate their results, have found it desirable to set a definite time and, for the purpose of this study, they chose the first 48 hours from the onset of the symptoms of the acute attack.

In a collection of 167 cases which were operated upon within 48 hours of the onset, there occurred six deaths, a mortality rate of 3:59 per cent. The authors were more concerned with the promptness of the operation than with the type of procedure, but cholecystectomy was the operation of choice in these cases, while cholecystostomy was reserved for the more critical cases.

They point out the fact that a cholecystectomy for acute cholecystitis is more difficult than one performed in the quiescent period. Several procedures which make for safety while doing operation in this stage are given. For instance, the authors prefer as a rule to remove the gallbladder from above downwards, controlling the bleeding from the liver bed by the pressure of a gauze pad and retractor. The cystic duct is carefully ligated, using traction toward the common duct instead of away from it. This prevents the possibility of pulling the cystic duct off accidentally at a lower level than was intended. If the cystic artery does escape and bleeds, they attempt to control this and secure a dry field by the use of a small angular retractor or the finger in the foramen of Winslow making pressure on the hepatic artery until the bleeding vessel has been clamped and ligated. When there is an oozing liver bed, that cannot be obliterated, they place a free omental graft with a few interrupted sutures.

It has frequently been said that acute cholecystitis is not like acute appendicitis, and that there is not the same necessity for prompt operative interference. The authors cannot agree with this statement. They graphically demonstrate their reason for disagreement with a table which shows the results in 100 consecutive cholecystectomies for acute cholecystitis on Dr. Graham's service at the Methodist Hospital in Brooklyn. This shows:

Acute cholecystitis operated upon within 48 hours —51 cases—two deaths—3.93 per cent.

Acute cholecystitis operated upon two to five days—27 cases—two deaths—7.40 per cent.

Acute cholecystitis operated upon five days or more—22 cases—five deaths—22.72 per cent.

Total mortality in 100 cases—nine deaths—9.0 per cent.

This shows that in their experience a delay of more than five days gives a high operative mortality, and raises the question of whether operation should be performed or delay advised. They feel that this decision must be made in the individual case. Also when an operation is done, the further question of what operation is indicated will always arise. Gangrenous and perforated gallbladders are seen within 48 hours after the onset of symptoms and it must be realized by surgeons generally that these conditions are not rare or unusual events. Most of the recently published series of cases of acute cholecystitis show an incidence of gangrene of about 20 per cent.

They quote a series by Pennoyer of Roosevelt Hospital in New York of 300 cases of acute cholecystitis in which the general policy was to delay whenever possible. Pennoyer's mortality was 10 per cent. This presents a striking contrast to the 3.59 per cent mortality in the cases operated upon within 48 hours of the onset and certainly seems to be a strong argument in favor of a determined effort to obtain these cases for operation within 48 hours.

They make the following statement: "It is difficult to see two sides to this question, when it is so evident that a lowering in mortality could be accomplished so easily by education of the laity and cooperation between the family physician and the surgeon to secure a prompt operation, early in the attack, for every person suffering from acute cholecystitis who is a proper operative risk."

LeRoy D. Long.

Regional Enteritis; Claude F. Dixon; Annals of Surgery; November, 1938; Vol. 108, No. 5; page 857.

The author feels that regional enteritis, terminal ileitis, or nonspecific granuloma of the intestine is either occurring more frequently or is being recognized more often than in the past. He reports a total of 69 patients with regional enteritis who have been treated at the Mayo Clinic.

The 14 cases reported by Crohn, Ginsberg and Oppenheimer, in 1932, gave the first classic description of what is known as ileitis, granuloma of the intestine, or segmental enteritis. In Crohn's original article he expressed the belief that this disease was confined to the ileum, but, in 1936, he and Rosenak reported a total of 60 cases, confirmed at operation, in nine of which there was involvement of some portion of the large bowel. It now seems certain, judging from reports by many others as well as from some of the cases in this series, that so-called terminal ileitis not infrequently involves the cecum and portions of the large intestine as well as the terminal ileum.

In this Mayo Clinic series the frequency of signs and symptoms encountered is interesting. The frequency and the order in which they occur in this series was as follows: Loss of weight 100 per cent; next in order came cramping pains, diarrhea, palpable mass (in 77 per cent), nausea and vomiting, anemia, external fistula, and blood in stools.

Dr. Dixon thinks that the rational treatment at the present time consists in resection of the diseased segment of intestine. A short-circuiting operation alone such as ileocolostomy often affords temporary relief and apparently, in isolated instances, may produce subsidence of all symptoms. A two stage operation, although impractical in some given cases, seems to be the procedure of choice because of safety. So-called spontaneous cures have been occasionally recorded but must be viewed with some skepticism.

Ulceration of the mucosa of the bowel and enlargement of the mesenteric lymph nodes may be the beginning of regional enteritis, and transillumination of the intestine may prove to be an aid in locating such early lesions. By placing a cold Cameron light behind the suspected segment of intestine and transilluminating it, one may be able to detect a small defect such as an ulceration or a polyp.

The etiology of regional enteritis is unknown. The concensus at present seems to place the cause of regional enteritis on an infectious basis. Up to the present time, however, studies of specimens which have been removed have failed to reveal a specific Bacterium as the cause of the disease. (A study of the literature on non-malignant disease of the intestines gives the impression that many such lesions have been incorrectly diagnosed as tuberculosis.)

It seems probable that when one is dealing with proved segmental enteritis, extensive recurrence of the disease is most likely to follow unless radical resection is carried out. Radical excision of the mesentery should be made if enlarged nodes are present.

Dr. Dixon feels (and I heartily agree with him) that the side-to-side anastomosis of the ileum to the transverse bowel is safer than end-to-end or end-to-side anastomosis which is done by many surgeons.

LeRoy D. Long.

---o---

EYE, EAR, NOSE AND THROAT

Edited by Marvin D. Henley, M.D.
911 Medical Arts Building, Tulsa

Use of Sulfanilimide in Otolaryngology. Harry P. Schenck, M.D., Philadelphia. Archives of Otolaryngology, November, 1938.

An extensive historical and experimental survey is given in the beginning of this article. The entire article is about 50 pages in length and is quite the most complete publication on this drug that has yet been published. Long and Bliss concluded that about 48 hours is the time elapsed before the maximum therapeutic effect is obtained. In far advanced infections or practically moribund patients spectacular results cannot be expected. "In man, absorption of sulfanilimide is apparently complete from the gastrointestinal tract in four hours." The initial and maintenance dose are discussed. The opinion is expressed that sulfanilimide by injection is not necessary except in cases of nausea, etc., because it produces no higher concentration in the blood than by oral administration alone. As soon as clinical improvement is noted, the dose of the drug should be decreased; if there is no clinical improvement and no untoward side effects are noted, then the dose of the drug should be increased. In recurrence of the same infection, increased dosage is indicated. The above investigators suggest: "that in cases of severe infection in which the immediate prognosis is grave both parenteral and oral administration of sulfanilimide may be used; for moderately severe infections either parenteral or oral administration may be employed; for mild or relatively chronic streptococcic infections, oral administration alone is adequate and frequently one-half to two-thirds the estimated dose is effective.

Some toxic manifestations are weakness, dizziness, tinnitus, lassitude, anorexia, general malaise, nausea, cyanosis, sulfhemoglobinemia and fever. Deaths have been reported repeatedly following the use of sulfanilimide. The administration of magnesium sulfate in conjunction with sulfanilimide is contraindicated because of the combination removing from the blood sulfhemoglobin and methemoglobin. Sulfhemoglobin "could be detected six weeks after the administration of sulfanilimide ceased, while methemoglobin disappeared in about 24 hours."

Pharyngitis and tonsillitis show a favorable effect when the infection is due primarily to hemolytic streptococci; the temperature becomes normal in a few hours to three days but the streptococci persists in the cultures for as long as four or five weeks. Streptococcus viridans is affected little, if any. Some report no better effects than from the use of sodium salicylate.

Vincent's Infection shows no effect from sulfanilimide topically or orally.

Ludwig's Angina: One author reports a case of a three-year-old child apparently cured by sulfanilimide; two other authors report two deaths in 20 and 35 hours after beginning treatment with sulfanilimide.

Other oral infections such as "dry socket," osteomyelitis of the mandible, peridontal and periapical infections, stomatitis aphthosa, subperiosteal abscess, parotitis and various other similar infections are reported to be favorably influenced by the giving of the drug.

Adenitis-suppurative seems not to be influenced by this drug but non-suppurative adenitis is acted on favorably.

Otitis Media: Watson-Williams are of the opinion that sulfanilimide is of definite value. Pediatricians in general seem to feel that there are fewer mastoid complications following a middle ear infection.

Mastoiditis: Especially of-value in those cases where there is a meningeal irritation present. Basman and Perley note that "the outstanding feature of sulfanilimide therapy in the treatment of mastoiditis is the smooth post-operative course with lack of complications."

Otogenic Meningitis: "The most convincing evidence of the effectiveness of sulfanilimide therapy in man has accrued from the clinical observations in cases of beta hemolytic streptococcic meningitis." The effect on staphylococcic infections is a moot question.

Pneumococcic Meningitis: The application here has not been widespread. The reports from various investigators are not uniform.

Other types of meningitis such as Bacillus proteus and influenza bacilli also show conflicting reports from different men.

Meningococcic Meningitis: One advantage of the sulfanilimide here over the anti-meningococcus serum is the absence of intraspinal and intravenous therapy, the danger of protein shock and the discomfort of serum sickness. The majority of reports concur in its efficacy here.

Abscess of the Brain: Two cases are reported with recovery with the use of sulfanilimide.

Cavernous Sinus Thrombosis: A case with a clinical picture of cavernous sinus thrombosis is reported with recovery with the giving of sulfanilimide.

Bacteremia: "Sulfanilimide appears to be strikingly effective against the types of bacteremia due to the beta hemolytic streptococcus, the meningococcus and, to some extent, the pneumococcus. It is ineffective against Str. viridans and the staphylococcus."

Erysipelas: The results are favorable—gives a reduction of the incidence of complications and diminishes the tendency to recur.

Infection of a wound due to hemolytic streptococcus reacts favorably to this therapy.

Infection of the Sinuses: Few reports are available but the majority of those available report favorably on the action of the drug.

The article closes with discussion of the use of sulfanilimide in other diseases such as acute rheumatic fever, tularemia, acute infectious mononucleosis, lymphatic leukemia, and post-traumatic gangrene (gas).

———

Nature of the Filtrable Agent of Trachoma. Phillips Thygeson, M.D., and Polk Richards, M.D. (Digested from the Archives of Ophthalmology, October, 1938.) Published in the Digest of Ophthalmology and Otolaryngology, Vol. 1, No. 2, December, 1938.

"It is now generally agreed that none of the bacteria found on trachomatous conjunctiva are the cause of the disease. It has, however, been demonstrated that the causative agent of trachoma is filtrable, has the characteristics of a virus and that it is identical with the elementary body of Halberstadter and von Prowazek. The available evidence indicates that the agent of trachoma is located in the epithelium of the conjunctiva, and the material yielding active filtrates contained substantial numbers of epithelial inclusions.

Halberstadter and von Prowazek noted bodies which they thought were the cause of the disease both free in the secretion and as inclusions in the cytoplasm of epithelial cells. A number of workers accepted these bodies as etiologic agents, but the evidence has been insufficient to gain universal acceptance, although the inclusion bodies are recognized as the most characteristic microscopic evidence of the disease.

Elementary b o d i e s from epithelial scrapings (Giemsa-stained) from persons with active trachoma were seen as minute, sharply defined, reddish blue bodies having a diameter of about 0.25 micron. There are no morphologic differences between them and the elementary bodies of vaccina or molluscum contagiousum, but they differ in staining qualities. They are almost identical in both morphologic structure and staining with the granules of inclusion blennorrhea and psittacosis.

It is believed that the elementary b o d i e s of trachoma are virus bodies like those of psittacosis and inclusion blennorrhea and except in staining qualities, to typical virus elementary bodies, such as those of vaccinia, fowl-pox and molluscum contagiousum. The examination of Giemsa-stained epithelial scrapings from 1,700 persons with conjunctivitis showed elementary bodies of Halberstadter and von Prowazek only in persons with inclusion blennorrhea and trachoma.

Filter tests showed that no elementary bodies were demonstrable in either trachomatous material or molluscum contagiousum after passing through Berkefeld V filters under ordinary conditions, but with Elford membranes 0.6 micron pore diameter elementary bodies were demonstrable in both. An inoculation experiment upon a human volunteer with material which had been passed through an Elford graded collodion membrane of 0.6 micron average pore diameter although free from bacteria produced typical trachoma.

Since the elementary bodies of trachoma and inclusion blennorrhea are indistinguishable by morphological or clinical means, epidemilogic data were used' to differentiate the two. Inclusion blennorrhea has a low degree of communicability, does not become epidemic, and cases in adults are rare. Inclusion blennorrhea has not been reported in many localities where trachoma is of common occurrence. Rotth observed that inclusions are not found in inclusion blennorrhea after the first few months, whereas trachoma inclusion bodies are present over a period of years.

Elementary bodies are found in practically all cases of active trachoma, the number decreasing proportionately with the degree of activity of the disease. In cases of cicatricial and healed trachoma they were usually absent. In those of over 10 years duration which were undergoing acute exacerbation inclusion bodies and free elementary bodies were found in large numbers. Experiments indicated that the bodies develop in the epithelial cells when transferred to monkeys and to one human volunteer.

The virus of trachoma apparently cannot be cultivated by ordinary methods. It is difficult to demonstrate elementary bodies in patients who have extensive treatment. A test upon 10 cases was made to determine the effect of sulfanilimide treatment with the result that after 15 days of treatment no inclusions were found.

The Diagnosis and Treatment of Meniere's Disease. S. H. Mygind and Dida Dederding, Copenhagen. Annals of Otology, Rhinology and Laryngology, September, 1938.

Mentioned in the differential diagnosis are: collateral labyrinth edema; middle ear catarrh and tubal stenosis; neuro-labyrinthitis; otosclerosis; intracranial affections such as epidemic encephalitis, disseminate sclerosis, cerebral tumor, and acoustic nerve tumor.

The examination of these patients should include the otologist, the internist, the neurological and the ophthalmological inspection and examination of the cerebrospinal fluid.

Very little medication is advocated by the authors, either in the acute attack or in the treatment proper. The aim of the treatment is to reduce the intake of fluid and the consumption of salt. Their routine of so doing is outlined. An exact dose or amount of liquids and salt is not given, but the patient is observed very closely for some time and his daily habits as to food are recorded and then he is put on their schedule. If possible it is best to hospitalize these patients for about a month until they learn their routine thoroughly. Daily intake and output of fluid is measured. If the weight is too high or too low this is controlled by the proper foods. Care is taken that there is not a deficiency of vitamins or calcium. The aim is "to empty the abnormal water depots in the ear and elsewhere." It is also important to ward off factors that tend towards this retention. Stimulation of circulation in the skin, muscles and lungs is advocated. Irradiation with a carbon arc light is used for this purpose. Other forms of physiotherapy are used advantageously. These must be used cautiously at first, increasing in length and severity only when it is known that the patient tolerates it well. "On the whole it is essential not to overdo the treatment but to apply a suitable mixture of stimulation and rest during cautious training."

The authors question Gothlins suggestion that a C-Avitaminosis is a frequent cause of Meniere's disease.

Local treatment of regular catheterization of the eustachian tube is recommended, for prevention of stenosis as well as for mobilization of the auditory ossicles. The content of the labyrinth may also be influenced by this manipulation via fenestrae.

After a month's hospitalization and three to six months on the routine out of the hospital the patient is allowed to resume his ordinary means of living. The giddiness is many times cured and the hearing improved. At the end of three years 81 per cent of the patients treated were still permanently free from giddiness. The series treated included 157 patients. Sixty-one patients showed improvement in hearing during the time of treatment. At the end of three years about half of these said their improvement in hearing was permanent. These results might be termed as satisfactory.

"Isolated cases defy all treatment, but in the majority of cases the bad result must be ascribed partly to inefficient control of the patient and partly to insufficient individualization of the treatment. What matters is to find out the combination of casual agents, exogenous and endogenous, physical and psychical, which are at the bottom of each individual case."

---o---

INTERNAL MEDICINE
Edited by Hugh Jeter, M.D., 1200 North Walker, Oklahoma City

Histologic Study of the Endometrium During Pregnancy. Albert C. Broders and John R. McDonald. Section on Surgical Pathology, The Mayo Clinic, Rochester, Minnesota. (American Journal of Clinical Pathology, September, 1938, Vol. 8, No. 5.)

It has been known since 1899 when Opitz stated that endometrial glands undergo certain changes during pregnancy. He found that early in pregnancy the glands form papillary processes which projected into the lumens and that the intervening stroma was scanty. Later in the course of pregnancy, the papillary projections and greater part of the epithelium disappear and the glands are lined by one layer of cells. It is thought that decidual tissue is present in the uterus in all cases of ectopic pregnancy but this author did not find it present in all cases.

The findings are based on the study of the endometrium in 111 cases of intra-uterine pregnancy, 27 cases of extra-uterine pregnancy and two cases in the agravid uterus. The menstrual cycle is divided into early and late proliferated phases and differentiative phases. The results are as follows: In the 111 intra-uterine cases, 99 showed either decidual formation changes or endometrial glandular changes. The glands were most typical in cases where the decidual formation was minimal. Therefore, the glandular changes are comparable to the late differentiative phases of the menstrual cycle and occur in early pregnancy.

In 27 cases of extra-uterine pregnancy, 11 cases revealed typical decidua or glands of pregnancy or both and correspond to the late differentiative phases or early pregnancy.

In two cases of agravid uteri, one showed glands of pregnancy and was comparable to the late differentiative phase.

Conclusion:

1. The endometrial glands are present in a large proportion of cases of early pregnancy, a smaller number of extra-uterine pregnancy and occasionally in agravid uteri and that these glands have the same significance as decidual tissue.

2. The endometrium usually shows late differentiative phases in early uterine pregnancy. It is less common in extra-uterine pregnancy.

The Early Diagnosis of Acute and Latent Plumbism. Frederick L. Smith, 2nd, Thomas K. Rathmell and George E. Marcil. (American Journal of Clinical Pathology, September, 1938, Volume 8, Number 5.)

In this the authors evaluate the laboratory findings in cases of absorption into the body of a substance which in excessive amounts may cause an acute toxic condition, or produce such an effect at a later date by its accumulation in the body and its subsequent release due to a lowering of a normal tolerance and some uncontrollable change in the equilibrium of physiological and biological factors. Especial attention is given to the early diagnosis of acute and latent plumbism although the differential diagnosis is well discussed.

Further, in this, the authors present a diagnostic procedure for all types of lead intoxication, including incipient, latent, acute and c h r o n i c phases of the disease. This procedure is based upon the lead content of the serum, cells and fibrin fraction and whole blood from the patients.

The a u t h o r s maintain that a differentiation could be made between any stage of lead poisoning and other pathological conditions in which the clinical signs and symptoms might be confused with those of lead toxics. In addition to the diagnostic procedure the authors have followed the progress of cases of plumbism by daily shiftograms and hemograms and by making additional lead blood analyses when hemographically or clinically indicated.

The range of lead values for the healthy normal individual is given and appears to be independent of sex, age, climatic conditions, daily fatigue, violent exercise, meals, menstruation and ovulation.

The authors in this paper point out that the lead anemia is due to abnormal destruction of red blood cells in the circulating blood and not due to a diminished production of blood, except in the last stages of plumbism when a degeneration of the bone marrow may occur. The chief characteristics of the immature cells is the presence of a basophilic substance and this may be produced by many substances such as lead, arsenic, Benzol and the effects of high altitudes. The authors conclude that stipple cells are not pathognomonic of plumbism but are present and increase in many other diseases. They maintain that the stippling of red blood cells may occur whenever the productions of red blood cell destruction are retained in the body.

Many interesting tables are presented including (1) clinical signs and symptoms of plumbism with differential diagnosis, (2) relation of basophilic stippling, reticulocyte count and basophilic aggregation to the development of clinical symptoms in acute, chronic, and induced plumbism, (3) leukocytic shifts during the various stages of plumbism, (4) lead content of the blood of healthy and normal individuals, (5) distribution of lead in the blood associated with pathological processes other than plumbism, (6) distribution of lead in the blood during acute lead poisoning and active periods of chronic plumbism and (7) the distribution of lead in the blood during periods of acute exacerbation of plumbism and the relation to clinical crisis.

In summary, the authors present a diagnostic procedure pathognomonic for lead in any of its clinical forms and manifestations.

---o---

PLASTIC SURGERY
Edited by
GEO. H. KIMBALL, M.D., F.A.C.S.
404 Medical Arts Building, Oklahoma City

A Principle To Be Considered In Transplanting Costal Cartilage for Repairing Deficiencies of the Nasal Skeleton. Forrest Young, M.D., Rochester, N. Y.

The author has called attention to a new principle not commonly used in the reconstruction of the nasal skeleton. Instead of using the long strut of cartilage along the dorsum together with the hinged section for the septal portion, he recommends using a section of cartilage shaped in such a way as to simulate not only the septum but also the alar cartilages.

The author states in his operative technique procedure, that the method which he has gradually evolved in a rather crude attempt to replace not only the dorsal edge of the septal cartilage but the alar cartilages as well. Instead of placing a long strut of cartilage along the dorsum, appro-

priately shaped to fill in the depression, as is the usual practice, a section of costal cartilage is removed with its perichondrium intact. This section is selected with the curve or straight line desired for the dorsal like of the nose. If a columellar support is needed, the first cut provides for a vertical post hinged to the main mass. Parallel longitudinal cuts are made on the edge opposite that selected for the dorsal ridge. These cuts go down or almost to the perichondrium and the thin wings are fractured outward so that they remain hinged by perichondrium. The median mass is thinned and shaped to a pattern previously determined from a cast of the face upon which the desired nose has been built in clay and half removed. The wings are thinned and shaped.

Modeling such a transplant we believe is superior to the usual cantilever strut. If carried out according to indications and well conceived preoperative plans, it produces more normal appearing side walls of the nose and allows a larger airway below, because the nasal lining is not held downward by a large mass of cartilage designed merely to rest upon it in its depressed position.

The author favors autogenous cartilage. He advises against rubber, paraffin, celluloid and metals.

COMMENT: The author presents a very well written as well as completely illustrated technique for his new principle. Part of this plan has been suggested by Gillies and McIndoe.

From the description of the author's technique together with his end results as shown, he has evidently a worthwhile principle.

Total Reconstruction of the Auricle. Earl C. Padgett, Kansas City, Mo. S. G. & O., December, 1938.

The author has worked out a technique for total reconstruction of the auricle. It is well known that this operation has always been particularly difficult, the end results have often been discouraging.

Reasons for reconstruction of auricle: (1) to promote economic efficiency, (2) to alleviate a psychiatric defect, and (3) to give personal satisfaction. The prejudiced attitude of employers and associates often promotes an economic impasse. Whipping the defense reaction against the onslaught of a cruel environment is not a pleasurable pastime even if one is capable of such a reaction. But if one be so unfortunate as to fail in readjustment and the negative surmounts the positive ego, inadequacy to environment follows. The knowledge that one is presentable socially may be a great boon to a sensitive, tried and sore spirit. Therefore, it cannot be said that an adequate procedure which tends to abrogate these reactions, even without other objectives, does not entail in its accomplishment a beneficent craft.

The author presents a plan which he states can be done with safety in three stages, hospitalization not to exceed three weeks.

Material Required: The author uses cartilage from the patient and trims the material to the shape of the helix and anti-helix. These sections are then buried under the skin of the scalp at the level of the opposite ear. He then fashions a flap on the neck, the posterior part of which is tubed to make the rim of the auricle and the bulk is used to cover the raw surface behind the reconstructed ear.

The technique is carefully described so that it can be followed without difficulty.

The indications for the operation are considerably different in the female than in the male. The female can, if she wishes, hide the missing auricle or a deformed one with her hair. Before an attempt is made to reconstruct the auricle, the individual should have attained his full growth, first, because one uses the size of the opposite ear as a pattern and, second, because if the individual has not attained an adult age, the reconstructed ear will not become larger while in all probability the opposite one may grow somewhat.

Requirements and causes of failure: The requisites for good imitation of the normal ear are correct size, similar outline, nearly equal divergent angle from the head, the same relative height and the same position in an anterior posterior direction and that the new auricle retain its size and shape more or less permanently.

In attempts to reconstruct the auricle satisfactorily, the causes of an unsuccessful outcome, barring infection or failure of the material used for structural support to remain imbedded within the tissues without reaction, have been: (1) the inability to obtain structural support of the proper shape and size, (2) the failure to obtain adequate covering of the proper thickness, texture, color, (3) difficulty in maintaining the new auricle at an upright level in comparison with the opposite ear, (4) the development of an improper divergent angle of the auricle from the head, and, finally (5) a tendency for folding, shrinkage, and dimunition in size. When one of these stumbling blocks to success was present, the new auricle could not be considered a glaring success but if more than one or all were present, the qualitative result was decreased progressively, in accordance with the degree of the enumerated defects.

The author suggests that on formulating a plan one should err on the side of too much ear than too little ear, both as to cartilaginous as well as to soft tissue requirements. The flaps should be larger than necessary as it is easier to discard than to go after more tissues.

This in recapitulating the author says: The following desiderata are i m p o r t a n t: A sufficient amount of soft tissues; a type of soft tissue which can be molded to give certain contours that cannot be given by rigid tissues; a sufficient amount of rigid tissues; rigid tissue of a size and shape which simulates most of the larger basic contours of the auricle; the rigid tissue that is more or less permanent; a rigid tissue that is easy to transplant; will stand trauma; maintenance of the proper elevation and preservation of the proper divergent angle from the head.

The author mentions two t y p e s of deformity which present in reconstruction: The congenital rudimentary or absent auricle and the individual in whom some trauma or disease has destroyed the auricle. The author states that he has had 86 cases of congenital absence or defect of the auricle. He presents very well the first, second and third stages of the operative procedure with illustrations.

In the four individual cases which are herein presented the defect in two instances was of congenital origin. The oldest of these was built in 1928. At the present time the shrinkage has been only slight. The other congenitally malformed ear was constructed in 1933. Case two suffered traumatic destruction of the auricle. It was built in 1932. Case four following the application of a 'cancer paste' had suffered almost total destruction of the auricle along with the soft structures about the ear. The depth and extent of the slough may be appreciated when it is noted that the patient had a seventh nerve paralysis because of it. The base upon which the new ear was to rest was repaired and the new auricle was rebuilt in 1936.

The operation presented is one developed from an experience which necessarily entailed some trial and error.

COMMENT: The total reconstruction of the auricle has been tried by many surgeons, the results of most have been somewhat unsatisfactory. Dr. Sheehan sometimes uses the cartilage of the mother which is buried under the skin of the child

in order to make an auricle. The mother subsequently covered her ear region by her manner of hair dress.

The author is to be complimented and congratulated on his clear cut description of this operation.

---------o---------

UROLOGY
Edited by D. W. Branham, M.D.
514 Medical Arts Building, Oklahoma City

Facts Behind the Laws. Mary S. Edwards, Statistician, American S o c i a l Hygiene Association. Journal of Social Hygiene, November, 1938.

The following facts have been gleaned from this article and may be interesting to the profession in view of the approach of the legislative year.

1. Over 95 per cent of syphilis infections are due to sexual contact.

2. Approximately five per cent of all men, women and children (1,650,000 persons) in this country are afflicted with syphilis. Dr. Thomas Parran states he has estimated one in ten adults are stricken with syphilis during his or her lifetime.

3. Seventy-five per cent of infections are contracted before 30 years of age, which brings this group within the marriagable age and the age of the greatest frequency of child bearing. According to the United States Public Health Service 1,000,000 woman who may become mothers have syphilis.

4. Each year 60,000 babies are born with congenital syphilis; one-third of these will suffer from total or partial loss of vision and a considerable percentage will develop mental disturbances or various bone and skin deformities. Less than half of these treated will show satisfactory results.

5. Congenital syphilis is practically 100 per cent preventable if the mothers infection is diagnosed and treated before the fourth prepartum month.

6. A positive Wassermann is usually the only evidence of the disease.

A careful consideration of such facts throw overwhelming weight on the side of carefully written adequately administered and properly understood laws to prevent syphilis in marriage and in unborn children.

Studies on Cystocele and Urinary Incontinence In The Female by Use of Cystograms and Urethrograms. J. Duane Miller. Journal of Urology, November, 1938.

The author has written an excellent article incorporating many illustrations of cystograms and urethrograms in the various deformities incident to perineal pathology occuring in women.

He states that:

Cystograms in the antero-posterior and oblique views in the dorsal, erect and erect straining positions have yielded information valuable in the selection of operative procedure for repair of individual cases of cystocele. They have also served as a method for the evaluation of the repair.

Urethrograms have proved an aid in the investigation into the causes of incontinence and residual urine and have indicated the need, during repair, for special attention to—narrowing the bladder neck and urethra, correcting injuries to the M. trigonalis, and/or providing adequate fixation at the level of the internal sphincter.

Urethrograms may furnish the clue to diagnosis in some cases of chronic urethritis.

OFFICERS OKLAHOMA STATE MEDICAL ASSOCIATION

President, Dr. H. K. Speed, Sayre.

President-Elect, Dr. W. A. Howard, Chelsea.

Secretary-Treasurer-Editor, Dr. L. S. Willour, McAlester.

Executive Secretary, Mr. R. H. Graham, McAlester.

Speaker, House of Delegates, Dr. J. D. Osborn, Jr., Frederick.

Vice Speaker, House of Delegates, Dr. P. P. Neabist, Medical Arts Building, Tulsa.

Delegates to the A. M. A., Dr. W. Albert Cook, Medical Arts Building, Tulsa, 1938-39; Dr. McLain Rogers, Clinton, 1937-1938.

Meeting Place, Oklahoma City, May 1, 2, 3, 1939.

SPECIAL COMMITTEES 1938-39

Annual Meeting: Dr. H. K. Speed, Sayre; Dr. W. A. Howard, Chelsea; Dr. L. S. Willour, McAlester.

Conservation of Hearing: Dr. H. F. Vandever, Chairman, Enid; Dr. J. B. Hollis, Mangum; Dr. Chester McHenry, Oklahoma City.

Conservation of Vision: Dr. W. M. Gallaher, Chairman, Shawnee; Dr. Frank R. Vieregg, Clinton; Dr. Pauline Barker, Guthrie.

Crippled Children: Dr. Earl McBride, Chairman, Oklahoma City; Dr. Roy L. Fisher, Frederick; Dr. M. B. Glismann, Okmulgee.

Industrial Service and Traumatic Surgery: Dr. Cyril C. Clymer, Medical Arts Bldg., Oklahoma City; Dr. J. Wm. Finch, Hobart; Dr. J. A. Rutledge, Ada.

Maternity and Infancy: Dr. George R. Osborn, Chairman, Tulsa; Dr. P. J. DeVanney, Sayre; Dr. Leila E. Andrews, Oklahoma City.

Necrology: Dr. G. H. Stagner, Chairman, Erick; Dr. James L. Shuler, Durant; Dr. S. D. Neely, Muskogee.

Post Graduate Medical Teaching: Dr. Henry H. Turner, Chairman, Oklahoma City; Dr. H. C. Weber, Bartlesville; Dr. Ned R. Smith, Tulsa.

Study and Control of Cancer: Dr. Wendell Long, Chairman, Oklahoma City; Dr. Paul B. Champlin, Enid; Dr. Ralph McGill, Tulsa.

Study and Control of Tuberculosis: Dr. Carl Puckett, Chairman, Oklahoma City; Dr. W. C. Tisdal, Clinton; Dr. F. P. Baker, Tallihina.

ADVISORY COUNCIL FOR AUXILIARY

Dr. H. K. Speed, Chairman..Sayre

Dr. C. J. Fishman......................................Oklahoma City

Dr. W. S. Larrabee...Tulsa

Dr. J. M. Watson...Enid

Dr. T. H. McCarley...McAlester

STANDING COMMITTEES 1938-39

Medical Defense: Dr. O. E. Templin, Chairman, Alva; Dr. L. C. Kuyrkendall, McAlester; Dr. E. Albert Aisenstadt, Picher.

Medical Economics: Dr. C. B. Sullivan, Cordell, Chairman; Dr. J. L. Patterson, Duncan; Dr. W. M. Browning, Waurika.

Medical Education and Hospital: Dr. V. C. Tisdal, Chairman, Elk City; Dr. Robert U. Patterson, Oklahoma City; Dr. H. M. McClure, Chickasha.

Public Policy and Legislation: Dr. Finis W. Ewing, Surety Bldg., Chairman, Muskogee; Dr. Tom Lowry, 1200 North Walker, Oklahoma City; Dr. O. C. Newman, Shattuck.

(The above committee co-ordinated by the following, selected from each councilor district.)

District No. 1.—Arthur E. Hale, Alva.

District No. 2.—McLain Rogers, Clinton.

District No. 3.—Thomas McElroy, Ponca City.

District No. 4.—L. H. Ritzhaupt, Guthrie.

District No. 5.—P. V. Annadown, Sulphur.

District No. 6.—R. M. Shepard, Tulsa.

District No. 7.—Sam A. McKeel, Ada.

District No. 8.—J. A. Morrow, Sallisaw.

District No. 9.—W. A. Tolleson, Eufaula.

District No. 10.—J. L. Holland, Madill.

Scientific Exhibits: Dr. E. Rankin Denny, Chairman, Tulsa; Dr. Robert H. Akin, Oklahoma City; Dr. R. C. Pigford, Tulsa.

Scientific Work: Dr. W. G. Husband, Chairman, Hollis; Dr. J. S. Rollins, Prague; Dr. J. L. Day, Supply.

Public Health:

Chairman—Dr. G. S. Baxter, Shawnee.

District No. 1.—C. W. Tedrowe, Woodward.

District No. 2.—E. W. Mabry, Altus.

District No. 3.—L. A. Mitchell, Stillwater.

District No. 4.—J. J. Gable, Norman.

District No. 5.—Geo. S. Barber, Lawton.

District No. 6.—C. E. Bradley, Tulsa.

District No. 7.—G. S. Baxter, Shawnee.

District No. 8.—M. M. De Arman, Miami.

District No. 9.—T. H. McCarley, McAlester.

District No. 10.—J. B. Clark, Coalgate.

SCIENTIFIC SECTIONS

General Surgery: Dr. F. L. Flack, Chairman, Nat'l Bank of Tulsa Bldg., Tulsa; Dr. John E. McDonald, Vice-Chairman, Medical Arts Bldg., Tulsa; Dr. John F. Burton, Secretary, Osler Building, Oklahoma City.

General Medicine: Dr. Frank Nelson, Chairman, 603 Medical Arts Bldg., Tulsa; Dr. E. R. Musick, Vice-Chairman, Medical Arts Bldg., Oklahoma City; Dr. Milam McKinney, Medical Arts Bldg., Oklahoma City.

Eye, Ear, Nose & Throat: Dr. E. H. Coachman, Chairman, Manhattan Bldg., Muskogee; Dr. F. M. Cooper, Vice-President, Medical Arts Bldg., Oklahoma City; Dr. James R. Reed, Secretary, Medical Arts Bldg., Oklahoma City.

Obstetrics and Pediatrics: Dr. C. W. Arrendell, Chairman, Ponca City; Dr. Carl F. Simpson, Vice-Chairman, Medical Arts Bldg., Tulsa; Dr. Ben H. Nicholson, Secretary, 300 West Twelfth Street, Oklahoma City.

Genito-Urinary Diseases and Syphilology: Dr. Elijah Sullivan, Chairman, Medical Arts Bldg., Oklahoma City; Dr. Henry Browne, Vice-Chairman, Medical Arts Bldg., Tulsa; Dr. Robert Akin, Secretary, 400 West Tenth, Oklahoma City.

Dermatology and Radiology: Dr. W. A. Showman, Chairman, Medical Arts Bldg., Tulsa; Dr. E. D. Greenberger, Vice-Chairman, McAlester; Dr. Hervey A. Foerster, Secretary, Medical Arts Bldg., Oklahoma City.

STATE BOARD OF MEDICAL EXAMINERS

Dr. Thos. McElroy, Ponca City, President; Dr. C. E. Bradley, Tulsa, Vice-President; Dr. J. D. Osborn, Jr., Frederick, Secretary; Dr. L. E. Emanuel, Chickasha; Dr. W. T. Ray, Gould; Dr. G. L. Johnson, Pauls Valley; Dr. W. W. Osgood, Muskogee.

STATE COMMISSIONER OF HEALTH

Dr. Chas. M. Pearce, Oklahoma City.

COUNCILORS AND THEIR COUNTIES

District No. 1: Texas, Beaver, Cimarron, Harper, Ellis, Woods, Woodward, Alfalfa, Major, Dewey—Dr. O. E. Templin, Alva. (Term expires 1940.)

District No. 2: Roger Mills, Beckham, Greer, Harmon, Washita, Kiowa, Custer, Jackson, Tillman—Dr. V. C. Tisdal, Elk City. (Term expires 1939.)

District No. 3: Grant, Kay, Garfield, Noble, Payne, Pawnee—Dr. A. S. Risser, Blackwell. (Term expires 1941.)

District No. 4: Blaine, Kingfisher, Canadian, Logan, Oklahoma, Cleveland—Dr. Philip M. McNeill, Oklahoma City. (Term expires 1941.)

District No. 5: Caddo, Comanche, Cotton, Grady, Love, Stephens, Jefferson, Carter, Murray—Dr. Walter Hardy, Ardmore. (Term expires 1941.)

District No. 6: Osage, Creek, Washington, Nowata, Rogers, Tulsa—Dr. James Stevenson, Medical Arts Bldg., Tulsa. (Term expires, 1941.)

District No. 7: Lincoln, Pontotoc, Pottawatomie, Okfuskee, Seminole, McClain, Garvin, Hughes—Dr. J. A. Walker, Shawnee. (Term expires 1939.)

District No. 8: Craig, Ottawa, Mayes, Delaware, Wagoner, Adair, Cherokee, Sequoyah, Okmulgee, Muskogee—Dr. E. A. Aisenstadt, Picher. (Term expires 1939.)

District No. 9: Pittsburg, Haskell, Latimer, LeFlore, McIntosh—Dr. L. C. Kuyrkendall, McAlester. (Term expires 1939.)

District No. 10: Johnson, Marshall, Coal, Atoka, Bryan, Choctaw, Pushmataha, McCurtain—Dr. J. S. Fulton, Atoka. (Term expires 1939.)

International Post-Graduate Medical Assembly

Following is the program of the International Post-Graduate Medical Assembly of Southwest Texas, to be held at San Antonio, Texas.

Data on the meeting:

1. Dates: January 24, 25, 26, 1939.
2. No registration fee for doctors living outside of Bexar county.
3. Complimentary stag smoker, Tuesday night, January 24.
4. Dutch treat dinner-dance, Wednesday night, January 25.
5. Public health lectures, January 25.
   Topics: Dr. J. A. Myers on Tuberculosis.
   Dr. Karl A. Menninger on Insanity.
6. Short trip into northern Mexico for the guest speakers.

Guest speakers:

Dr. Fred L. Adair, University of Chicago.

Dr. G. H. Belote, University of Michigan.

Dr. Russell L. Cecil, Cornell University.

Dr. James B. Costen, Washington University.

Dr. Harry S. Gradle, Northwestern University.

Dr. D. Nelson Henderson, University of Toronto.

Dr. Arthur E. Hertzler, University of Kansas.

Dr. Roy R. Kracke, Emory University.

Dr. W. Russell MacAusland, Tufts Medical College.

Dr. Karl A. Menninger, The Menninger Clinic.

Dr. J. A. Myers, University of Minnesota.

Dr. Howard C. Naffziger, University of California.

Dr. H. G. Poncher, University of Illinois.

Dr. Alexander Randall, University of Pennsylvania.

Dr. Charles G. Sutherland, Mayo Foundation.

Dr. Ismael Cosio Villegas, National University of Mexico.

Exploitation of the Medical Profession

Everywhere it is rampant — newspapers, magazines, billboards, radio. "Your doctor will tell you that. . . ." "Medical science has found that. . . ." "The greatest specialists in Timbuctoo say that. . . ." And the rest of the story is of course, "Use our pills or our vitamins three times a day; ask your doctor."

You are forced to compete with those who offer your patients free advice regarding medical treatment. You deliver Mrs. Blank's baby today, and tomorrow she will receive by mail samples of baby foods with complete directions how to use them. Indeed, some physician representing a commercial organization and knowing that the case is in your hands may address a personal letter to your patient offering his services free.

It has been said that 10 more years of the present trend of indifference in medical practice will do away with the need for private practice of infant feeding and other branches of medicine.

Mead Johnson & Company have always believed that the feeding and care of babies and growing children is an individual problem that can best be controlled by the individual physician. For over 20 years and in dozens of ethical ways we have given practical effect to this creed. We hold the interest of the medical profession higher than our own, for we too, no doubt, could sell more of our products were we to advertise them directly to the public.

So long as medical men tacitly encourage the present trend, so long will serious inroads continue to be made into private medical practice. When more physicians specify MEAD'S Products when indicated, more babies will be fed by physicians because Mead Johnson & Company earnestly co-operate with the medical profession along strictly ethical lines and never exploit the medical profession.

Report of Licenses Granted to Practice Medicine

NAME	Year of Birth	Place of Birth	School of Graduation	Year of Graduation	Permanent or Present Address
Raines, Morris McKay	1914	Enid, Okla.	Oklahoma University	1937	Hinton, Okla.
Hollingsworth, Rob't. S.	1911	Springfield, Mo.	Oklahoma University	1937	Decatur, Ill.
Loughmiller, Robert Farris	1912	Oklahoma City, Okla.	Oklahoma University	1937	Oklahoma City, Okla.
Hamra, Henry M.	1913	Henryetta, Okla.	Oklahoma University	1937	Henryetta, Okla.
Van Hoesen, Daisy G. (F)	1910	El Reno, Okla.	Oklahoma University	1937	Weehawken, N. J.
LaFon, William F.	1913	Edmond, Okla.	Oklahoma University	1937	Wichita, Kansas
Stuard, Charles Goodson, Jr.	1909	Waurika, Okla.	Oklahoma University	1937	Kansas City, Mo.
Baumann, Milton Charles	1911	Springfield, Ill.	University Illinois	1937	Ada, Okla.
Deutsch, Harry Louis	1911	Steger, Ill.	University Illinois	1938	Stilwell, Okla.
Deutsch, Hobert Eugene	1904	Lake City, Mich.	University Illinois	1936	Lake City, Mich.
Ewell, Wm. Carl	1909	Welty, Okla.	University Arkansas	1937	Tulsa, Okla.
O'Brien, John Emmet	1896	Burlington, Vt.	University Vermont	1923	Rutland, Vermont
Perry, James Hardin	1912	Canadian, Texas	Univ. Tennessee	1937	Healdton, Okla.
Platt, Arnold David	1909	Columbus, Ohio	Ohio State Medical	1938	Tulsa, Okla.
Puckett, Howard Louis	1908	DeKalb Co., Tenn.	Univ. Michigan	1931	Stillwater, Okla.
Tuttle, Arthur Dale	1904	Kansas City, Mo.	Col. Med. Evangelists	1935	Weatherford, Okla.
Walker, William Kenneth	1909	Weleetka, Okla.	Baylor University	1936	Marlow, Okla.
Bond, Ira T., Jr.	1906	Rush Springs, Okla.	Oklahoma University	1927	County Line, Okla.
Hammond, Jas. Harold	1911	Edmond, Okla.	Oklahoma University	1937	Oklahoma City, Okla.
Berry, John Curtis	———	Washington, Okla.	Oklahoma University	1937	Norman, Okla.
Dyer, Isadore	1909	New Orleans, La.	Tulane Med. School	1933	Tahlequah, Okla.
Hassler, Ferdinand Rudolph	1901	Pittsburgh, Pa.	Oklahoma University	1937	Muskogee, Okla.
McBride, Ollie	1902	Lexington, Okla.	Oklahoma University	1937	Ada, Okla.
Royer, Charles Abraham	1907	Coffeyville, Kans.	Kansas University	1932	Alva, Okla.
Kaeiser, William Henry	1906	Buck, Okla.	University Illinois	1936	McAlester, Okla.
Wilson, Charles Hugh	1911	Oklahoma City, Okla.	Oklahoma University	1927	New Rochelle, N. Y.
Wells, Lois Lyon (F)	1894	Selma, Calif.	Vanderbilt Univ.	1935	Oklahoma City, Okla.
Battenfield, John Y.	1912	Pryor, Okla.	Oklahoma University	1937	Muskogee, Okla.
Dargatz, Fred Edward	1886	Osborne, Kans.	U. Kansas City Mo.		Ardmore, Okla.
Zampetti, Herman Anthony	1910	Wilkes-Barre, Pa.	Creighton Univ.	1937	Drumright, Okla.
Tidwell, Robert A.	1913	Miami, Okla.	Oklahoma University	1937	Detroit, Mich.
Brewning, Robert Leroy	1883	——— Ala.	Birmingham M. Col.	1911	Pawnee, Okla.
Calef, Victor	1913	Alexandria, Egypt	St. Louis Univ.	1937	Enid, Okla.
Tracewell, George Logan	1909	Valentine, Nebr.	University Nebraska	1935	Okmulgee, Okla.

THE JOURNAL
OF THE
OKLAHOMA STATE MEDICAL ASSOCIATION

VOLUME XXXII	McALESTER, OKLAHOMA, FEBRUARY, 1939	Number 2

The Surgical Diabetic

GREGORY E. STANBRO, M.D.
OKLAHOMA CITY, OKLAHOMA

This paper discusses certain phases of a disease which affects over one per cent of our p o p u l a t i o n. There are more than 1,000,000 diabetics in the United States to-day. This number is not decreasing, but the incidence is progressively increasing. Diabetic children are living, 100 having passed the 10-year mark in Joslin's Clinic in 1933. In the pre-insulin era, the average diabetic lived six years; today he lives five times as long. The living diabetics of to-day are the dead diabetics of pre-insulin days. Their l i v e s have been saved and carried on by the three diabetic horses, namely, diet, exercise and insulin.

Great strides have been made and are being made in the understanding and care of the diabetic. We have learned the importance of heredity, that artereosclerosis occurs in the neglected and neglectful patient and we are b e c o m i n g cholesterol minded. No specialty e s c a p e s contact with the diabetic and it is frequently every specialist's duty to diagnose and perhaps treat some manifestation of this disease of metabolism, which l e a d s tuberculosis in mortality. Consequently, as a result of the reduction of the death rate in diabetic children to almost zero and through improved care, the diabetic is allowed to live a longer and less burdensome life and there is an increasing number of diabetics who are more prone to develop conditions requiring surgery. This large group is liable to all surgical diseases and in addition, is particularly susceptible to two special surgical diseases, namely, gangrene, chiefly of the lower extremities, and infection, as carbuncles and furunculosis.

The subject "Surgical Diabetes" is consequently of outstanding importance to the surgeon on account of its accelerated frequency and because of the fact that the surgical diabetic is the serious diabetic. Every other diabetic is a surgical diabetic before he dies, and as a surgical diabetic he is six times more liable to die than the medical diabetic. He, therefore, deserves six times the attention. Although the diabetic is susceptible to all surgical diseases throughout the span of life, 50 is the average age. He is not only susceptible to the usual diseases demanding surgery, and the complications likely to occur in any individual, but he is more prone to develop degenerative changes on account of his disturbed metabolism. S c l e r o s i s of his arteries is 10 years in advance of his years, and he is probably more susceptible to infection and to trauma. Even if he is not, any infection raises the blood sugar, delays healing, and reduces the potency of insulin from 50 to 75 per cent. The infection that induces a constitutional reaction, augments the severity of the diabetes and, as the diabetes grows worse, tissue resistance decreases, and infection progresses. Neglected infection spreads and the diabetes grows more and more difficult to control. There is an unexplained diminution in the ability of the body to utilize carbohydrates, the potency of insulin is markedly decreased, and otherwise diagnostic signs and symptoms are masked by the acidosis and impending coma. A mild diabetic becomes temporarily a severe one. Keen judgment and q u i c k decision are necessary. Early removal of local infection stops the vicious circle and insulin regains its potency. Therefore, the surgical diabetic should always be looked upon as a surgical emergency. The surgeon should have a thorough understanding of diabetic pathology and he should have the continuous cooperation of the internist, for the surgical problems are also medical problems.

To state that a surgical patient has diabetes gives as little information regarding that patient's fitness for surgery and his prognosis, as to say that a non-diabetic patient has appendicitis. In addition to the routine examination of the surgical patient, a complete and detailed history of his diabetes is essential.

The length of time he has been a diabetic, the severity of the disease, and the treatment he has received, are all essential. Has his diabetes been neglected, or has he been neglectful? Diabetes is not only a disease of carbohydrate metabolism, but also of protein and fat metabolism. It is now known that this r a p i d l y developed arteriosclerosis is due to inadequate dietary measures. It should be realized that, on account of this sclerosis, the average surgical diabetic has myocarditis. He is a potential coronary thrombosis case. There is an abnormal deposition of glycogen in the heart, in the kidneys, and in the skin.

Realizing the foregoing, the best surgical treatment is prophylaxis, for the diabetic's greatest enemy is surgical disease, and in the majority of instances preventive measures prevent death. Gangrene is the m a j o r surgical complication today and usually occurs in the untreated or poorly treated c a s e s. Ketosis, hyperglycaemia, arteriosclerosis, and malnutrition, increase diabetic liability to infection. Scrupulous cleanliness, a v o i d a n c e of the slightest trauma, postural exercises and the avoidance of hot and cold extremes are some of the measures of prevention. Tight shoes should not be worn. Corns and bunions should receive meticulous c a r e. Joslin says "He taught the Jew and the Gentile to wash his feet." Pain in the legs and cold extremities are premonitory signs and should be signals of danger and preventive measures t a k e n. Furunculosis and carbuncles are a constant bugaboo to the diabetic. Carbuncles are s e p t i c, the worst class of diabetic infection, and carry the highest mortality.

Notwithstanding instruction, care, and prophylaxis, a definite percentage of diabetics are coming to surgery each year. There is the patient who is to be subjected to an operation either for a condition primarily diabetic, s u c h as gangrene, carbuncle, or furunculosis, or, there is the group made up of surgical diseases, which occur independently of, but simultaneously with diabetes, as appendicitis, cholelithiasis, thyroid disease, etc.

Before 1921 and the advent of insulin, diabetes was a contra-indication to elective surgery and the mortality was 40 to 80 per cent. Today the presence of diabetes is of definite consequence, but u n d e r proper management, the prognosis is good. It has even been said that mild diabetes is an asset to the patient, in that it warns the surgeon to thoroughly prepare the patient, who otherwise m i g h t be operated upon following casual pre-operative measures. Mortality is not higher than 10 per cent, and in some clinics as low as 2.5 per cent. In Bazin's clinic, the mortality in a series of surgical diabetics was 2.7, while in the non-diabetics it was 2.4.

The general pre-operative rules are the same, whether the case be one of primarily diabetic surgery, or a surgical disease occurring in the p r e s e n c e of diabetes. If possible, the patient should be under the care of an internist. Surgery tends to dehydration, acidosis, elevation of the blood s u g a r, and the reduction of the nitrous oxide combining power of the blood plasma. Local power of resistance is diminished and degenerative changes are more prone to develop on account of the disturbed metabolism. The patient is over 40, and usually 50 years old. He must be prepared thoroughly and watched closely. If the s u r g i c a l infection is not treated, there will be no diabetic to treat.

If the operation is one of choice, several days of pre-operative care is advantageous. An attempt is made to have the patient's urine sugar free and the blood sugar as near normal as possible, and at least below 250. Preparation should be carried out with the patient in bed; it cannot be accomplished otherwise. The diet should be liberal in carbohydrates, containing at least 100 grms., and a more liberal diet is necessary in the infectious case than in the non-infectious case. Any diet necessary may be given to build up the patient, said diet being b u f f e r e d with insulin. Clark (John Hopkins Bulletin) found that wounds heal faster when the diet is adequate in carbohydrates, and fasting diets delay healing. Joslin says "Feed the patient up to the last hour possible before operation. He will most likely fast altogether too much afterward." When there is much glycosuria, there is dehydration, a dry tongue, thirst, and a soft eye. At least 3,000 cc. of fluids should be given every 24 hours by mouth, per rectum, or subcutaneously. Be guarded in giving intravenous fluids on account of c a r d i a c changes. Give 30 to 50 grms. of glucose in the form of oatmeal or orange juice, at least two hours before the operation, with the usual dose of insulin. Soda bicarbonate g i v e n by some is unnecessary and valueless. Joslin says "I believe that often a patient threatened with diabetic coma is sent into actual coma by the careless administration of soda." Acetone lies dormant in union with protein or the amino acid group. Soda results in a splitting off of the Ketones, overwhelming the vital centers, coma, and perhaps death resulting. A marked loss of weight precedes surgery in the diabetic, an average of 54 pounds in a s e r i e s of McKittrick. Therefore, be guarded in giving morphine and scopolamine. Laxatives should not be used and only enemeta given, thereby avoiding possible diarrhea and further dehydration.

If the case is an urgent one, indicated surgery should not be delayed long because of the diabetes, even t h o u g h the blood sugar be high and there be acetone and diacetic in the urine. Infection increases the severity of diabetes and delay means death of the patient.

Examine the urine and give 50 grms. of glucose by some means, by mouth, per rectum, or intravenously. Give 30 to 50 units of insulin. Operate and stop the vicious circle, namely; infection—reduction of potency of insulin—lowering of tissue resistance — advance of infection — slough — lymphangitis—septicaemia—death.

Anaesthesia: Ether and c h l o r o f o r m should be avoided, as they are lipin solvents. Ether causes a blood sugar rise of 300 milligrams the first hour, which means glycosuria, acetonuria, and diacetic acid. Nitrous oxide and oxygen is less damaging,

b u t is dehydrating. Cyclopropane a n d ethylene probably are the best inhalation anaesthetics. Infiltration anaesthetic is satisfactory, though there is the possibility of devitalization of tissues already suffering from metabolic derangement. Spinal anaesthetic is the anaesthetic of choice in surgery, below the diaphragm.

Operation: Strictly speaking, d i a b e t i c surgery rests upon arteriosclerosis and infection. During the operation, the general rules are the same, whether the operation be one of choice or emergency. Time is an important factor. The simplest operation which will relieve the patient is the best. No secondary operation s h o u l d be performed. The patient should be kept warm, and fluid loss prevented. Subcutaneous fluids should be given if necessary. One may give the patient glucose and fluids through a Lyon tube before, during, and after surgery.

In the care of carbuncles, furunculosis, and similar infections, the standard surgical treatment is indicated, remembering that carbuncles are of the septic group and diabetically speaking, are of the w o r s t class, and the mortality is high.

Incision, debridement, d r a i n a g e, wet dressings, elevation, etc., should be instituted without delay. Baking and ultra v i o l e t ray are helpful adjuncts. Delay means coma or septicaemia, or both, control of n e i t h e r and death. Gangrene, which is the major surgical complication today, is negligible under 40, but occurs in 31 per cent of diabetics over 60 years of age. Add infection with its swelling and loss of local power of resistance, and the serous and cellular exudate pinches still further the blood supply, resulting in necrosis and death.

The local treatment depends on the circulatory response and the presence or absence of sepsis. The presence of gangrene without infection is unusual and means the absence of putrefactive bacteria and sloughing. A few cases may continue, as dry gangrene. If the surgeon w a i t s, he must watch closely, remembering that the highest mortality is in amputation cases and control is much easier after amputation than before. The limbs should be X-rayed. High amputation means better collateral circulation, therefore amputation should be high, below the knee, or in mid-thigh. Do not use a tourniquet, as it traumatizes the tissues and the sclerosed vessels. The Kocher amputation, layer by layer, is the most satisfactory. It is simple and rapid. The technique must be scrupulous. Hemostasis must be exact. The operation is completed with t h r o u g h and through simple closure, under very little tension and without drainage. When the operation is elective, or one of choice, complete preparation can be carried out, but if the condition is infectious, it is a surgical emergency.

Gall Bladder: G a l l bladder disease is nine times as frequent in the diabetic as in the non-diabetic, and cholecystostomy is usually the wiser operation. Remove the gall bladder and the patient improves and the diabetes moderates. This is a frequent occurrence in diabetes. Joslin says "Remove the g a l l stones as a preventative."

Hyperthyroidism is as harmful as an infection. The increased metabolism drives the diabetic down hill and he becomes the severest of the severe. The endogenous eating of the thyroid goes on day and night while the exogenous eating of the diabetic only occurs T. I. D. The endogenous diet c a n n o t be controlled. The symptoms of goiter and diabetes are very similar, namely; red cheeks—overeating—emaciation—leucocytosis—glycosuria and uncontrolled metabolism is high in each. The b l o o d sugar reading decides. Never fail to save the diabetic the burden of hyperthyroidism.

The acute abdomen in the diabetic is insidious in its onset, frequently simulates coma, and surgical symptoms are often obscured. When acidosis is present, the surgeon must differentiate between the signs and symptoms due to acidosis and those due to an intra-abdominal lesion. In each there may be: (1) Pain and cramping, (2) nausea and vomiting for hours or days, (3) obstipation, (4) some fever because slight infection may initiate acidosis, (5) rapid pulse, (6) dry tongue, (7) abdominal cramps and tenderness not usually localized, (8) leucocytosis from 12,000 to 40,-000. A careful history is therefore paramount in importance. The pain is more definite and localized in the surgical abdomen. Nausea and vomiting usually *follow* pain in the surgical belly. Local tenderness is the most important single symptom. Pain may disappear, but tenderness remains. Logical relationship of signs and symptoms should be present. Special examinations may be helpful, as the Graham dye test and the van den Bergh in differentiating gall bladder involvement.

Appendicitis: Appendicitis is difficult to differentiate. Quoting McKittrick, "Acute appendicitis is i n s i d i o u s in its onset, treacherous in its course and uncertain in its outcome." If carefully sought for, the local tenderness persists. Rectal and vaginal examinations may clinch the diagnosis. As a rule, the older the patient, the more indefinite are the signs and symptoms of appendicitis. A careful history, thorough examination, urine and b l o o d examinations in a known diabetic, u s u a l l y make the decision. When in doubt, an appendectomy should be done under local anaesthesia, and no harm will be done. Delay m e a n s disaster. In the unavoidable interim, glucose and insulin should be given, moderating the acidosis and possibly clarifying an otherwise doubtful diagnosis.

Post-operative Care: Post-operative care is a continuation of the pre-operative preparation, remembering that with relief of infection the insulin dosage is reduced.

Test the urine every two hours for the first 24 hours, and give insulin accordingly. Test the blood sugar within six hours. Do not worry over sugar in the urine, but watch for diacetic acid, for "When Ketosis comes with infection, coma is not far off." Start fluids by mouth as soon as possible, in the form of cereal gruels, milk, ginger ale, etc. If the patient cannot take sufficient fluids by mouth and per rectum, give glucose solutions subcutaneously. The patient should get at least 50 gms. of glucose the first 24 hours, and it may be necessary to give a liberal diet buffered with sufficient insulin. Late in the convalescent period, postural exercises in bed will be helpful. They preserve the carbohydrates, prevent pneumonia, improve the circulation, stop pains, and heal u l c e r s and wounds.

Remember! Continued loss of weight in a well treated diabetic means one of three things—malignancy, pus, or tuberculosis.

Dual Etiology of Intractable Asthma*

RAY M. BALYEAT, M.D.
L. EVERETT SEYLER, M.D.
OKLAHOMA CITY, OKLAHOMA

Of 200 cases of intractable asthma which we have treated during the past few years, about one-fourth of all cases was unable to work and another fourth was 75 per cent disabled. Many others had difficulty in carrying on a gainful occupation. The degree of disability in intractable asthma certainly justifies careful consideration of all etiologic factors.

During the last quarter of a century, much has been written by Rowe[1], Duke[2], Vaughan[3], Coca[4], Feinberg[5], one of us[6] (R. M. B.), and others, concerning sensitization factors in all types of asthma. For many years, we have believed that there is another group of factors in these cases, but only during the last two years have we been able to demonstrate definitely that it existed. Our study leads us to believe that over 90 per cent of all cases of intractable asthma has a dual etiology.

ETIOLOGIC FACTORS IN INTRACTABLE ASTHMA

1. Sensitization factors
   (a) Food
   (b) Animal emanation and various dusts
   (c) Pollen
   (d) Miscellaneous

2. Mechanical factors
   (a) Mucus plugs
   (b) Purulent bronchial secretions
   (c) Asthmatic bronchiectasis
   (d) Usual form of bronchiectasis

Much has been written concerning the sensitization factors, and there is no question about the importance of that group in this type of asthma. Our recent work leads us to believe that the mechanical group of factors is of equal importance in the majority of cases, and in many, of greater importance than the sensitization

*Read before the Annual Meeting of the Oklahoma State Medical Association at Oklahoma City, Oklahoma, May 14, 1935.
*From the Balyeat Hay Fever and Asthma Clinic, and the University of Oklahoma Medical School, Oklahoma City, Oklahoma.

factors. This evening I wish to discuss primarily the mechanical factors.

COURSE OF DEVELOPMENT OF MECHANICAL FACTOR IN INTRACTABLE ASTHMA

Practically all cases of intractable asthma start with periodic attacks of asthma due to local edema of the mucosa of the bronchial tubes, produced by contact with some substance to which the patient is specifically sensitive. Later these

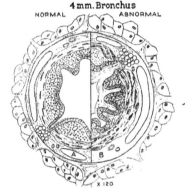

Fig. 1.—Cross section of 4 mm. bronchi— A, normal; B, asthmatic.

Note in B folds of mucous membrane filled with mucus, also, hypertrophy of muscles and mucous glands. Note decrease in size of lumen of asthmatic bronchus compared with the normal.

patients develop a superimposed infection, which leads to the production of mucus or purulent material. The plugging of the bronchial tubes with mucus or purulent exudate mechanically produces attacks of asthma.

Seasonal hay fever patients not uncommonly have typical hay fever over a period of 15 or 20 years without asthma, and then, at the end of the season, develop a cold and have slight asthma. The asthmatic attacks will cease at frost or with the disappearance of the specific pollen to which they are sensitive. There comes a time in many cases when, due to pollen, the local edema of the bronchial mucosa becomes complicated with an infectious process following a cold, and then the patient continues to have asthma after the

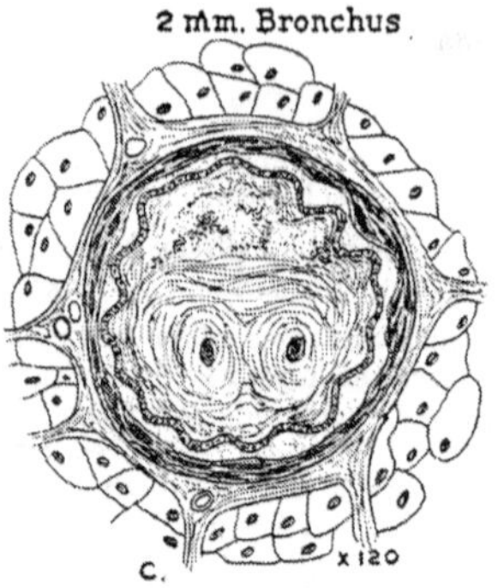

2 m̂m. Bronchus

Fig. 2.—Portion of transverse section of a bronchial tube in a case of chronic asthma. (2 mm. in diameter. Magnified 120 x.) Note the lumen is filled with mucus and purulent material.

time of pollination or after frost. This infection may or may not clear up. If it does not clear up, the patient continues to have asthma at any time during the year, frequently accentuated at times during which he has an acute cold. Finally, he may have asthma, severe in type, at any time during the year and never be entirely free from raising ropy or purulent mucus.

Why Asthmatic Attacks in Cases of Intractable Asthma Occur About The Same Time Each Night

For one patient to say that his attacks of asthma occur about 1:30 each morning, the second to tell you that his t r o u b l e comes on at 3, and the third to insist that his paroxysms start at 5 or 5:30, is not uncommon. A satisfactory explanation for the regularity of the attacks and the variation in the time of night in which they occur in different individuals has never been given. It appears to us that the thing that probably happens is as follows: In one individual the amount of mucus secreted and the amount of pus that collects in the bronchiectatic areas is fairly great; therefore, three hours after retiring—for example, at one o'clock—so many of the bronchial tubes are filled that nature re-

quires them to be cleaned out. This operation initiates, or is accompanied by, an asthmatic attack. In another individual the lumina of the bronchial tubes are occluded more slowly so that ejection of m u c u s is postponed until about three o'clock in the morning, while in the third individual it is five o'clock b e f o r e the cleansing process takes place.

Chief Cause of Death in Intractable Asthma—Chronic Sepsis

In many cases of asthma it is difficult to determine what actually causes death. A number of authors have written concerning the possibility of myocardial changes as an important factor in the cause of death in the asthmatic, but histories, physical findings and electrocardiographic studies offer little evidence that death in the average case of intractable asthma is due to cardiac failure. During the last two years, we have made bronchograms on about 200 cases of intractable asthma, and we find the majority suffering from some type of bronchiectasis. The bronchiectatic areas remain f i l l e d with purulent secretions. Most of these patients have WBC counts of from 12,000 to 18,000, which is evidence of toxin absorption. We believe, therefore, that death in the majority of cases of intractable asthma is due to chronic sepsis.

References

1. Rowe, Albert H.: Food Allergy, Philadelphia, Lea & Febiger, 1931.
2. Duke, Wm. W.: Asthma, Hay Fever, Urticaria and Allied Manifestations of Allergy, St. Louis, The C. V. Mosby Co., 1925.
3. Vaughan, Warren T.: Allergy, St. Louis, The C. V. Mosby Co., 1931.
4. Coca, Arthur F., Walzer, Matthew, and Thommen, August A.: Asthma and Hay Fever in Theory and Practice, Baltimore, Charles C. Thomas, 1931.
5. Feinberg, S. M.: Allergy in General Practice, Philadelphia, Lea and Febiger, 1934.
6. Balyeat, Ray M.: Allergic iDseases: Their Diagnosis and Treatment, Philadelphia, F. A. Davis Company, 1930.

---o---

Doctors In Music

Do you or any of your medical friends play any musical instrument? Mead Johnson & Company is now preparing a new publication devoted to the hobbies and achievements of physicians, past and present, in the field of music. Doctors' orchestras, doctors' glee clubs, historical or biographical items, with or without illustrations, will be welcomed. Please send your item to Mead Johnson & Company, Evansville, Ind. (If you have not received your free copy of their recent publication "Parergon," devoted to fine art by doctors, send for it now.)

Experience With the Use of Prontylin
Case Report

HAYS R. YANDELL, M.D.
PONCA CITY, OKLAHOMA

PATIENT

Mr. A. B. Age 23. Single. Hospital No. 22,798.

HISTORY

On October 20, 1937, patient developed a gonorrheal urethritis with the usual discharge and burning. He gave a history of exposure four or five days before the onset of his symptoms. He was treated by his f a m i l y physician with G.C. vaccine, three injections per week for three weeks; discharge persisted for three weeks. He was given no irrigations. On November 10 he developed severe, constant pain in his right shoulder, which was greatly aggravated on motion. For two weeks he had noticed swelling and exquisite tenderness in the region of this joint. Pain was severe enough to keep him awake at night. He was unable to abduct the right arm. He had been running a temperature and noticed that he perspired profusely. On November 14 he developed pain in the left index finger at the metacarpal-phalangeal joint; joint was swollen, red, and tender; this persisted for two days, and then subsided. Patient was admitted to the Ponca City Hospital on December 1, 1937.

The past history and physical findings were essentially negative as far as they pertained to this specific condition, except for marked swelling, some redness, and exquisite tenderness in the region of the right shoulder joint. Patient was unable to abduct his arm without severe pain; no involvement of other joints. Temperature was 101; pulse, 90, respirations, 20; blood pressure, 140/90.

LABORATORY

Urinalysis: Cloudy, acid reaction, Sp. gr. 1.010, trace of albumin, no sugar, occasional R.b.c., few W.b.c., few epithelial cells.

W.b.c. 12,100.

Polymorphonuclear neutrophils, 84 per cent.

Lymphocytes, 15 per cent.

Monos, one per cent.

X-ray: X-ray of right shoulder revealed a marked effusion.

The Wassermann was negative.

DIAGNOSIS

Gonorrheal arthritis of the right shoulder.

COURSE

Patient was put at bed rest; right arm was immobilized by means of a sling. He was given codeine for immediate relief of his pain, and p r o n t y l i n, gr. 15, and s o d i u m bicarbonate, gr. 15, every four hours for three days, making a total of 90 grains of prontylin every 24 hours. After the first 24 hours of this treatment the pain was almost completely relieved, and he continued to remain free from pain in of his pain; and p r o n t y l i n, gr. 15, and the right shoulder from then on. His temperature was 101 on the day of admission; the maximum on the following day was 99.2. It then remained normal.

On December 4 the blood counts were as f o l l o w s: Hemoglobin, 80 per cent (Sahli); R.b.c. 4,440,000; W.b.c. 18,450. Differential: Polymorphonuclear neutrophils, 91 per cent; lymphocytes, nine per cent.

On this date the prontylin and sodium bicarbonate were reduced to gr. 10 every four hours, making a total dosage of 60 grains of prontylin every 24 hours. Patient continued to have complete symptomatic relief.

On December 6, the prontylin and sodium bicarbonate were reduced to gr. 10, t.i.d He was dismissed from the hospital on this date. Examination of the shoulder showed no swelling; no tenderness. Active m o t i o n was started, and abduction was limited to an angle of about 45 degrees. He was dismissed and instructed to take prontylin, gr. 5, and sodium bicarbonte, gr. 5, three times daily.

He returned to the clinic for examination on December 8. He stated that he had had no more pain and that the motion in his right shoulder was greatly increased. He had had no u r e t h r a l discharge, frequency, or burning. The findings were as follows: Temperature, 98; pulse, 88; blood pressure, 140/90. Patient was somewhat nervous. There was an erythematous mottled rash over the anterior c h e s t wall. There was no swelling or tenderness of the right shoulder joint. He was able to abduct his arm to 90 degrees without pain.

Examination of the prostate was negative.

X-ray of the right shoulder was negative.

Two glass specimens of u r i n e showed both to be slightly cloudy.

Prostatic smear showed 25 w.b.c. per high power field; it was negative for gonococci.

Urinalysis: Alkaline r e a c t i o n, Sp. gr. 1.016, no albumin, no sugar, microscopic examination of the sediment was negative. R.b.c., 3,360,000. W.b.c., 11,550. Hemoglobin 68 per cent (Sahli).

Prontylin was discontinued. Patient was instructed to take 15 gr. of sodium bicarbonate daily. He was also given Feosol tablets, 1 t.i.d.

December 15: Nervousness much less.

Rash practically cleared up. Ten pounds gain in weight the past week; absolutely free from pain in right shoulder, with complete function. No urinary symptoms.

R.b.c., 4,370,000. .

Hemoglobin, 78 per cent (Sahli).

CONCLUSIONS

The points of interest in this case are:

First: After three weeks of unusually severe pain, with a daily temperature of 101, and considerable loss of weight, within 24 hours patient was entirely relieved of pain and temperature.

Second: T h e improvement continued, without any recurrence of symptoms, and patient was completely and entirely recovered in less than two weeks after the treatment with prontylin was instituted. Furthermore, there was no evidence of gonorrheal urethritis.

Third: His red blood count, after eight days of prontylin treatment, dropped from 4,440,000 to 3,360,000, and hemoglobin from 80 per cent to 68 per cent. However, by December 15, just one week after prontylin was discontinued, his red blood count was back to 4,370,000 and hemoglobin 78 per cent. With the discontinuance of the prontylin the erythema on his chest cleared up and the blood picture came back to normal.

---------------0---------------

Experience With the Use of Larostidin
Case Report

GEO. H. NIEMANN, M.D.
PONCA CITY, OKLAHOMA

PATIENT

Mr. R. C. H. Age 53. Married 21 years. Occupation: manager of cafe. Hospital No. 21,959.

At the age of 15 the patient began to have attacks of gnawing pain localized in the mid-epigastrium, which a p p e a r e d about two hours after eating, and which were always relieved by milk, food, or soda. The attacks lasted on the average of one to two months, and always occurred

in the fall and in the spring of the year. These persisted until he was 41 years of age, at which time they became more prolonged and more severe in nature. He placed himself on a milk diet for a year. Following this he was symptom free for one year. At the end of this time, however, he developed a recurrence of his pain, which occurred after every meal, and also at night. He became extremely nervous and began to lose weight. These symptoms persisted for four years, during which time he obtained most relief from soda bicarbonate.

When he was 47 years of age, in 1932, a perforation occurred in the region of the pylorus. He was operated upon 12 hours after the perforation. P l a s t i c was performed at the site of the perforation. The patient made an uneventful recovery, except for a post-operative ventral hernia. He was then s y m p t o m free for three months, at the end of which time he again developed a recurrence of his former symptoms, with remissions and exacerbations up to October, 1936, at which time he was 51 years of age. At this time he was having attacks of weakness and passing black, tarry stools. There was progressive weight loss and pallor. In December, 1936, he vomited about one q u a r t of bright red blood. In February, 1937, he again had a large hematemesis and passed bloody and tarry stools.

He was admitted to the Ponca City Hospital on March 5, 1937, at which time he was semi-comatose. Blood counts at that time were: H e m o g l o b i n, 30 per cent (Sahli); R.b.c., 1,700,000; W.b.c., 6,100; differential, polymorphonuclear neutrophils, 65 per c e n t; lymphocytes, 32 per cent; monocytes, three per cent. He was given a direct blood transfusion of 560 c.c. from a suitable donor. Following the transfusion, he was given 24 daily intravenous Larostidins, 5 c.c., with instructions as to diet, which consisted of soft foods, cereals, tender vegetables, and milk. Following several intravenous treatments of Larostidin, he became symptom free and all hemorrhage ceased. He gained 25 pounds in weight.

In April, 1937, following the completion of the course of Larostidin, he developed symptoms of pyloric obstruction. He was unable to retain any food. X-ray of the stomach at this time confirmed the diagnosis of complete obstruction due to stenosis at the pylorus. On July 10, 1937, a routine posterior gastro-enterostomy and repair of a ventral hernia were performed.

Operative findings: At the gastric side of the pyloric ring there was scar tissue which caused a complete stricture in this region. No e v i d e n c e of previous ulcer could be found; it was taken for granted

that the ulcer was in the region of the stenosis. There was no evidence of malignancy. No pathologic mesenteric glands were found.

This was followed by an unusually rapid recovery, and patient was dismissed from the hospital on July 18, 1937, eight days after his operation. Since that time he has been absolutely symptom free and has gained 45 pounds in weight.

Examination on December 18, 1937, revealed the patient to be in excellent condition; weight 170. Abdominal examination revealed no masses or tenderness. Incision was well h e a l e d. Blood counts: R.b.c., 4,030,000; hemoglobin, 75 per cent; W.b.c., 7,200.

CONCLUSIONS

First: This man evidently suffered from the effects of a recurrent g a s t r i c ulcer since the age of 15, or for 38 years.

Second: He has remained on an exclusive milk diet for as long as a year at a time.

Third: He has been placed on sippy diet and modified gastric ulcer diets at various times. During this period he used soda most of the time for relief.

Fourth: Recently he had several severe hemorrhages.

Fifth: He has had one definite perforation.

In this particular case 24 treatments of Larostidin firmly and completely healed the ulcer to the extent of causing a complete stenosis as a r e s u l t of scar tissue formation.

---o---

Sulfanilamide Derivative Named

Recent reports from investigators indicate that a pyridine derivative of sulfanilamide [2(-amino-benzene-sulphamido) pyridine or sulfanilamidopyridine] is apparently more promising in the treatment of certain types of pneumonia than sulfanilamide itself, the Council on Pharmacy and Chemistry of the American Medical Association says in The Journal of the American Medical Association for January 7.

A number of investigators, and manufacturers as well, requested the Council to coin a nonproprietary designation for this product. The Council has therefore adopted the term "sulfapyridine" (sulf-a-pyr-i-dine).

The product is in an experimental stage and according to present information the government has not licensed it for interstate sale. The Council will publish a preliminary report on this product in the near future.

Social Diseases at the Cross Roads

HORACE H. PORTER, M.D., ROBERT B. WITCHER, M.D.
AND CECIL KNOBLOCK
TULSA, OKLAHOMA

About three decades ago a golden era of experiment and discovery permeated scientific mind and science. One need only ponder momentarily on master minds such as Metchnikoff, Roux, N e i s s e r, Bruck, Schaudinn, Wassermann, B o r d e t, Hoffmann, Fournier and Ehrlich. Too often the name of the young fourth year medical student, Maisonneuve, is omitted from this illustrious g r o u p. One need tarry briefly to realize that in this period (1900-1910) the attack on venereal diseases made great advances, diagnostically as well as therapeutically. The identification of the causative organism, the development of the serological t e s t, the transmission of the disease by a n i m a l experimentation, and the differentiation of gonococcus and treponema pallidum, associated with means of chemotherapeutically preventing transmission, led to a crowning event; namely, the use of arsenic and mercury therapeutically.

The venereal disease problem is as old as civilization, and Moses, the lawmaker, was probably the first public health administrator and sanitarian. R e l i g i o u s laws and moral issues have been handed down through the centuries, and regulatory themes have always followed a well formulated policy emphasizing the moral attack and appealing to the finer instincts related to the doctrine of sexual abstinence before marriage and later faithfulness.

Public health measures for control and attacks on commercial prostitution h a v e opened the way for careful consideration of the issues involved. Nature will have its way, but regulation and persuasion appeal only to the minority. It would thus appear that some element is being omitted from this large program. Social diseases instead of diminishing have spread to other strata of society. It is far more important to prevent these diseases than to impotently attempt to treat and cure them.

A large university clinic, with all its intellectual setting and prowess, admits that, roughly speaking, only 15 per cent of the patients r e t u r n for adequate continued treatment. What has happened to the 85 per cent who, in later years, will become economic burdens to society? Social diseases cannot be eradicated by inflicting extremely painful therapeutics on the unfortunate victims. The chief difficulty lies in the fact that the initiation of treatment is too late—even in a vast majority of early cases. The most expert clinician would not minimize the dangers associated with anti-syphilitic therapy. One need only turn hastily to the writings of Stokes, and also Kolmer, to appreciate the apprehension in the minds of experts. These apprehensions soon permeate the minds of the patients and offer sufficient reason for the poor follow-up.

Our contention has a l w a y s been that those who are infected should be gently and adequately treated by the best methods known to medical science. On the other hand, it has been our opinion that preventive measures should be used by the uninfected. We, therefore, feel that social hygiene is at the crossroads. One must not become blinded to the fact that society is living in an age of preventive medicine, and it should be a simple matter of educational appeal and regulatory laws for marriage and pregnancy. Certainly, in this day and age, one would not suggest pasteurization *after* a milk-borne epidemic, or vaccination *after* an epidemic of small pox, or antitoxin *after* an e p i d e m i c of diphtheria, or treatment of the water supply *after* an epidemic of typhoid. What has been responsible for this state of improved health? *Preventive medicine and sanitary codes!*

The social d i s e a s e program has been most thoroughly presented, and adequate funds have been available for educational purposes. It should be emphasized that a most thorough task has been accomplished, notwithstanding the fact that the "spirit is willing but the flesh is weak." However, regarding therapy the situation is much beclouded and the end results uncertain. Then, too, much is to be desired in regard to prognosis.

Prophylaxis is not a new thought, immature, or even mellow with age. It is one that comes into every mind day in and day out. Youth, in particular, carries with it that spirit of adventure and daring, always hoping that, just this once, escape is still within its reach. So youth and middle age present a serious problem—one that must be met and solved to safeguard the citizenry.

Many prominent thinkers along public health aspects have presented their views in the medical literature. Carrier[1] as early as 1905 stated "Venereal diseases exist in every community to such an extent that an imperative demand is made for prophylaxis. Medical pessimism in this matter of prophylaxis must be eliminated." Eytinge[2] in 1909 reported from the U.S.S. Ranger and C o n c o r d, that it was conclusively shown when the ointment (calomel) was used, venereal diseases were avoided. On the U.S.S. Ranger there were 256 exposures and no infections.

During the war the prophylactic package gave excellent results. However, the statement is always emphasized that these results only occurred in military organizations and c o u l d not be obtained among civilians. This particular p o i n t will be taken up in our discussion. The fact remains, however, that preventive measures are scientifically and logically c o r r e c t when these measures are used. It is the system that is wrong and not the sanitation.

P h e l p s, Commander, U.S.N.[3], in 1925 comprehended the fault in the preventive plan of the naval personnel and indicated that often solutions injected into the urethra are irritating and cause much pain which militates against their use. This, naturally, cuts down the effective control of venereal infections.

Vonderlehr, et al[4], state "It is recognized that local chemical or mechanical prophylactic measures scientifically applied may be important factors in the prevention of syphilitic and gonococcal infections. Physicians in clinics and p r i v a t e practice should be encouraged to i n c l u d e such measures in their practices. In view, however, of actual experience which thus far has shown difficulties in the way of the general application of these measures, it is further suggested that the Public Health Service continue experimental studies of such procedures for effectively incorporating prophylactic measures in the general program."

Later, Vonderlehr[5] further states "Studies pertaining to the prophylaxis of syphilis have also been prosecuted. R e c e n t work on laboratory animals demonstrates not only the effectiveness of prophylaxis when properly applied, but proceeds a step further to indicate the mode of action of the prophylactic agent. It has been shown that the prophylactic action of mercury, for instance, is dependent not only upon the local spirocheticidal action of the drug but also upon the fact that the mercury through absorption has a systemic action which i n h i b i t s the development of the causative organism of syphilis. This point was proved by failure to produce a chancre in rabbits in which the glans penis had been exposed to virulent spirochete emulsions without the subsequent application of the mercury to this area. The drug was applied to the skin of the back and protected a large percentage of the exposed animals."

The Advisory Committee of the U. S. Public Health Service[6] r e c e n t l y stated "Gonorrhea and syphilis are so closely related, epidemiologically, that the administration of programs for their control may be considered as one problem. There is, in our opinion, every reason for proceeding as rapidly as possible with the control of both diseases. The incidence of gonorrhea is at l e a s t twice and probably three or four times that of syphilis. What it may lack in ability to kill, it makes up in morbidity and numbers. Since it may be acquired repeatedly, it is often a recurring cause of poor health and economic loss. The complications of gonorrhea are neither rare nor lacking in seriousness. Gonococcal ophthalmia neonatorum, gonococcal infections in girl children, and gonorrhea in married women account for almost as high a proportion of innocent infections with gonorrhea as with syphilis. The sterility which follows gonococcal infection is permanent, whereas men and women with syphilis can have healthy children."

This committee o f f e r e d the following specific recommendations: "It is recommended that physicians in clinics and private practice be encouraged to promote local chemical or mechanical prophylaxis; that the United States Public Health Service determine what constitutes a reliable prophylactic; and that the recommendations of the United States Public Health Service be given support of national legislation in order that only approved material may be o f f e r e d for sale. It is likewise recommended that the prophylaxis of gonococcal ophthalmia neonatorum be completely reviewed to determine whether or not it should be the subject of national legislation and whether the simple application at birth of any prophylactic is sufficient for the prevention of ophthalmia neonatorum."

Moore[7] states "Unlike many other infectious diseases, syphilis is not preventable by elimination of the contact which causes it, by experimentation of an intermediate host, by immunization, or by quarantine. Efforts to control the disease by reducing the number of sexual contacts of human beings have failed." In discussing mechanical, chemical, and chemotherapeutic prophylaxis he believes that "all of t h e s e methods are effective in experimental animals, and three of them, m e c h a n i c a l, chemical and chemotherapeutic (with bismuth) prophylaxis h a v e demonstrated their value in men." Moore further points out that these measures offer protection for the men only, and that owing to ignorance, laziness or carelessness syphilis in civilian life cannot be controlled. However, he believes that mass prophylaxis of social diseases can be accomplished and is the best solution now available. "I may p e r h a p s be forgiven if I emphasize the point that the value of prophylaxis and treatment in the control of syphilis depends almost entirely on the state of mind of the public health officer."

Wolbarst[8] makes a constructive suggestion in his statement: "If we cannot make men virtuous let us at least try to make them cautious." He believes that the one vital measure of defense against social diseases which offers the greatest promise of success has been almost entirely neglected.

Also, that an attack at the source is the method of choice and that a totally new method of attack must be developed and put into operation. He further believes that chemical and pharmaceutical ingenuity will produce an ointment or vaginal suppository that will protect against gonococcus and other living organisms alike, and that "the medical profession, public health officials, social workers, and the public generally must accept the fact that it is *just as moral to prevent venereal disease as it is to cure it—and it is much less expensive."*

In an introductory manner, it is important to quote Chesney[9]:

"If the detection of the infectious carrier of syphilis is difficult, and that fact everyone would grant, then one naturally turns to the question of protecting the individual who runs the risk of infection. Can the laboratory c o n t r i b u t e anything to this problem?

"As everyone knows, it has been clearly demonstrated that there are chemical substances which when properly used under controlled conditions will actually prevent syphilis from being contracted even when exposure has occurred. The universal experience has been that this type of prophylaxis works well in military organizations but loses its effectiveness in civilian life. We need not here go into the reasons for that failure, but at the same time we should not let it keep us from studying the subject further in order to obtain a clear understanding of the limitations of any particular method of prophylaxis. Moreover, we may profitably seek b e t t e r methods than those in our possession at the present time, and in this search the laboratory can be of the greatest assistance. It is well at this point to remind ourselves that practically no attempt has been made to discover a m e t h o d of prophylaxis against syphilis which would be effective in women. Is the problem insoluble? I doubt it."

Chesney's comments represent one of the first occasions on which a new approach to the elimination of social diseases has been presented.

Much has been written on the ways and means of preventing venereal diseases. In fact, more than three decades ago Weiss[10], Chairman of the Committee on Prophylaxis of Venereal Diseases said "the dangers of venereal disease to the people, their socio-economic importance, their causing premature invalidism, are of sufficient moment for all governments to exert their utmost to cope with them."

What have the governments been doing in 35 years? From a therapeutic point of view, nothing has been done. The meager answer has come from p r i v a t e sources. With the exception of Chesney, no one has at anytime proposed the protection of the female and thus break the chain of infection.

In an e d i t o r i a l by Moore[11], one is impressed with the remark "Syphilis is an entirely preventable disease." This author, as well as many other prominent public health investigators who h a v e endorsed and urged the use of prophylaxis, neglected to consider the f e m a l e as a vehicle whereby syphilis and gonorrhea could be stamped out. As dogmatic as many of the moralists may be, few, if any, are cognizant of the real suffering associated with these social aspects of life, and it must be agreed that woman suffers most.

With these ideas in mind, our attack on this problem led us to consider the insecurity of mechanical devices. Moore[7] reported that these devices are more or less imperfect. Many preparations u s e d are toxic and accumulate poisons as . well as being relatively inert in preventing syphilis and gonorrhea. Unfortunately preventives are few, and insofar as is known not effective for both diseases. This a serious drawback because the two diseases are often concurrent.

Years of experience have s h o w n that these practices are unsatisfactory, and the question arose concerning the properties required of a preventive. It was felt that a preventive for syphilis and gonorrhea must exhibit the following properties:

1. Effective for male and female simultaneously.
2. Nontoxic to the human being, showing no irritation to the exposed tissues, either immediate or delayed.
3. Its protective action must be immediate, not localized but spreading over all the surfaces that are subject to *genital* infection.
4. The action must be so prolonged that the causative organism will be destroyed.

5. It must be used in such a quantity that both the male and female genitalia will be completely covered by a film necessary for protection.

Beside the above, the p r o d u c t would have to be easily applied and available to patients in all walks of life.

A f t e r considerable physical, chemical, and bacteriological s t u d i e s, progonasyl was devised. This is a combination of triethanolamine, mineral oil, oleic acid, vegetable oil and organic iodine.

Most products to be i n d u c e d into the vaginal vault are introduced at their *maximum* germicidal value and rapidly lose this quality. This product is in direct contrast. It is a very light oil adhering to and rapidly covering all mucous membrane surfaces, soon forming a tenacious jell. This jell is developed by the admixture of moisture from the mucous membranes. Its viscosity is low, and it spreads to all the surfaces rapidly, t h u s enmeshing and absorbing from diseased surfaces all debris and protozoal life, causing devitalization by means of desiccation or osmosis. This point can be shown by dark field examination. The effect lasts from seven to 15 hours, thus offering protection to both the *male* and *female before* infection takes place.

Due to the fact that progonasyl is used in its natural state, and upon its introduction into the vaginal vault it absorbs moisture until a definite jell is formed, the following findings were based upon the action of the jell and not upon the clear oil base, and timed from the formative period.

Thirty seconds are required to mix the oil with the organisms (with slight additional moisture) to produce a jell of maximum value. This time value is constant for the following tests:

Temperature of admixture............................20°C.
Temperature of incubation.............................37°C.
Incubation time...................................48 hours
Media used............................Beef Infusion
    Nutrient agar, blood agar and Gradwohl medium.
1 loop of bacteria (from slant) to 10 loops progonasyl.
Reaction ....6.7—7.6

Name of Organism	Time to Inhibit Growth
B. typhosis	2 minutes
B. para typhosis A	2 minutes
B. para typhosis B	2 minutes
Gonococcus	2 minutes
B. dysentery flexner	5 minutes
Staphylococcus aureus	5 minutes
Staphylococcus citreus	8 minutes
Streptococcus pyogenes	8 minutes
B. coli	8 minutes

Attempts to culture the treponema pallidum in all time intervals were negative in the anaerobic methods, and dark field illuminations were m a d e to determine what effects, if any, were produced upon the physical body.

Fresh serum from a primary syphilitic lesion was covered lightly with a cover glass and brought into proper focus. At the edge of the cover glass was placed a few drops of progonasyl and, upon bringing the dark field again into view, the oil was allowed to contact the edge of the cover glass and to become mixed with the serum c o n t a i n i n g the T. pallida. Upon contact there is an immediate and rapid flow of the serum to the oil, carrying all organisms with it. This movement then slows down and a slight reverse action takes place when a portion of the iodine (?) value is released to give a very pale yellow stain to the blood cells. At one and a half minutes after this reverse play is started, the treponema becomes immobile.

The second step is the a c t i o n of the *oily emulsion* upon the treponema body. Upon contacting the advancing jell formation the treponemata are pulled into the jell body and at this time relax their spiral formation (as in a stained specimen or section). The action of this advancing jell formation presents a constant molecular bombardment for a period of 30 minutes in the very thin layer of material contained between the slide and the cover g l a s s. This molecular bombardment is not noted when brought into contact with water, but apparently results as an interchange with the p r o t e i n value of the exudate. After this molecular bombardment *front* of the jell f o r m a t i o n has passed, the fine emulsion remains holding the organisms enmeshed.

The rapid rate of a c t i o n of cultural methods proved the high germicidal activity in the colloid where there was an increasingly greater action developing in contra-distinction to u s u a l germicides which are a p p l i e d at their maximum value while their activity diminishes at a r a p i d rate accompanied by the high physiological toxicity. It is our belief that this is the first attempt to produce high germicidal activity as carried by a colloid, as well as to subject organisms to

hydrophilic action as a means of devitalization. The hydrophilic c o l l o i d thus formed will produce desiccation of all types of unicellular protozoa.

Toxic action was studied by means of oral administration of several tablespoonfuls of the oil to laboratory workers. This was repeated on several days and it was noted that mild catharsis was the only effect of the oil.

Ultramicroscopic tests showed that this s u b s t a n c e, designated as progonasyl, readily took up moisture developing a cloud which was shown later to possess the ability to enmesh protozoal organisms. The dark f i e l d microscope also clearly demonstrates this tenacious jell formation based on the principles of osmosis. This jell is thirsty for moisture and consequently withdraws moisture from protozoan forms of life, or from simple protoplasm. Organisms are enmeshed in the jell and are s o o n devitalized. The oil shows no surface germicidal action and in this respect differs from all other prophylactic agents.

In order to ascertain its irritating action, it has been a p p l i e d as an ointment on eczematous lesions with a soothing effect on the broken skin surfaces. Following this, it was used on more than 200 cases in which there was present marked vaginal discharge as well as local irritation. The duration of this condition varied from a few weeks to several years. Laboratory examination before treatment showed the presence of trichomona, B. coli, and other nonspecific organisms. Much to our surprise, the bacterial irritation present at f i r s t examination gradually subsided. In a great many cases it completely cleared, and the m u c o u s membranes became negative bacteriologically. Needless to say most of these cases were still clear after a lapse of several months. These clinical observations have been confirmed by several of our colleagues. In our opinion there was a complete absence of irritating action. Furthermore, it is believed that the product was efficacious in removing much of the debris and discharge.

The above experiments were repeated on a group of p a t i e n t s suffering with vaginitis. In this group more than 75 patients were examined and treated. In most instances 5 cc. of oil were injected into the vaginal vault for a period of 10 days. A daily douche was employed, and in every instance the mucous membranes became h e a l t h y and entirely normal. Certainly, if the oil had any irritating action it would have caused increased irritation or ill effect. This last experiment was checked by at least four clinicians. It is our firm belief that this oil can be used indefinitely without irritation or ill effect. Furthermore, it is our opinion that daily instillation of the oil, followed by douches on the next morning, constitutes a b l a n d, safe, and efficient m e t h o d of treating trichomonal infections.

Our success with this type of case led us to make a study of all types of vaginal disorders. Among these, 30 cases of acute and chornic gonorrhea (police characters obtained from the clinic) were treated d a i l y with progonasyl. No. thought of cure was in our minds. The above mode of treatment was applied to this group with encouraging results, insofar as relieving the discharge was concerned. It was later learned that several of these women had returned to their usual mode of living and that, when this product was previously applied to the vaginal vault, the males with whom they had contact did not become infected.

It occurred to us that by this method a break in the chain of infection might be obtained, thus preventing the spread of social diseases. Earlier in this report, attention was called to the suggestions of Chesney[9] and it appeared to us that this solution of the problem was at hand. Insofar as the literature at our disposal is known, the female has not previously been used successfully as the vehicle whereby the spread of venereal diseases may be curbed.

Our thoughts then turned to the historic Metchnikoff experiments on syphilis. In our experiment with gonorrhea, there was the added knowledge that it could be cured in a large percentage of cases if infection should result. Our experiments and observations in previous cases have been so favorable that protection was almost certain. On this basis it was decided to seek volunteers for carrying out this more crucial test. As stated above, the females who were i n f e c t e d with gonorrhea and who used this oil did not infect their male partners and, therefore, it seemed plausible that the reverse should likewise follow.

Four women and two men volunteered for this experiment. The f o u r women, designated as patients A, B, C, and D, were first carefully examined clinically, smears were taken and examined microscopically, and these four women were found to be free from gonorrhea. They were further questioned as to whther they had previously had any infection. The tests and clinical history were negative and they were confined in locked apartments that had been carefully searched, and the w a t e r supply had been turned off. They were under the constant supervision of at least one of the clinicians and a maid. The clinical and microscopical examinations were repeated with n e g a t i v e results. Their meals and other necessary articles (newspapers, drinking water, magazines, cigarettes, candy, etc.) were brought to them by the maid under our supervision. Careful search was made to prevent access to any drugs or medicaments. No accessories of any kind were permitted except sleeping apparel.

The two males, designated as "E" and "F," were examined and found to have acute gonorrhea. One had the disease for seven days, and the o t h e r for ten days. Microscopic examination from e a c h of these men showed an abundance of characteristic intracellular and extracellular gram negative diplococci. Clinically, the condition of both men was that of severe gonorrhea.

Injection into the vaginal vault of 4 cc. of the oil was made by one of us in the presence of the others. Male E and female A, and male F and female B were permitted to indulge in sexual relations. After a few hours, the two men were permitted to return to their apartment, and the women were confined to their apartment for ten days, a clinician and a maid being in constant supervision.

After a few hours rest, the same two men were permitted to have sexual relations with females C and D. These latter two patients were similarly maintained in their apartments and the two men discharged. In all four instances examination of the females showed the p r e s e n c e of spermatozoa. During the period of detention the women were not permitted to take any baths, and only had water for drinking purposes and for washing their faces and hands. On the ninth day a vaginal douche of plain warm water was permitted for cleansing purposes. On the tenth day, clinical and microscopical examinations of the four women were made and the vaginal smears examined by each of us were found negative. Later examination similarly showed the absence of gonococcus and gonorrhea.

In our many years of experience, an occasional exposure fails to show the presence of a suspected infection. However, it is our belief that such could not have happened in the case of all four of these women. It is our opinion that the oily preparation was solely responsible for the protection of these women against infection.

It was realized that the experiment carried out above might be criticized from the point of view that no control was employed in which the injection of the oil was omitted before mating with one of the infected men. To answer this criticism, an additional set of experiments was made with an entirely different group of patients. For this purpose two women, hereafter known as G and H, were carefully examined clinically and smears were taken and examined microscopically by three observers. G and H were found to be free of gonorrhea, and their clinical history showed that there had been no previous infection. One man, hereafter referred to as I, was examined and found to have an acute gonorrhea of six days duration, and showed clinical symptoms of the acute stage. Microscopic examinations of the discharge, made separately by each of us, showed an abundance of characteristic intracellular and extracellular gram negative diplococci. Clinically, the condition was that of a severe, acute, gonorrhea. The two women were maintained in constant supervision of one or more of us and a maid in a locked apartment, under the same conditions heretofore described. G and H were again examined clinically and microscopically for any possible evidence of gonorrhea, but were found negative. Four cc. of the oily medicament was injected into the vagina of woman H, whereas woman G received no medication whatever. I and G were

permitted to have intercourse and the spermatozoic discharge was found.

After four hours woman H had intercourse with male I and again spermatozoic discharge was found. The man was dismissed but the two women were confined under lock and key in the apartment for ten days. Their meals and other necessary articles were brought to them in the same manner as described in the first set of experiments. At the end of the third day female G, who had not been injected with the oily medicament, was examined and the microscopic study showed gram-negative, extracellular diplococci. Clinically, there was no evidence of gonorrhea. At the end of the fourth day examination was again made and a slight discharge noted. Microscopic examination of the discharge showed gram-negative, intracellular diplococci, and the clinical condition was that of gonorrhea. On the day following the patient was treated with sulfanilamide, according to the method of Van Slyke and Mahoney[12] from the U. S. Public Health Service. She responded promptly at the end of ten days, and has since remained cured.

Female H was kept under supervision for ten days and at no time showed any evidence of discharge or any microscopic condition simulating gonorrhea. At the end of the eleventh day she was examined clinically, and by means of vaginal smears and then released as not having contracted the disease. Further observation of this patient showed no infection.

It is our opinion that, in this set of experiments, the most exacting requirements of science have been made, proving that the oily medicament, without question, protects against gonorrheal infection.

As a result of our experiments, it is believed that the oil employed by us exerts real germicidal action on various types of unicellular organisms. It has the power to destroy gonococcus and similar organisms promptly, and at the site of infection. It forms a hydrophilic colloid when exposed to the moisture from the mucous membranes and produces its germicidal action by virtue of its desiccating effect on organisms. This is in contrast to the action of most germicides which act at maximum concentration at the surface.

According to our information, this is the first time that the female has been offered the protection of prevention by physical chemical means in relation to social diseases. Our experiments indicate that the oil is non-irritating when applied to the mucous membranes even over a long period of time and that it in no way disturbs the normal sexual functions when its use is discontinued. It offers a mode of protecting the male and female simultaneously, and yet it is so nontoxic that one can take large doses by mouth without any injury.

In the various types of experiments that have been carried out, its use has been applied to approximately 400 females, and in no instance has there b e e n the slightest deleterious a c t i o n. These experiments have proved conclusively that it protects non-infected females from infection even though they may be exposed to infected males, and vice versa.

It further appears that it is simultaneously a preventive for both syphilis and gonorrhea and economically w i t h i n the reach of all. As a contribution to diminishing the incidence of venereal disease, it seems to offer many possibilities.

Recognition is g i v e n to Dr. Allen C. Kramer, Dr. W. A. Dean and to Dr. Samuel J. Bradfield for t h e i r collaborative work.

BIBLIOGRAPHY

1. Carrier, A. E.: Venereal Prophylaxis. J. Michigan State Medical Society, September, 1905.

2. Eytinge, E. O. J.: System of Venereal Disease Prophylaxis and Its Results. Military Surg., August, 1909, p. 170.

3. Phelps, J. R.: U. S. Naval Med. Bull., July, 1925.

4. Vonderlehr, R. A., et al: Recommendations for a Venereal Disease Control Program in State and Local Health Departments. Report of an Advisory Committee to the U. S. Public Health Service. Am. J. Syph., Gon., and Ven. Dis., 20:1, January, 1936.

5. Vonderlehr, R. A.: The Relationship of Venereal Disease Control Work in the U. S. Public Health Service to the Physician in Private Practice. Am. J. Syph., Gon. & Ven. Dis., 21:32, January, 1937.

6. Report of an Advisory Committee: Recommendations for a Gonorrhea Control Program. Ven. Dis. Inf., 19:1, January, 1938.

7. Moore, J. E.: Prophylaxis and Treatment in the Control of Syphilis. Southern Med. J., 30:149, 1937.

8. Wolbarst, A. L.: Suggestions for More Effective Venereal Disease Prophylaxis. Medical Record, August 18, 1937, p. 149.

9. Chesney, A. M.: Research Needs in the Control of Syphilis. Am. J. Syph. Gon. & Ven. Dis., 21:121, March, 1937.

10. Moore, J. E.: Editorial—The Prophylaxis of Syphilis. Am. J. Syph. Gon. & Ven. Dis., 20:683, November, 1936.

11. Weiss, Ludwig: Report of Committee on Prophylaxis of Venereal Diseases. J.A.M.A., 40:1317, May 9, 1903.

12. Van Slyke, C. J., Mahoney, J. F., and Taylor, J. D.: U. S. Public Health Service. Ven. Dis. Bull. Vol. 18, No. 12, December, 1937.

———————o———————

Lymphopathia Venereum*

J. V. Van Cleve, M.D.
WICHITA, KANSAS

Lymphopathia venereum is a specific, indolent infectious disease due to a filterable virus which is transmitted by sexual intercourse, and for that r e a s o n many have termed it the "fourth venereal disease."

The term "lymphopathia venereum" if universally adopted is preferable to lympho-granuloma-inguinale and will lead to less confusion for it will give a more accurate conception of the disease, and yet will embrace the various extra-inguinal localizations that are now recognized as being of identical etiology.

There is no doubt as to the prevalence of this infection in the United States, and, quite contrary to past belief, it occurs with about the same frequency in the temperate and sub-tropical climates as it does in the tropics. Undoubtedly in the past the failure of recognition was the inability of the physician to diagnose the condition.

Lymphopathia venereum affects young male adults more often than females and is characterized as a sub-acute, resistant inflammation of the inguinal lymph glands, o f t e n resulting in suppuration, abscess formation and chronic fistulas, with a tendency toward healing by retractile scarring and fibrosis. The incubation period, according to Hellerstrom, is from 10 to 30 days and dates from the time of exposure to the appearance of lymph gland involve-

*Read before the Section on Dermatology and Radiology, Annual Meeting, Oklahoma State Medical Association, Tulsa, Oklahoma, May, 1937.

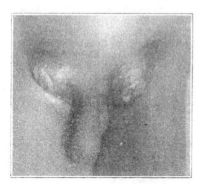

Fig. I—Bi-lateral inguinal involvement
with draining sinuses.

ment. Because of anatomic differences in
male and female lymphatic structures, superficial and intermediate inguinal disorder in the female are the exception rather than the rule.

The lymph drainage of the male genitalia is directed almost entirely into the
inguinal lymph spaces and then into the
deep i l i a c s. Therefore, when the initial
lesion is on the external g e n i t a l, these
nodes become affected. In the female the
anatomy of the lymph drainage is quite
different. Only the lymph from the vulva
is directed into the inguinal lymphatics
while that from the v a g i n a and cervix
drains into the lymphatics around the rectum. This explains the frequent dissimi-
larities of the disease in the two sexes.

In women the disease more often presents itself in the deep pelvic and peri-
anal lymphatics, therefore the later manifestations are more commonly seen. After
running an indolent, chronic course, the
d i s e a s e resolves itself into esthiomene
(chronic ulceration of the v u l v a with
elephantiasis and sclerosis), and the gen-
ito-ano-rectal syndrome (ano-rectal syph-
iloma with stricture of the bowel). There
may be no subjective symptoms in the female during the active stage of the infection until the appearance of the adenitis.

A careful history and physical examination will elicit the presence of a primary
sore in about 50 per cent of cases. The history of a s m a l l, painless, non-indurated
lesion on the genitals, appearing from three
days to three weeks after exposure, which
r a p i d l y disappears in from five to ten

days, followed by inguinal glandular involvement, should immediately lead one
to suspect lymphopathia venera.

This primary erosion is usually dry with
sharply defined edges and in the male
usually presents itself on the glans penis
or prepuce. In the female the portal of
entry is often difficult to determine. Primary lesions of the external genitalia are
rare, but when they do occur, they present
themselves in the region of the fourchette
or the vagina. Many of the infections in
females undoubtedly occur through the
vagina or cervix, in which case primary
lesions would be unnoticed. Four types of
primary lesions have been described: the
ulcerated, nodular, herpetic and the lym-
pho-granulomatous urethritis.

The onset of the disease is rather insidious and favors the appearance of a systemic infection resembling the symptoms
so commonly noted in cases of a mild septicemia. A few days prior to the swelling
of the lymph nodes, the patient suffers
from s l i g h t headache, anorexia, dorso-
lumbar pains and generalized discomfort.
These symptoms are followed in a few days
by an inflammatory involvement of the
lymph nodes. In men the first glands to
be affected are t h o s e of the superficial
group in the inguinal region, either the
pubic glands or the medial group of the
proximal sub-inguinal lymph glands, which
lie in close proximity to Poupart's ligament. The disease progresses very slowly
and extends from gland to gland, finally
producing a peri-adenitis. Swelling of the

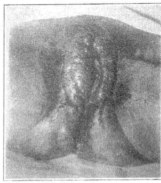

Fig II—Elephantiasis of the vulva with
rectal stricture and fistulas.

glands is constant and variable, and tenderness becomes more pronounced as the s w e l l i n g increases. The skin over the glands becomes reddened and, as the peri-adenitis develops, it becomes attached and fixed; matting of the glands is elicited as the disease progresses, usually after five weeks from the onset of symptoms. The iliac glands also become involved, and at this stage the skin over the affected glands takes on a purplish hue.

Along with the gradual development of peri-adenitis, chills, fever and night sweats are generally noted. There also develops a m o d e r a t e leukocytosis, varying from 10,000 to 12,000, with a definite increase in mononuclears. Eosinophilia is more or less constant. Walking b e c o m e s more and more difficult, even though pain is not an outstanding symptom.

Eventually softening of the glandular masses occurs and definite fluctuation is noticed. This is usually followed by the appearance of one or more fistulas, which become inter-communicable. These . interlacing channels give the affected area the usual honeycomb appearance. Thick, viscid, creamy, yellow pus may exude for a long period, which later becomes sero-sanguineous. Systemic symptoms often disappear long before the fistulas cease draining.

A most careful h i s t o r y and physical examination, together with the positive diagnostic test of Frei, are paramount to the c o r r e c t diagnosis of lymphopathia venereum. The discovery by Frei in 1925 of the specific diagnostic intradermal test, which has been given his name, has greatly simplified the establishing of this clinical disease entity and has paved the way for all the successful research that has since been done in linking these various syndromes under one disease entity. The Frei test is extremely sensitive and most reliable, and if properly interpreted, is one of the most specific test substances in immunological use.

Histologically the principal p i c t u r e is that of a sub-acute or chronic infectious granuloma with multiple abscess formation, the abscesses varying greatly in size and shape. The normal lymph node structure appears to be replaced by a diffuse granulomatous hyperplasia, composed of lymphocytes, plasma cells, epithelioid cells,

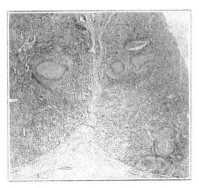

Fig. III—Histopathology of lymph glands.

fibroblasts and an occasional multinucleated giant cell of the L a n g h a n s type. Sharply demarcated from the hyperplastic surrounding pulp are numerous necrotic areas of varying size and shape, which appear both ramified and discrete. In the center of the abscesses are g r a n u l a r detritus, collections of polymorphonuclear leukocytes and small round cells. Surrounding these centers is a palisading of epitheloid cells and a few mononuclears. The capsule of the n o d e s shows great thickening and consists of dense, moderately hyalinized fibrous tissue, with little evidence of inflammatory reaction.

Numerous remedies have been advocated, but no single remedy is known to have specific therapeutic value, and, more certainly, no routine treatment can be recommended. The measures selected and resorted to will necessarily depend on a number of factors such as the form, stage of the disease, age and economic status of the patient. In patients where the diagnosis is made early before fistulas are formed, the treatment of choice is graded sub-cutaneous doses of the antigen; although intravenous injections of t a r t a r emetic have also influenced the course of the disease. It is now generally accepted that surgical excision of the glands and fistulas is the therapeutic measure of choice in all cases of suppurative adenitis. This procedure in almost all cases results in a cure in from four to eight weeks, even though there is involvement of the deep glands.

My purpose in this paper is to show that lymphopathia venereum is a definite disease entity of venereal origin and has the possibility of grave consequences.

It should be handled with the same administrative methods and control as are gonorrhea and syphilis. It is hoped that the medical profession wil become more interested in this condition, so that fewer cases will pass undiagnosed. The prob-

lem is more than a dermatological or urological one for it involves greatly the field of internal medicine, surgery, and pathology. With regard to this disease, the surface has only been scratched as far as present knowledge is concerned, and with the proper stimulation and interest on the part of the medical profession at large much may be attained.

————————O————————

Individuality in the Treatment of Fractures Into or Near Joints

FRANK A. STUART, M.D.
TULSA, OKLAHOMA

The purpose of this paper is to stress upon you the importance of (1) individuality in the treatment of fractures into or near joints, (2) promptness, (3) gentleness, and (4) thoroughness. It is prompted by the fact that my own child when three years of age, fell from my fast moving car and sustained a fracture of the humeral condyles.

It is not within the scope of this paper to discuss in detail each type of fracture into or near a joint, but to bring to your attention some of the startling facts about a few of our larger joints that have been learned through a c t u a l experience and through the statistics of the men who have treated these types of fracture.

Fractures into the Shoulder Joint: A not unusual t y p e is the so-called "fracture-dislocation at the shoulder." Here again the greater tuberosity may be fractured or the head of the humerus may be badly comminuted or the fracture occur through the surgical neck accompanied with dislocation of the head. C l o s e d reduction usually fails to reduce the dislocated head and it becomes necessary to open up the joint, reduce the dislocated head and suture, preferably by stainless steel wire, the detached head or comminuted fragments after the fracture has been reduced. Some form of internal fixation "must be carried out," otherwise the fracture will slip,

necessitating another operation. R i g i d immobilization with arm at 45 or 90 degrees abduction is necessary. Early physiotherapy and passive motion is essential. The other fractures about the shoulder joint need only be placed on a traction humerus abduction arm splint, of course using skin traction.

Fracture of Humeral Condyles in Children and Adults: If complications are to be avoided here, immediately accurate reduction of the fracture with close alignment of the fractured surfaces must be accomplished. Such complications are (1) distortion of the epiphysis which will in years to come lead to a cubitus varus or valgus deformity, unstable joint and sometimes a tardy ulna nerve palsy, (2) if nutrition to the fragment is impaired, non-union or mal-union is likely to occur, and does usually with the closed method.

J. S. Speed reviewed 120 cases of fractures of the humeral condyle recently and concluded that (1) "Serious disability follows these fractures in children much more than is appreciated by the average surgeon treating fractures," (2) "Closed reductions are at best uncertain," and (3) "Immediate open reduction using wire nail (small finishing nails) gives the highest percentage of satisfactory results." His conclusions are borne out by the fact that I let sympathy stand in my way and tried closed reduction on my child's arm and later resorted to open reduction. In compound fractures in this area, the method described by Dunlop in the Bone & Joint Journal, January, 1939, is recommended. Proper application of physiotherapy is of great value in restoring motion to these joints. Sometimes one may expect months to elapse before full range of motion is restored.

In adults this type of fracture is usually treated by resuturing the detached fragment, or if badly comminuted, by manipulation or skeletal traction, the Kirchner wire being put through the olecranon. The method introduced by Hugh Owen Thomas and popularized by Sir Robert Jones gives fair results and consists of flexing the elbow to 60 degrees and letting the fracture fall into alignment by its own hanging weight. Usually, however, we have impaired motion in these comminuted fractures through the condyles in adults and the ultimate amount of permanent disability cannot be determined for six months to one year. Physiotherapy here also is of great value.

Fractures of the capitellum are very rare. When they do occur the joint should be opened and the fractured piece either removed or nailed in place.

Fractures of the Head of the Radius: These may be treated either (1) conservatively, that is, when only a crack or a small fissure occurs and where there is no displacement, or (2) by surgical removal of the head of the radius in those cases where the head is comminuted or where a piece is broken off and where the head is fractured and tilted. The end results in either are satisfactory provided early physiotherapy is employed.

Fractures of the Wrist: The point that should be stressed here is not one of the various accepted methods dealing with the reduction of the most common type in this locality, namely, the "Colles' fracture," but rather to urge you the next time you reduce one of these fractures, not to be satisfied with the final position of the fracture until you have the radial side of the radio-carpal joint leaning forward about 10 to 15 degrees. This insures a normal return of flexion at the wrist. We know of no way yet to overcome the radial shortening we so frequently get in the Colles' fracture, therefore, the patient should be forewarned that this might occur.

Physiotherapy begun at the end of the fourth or fifth week, at first using heat and light massage, later passive and still later active motion, is of great value in these cases.

Fracture in the Hip Joint: Fractures of the neck of the femur usually occur within the joint capsule, which naturally makes them be classed as "into the joint."

Prior to the revived methods of "internal fixation," these fractures of the hip were either left alone or treated by Whitman's abduction method and cast. Since Smith-Peterson's paper in 1931 internal fixation or nailing of this fracture has again been widely used and the early end results show a decided advantage in favor of the latter method. By the Whitman method we got only about 50 per cent bony unions, but by the use of some type of internal fixation the results are as high as 90 per cent bony union. No casts are used after the hip is fixed by internal fixation and the patient is walking on crutches as early as three months, in our cases, with no ill effects.

Fracture of Tibia and Femur Involving the Knee Joints: When the fracture lines extend into the joint surface, either from the femoral or tibial side, it has long been known that the function of the knee joint is seriously if not permanently impaired.

Of 13,000 fracture cases on record at the University of Pennsylvania only 186 involved the knee joint. One hundred and thirty-four involved the upper end of the tibia while 28 involved the condyles of the femur. The outer condyles of the femur and tibia were the most frequently affected.

Here again the individuality in the treating of fractures must be borne in mind. Most men have in the past advocated closed reduction of these fractures, however, in some of the cases on which I have done a closed reduction, I have later wished I had done an open. The knee joint is one of our weight bearing joints, and any irregularity in the weight bearing surfaces usually produces either pain or instability or perhaps both, which, if present, means permanent disability.

Recently Thompson has brought f o r t h what he calls the "beaded wire." This is nothing more than a Kirchner wire that has a knob of metal on it. We have used this with pleasing success in fresh fractures of either the condyle of the tibia or both condyles. The fracture is reduced, the beaded wire placed so that the head is against the loose fragment, and traction made by means of a special nut that pulls the bead up tight a g a i n s t the detached fragment which in turn h o l d s the bone fragment against the shaft of the bone. Then the wire is incorporated in a plaster of paris cast. Here again early physiotherapy is very important and the mental attitude of the patient is greatly improved. Since the advent of a new metal, "vitalium," long screws or nails may also be used to a great advantage here. This metal never has to be removed.

Fractures of the Patella: If the fragments are separated or l o o k as if they might easily pull apart, it is generally conceded that open reduction with resuture and close approximation of the surfaces should be done. Some men prefer chromic catgut or fascial lata, however, we prefer to use stainless steel wire. By the use of wire we find we are able to institute passive motion much sooner, without fear of separation of the fragments as the wire causes no trouble whatsoever and it may be left in indefinitely. The leg should be placed in full extension in a cast. Physiotherapy s h o u l d be instituted relatively early in these cases in order to restore as much motion as possible.

Fractures of the Ankle: Here again is one of our weight bearing joints that literally bristles with trouble, due to the fact that a relatively small amount of limitation of motion may mean quite a high percentage of permanent d i s a b i l i t y. The causes of disability usually are (1) pain and tenderness, (2) weakness of ankle and foot and (3) stiffness.

There are many classifications of fractures of the ankle joint, but the ones of (1) external rotation, (2) abduction (fibula flexion), (3) adduction (t i b i a flexion), (4) compression, seem the simplest.

(1)—Fractures produced by an external rotation force, gives an oblique fracture or spiral fracture of the lower third of the fibula.

(2)—Fractures produced by abduction results in a fracture of the internal malleolus plus a fracture of the fibula in its lower third.

(3)—Fractures produced by adduction results in a fracture of both the external and internal malleoli.

(4)—Compression fractures of the ankle joint are produced by a fall. The most common types are what Henderson describes as (1) "The tri-malleoli" or (2) "Marginal type of fractures."

In order to properly treat fractures of the ankle, one must understand just how they are produced. Usually conservative methods give satisfactory r e s u l t s in all fractures of the ankle except the "compression types" where open reduction may be necessary in order to r e s t o r e a smooth joint surface. Reduction u n d e r general anaesthesia of the fracture and its retention in a plaster of paris cast usually suffices. Physiotherapy in the form of light massage at first, then passive motion and later active motion is most essential in concluding the treatment of f r a c t u r e s about the ankle joint because if we get a small amount of stiffness in the ankle joint, it results in a much larger percentage of permanent disability than in other joints. Properly a p p l i e d physiotherapy to this joint also reduces swelling about the joint and minimizes residual pain.

In conclusion, I should like to stress the importance of:

1. Individuality of t r e a t i n g fractures near or into a joint. You cannot read a text book and then treat a fracture exactly as it says for each fracture case is a separate problem. Only very rarely do we see two fractures exactly alike.

2. Accurate anatomic reduction must be attained if an end r e s u l t you would be proud of is obtained.

3. The fracture surfaces must be held rigid and when these fractures occur near a joint, the fracture can best be held by internal fixation then motion in the nearby joint can be begun much earlier.

4. Early passive m o t i o n preceded by heat and proper massage is not being done enough in our fracture work. Too often

we just put the patient under the lamp for 30 minutes, replace him in the cast and let him leave the office.

5. It is wise always to X-ray a fracture on the tenth day after reduction and if it has slipped it can be again reduced before callus has become deposited at the fracture site.

BIBLIOGRAPHY

Henderson, M. S.: The Open Treatment of Fractures, Illinois Medical Journal, January, 1927.

Moffat, Barclay W.: Bimalleola Fractures, Journal of American Medical Association, Vol. 90, P. 690, March 3, 1928.

Hendrson, M. S.: Fractures of the Ankle, Wisconsin Medical Journal, October, 1932.

Gill, A. Bruce: Injuries of the Foot and Ankle, Atlantic Medical Journal, May, 1928.

Eliason & Ebling: Non-Operative Treatment of Fractures of Tibia and Femur Involving the Knee Joint, Surgery, Gynecology and Obstetrics, November, 1933, Vol. LVII, 658-667.

Speed & Macey: Fractures of Humeral Condyles in Children, Journal of Bone and Joint Surgery, Vol. XV, No. 4, pp. 903-919, October, 1933.

Eliason, Eldridge L.: Individuality in Treatment of Fractures, Northwest Medicine, Seattle, Vol. XXXIII, No. 3, pp. 73, March, 1934.

American College of Surgeons: An Outline of the Treatment of Fractures, 1933.

John Dunlop, M.D.: Transcondylar Fractures of the Humerus in Childhood, Journal of Bone and Joint Surgery, January, 1939, p.p. 59.

———o———

Art Tells History of American Medicine

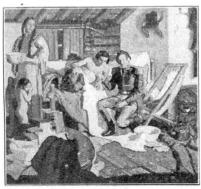

"Beaumont and St. Martin"

"Beaumont and St. Martin" is the first of six large paintings in oil memorializing "Pioneers of American Medicine" which artist Dean Cornwell will complete in the next few years. Others in the series are: Dr. Oliver Wendell Holmes, Dr. Ephraim McDowell, Dr. Crawford W. Long, Dr. William T. G. Morton, and Major Walter Reed, and one woman, Dorothea Lynde Dix who, while not a physician, stimulated physicians to study insanity and feeblemindedness.

Arrangements to supply physicians with free, full color reproductions of "Beaumont and St. Martin" without advertising, and suitable for framing, have been made with the owners, John Wyeth & Brother, 1118 Washington Street, Philadelphia, Pa.

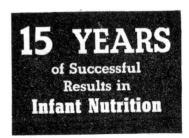
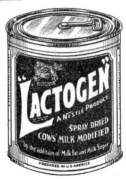

THE JOURNAL
OF THE
Oklahoma State Medical Association

Issued Monthly at McAlester, Oklahoma, under direction of the Council.

Copyright, 1938, by Oklahoma State Medical Association, McAlester, Oklahoma.

| Vol. XXXII | FEBRUARY | Number 2 |

DR. L. S. WILLOUR.................................Editor-in-Chief
McAlester, Oklahoma

DR. T. H. McCARLEY.................................Associate Editor
McAlester, Oklahoma

Entered at the Post Office at McAlester, Oklahoma, as second-class matter under the act of March 3rd, 1879.

This is the official Journal of the Oklahoma State Medical Association. All communications should be addressed to The Journal of the Oklahoma State Medical Association, McAlester Clinic, McAlester, Oklahoma. $4.00 per year; 40c per copy.

The editorial department is not responsible for the opinions expressed in the original articles of contributors.

Reprints of original articles will be supplied at actual cost provided request for them is attached to manuscripts or made in sufficient time before publication.

Articles sent this Journal for publication and all those read at the annual meetings of the State Association are the sole property of this Journal. The Journal relies on each individual contributor's strict adherence to this well-known rule of medical journalism. In the event an article sent this Journal for publication is published before appearance in The Journal the manuscript will be returned to the writer.

Failure to receive The Journal should call for immediate notification of the Editor, McAlester Clinic, McAlester, Oklahoma.

Local news of possible interest to the medical profession, notes on removals, changes of addresses, births, deaths and weddings will be gratefully received.

Advertising of articles, drugs or compounds unapproved by the Council on Pharmacy of the A. M. A., will not be accepted.

Advertising rates will be supplied on application.

It is suggested that wherever possible members of the State Association should patronize our advertisers in preference to others as a matter of fair reciprocity.

Printed by News-Capital Company, McAlester.

EDITORIAL

POSTGRADUATE MEDICAL PROGRAM

The postgraduate program in obstetrics is still progressing into sections of Oklahoma where medical courses for doctors have never yet been given. The fourth circuit in the centers of Ponca City, Blackwell, Tonkawa, Tulsa, Cushing, Stillwater, Bristow and Sapulpa has just been completed. One hundred and twenty-five doctors took the course. Over 40 took it in Tulsa. Physicians are advising the Committee, so states Dr. Henry Turner, Committee Chairman, that it is the best course ever offered to doctors in Oklahoma. In addition, Doctor Edward Smith, the instructor, has given instruction on antepartum care to 14,700 women and high school and college girls. Some of the warmest letters of praise have been received by the Committee from Superintendents and Principals of high schools, Presidents of colleges and Deans of Women about the practical value of these lay lectures and asking, in fact pleading, for more of them and insisting that boys also should have them. Of course all these cannot be supplied, for the first object of the program is postgraduate instruction, and the instructor's time is therefore limited for this secondary part of the program. Such lay lectures are always arranged through the local medical profession. Many women have come into the doctors' offices, as result of being better informed about symptoms of danger described in Dr. Smith's lay lectures. One Payne county physician had 20 new cases in one week.

In Tulsa, the Tulsa County Medical Society thought so much of the value of these lay lectures that they "hired" Convention hall and set up a Public Health forum at the close of the course, having Doctor Smith hold a forum on antepartum care. This is unique in the history of Oklahoma, and a challenge to all other live-wire county societies.

During the week of January 30, the fifth circuit was opened in southwest Oklahoma and includes the teaching centers of Lawton, Frederick, Hollis, Altus and Hobart. This is the first time in history of postgraduate medical study under this circuit plan, that courses have ever been organized in Frederick and Hollis. Funds of the Commonwealth and State Health Department made this possible, for the limited doctor population of this area made self-supported courses in the past impossible. Naturally doctors of those centers and counties are most appreciative. In Harmon County every doctor in the county is enrolled. In Tillman county every doctor except one specalist in eye, ear, nose and throat, enrolled.

One hundred per cent enrollments in these counties shows the appreciation of the physicians over the program being brought to them. Doctor Smith states he has done $40,000 worth of consultations if it were placed upon a pay basis among members of his courses. But these are free private consultations with the doctors who are registered in the courses, and a part of the program outlined by the Committee. Doctors frequently realize f e e s from the outlined courses of treatment, agreed upon between the instructor and himslf, which pay many times his fee for the course, and in addition brings many patients back to health and earning capacity.

The Postgraduate Committee h e l d a meeting in Oklahoma City Sunday, January 29, and Dr. Turner in his Chairmanship report of the first year's activities revealed: that 375 doctors had taken the course, that 14,700 laity had listened to instruction on antepartum care, that over 400 free and private consultations had been made by the instructor among doctors of the postgraduate groups. Further, that instruction had covered 38 of the 77 counties for the first year and that 24 teaching centers had been used. Virtually the entire east part of Oklahoma has now been covered. The instructor has driven 34,844 miles in his intensive efforts, as shown by his car speedometer. All in all this postgraduate course and program promises to be one of the most beneficial to doctors and people, of any during the past 12 years of postgraduate medical education in Oklahoma. A booth at the Annual State meeting this year will furnish statistical accomplishments and give doctors of sections not yet visited, exact information when their area will be reached. Visit your booth this year at the state meeting on Medical Education.

L. W. KIBLER, Field Director,
Post graudate Medical Education,
Oklahoma State Medjcal Assn.

---o---

PROTECTION FOR THE NEW-BORN

The Oklahoma H e a l t h Department is contemplating the introduction of a bill during the present session of the Legislature on Prenatal Serological Examination and the suggested form of the law follows:

OKLAHOMA HEALTH DEPARTMENT
State Prenatal Examination Law

The following model prenatal examination law based upon the laws passed by the states of New York and New Jersey has been prepared by experts under the auspices of the American Social Hygiene Association and is recommended for all states in the Union.

Detailed information regarding this law may be found in the November, 1938, issue of the Journal of Social Hygiene, 50 West Fiftieth Street, New York City (35 cents per copy while they last).

Additional copies of this law may be secured without charge by addressing Dr. Chas. M. Pearce,

Commissioner, Oklahoma Health Department, Oklahoma City, Oklahoma.

"A Suggested Form of State Prenatal Examination Law"

Section I. Serological blood test for syphilis of pregnant women.—Every physician attending a pregnant woman in (name of state) during gestation shall, in the case of each woman so attended, take or cause to be taken a sample of blood of such woman at the time of first examination, and submit such sample to an approved laboratory for a standard serological test for syphilis. Every other person permitted by law to attend upon pregnant women in the state but not permitted by law to take blood tests, shall cause a sample of the blood of such pregnant woman to be taken by a duly licensed physician and submitted to an approved laboratory for a standard serological test for syphilis. The term "approved laboratory" means a laboratory approved for this purpose by the state department of health. A standard serological test for syphilis is one recognized as such by the state department of health. Such laboratory tests as are required by this act shall be made on request without charge by the state department of health.

Section II.—In reporting every birth and stillbirth, physicians and others permitted to attend pregnancy cases and required to report births and stillbirths shall state on the birth certificate or stillbirth certificate, as the case may be, whether a blood test for syphilis has been made during such pregnancy upon a specimen of blood taken from the woman who bore the child for which a birth or stillbirth certificate is filed and, if made, the date when such test was made, and, if not made, the reason why such test was not made. In no event shall the birth certificate state the result of the test.

Should this measure appeal to you as being proper and advantageous it might be well for the medical profession in this state to support its passage. Please take the time to read and evaluate this proposed law.

---o---

Editorial Notes—Personal and General

The following Oklahoma Doctors attended the meeting of the American Academy of Orthopedic Surgeons which was held in Memphis, January 15-19: Doctors D. H. O'Donoghue, C. R. Rountree, Earl D. McBride, E. Margo, R. L. Noell, L. S. Willour, J. E. McDonald, and Paul C. Colonna.

Doctor Colonna appeared on the program presenting his "hip-joint reconstruction" operation. Drs. Colonna and Harte, of the Departments of Orthopedic Surgery and Pathology, Oklahoma Medical School, presented a scientific exhibit on "A Critical Analysis of 40 Registered Primary Malignant Bone Tumor Cases." Dr. Earl D. McBride, Oklahoma School of Medicine, presented a Scientific Exhibit on "Absorbable Metal in Fractures."

DR. GRADY F. MATHEWS, Tahlequah, has been appointed as State Health Commissioner, to succeed Dr. Chas. M. Pearce. His name was selected from four submitted by the Oklahoma State Medical Association. As h e a l t h commissioner, Dr. Mathews automatically becomes a member of the State Welfare Board. He has been a field worker of the State Health Department.

DR. MORRIS FISHBEIN, Editor, Journal American Medical Association, Chicago, will be the guest of Pottawatomie County Medical Society, March 14, 1939, at Shawnee.

News of the County Medical Societies

HARMON County Medical Society elected the following officers for 1939 at their meeting in December: President, Dr. W. G. Husband, Hollis; Vice-President, Dr. S. W. Hopkins, Hollis; Secretary-Treasurer, Dr. L. E. Hollis, Hollis.

CREEK County Medical Society elected Drs. George C. Croston, Sapulpa, President; Wendell L. Smith, Drumright, Secretary; John M. Wells, Bristow, Censor; W. P. Longmire, Sapulpa, Delegate; E. W. King, Bristow, Alternate, for 1939.

HUGHES County Medical Society elected the following officers for 1939: President, Dr. W. L. Taylor, Holdenville; Vice-President, Dr. R. B. Ford, Holdenville; Secretary-Treasurer, Dr. Imogene Mayfield, Holdenville.

McCURTAIN County Medical Society met in January, 1939, and elected the following officers: Dr. R. D. Williams, Idabel, President; Dr. A. W. Clarkson, Valliant, Vice-President; Dr. R. H. Sherrill, Broken Bow, Secretary.

NOBLE County Medical Society elected the following officers for 1939 at their meeting January 22: President, Dr. J. W. Francis, Perry; Secretary, Dr. C. H. Cook, Perry; Delegate, Dr. T. F. Renfrow, Billings; Alternate, Dr. A. M. Evans and Dr. C. H. Cook, Perry.

KAY County Medical Society elected the following officers at their meeting in January: Dr. George Niemann, Ponca City, President; Dr. Merle Clift, Blackwell, Vice-President; Dr. R. G. Obermiller, Ponca City, Secretary.

GREER County Medical Society met in January and elected the following officers for 1939: President, Dr. G. F. Border, Mangum; Vice-President, Dr. J. T. Lowe, Mangum; Secretary, Dr. J. B. Hollis, Mangum; Delegate, Dr. Hollis; Alternate, Dr. J. B. Lansden, Granite.

PITTSBURG County Medical Society held their annual inaugural banquet January 20, McAlester, for their members. Following the banquet Dr. Geo. A. Kilpatrick was installed as President, succeeding Dr. A. R. Russell; Dr. C. O. Williams as Vice-President; Dr. E. D. Greenberger, Secretary-Treasurer; and Drs. E. H. Shuller and T. H. McCarley, as Delegates. The principal address of the evening was given by Mr. H. M. Armstrong, of the Extension Department of the University of Oklahoma. His subject was "America and the Social Scene." Mr. Herman Larson, Associate Professor of voice at the University, and Mr. Spencer H. Norton, Associate Professor of Music at the University, entertained with several musical selections.

OKFUSKEE County Medical Society elected the following officers for 1939: President, Dr. A. S. Melton, Okemah; Vice-President, Dr. J. M. Pemberton, Okemah; Secretary, Dr. C. M. Bloss, Jr., Okemah.

ALFALFA County Medical Society elected the following officers for 1939 at their regular meeting in January: President, Dr. Z. J. Clark; Vice-President, H. E. Huston; Secretary, Dr. L. T. Lancaster, all of Cherokee.

OSAGE County Medical Society met in January and elected the following officers for 1939: President, Dr. M. E. Rust, Pawhuska; Vice-President, Dr. B. E. Dozier, Shidler; Secretary, Dr. George K. Hemphill, Pawhuska; Delegate, Dr. Paul H. Hemphill, Pawhuska; Alternate, Dr. R. S. Smith, Hominy.

McINTOSH County Medical Society elected the following officers for 1939: President, Dr. J. W. Stoner, Checotah; Vice-President, Dr. D. E. Little, Eufaula; Secretary, Dr. W. A. Tolleson, Eufaula.

CLEVELAND County Medical Society was entertained at dinner by Dr. and Mrs. O. E. Howell, Norman, and following dinner officers for 1939 were elected as follows: President, Dr. W. H. Atkins; Vice-President, Dr. George Wiley; Secretary-Treasurer, Dr. Elizabeth Dorsey; Delegate, Dr. D. W. Griffin, all of Norman.

BRYAN County Medical Society elected Dr. Alfred Baker, President, and Dr. Jas. L. Shuler, Secretary, both of Durant, for 1939.

CARTER County Medical Society met December, 1939, and elected the following officers for 1939: President, Dr. Emma Jean Cantrell, Wilson; Vice-President, Dr. David Cantrell, Wilson; Secretary-Treasurer, Dr. J. Hoyle Carlock, Ardmore.

KIOWA County Medical Society elected the following officers for 1939: President, Dr. J. M. Bonham; Vice-President, Dr. H. B. Watkins; Secretary-Treasurer, Dr. J. Wm. Finch, all of Hobart.

WOODS County Medical Society met December 5, 1938, and elected the following officers for 1939: President, Dr. Clifford A. Traverse, Alva; Secretary, Dr. O. E. Templin, Alva; Delegate, Dr. Daniel B. Ensor, Hopeton.

JACKSON County Medical Society elected the following officers for 1939: President, Dr. J. R. Reid, Altus; Vice-President, Dr. R. F. Brown, Altus; Secretary-Treasurer, Dr. J. M. Allgood, Altus; Delegate, Dr. Wayne Starkey, Altus; Alternate, Dr. E. A. Abernethy, Altus.

OKMULGEE-OKFUSKEE County Medical Societies met December 19, 1938, at Henryetta for their annual dinner. The program was devoted to a discussion of the care of the indigent, with Dr. A. W. Pigford, Tulsa, describing the Tulsa set-up. The following officers were elected for 1939: President, Dr. H. D. Boswell, Henryetta; Vice-President, Dr. J. R. Cotteral, Henryetta; Secretary-Treasurer, Dr. C. E. Smith, Henryetta; Censor, Dr. I. W. Bollinger, Henryetta; Delegates, Dr. J. C. Matheney, Okmulgee, and Dr. G. Y. McKinney, Henryetta; Alternates, Dr. J. G. Edwards, Okmulgee, and Dr. R. W. Hubbard, Oklahoma City.

OTTAWA County Medical Society elected the following officers for 1939 at their meeting in December: President, Dr. Matt A. Connell, Picher; First Vice-President, Dr. J. S. Jacoby, Commerce; Drs. W. G. Chesnut of Miami and H. K. Miller, Fairland, Second and Third Vice-Presidents, respectively; Secretary-Treasurer, Dr. W. Jackson Sayles, Miami, re-elected.

CARTER County Medical Societ met January 23, 1939, at Ardmore with the following program:

"Plans of Committee on Medical Policy and Legislation," Dr. Finis W. Ewing, Chairman, Muskogee; "Program of State Medical Executive Secretary," Mr. R. H. Graham, McAlester, Executive Secretary; "Discussion of State Legislative Policy,"

Dr. J. S. Fulton, Atoka; "Presentation and Discussion of Farm Group Proposal," by Drs. Walter Hardy, F. P. Von Keller and J. Hobson Veazey.

WOODWARD County Medical Society met in December as guests of the Staff of the Western State Hospital at Supply with dinner at 6:30 and the following program:

Report of Dr. Johnson of the Staff on "Results With Insulin Treatment, Covering One Year."

Doctors Coyne Campbell, Oklahoma City, and H. K. Speed, President, of the State Association, Sayre, were guest speakers.

The following officers were elected for 1939: President, Dr. C. E. Williams, Woodward; Vice-President, Dr. Floyd Newman, Shattuck; Secretary-Treasurer, Dr. C. W. Tedrowe, Woodward.

OBITUARIES

Harry J. McGuire, M.D., 1900-1938

Ushered in on the crest of Christmas chimes and carols commemorating the birth of the Prince of Peace, good will, good cheer and brotherly love to all, and when our hearts and minds were filled with a buoyancy of Yuletide season, it was likewise ushering out the realities of a departed life in the person of our good member, Harry McGuire. Harry was a likeable chap, friendly, a pleasant smile, and a host of friends, with a "Hello, so-and-so, how are you?"

The grim fates of life are hard to reckon with when men in the prime of life with a promising future are plucked from their field of toil and pursuit to the consummation of it all—eternity.

Harry worked hard and well at his job as county surgeon, rendering unto many an aching heart of the needy entrusted to his care the skill and marvel of modern surgery.

Is not that a gracious service?

It is hard for the tongue and pen of man to utter a kind word or deed that will soothe an aching heart caused by the departure of a loved one. But the County Medical Society one and all would kindly like to say, we extend to the family our heart felt sympathies in the greatest of human sorrow and sadness.

John C. Perry, Chairman.

Burtis W. McLean, M.D., 1875-1939

Gentlemen, again in the field of activity a sturdy oak has been plucked from our midst, in the life of Dr. Burtis W. McLean of Jenks, Oklahoma. It was an inspiration and an honored privilege to the members of the Tulsa County Medical Society that attended the simple and plain service which was the desire of our departed member, in the little church house across the street from his home, in the little city of his choice where he gave 39 years of active toil in the profession that we most dearly cherish.

There was many a tear-stained eye that passed the floral be-decked bier of this humble apostle of the healing art, no doubt the devoted, honored, respected, true and loyal friends and former patients, with saddened faces and aching hearts, representative of families whose hand he had grasped when they entered this world, and likewise calmly held as they departed from it.

It has well been said and worthy of repetition, that there are good qualities, merits, morals, examples and sterling characters in all mankind if you will only seek it out.

And to the membership of this society I wish to extend to you and call to your attention a beautiful example and loyalty and devotion to our honored profession, as this man gave his life by the roadside, no doubt the cause of a road hog: trying to reach our meeting place some 18 miles away. He was quiet, unassuming, loved solitude, entered our meetings taking his seat, never entering into discussions, and when the meeting was over silently steal away, always leaving the expression of Solomon, "A silent tongue is the key to wisdom."

If this sacrifice of life to the devotion and good of our cause and society in a man of his attained age, picked up by the side of the highway, sittng on the bumper of his car grasping for breath and mortally dieing, trying to reach the meeting place of his society means anything to us: it must surely be a beautiful example of loyalty and devotion. And the security of medicine and our profession in Oklahoma would be well founded, and our good member's life would have not been in vain.

To the devoted wife and life companion the Tulsa County Medical Society humbly says, "May God's blessings be your solace and comfort in your hour of sorrow, in this reality of realities that all the living must sooner or later meet."

Robert Allen Cavitt

Robert Allen Cavitt, Morrison, Oklahoma, age 67. Graduate of College of Physicians and Surgeons at St. Louis, 1898. County Health Officer of Noble County and member of the 13th legislature. Died December 24, 1938.

Recent Deaths
(Insufficient Data for Obituary)

Dr. B. F. Moreland, Idabel, January 16, 1939.
Dr. W. G. Wainright, Tulsa, January 18, 1939.
Dr. J. C. McNees, Ardmore, December 14, 1938.
Dr. Harvey A. Dever, El Reno, December 26, 1938.
Dr. Arthur E. Hale, Alva, January 11, 1939.
Dr. W. R. Black, Seminole, December 22, 1938.

Annual Spring Clinic of the St. Joseph Clinical Society

The St. Joseph Clinical Society will hold its eighth annual spring clinic on March 28 and 29, at the Hotel Robideaux, St. Joseph, Mo. There will be no registration fee. The purpose of the meeting is to offer a concentrated post-graduate course in recent advances in clinical medicine and surgery as interpreted by eminent clinicians who will be our guest speakers.

Over 60 such guest speakers have already honored the Society in the past. This year's speakers offer an especially attractive series of clinical lectures. Aware of the ever increasing importance of more recent social trends as they affect organized medicine, we have secured Dr. Morris Fishbein who will deliver an address to which the general public will be invited. Two luncheons and banquets will be reserved for relaxation and entertainment. The St. Joseph Clinical Society extends a cordial invitation to all members of the medical profession who may wish to be our guests at this clinical gathering.

The speakers and their subjects:

Dr. Gershom J. Thompson: "Transurethral Prostatic Resection."

Dr. Q. W. Newell: "Cancer of the Uterus."

Dr. Fred J. Taussig: "Treatment of Septic Abortion." (Round table discussion.)

Dr. F. J. Taussig: "The Co-ordination of Radium with Surgery in the Treatment of Cervix Cancer."

Dr. Willis C. Campbell: "Some aspects of Surgery of the Hip Joint."

Dr. Heyworth N. Sanford: "Jaundice in the New Born."

Dr. Heyworth N. Sanford: (Banquet) "Some Observations on Disturbances of Blood Coagulation."

Dr. August A. Werner: "The Effect of the Ductless Glands in Growth and Development."

Dr. Ralph A. Kinsella: "The Pneumonias."

Dr. Walter C. Alverez: "Useful Hints in the Treatment of Indigestion."

Dr. Maurice C. Howard: "Problems in Gastric Hemorrhage."

Dr. Morris Fishbein: (Noon luncheon) "American Medicine and the National Health Program."

Dr. Morris Fishbein: (Open public address) "The Social Aspects of Medical Care."

Dr. J. A. Myers: "Modern Methods in Diagnosis and Therapy of Tuberculosis."

Dr. Coyne H. Campbell: "Practical Points in the Management of Neurotic Symptoms, Inhibitions and Anxiety."

Dr. Manuel Grodinsky: "Pyogenic Infections of the Hand and Foot."

---o---

MOTION PICTURES AVAILABLE

The following films are available for use for County Medical Societies or other scientific organizations. You will notice that some of the films are for lay audiences. Requests for films should be instituted as far in advance as p o s s i b l e, so that the p r o p e r reservations can be made. The exact shipping address and dates should be given at the time of the request; also the type of apparatus in which the film is to be run. Responsibility for the projection and care of the film must be borne by the individual or organization which is borrowing it. The American Medical Association does not have projectors available for loan. The only expense incurred is that of transportation both ways. C a r e l e s s handling, resulting in serious damage may be charged to the borrower. A brief description of each film is given in the following list.

Application for these films should be made to the Committee on Post Graduate Medical Teaching of the Oklahoma State Medical Association, 217 Plaza Court, Oklahoma City. These applications will be forwarded to the American Medical Association for distribution of the films. List:

(1)—MOTION PICTURES FOR MEDICAL SOCIETIES AND OTHER SCIENTIFIC ORGANIZATIONS

Syphilis—A Motion Picture Clinic

Sound. 35 mm., 9 reels; also 16 mm., 2 large reels, 1,600 ft. each. Running time, about 1½ hours.

The diagnosis and treatment of syphilis presented by the following individuals:

Dr. John H. Stokes—Diagnosis of early syphilis.

Dr. Harold N. Cole—Treatment of syphilis.

Dr. Paul A. O'Leary—Latent syphilis.

Dr. James R. McCord—Treatment of syphilis in pregnancy.

Dr. Philip C. Jeans—Congenital syphilis.

Dr. Joseph Earle Moore—Late manifestations and neurosyphilis.

Short talks also given by: Dr. Charles Gordon Heyd, Dr. Morris Fishbein, Dr. Thomas Parran, Dr. R. A. Vonderlehr.

(Script is available in a pamphlet—40 pp., price 10c.)

Sponsored jointly by the American Medical Association, 535 N. Dearborn street, Chicago, and the United States Public Health Service, Washington, D. C.

Produced by Burton Holmes Films, Inc., 7510 N. Ashland Ave., Chicago.

Audience: medical.

Cancer—(Canti Cancer Film)

Silent. 35 mm., 3 reels. Running time, about 45 minutes.

A film demonstrating the proliferation of cell tissue and the formation of cancers.

Produced by Dr. R. G. Canti, London, England.

Audience: medical.

Blood Circulation (Harvey Blood Film)

Silent. 35 mm., 3 reels. Running time, about 45 minutes.

An attempt has been made to reproduce the dissections and experiments performed and described by Harvey himself, and here explained in the main by extracts from Robert Willis' translation of Harvey's book.

Audience: medical.

Blood Transfusion

Silent. 16 mm., 1 large reel, 1,200 feet. Running time about 45 minutes.

Three methods of blood transfusion, illustrated in detail.

Sponsored by the Blood Transfusion Betterment Association, 39 E. 78th St., New York, N. Y.

Produced by Mr. Joseph P. Hackel, New York, N. Y.

Audience: medical.

Comparative Physiology of Labor

Silent. 16 mm., 4 reels, total about 1,400 feet. Running time, about 1 hour.

Demonstration of normal labor in the human, the horse, the cow, the sheep, the dog, the pig, and rabbit.

Produced by Professor K. de Snoo, Obstetrical and Veterinary Clinics, University of Utrecht, Netherlands.

Audience: medical.

Effects of Heat and Cold on the Circulation of the Blood

Silent. 16 mm., 1 reel, 300 feet. Running time, 12 minutes.

Demonstration of the effect of heat and cold on circulation as seen through a glass chamber installed in a rabbit's ear.

Produced by Dr. E. R. Clark, University of Pennsylvania, School of Medicine, Philadelphia.

Audience: medical.

Effects of Massage on Circulation of Blood

Silent. 16 mm., 1 reel, 200 feet. Running time, 8 minutes.

Demonstration of the effect of massage on circulation as seen through a glass chamber installed in a rabbit's ear.

Produced by Dr. E. R. Clark, University of Pennsylvania, School of Medicine, Philadelphia.

Audience: medical.

Contraction of Arteries and Arterio-Venous Anastomoses

Silent. 16 mm., 1 reel, 250 feet. Running time, 10 minutes.

This film visualizes the contraction of arteries and arteriovenous anastomoses as seen through a glass chamber installed in a rabbit's ear.

Produced by Dr. E. R. Clark, University of Pennsylvania, School of Medicine, Philadelphia.

Audience: medical.

Therapeutic Exercises for the Shoulder Joint Following Dislocation

Silent. 16 mm., 1 reel, 250 feet. Running time, 10 minutes.

Demonstration of static, passive, active and resistive exercises for the shoulder joint, using simple apparatus.

Produced by the Council on Physical Therapy, American Medical Association, 535 N. Dearborn St., Chicago.

Audience: medical.

Treatment of Compression Fracture of the First Lumbar Vertebra

Silent. 16 mm., 1 reel, 300 feet. Running time, about 12 minutes.

This film shows physical therapy procedures to be administered to a fracture of the first lumbar vertebrae during a patient's confinement in bed and immediately following.

Produced by Dr. Harry E. Mock and Dr. John Pribble, 122 S. Michigan Ave., Chicago.

Audience: medical.

Aids in Muscle Training

Silent. 16 mm., 1 reel, 300 feet. Running time, about 12 minutes.

Demonstration of sling suspension exercises for the upper and lower extremities, graded exercises on a powdered board for the lower extremities, and three kinds of "walkers" for reeducation exercises.

Produced by the Council on Physical Therapy, American Medical Association, 535 N. Dearborn St., Chicago, Ill.

Audience: medical.

Underwater Therapy

Silent. 16 mm., 1 reel, 400 feet. Running time, about 16 minutes.

Presentation of therapeutic use of large and small exercise pools, Hubbard tanks, and home-made tanks, and demonstration of types of exercises given in cases such as infantile paralysis, cerebral palsy and postoperative congenital dislocation of the hip.

Produced by the Council on Physical Therapy, American Medical Association, 535 N. Dearborn St., Chicago, Ill.

Audience: medical.

Occupational Therapy

Silent. 16 mm., 1 reel, 300 feet. Running time, 12 minutes.

This film demonstrates occupations that may be prescribed by physicians to motivate and control the desired physical or mental activity of the patient and assist in his adjustment to long hospitalization. A section on cerebral palsy is included, picturing indirect muscle training through prescribed activity and stressing the importance of early treatment to prevent growth of faulty habit patterns.

Produced by the Council on Physical Therapy, American Medical Association, 535 N. Dearborn St., Chicago.

Audience: medical.

Massage

Silent. 16 mm., 1 reel, 100 feet. Running time, 4 minutes.

Demonstration of technic of massage, describing the various movements and why they are performed in a given way.

Produced by the Council on Physical Therapy, American Medical Association, 535 N. Dearborn St., Chicago.

Audience: medical.

(2)—MOTION PICTURES FOR THE PUBLIC
A New Day

Sound. 16 mm., 1 reel, 400 feet. Running time, about 12 minutes.

A dramatized film on the prevention and treatment of pneumonia.

Produced by Metropolitan Life Insurance Company, 1 Madison Ave., New York, N. Y.

Prevention of Burns

Silent. 16 mm., ½ reel. Running time, about 7 minutes.

A dramatized picture depicting the prevention of burns in children, with a short presentation of tannic acid treatment.

Produced by the Milwaukee Children's Hospital, Milwaukee, Wis.

Men of Medicine

Sound. 16 mm., 1 reel, 800 feet. Running time, about 30 minutes.

THE MARCH OF TIME—produced by the Editors of Time and Life, 369 Lexington Ave., New York City.

Released by RKO Radio Pictures.

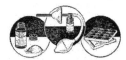
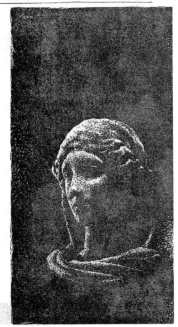

ABSTRACTS : REVIEWS : COMMENTS
and CORRESPONDENCE

SURGERY AND GYNECOLOGY
Abstracts, Reviews and Comments from
LeRoy Long Clinic
714 Medical Arts Building, Oklahoma City

Pancreatic Extract (Enzyme-Free) In the Treatment of Diabetic and Arteriosclerotic Gangrene; Joseph B. Wolffe; The American Journal of Surgery; January, 1939; page 109.

The author says that he has obtained very favorable results by treating cases of diabetic and arteriosclerotic gangrene with various enzyme-free pancreatic extracts prepared and standardized according to previous publications by him. The early rationale for using this substance was based mainly on the work of Frey and Kraut and of Vaquez and his co-workers, who showed that the pancreas contains a vasodilator substance. The author and his associates have since discovered and reported that it possesses many other pharmacologic properties:

(A) They believe it contains a parasympathetic stimulant (perhaps a cholinergic hormone) for the following reasons: (1) it neutralizes the rise in blood pressure produced by epinephrine; (2) topical application to the bullfrog eye constricts the pupil and neutralizes the dilator effect of epinephrine; (3) it increases peristalsis.

(B) This substance aids in fat metabolism, that is, it lowers blood cholesterol and phospholipids after parenteral administration.

(C) In depancreatized dogs it prevents fatty degeneration of the liver and prolongs the life of the animal.

(D) It causes appearance or increase in human urine of a substance related to choline, which is detected, like choline, by adding a solution of bismuth iodide in nitric acid to the urine. After injection of pancreatic extract, the quantity of brick red precipitate increases over a period of a few hours. In their experience there is a relationship between the quantitative appearance of this substance and actual clinical results.

(E) Their clinical impressions suggest that pancreatic extract prevents certain trophic changes.

In this article the author summarizes a series of 100 cases treated with pancreatic extracts. This series comprises 60 cases of diabetic-atherosclerotic gangrene and 40 cases of non-diabetic-atherosclerotic gangrene. The age range of the patients was from 44 to 78 years.

They divided all their diabetic cases treated with pancreatic extracts into two groups. The first consisted of those with beginning dry gangrene and the second group, consisting of diabetics, comprised 27 cases of more extensive gangrene.

Patients in their series of 100 cases seemed to do very well, presenting about 75 per cent of complete healing. Most of them were treated conservatively. The author stresses that injections of pancreatic extract did not constitute the sole treatment in all the cases. The extract was administered in doses of from one to three cc., either daily or on alternate days, depending on indications, in addition to an adequate diabetic regimen. Nor were other measures neglected, such as proper hygiene, asepsis, short wave diathermy, low fat diet, etc.

The usual diabetic management fails in many cases of gangrene, necessitating radical surgery. The author attributes this to the lack in insulin of some substance present in the pancreatic extract (desympatone).

The active substance present in the enzyme-free pancreatic extract, which is neither histamine nor choline, exerts a beneficial influence upon lipoid metabolism, as well as upon muscle metabolism in general. As a corollary to this, it may be that the combination of insulin, pancreatic extract and a diet low in fats, will prevent the early appearance of atherosclerosis in diabetics. If this is true, it is possible to expect a decreased incidence of diabetic gangrene.

The author's conclusion is that pancreatic extract (enzyme-free) proved of great value as an additional therapeutic agent in the management of diabetic and arteriosclerotic gangrene. It not only produces an early arrest of pathologic processes, but seems to stimulate repair more rapidly and more completely than any other conservative method in his experience.

LeRoy D. Long.

Clinical Aspects of the Blood Chemistry in Intestinal Obstruction; M. A. Falconer; Proceedings of the Staff Meetings of the Mayo Clinic; July 20, 1938; page 460.

The variations in the blood chemistry toward hypochloremia, azotemia, alkalosis and dehydration, which occur constantly in cases of experimental high intestinal obstruction among animals, do not occur uniformly in cases of obstruction observed clinically among human beings. Clinically, alterations in the blood chemistry when obstruction is present seem to be secondary to the onset of intoxication, for often cases of either high or low intestinal obstruction are encountered in which the obstructing lesion has been present for some time without the development of significant variations in the blood chemistry.

No uniformity characterizes the biochemical changes which may occur in the blood during obstruction at any given level of the intestine. Often, cases of obstruction are encountered which are caused by similar lesions and at similar sites, yet showing differing biochemical variations. A rise in the concentration of blood urea is the most constant change and is associated with a high urinary output of urea (and urinary nitrogen) in all cases except those associated with nephritis. This combination of a high concentration of blood urea and a high urinary output is the result of increased endogenous metabolism of protein.

Cases of intestinal obstruction may be associated with a normal concentration of chloride of the plasma during obstruction and even with ample chloride of the urine. The decrease in chloride is influenced by the duration and severity of the vomiting and tends to be severe in those cases in which vomiting is profuse. However, exceptions are encountered. The carbon dioxide combining power of the plasma may be variable. Usually, when the plasma chloride is low, the carbon dioxide combining power is high and when the plasma chloride is normal, the carbon dioxide combining power is either normal or decreased. Evidence of dehydration is furnished by repeated hematocrit determinations and erythrocyte counts which indicate a decrease in the concentration of the blood during recovery. Occasionally, pronounced dehydration is the most prominent finding.

The author divides cases of intestinal obstruction associated with changes in the blood into two syndromes: (1) cases associated with azotemia, hypochloremia, alkalosis and dehydration; (2) cases associated with azotemia, and dehydration, a normal concentration of chloride in the plasma and a variable acid base equilibrium. The first syndrome (the classical one) occurs in practically all cases of pyloric and duodenal obstruction, in the majority of cases of obstruction of the small bowel and in a few cases of obstruction of the large bowel. The second syndrome rarely is associated with pyloric and duodenal obstruction but is encountered in some cases of obstruction of the small bowel and in the majority of those of the large bowel.

Repeated examination of the blood in the author's cases enabled him to observe the effects of operation and saline therapy on the blood. He summarizes his conclusions as follows:

1. "Following release of the obstruction, there is a natural tendency toward restitution of the various constituents of the blood to normal. This tendency can be observed in every case in which recovery ensues. It commences simultaneously with clinical improvement but does not reach completion until some days after clinical recovery is manifest.

2. "In cases of hypochloremia in order to replace that which is lost from the body, sodium chloride is required in amounts of 15 to 25 gm. for each 100 mg. per cent that the plasma chloride is below normal. We have found that more marked responses occur in the plasma chloride values when sodium chloride is given as a physiologic solution either subcutaneously or intravenously rather than as a 10 or 15 per cent solution intravenously. When sodium chloride is administered in these amounts after the release of obstruction, the plasma chloride recovers at its own natural rate and it is often impossible to accelerate this rate of recovery by the administration of larger amounts of sodium chloride.

3. "Alterations in the concentration of blood urea afford better criteria of a patient's progress than alterations in the concentration of plasma chloride. Hypochloremia may be corrected by means of saline therapy without appreciably improving the patient's condition or modifying the azotemia. On the other hand, a steady and rapid rise in the concentration of blood urea is of grave prognostic significance.

4. "Dehydration is present in practically all cases of intestinal obstruction and may be severe. It is necessary to administer fluid until a daily output of 1,000 to 1,500 c.c. of urine is established. The most satisfactory method of determining the correction of dehydration is measurement of the total daily output of urine.

5. "In clinical cases of obstruction, parenteral fluids usually are required because of vomiting and because of the disturbed function of the bowel. Occasionally cases of uremic intoxication (alkalosis) complicating pyloric stenosis are encountered, in which owing to the persistence of symptoms of retention, little or no improvement follows the administration of solutions of saline and glucose parenterally. In such cases the administration of these solutions by jejunostomy is feasible and leads to more rapid improvement clinically.

"These biochemical variations are not the only changes which may occur in the blood of patients who have intestinal obstruction although they are probably the most important changes. Further work on these chemical changes is at present in progress."

Dr. J. F. Weir made a very able discussion of this paper and in general agreed with the author's conclusions.

In addition, Dr. Weir pointed out that surgeons had for some time been recognizing such cases on the basis of the occurrence of gastric retention and decreased excretion of urine before any chemical changes occurred in the blood and that adequate therapy relieved the condition. Thus, in an illness that could be recognized and satisfactorily treated before alteration of chemical constituents of the blood occurred, the condition could not be ascribed to this alteration. In other words, failure of motor function precedes depletion of fluids and electrolytes in the blood and tissues, increased tissue catabolism, and the severe coincidental clinical symptoms. It seems wise, therefore, in the light of our present knowledge, to attribute the condition to some unknown factor which gives rise to inhibition of motor function.

LeRoy D. Long.

X-Ray Demonstration of Submucous Myomas by Combined Use of Hippuran and CO2 Injections. I. C. Rubin, M.D., F.A.C.S., New York, N. Y. American Journal of Obstetrics and Gynecology, January, 1939, Vol. 37, No. 1, page 75.

Dr. Rubin has devised a refinement in the method for diagnosis of submucous myomas. He has employed intra-uterine injections of hippuran which leaves a crystalline deposit upon the uterine mucosa and the mucosa covering the submucous tumor. The hippuran is allowed to drain from the cavity of the uterus and thereafter CO_2 is injected and an X-ray made. Neither by itself is adequate for diagnosing fibroid tumors but the transparent contrast of CO_2 to the densely opaque hippuran outline causes the tumors to stand out in relief. The author reports that the media is innocuous, that there is no irritation and no residue or foreign body reaction. He advises it in selected patients where recognition of submucous myoma is important from the view-point of choice of therapy.

Comment: This is an additional feature to the already excellent work done by Dr. Rubin in connection with the intra-uterine injection of gases and oils. It will have very little general usage but in the instances where an attempt is being made to preserve the maximum function of the uterus in young women, this additional diagnostic assistance will be of extreme importance.

Wendell Long.

The Degree of Normal Menstrual Irregularity. An Analysis of 20,000 Calendar Records from 1,500 Individuals. Leslie B. Arey, Ph.D., Sc.D., Chicago, Ill. American Journal of Obstetrics and Gynecology, January, 1939, Vol. 37, No. 1, page 12.

This is a statistical study of a collection of reported series where the records of consecutive menstruations were set down on a calendar at the time of occurrence.

It reports 20,000 calendar records from about 1,500 women and girls as given in 12 different studies.

The author feels that such records are the only reliable ones and that ordinary hospital histories, oral testimony and similar data which depend on unaided memory have proven entirely unreliable.

"The average length of all cycles is 33.9 days for girls and 28.4 days for women."

"The mean length of cycle based on individual averages is 33.6 days for girls and 29.5 days for women."

"The maximum departures of individuals from

their means extends from 1 to 69 days in adults and from * to 211 in pubertal girls."

"In the first few years of menstrual function the cycle length is extremely variable (seven to 256 days)."

"From the menarche to the twentieth or twenty-fourth cycle, only two-thirds of the total cycles of an average individual kept within a 20-day range above and below her mean. Yet in middle adolescence, occupied by cycles 25 to 39, the regularity improved to such an extent that, on the average, two-thirds of all the cycles kept within a 10-day range."

In adults over 21 years of age there was a variation of plus or minus 2½ days on the average from the mean. "Expressed differently, an average adult woman must expect one-third of all of her cycles to depart more than two days from her mean cycle length." "The amount of variability shown by adults is greater than ordinarily is credited." "In the records of more than 500 women, 27 per cent never showed their own means during the observation period which averaged 11 cycles in length. Only 20 per cent experienced their own mean in at least one-third of their recorded cycles.

"The adults, reported in detail by 11 different investigators, represent all ages from late adolescence to approaching menopause. They include American, Canadian, British, German, and Hungarian subjects, and they sample various grades of society. In no instance did an example of perfect menstrual regularity appear over any significant period of time; this is all the more noteworthy since many individuals had previously declared themselves to be the acme of invariability. The most regular records are short ones. In a separate (unpublished) study of menstrual records extending as long as 20 years, it will be shown that temporary successions of atypical regularity (or irregularity) may occasionally interpose themselves in a rhythm of fundamentally different characteristics. It is these unrepresentative fragments of the true record that sometimes lead to erroneous conclusions concerning an individual rhythm; even a record extending for over a year may prove to be unrepresentative.

"In the face of all these facts it seems improbable that menstrual regularity, in any true sense of the word, ever will be encountered over significant periods of time. Certainly, not the slightest evidence pointing toward perfect regularity has so far been produced for even a single exceptional individual. Should such a person be found at some future time, she will constitute a true medical curiosity."

Comment: This is a well prepared statistical study which represents an important practical consideration, especially at the present time when ŕ great many endocrine products are rather promiscuously employed in order to correct an acquired or temporary irregularity of menstruation. It is well to remember that a mild degree of variation, while possibly due to endocrine dysfunction is basically caused by the patient's general poor health, variations in her mental and physical strain and to a certain degree upon the weather changes of seasons.

It is, therefore, wise to consider the individual very carefully from a general standpoint before offering specific endocrine therapy for irregularity, and also to take note of the fact that apparently normal individuals have a certain degree of variation in their so-called regularity.

Wendell Long.

EYE, EAR, NOSE AND THROAT
Edited by Marvin D. Henley, M.D.
911 Medical Arts Building, Tulsa

Parallel Study of the Pathogenesis of Rhinogenous Optic Neuritis and of Serous Iritis. Bela Waldman, M.D., Oradea (late Nagyvarad), Roumania. American Journal of Ophthalmology, January, 1939.

The opinions of American authors on this controversial question is so considerable that it results in confusion to the reader. This article is the opinion, experiences and case reports of one outside realm of the American investigators and so is quite interesting. In regard to optic neuritis of rhinogenous origin the author believes that it is a rare disease but that it does occur; also that when all other causes are excluded, even if the X-ray and nasal findings of the sinuses are negative, an explorative opening of the posterior sinuses is indicated.

He considers serous iritis of greater importance because of its greater incidence and because it often bilateral and consequently may result in a greater disability. This is called a seasonal disease because the author's cases have presented themselves from October to April; because of the good results obtained by nasal tamponade he considers the disease of **rhinogenous origin**; the causative agent most often found in the sinuses is the influenza bacillus. Catarrhal diplococcus is found normally on mucous membrane of the nasal cavities —its pathology is slight—but it is capable of bringing about a catarrh of the upper respiratory passages. The causative agents reach the eyeball by the hematogenous route or by direct passage. Hajek is quoted as to the extent the swelling may go in a sinus infection and its extension to the bone. The medullary cavities of the bony wall provide a straight path for the bacteria toward the optic canal; thence to the pia mater and the uvea.

The author's summary is as follows:

As can be seen from the foregoing, the pathogenesis of optic neuritis and of serous iritis displays considerable differences; they have, however, many points in common.

The optic neuritis of rhinogenic origin is the outcome of an aseptic process going on in the optic canal, and is brought about exclusively by mechanical factors. Its origin is the empyema of the posterior sinuses, or the chronic hypertrophic inflammation of the latter.

Spontaneous serous iritis, even in the presence of syphilis or tuberculosis, is in every instance the outcome of a catarrhal infection.

The source of infection is the catarrhal inflammation of the posterior sinuses, and pathogenic agents migrate directly from the sinus into the canal and thence, by way of the pia mater, into the uvea.

Studies on the Bacteriology of Hypopyon Ulcer. A report on the conjunctival flora of healthy coal mine workers. A. J. Rhodes, M.B., M.R.C.P.E., University of Edinburgh. The British Journal of Ophthalmology, January, 1939.

Cultures were taken from both conjunctival sacs as the men came off work and rubbed over blood agar in screw top bottles and sent to the laboratory for incubation. A total of 658 miners were examined from four different mines. It was thought that there might be a tendency for an organism, once having gained access to a group of workers to spread through that unit. On two occasions this theory was definitely proven to be true. Various tables accompany this article. The summary of the article is as follows:

1. The conjunctival flora of 658 healthy coal mine-workers has been examined, representing four different pits.

2. In two pits the oncost-worker evidently harboured a more profuse flora than the other workers.

3. Apart from this, below-ground workers did not harbour a flora essentially different from that of surface workers.

4. The following potentially pathogenic organisms may be found in all groups of workers in significant quantity: streptococcus viridans, pneumococcus, diplobacillus of Morax, haemophilic bacilli and B. Coli.

5. Streptococcus viridans occurred in 11.25 per cent of persons.

6. Fifty-four strains of pneumococcus were encountered (representing 8.1 per cent of the workers), but only one of these fell into a main type (type 3). The bulk of the remainder proved avirulent to the mouse, but showed typical reactions otherwise.

7. The distribution of diplobacillus of Morax was somewhat irregular, occurring in 2.3 per cent of all workers in pits L, V, and W, and in 6.76 per cent at pit A.

8. Haemophilic bacilli were isolated from 1.5 per cent of persons, and B. coli from 0.75 per cent.

9. It is considered that the conjunctival flora of coal mine-workers is potentially dangerous and that the source of infection in hypopyon ulcer is from organisms already present in the conjunctival sac. Those most liable to contract the disease are those most exposed to corneal trauma—the miners and brushers.

Retinitis In Diabetes. Henry P. Wagener, M.D., Thomas J. Dry, M.B., and Russell M. Wilder, M.D. Digested from New England J. Med., Vol. 211 and published in The Digest of Ophthalmology and Otolaryngology, January, 1939.

The material upon which this paper is based consists of the records of 1,052 cases of "run-of-the-mill" type of diabetes. While some patients suffer from both diabetes and severe hypertension, retinitis may be seen that is dependent entirely on the hypertensive disease. Constriction and sclerosis of the arterioles are present, with cotton-wool patches and superficial areas of hemorrhage, but such a picture is not suggestive of diabetes. However, in a large majority of cases of diabetes, characteristic retinal lesions are found irrespective of hypertension.

Five types may be described which represent progressive phases in the development of a common underlying process. "They are, (1) hemorrhages alone, with no other lesion, (2) hemorrhages with punctate exudates, (3) hemorrhages with both punctate and cotton-wool-like exudates, (4) hemorrhages or exudates associated with visible lesions in the veins, and (5) visible lesions in the veins with recurrent hemorrhages into the vitreous and proliferation of new vessels and formation of scar tissue.

"The earliest and mildest type of retinitis in diabetes consists of tiny punctate hemorrhages which are situated usually in the vicinity of dilated terminal venules in the macular region. In later phases of the disease these hemorrhages may be larger and more widely spread. Almost always, however, they are deeply situated and therefore more or less round in form.

"At a later but still early stage a few, shiny, irregularly-shaped punctate exudates are seen apparently lying in the deeper layers of the retina, either above or below the fovea centralis and usually in association with the minute hemorrhages just described. . . . In the more advanced stages the hemorrhages are very wide-spread, and many of them are large and of irregular form.

"Ophthalmoscopic examination in 1,052 cases in which patients had diabetes revealed hemorrhagic lesions of the retina in 187, or 17.7 per cent. Hemorrhage alone was observed in 5.5 per cent; hemorrhage associated with exudates, 12.2 per cent.

"The retinal lesions in question occur predominantly among patients more than 40 years of age. The lesions are usually but not always associated with hypertension or other evidence of general vascular disease.

"The retinal disease in question seems to pass progressively through successive stages, beginning with hemorrhages only and eventuating in a gross venous disease with nective tissue.

"It is our belief that diabetes injures the finer arterioles or venules of the retina, probably the latter; that the injury is insufficient in degree in most cases to bring about abnormalities that are visible with the ophthalmoscope; but that when a visible abnormality is produced, it is characteristic. When the patient is afflicted with other diseases of the vascular system, particularly hypertension, the lesion characteristic of diabetes is superimposed on the other lesion, giving a composite picture that is still characteristic, so that the trained observer can diagnose from it the presence of diabetes mellitus."

Tuberculosis of the Maxillary Sinus. Joseph H. Hersh, M.D., New York. Archives of Otolaryngology, December, 1938.

There is a review of the literature on this subject beginning in 1907. There have been only 26 cases reported. Six showed a favorable outcome.

The case reported is that of a female, age 26, Puerto Rican. She first had pain in her lower abdomen in the latter part of 1935; in February, 1936, had lobar pneumonia; at this time before she left the hospital she complained of pain in her cheek for which a radical operation for chronic suppurative sinusitis (maxillary) was done; this resulted in a fistulous tract from the right maxillary sinus to gingivolabial sulcus; the abdominal persisted with a mass increasing in size which was aspirated and the fluid obtained cultured tubercle bacilli; in March, 1937, the patient again entered the hospital with swelling over the right cheek, periorbital tissues; and right submaxillary region; right cervical and submaxillary glands showed enlarged and tender; she looked sick; creamy white pus exuded from above the right upper molar tooth; Wasserman was negative; X-ray of the facial region showed far advanced destruction of the right maxillary sinus; irrigation gave large amounts of foul smelling purulent material; granulations and polypi were removed and examined but were negative for malignancy; necrotic bone was also removed; histologically there was present tuberculosis of the bone and granulation tissue; eye symptoms developed in January, 1938; X-ray showed destruction of the floor of the orbit; extensive resection was not done because of the poor general condition of the patient.

The infection of the antrum was apparently hematogenous. If the mucosa of the sinus only is involved, the diagnosis is difficult; if there is destruction of the bone and fistulous formation, the diagnosis should be easy (ruling out malignancy). The author's opinion is that for a case to terminate successfully it must be diagnosed early and radical surgery done. The general condition of the patient must also be taken into consideration.

Foreign Bodies in the Air Passages, Causing Unilobar Obstructive Emphysema. P. G. Gerlings, Amsterdam. The Journal of Laryngology and Otology, January, 1939.

Symptoms of obstructive emphysema of the bronchi by Manges (roentgenologically) are:

1. Increased transparency of the affected side, especially on expiration.

2. Depression of the diaphragm on the affected side on expiration.

3. Displacement of the heart and mediastinal structures away from the affected side on expiration.

Obstructive emphysema of both lungs, according to Manges, have these characteristic symptoms:

1. Increased transparency of both lungs.

2. Depression of the diaphragm on both sides.

3. Rotation of the heart, with its apex forward (diminished transverse diameter), on expiration..

The literature shows nothing about unilobar obstructive emphysema except two cases by Gilse. The author's symptoms of this condition are:

1. Hypersonorous percussion.

2. Diminished breath sounds.

3. Increased transparency of one of the lung areas as proved by the X-ray picture.

4. Sometimes slight displacement of the heart towards the healthy side and depression of the diaphragm on the affected side.

The factors playing a part in the development of an obstructive emphysema are:

1. Foreign body.

2. Inspiratory and expiratory movement of the bronchus.

3. Bronchitis circumscripta.

Jackson names two types in obstructive emphysema, i.e., "check-valve type" and "ball-valve type." These are discussed.

The cases reported by the author producing this condition deal mostly with inspirated peanuts or portions of peanuts.

The author's summary is as follows:

The symptoms of unilobar obstructive emphysema are described. The diagnosis is important for the localization of a foreign body in the bronchus. Some cases are described to explain the factors playing a role in the case of an obstructive emphysema. The circumscribed bronchitis is considered to be important as may be seen from the case in which a piece of peanut kernel was found in the lower lobe bronchus and in which an obstructive emphysema of the whole lung existed.

------------------o------------------

PLASTIC SURGERY

Edited by

GEO. H. KIMBALL, M.D., F.A.C.S.

404 Medical Arts Building, Oklahoma City

The Use of Free Full Thickness Skin Grafts. J. Eastman Sheehan, M.D., New York. January 7, 1939, Journal American Medical Association.

The author points out that a skin graft to cover the defect in the face should ensure that the new skin will conform to its surroundings in texture, surface level, coloration and will incorporate imperceptibly with the skin adjoining.

He mentions the difficulty of a pedicle flap in this type of reconstruction as it leaves a visible disfigurement. The thin epidermic graft will not do either. The tubed pedicle flap, he states, undergoes its changes in its fat and fibrous tissues after its release from its pedicle and therefore texture, elevation and motility are not natural.

The author points out that the free full thickness graft has some of the above named disadvantages. He claims it does not take on a brownish tint that is different from the coloration of the face.

Not so long ago, a 50 per cent success was about all that could be expected of such a graft, meaning that they did not take. The author lists recent improvement in the following conditions:

1. The skin should be healthy. This applies not alone to the immediate vicinity of the area from which the graft is to be taken but to the body generally. Some of the deterrent conditions are obvious, as disease. Some of the danger signals, as pimples, which suggest delay until improvement has been effected. There may be a concealed infection, of which the skin itself gives no sign but which will prove disastrous when it is declared in the weakened condition of the cells after they have been deprived of their normal sustenance. Two highly useful tests can be applied by way of check on such unknown factors. One is the Schilling test. In the presence of infectious processes, immature neutrophils enter the circulation in increased numbers. As compared with a ratio of 10 in normal persons and of 25 in slight infection, there may be indicated an index of 50, 75 or more. By any such indication of infection the operator is put definitely on warning and must postpone until the index is suitably lowered. Again as the success of the graft is to be attained only when the bed on which it is placed is at its best, and as oozing will impair or destroy this condition, it is important to know what the probabilities are in this particular. Where, for example, the blood platelet count is much too low, such oozing is to be apprehended, with consequent danger to the success of the graft, as a whole or in part. In presence of these or any other warnings against haste, delay is instituted to allow of the conditions being corrected.

2. The graft area itself equally demands respect. It has a normal oxygen and sulfur content, and if either is below normal the impaired vitality of the cells will be reflected when the graft is transferred. Biochemical tests for these contents have been devised, and if the results are unsatisfactory there is reason for delay until correction is effected. Moreover, it has been found that these contents are reduced in the process of cleansing and preparing the area for operation. The cleansing, for this reason, is best done the night before the operation to allow time for recovery of the oxygen content. The skin is scrubbed with soap and water, further cleansed with sulfuric ether and left covered with antiseptic gauze overnight. The use of antiseptics with a view to bacterial destruction on and within the apertures of the skin has not survived trial and error. The most successful of them as germicides have been found to set up conditions difficult to deal with and in any event more importance attaches to having the skin in a healthy condition than to precaution against germs of infection in a skin not at its best.

3. A dry base at the defect area is absolutely essential. There must be close adherence of the graft to the base, and this there cannot be if there is oozing and consequent blood clots, even the smallest of which will be destructive as to the space it occupies. Obviously, the vessels in the base must have attention. If any are to be tied it must be by suture threads that will not promote infection. The finest Deknatel silk is used. Precautions having been taken against oozing by reason of conditions disclosed by the count of the blood platelets, it may be desirable to obtain further assurance by irradiation of the spleen by roentgen rays in amounts of from one-tenth to one-fifth erythems dose. About 24 hours after irradiation the coagulation time of

the blood is gradually materially reduced, a fact helpful to the restoration of the graft. Intravenous injection of calcium of a hemostatic preparation the day before operation may be of additional advantage.

4. In taking the graft, the lines of skin tension should be respected. The graft would be cut without bevels at the edges and be a little less than will cover the defect, as it is well to have the graft on stretch a little when it is sutured in place. There is no need for rough handling. The graft can be gently transferred by threads that are to serve as anchor sutures. It should not be washed in saline or other solution. Its own serums have the double utility of temporarily countering infection and of assuring adhesion between the graft and the base. The suturing in place must be done with great patience and with care to ensure that the resultant scar at the wound edges will have the least attainable visibility.

5. With this all done, there is still to consider the factors that govern the restoration of life and function in the graft skin. With a sound viable graft on a dry bed that phase begins on skin that has been detached from the normal agencies that supply life to the cells. There are two influences that make for recuperation from this moribund condition. One is the infiltration of minute vessels from the base into the corium; the other is the nourishment that may be derived by the cells from the pervading lymph. Vascular infiltration is a slow process and if the very lowest part of the skin is transferred as was formerly the practice it takes time for the vessels to reach the tissues of the subpapillary layer. Whereas the cells of the epidermis are not sustained by vessels but are nourished by the lymph from the base on which they are set, when it can be conveyed to them, the connective tissues of the corium must have sustenance from vessels to which they are accustomed. To mitigate the delays the lowest densest subcutaneous layer is removed. Whether it is that this results in more rapid infiltration of the remainder of the corium or that the subpapillary area shares with the epidermis the sustenance derived from the lymph fluid, or both, the fact is that restoration proceeds with greater rapidity and with increased assurance when this lowest stratum of the skin is discarded. To this may be attributed much of the recent advance in the ratio of success.

Comment: The author has given a detailed outline of the condition which must be followed before a full thickness graft can be successfully used. It has been my experience that such a graft should be put on in a dry sterile field, on slight tension, moderate pressure by marine sponge and left two or even three weeks. It is not always possible to leave a graft undisturbed because of, first, possible infection, second, immobilization apparatus may become loose or contaminated, third, when moulds or sutures are used and splinted to the graft, it may be necessary to remove them earlier.

These grafts do sometimes become pigmented. The coloration may be slight but it is present. Aside from its use about the face they are very valuable in the palms of the hands and the soles of the feet where weight bearing is to be expected.

This type of graft is much better than a large pedicle graft placed in the palm of the hand so that the patient is unable to flex his hand.

With the understanding of the principles brought out the percentage of success in this type of graft is increased markedly.

INTERNAL MEDICINE

Edited by Hugh Jeter, M.D., 1200 North Walker, Oklahoma City

The Present Incidence of Trichinella Spiralis in Man as Determined by a Study of 1,060 Unselected Autopsies in St. Louis Hospitals; by Thomas B. Pote, M.D., Washington University, St. Louis, Mo. (The American Journal of the Medical Sciences, January, 1939, Vol. 197, No. 802.)

In this the author reports the study of 1,060 unselected autopsies at Barnes and St. Louis City Hospital for the Trichinella larvae. All of the subjects were over 15 years of age and had died during hospitalization from some disease other than trichiniasis. Routine examinations of generous samples of muscles of election for trichinella, namely, the diaphragm, intercostals, pectorals and recti, were made. Over 12,000 examinations were made during the course of this study. The method for examining the material consisted of squeezing thin slices of muscle tissue between two pieces of plate glass in a compression frame. These fresh unfixed and unstained preparations were then examined microscopically for the larva.

The youngest member of the group was 17 years of age and the oldest 85. The author includes tables showing (1) the degree of infestation, (2) age distribution, (3) occupation and (4) incidence of infestation. In addition the author includes photomicrographs showing stained and unstained preparations of the larva. The author concludes from this study that a severe degree of infestation may exist without related clinical symptoms. In no case in the authors series was trichinella infestation diagnosed prior to postmortem examination.

The author further concludes that at least 15 per cent of the adult urban population is probably infected with trichinella spiralis in spite of the emphasis which has been placed upon meat inspection during the past four years.

Correlation Studies of Basophilic Aggregation and Reticulocytes in Various Clinical Conditions. Maurice D. Pearlman and Louis R. Limarzi, from the Department of Medicine, University of Illinois, Chicago, Ill. (American Journal of Clinical Pathology, November, 1938, Vol. 8, No. 6.)

In this the authors discuss the correlation between the basophilic aggregation counts and the reticulocyte counts in various clinical conditions. These show that the average reticulocyte count is somewhat higher than the basophilic aggregation count on the same blood. They feel that the reticulocyte count can be done more accurately and requires less experience than the basophilic aggregation count. Experiments conducted on six normal patients and 46 pathological conditions revealed that those conditions which cause an increase in the reticulocytosis also cause an increase in basophilic aggregation but that the correlation was not equal in all cases. In the article the techniques are fully described. Several charts are introduced to show that there is a divergence in the individual results of individual laboratory technicians which is greater when doing basophilic aggregation counts than when doing reticulocyte counts. In another chart they show that the same technician counting the same blood will himself obtain a larger variation in basophilic aggregation counts than he will when counting the reticulocytes. The authors conclude that the basophilic aggregation test is unreliable as a routine laboratory procedure because of the technical difficulties. They also conclude that in pathological conditions which ordinarily reduce the reticulocyte count, such as aplastic anemias and lead poisoning, the reticulocyte count is usually higher than the basophilic count. They emphasize the basophilic aggregation test is not uniquely diagnostic of lead poisoning, it is rather an index of marrow response. Finally they believe that the basophilic aggregation test should be abandoned in favor of the "vital" method for staining reticulocytes.

ORTHOPAEDIC SURGERY
Edited by Earl D. McBride, M.D., F.A.C.S.
717 North Robinson Street, Oklahoma City

Madelung's Deformity. Joseph I. Anton, George B. Reitz, and Milton B. Spiegel. Annals of Surg., CVIII, September, 1938.

This exhaustive review and critical analysis of the literature on this subject shows that there are many discrepancies in the cases reported as Madelung's deformity. The article contains a tabulation of analysis of relevant data of 171 cases of true Madelung's deformity reported in the literature between 1855 and the present time.

The authors report one case in minute detail. The pathology, predisposing factors and various etiological theories are discussed. They suggest calling the deformity dyschondroplasia of the distal radial epiphysis. They are inclined to believe that it belongs in the group of conditions which includes Calve' - Legg - Perthes, Osgood - Schlatter, Kohler's, and Kienbock's diseases.

The treatment which they recommend consists in palliative measures until the cessation of the growth. Then the deformity should be corrected by osteotomy. If the ulna is markedly longer, its projecting end must be resected.

The authors present the following classification of the various types of the deformity, which they believe is advantageous in view of the present state of the literature on this subject:

A. Presenting Radial Deformity:
  1. With interior bowing of the radius:
    a. Radial dyschondroplasia (genuine Madelung's deformity);
    b. Secondary static deformity; traumtic, luetic, inflammatory, tuberculous, osteitis, rickets, etc.;
  2. Without bowing:
    a. Radial dyschondroplasia;
    b. Secondary static deformity;
B. Presenting Ulnar Deformity:
    a. Ulnar dyschondroplasia;
    b. Secondary static deformity.

Subacromial Bursitis. A Clinical, Roentgenographic and Statistical Study. Samuel R. Rubert. Archives of Surgery, XXXVII, 619, October, 1938.

In a comprehensive article, Rubert presents the subject of subacromial bursitis from history to prognosis. A concise description of the anatomical picture and a consideration of the etiological factors are followed by a somewhat more elaborate description of the pathological picture. The roentgenographic observations are enumerated, and it is stressed that disease may be present without positive roentgenographic changes.

The author reports on a series of 288 cases seen in the orthopaedic department of the State University of Iowa. An analysis of these cases showed that the greatest incidence is between the ages of

40 and 70 years, that sex does not play an important role, and the right arm is more frequently affected than the left, and that there is an associated arthritic involvement in at least 16 per cent of the patients. Etiologically the cases were classified as traumatic, arthritic, and infectious.

The question of differential diagnosis is taken up fairly fully. The usual forms of treatment are enumerated, and it is reported that conservative measures give satisfactory results in 69 per cent of the cases; improvement in 19 per cent; and failure in 12 per cent. Operative treatment in 21 cases resulted in cure in about one-half of the cases. The author recommends that operative intervention should be reserved only for those patients in whom there has been a complete rupture of the tendon or in whom the condition does not respond to conservative measures.

Earl D. McBride, M.D.

UROLOGY
Edited by D. W. Branham, M.D.
514 Medical Arts Building, Oklahoma City

Gonadal Activity In Prostatic Hypertrophy. M. Muschat, M. Labess and D. Meranze, Philadelphia, Pa. Journal of Urology, December, 1938.

The administration of male sex hormone in the form of Oretone or Perandren is becoming a popular mode in the treatment of prostatic hypertrophy. Such therapy is based on the theory that these patients are afflicted with male sex hormone insufficiency. However, this contention is not supported by actual quantitative studies made on the amount of male sex hormone in the prostatic patient. Previous investigators have found normal amounts of male sex hormone in both men and animals by various methods.

By means of a new test, the creatinine utilization test, in which the peculiar ability of the body in normal individuals to utilize orally administered creatinine without increasing its output in the urine as compared to the creatininuria which occurs in nurslings and young boys when creatinine is ingested. Also, the administration of male sex hormone in castrated individuals will eliminate creatininuria, when creatinine is ingested. It has been found an efficient method to determine the amount of male sex hormone.

These studies proved that the creatinine utilization test is a correct indicator of gonadal activity in the male. They found the normal adult male shows creatinine retention below 15 per cent. The eunuchs and eunuchoids show marked creatinine retention from 35 to 50 per cent. There is a noticeable decline in the activity of the gonads after the age of 50. The cases with prostatic hypertrophy have the same creatinine retention as the normal male adults, indicating continued gonadal activity.

The authors feel that the administration of more male sex hormone appears not only useless but may be harmful in promoting further growth of the prostate. They feel that it would be more logical to attempt reduction of the testicular secretion instead of increasing it.

Renal Tuberculosis: Prognosis Following Nephrectomy. John L. Emmett, M.D., and John M. Kibler, M.D., Mayo Clinic, Rochester, Minnesota. The Journal of the American Medical Association, December 24, 1938.

A study of the records of 1,131 patients on whom nephrectomy had been performed for renal tuberculosis at the Mayo Clinic between the years 1912 and 1932 inclusive. A letter of inquiry was sent to all known to be alive. There were four groups of patients studied in this series.

Group 1, patients whose good kidney was not catheterized prior to operation. Group 2, patients whose good kidney was catheterized prior to operation, and microscopic examination of the centrifuged ureteral specimen of urine revealed either no pus cells or not more than three pus cells per high power field. Group 3, patients whose good kidney was catheterized prior to operation and microscopic examination of the ureteral specimen of urine revealed from three to ten pus cells per high power field. Group 4, patients whose good kidney was catheterized prior to operation and microscopic examination of the ureteral specimen of urine revealed more than ten pus cells per high power field.

Dr. John Hand of Portland, Oregon, aptly sums up the information obtained in the following discussion: "1. That of a kidney not excreting pus or acid-fast bacilli. The patient with this type may expect a 50 per cent chance of cure, a 75 per cent chance of improvement and a 13 per cent chance of death within five years. 2. That of a kidney not excreting pus but excreting acid-fast bacilli. There is an area of caseous necrosis in which acid-fast organisms are escaping through the tubules but in which a pyogenic reaction has not yet occurred at the papilla. The patient stands a 21 per cent chance of cure, a 36 per cent chance of improvement and a 51 per cent chance of death within five years. (These pictures make one realize that the acid-fast bacilli obtained in the specimen from the good kidney are in most instances not due to contamination). 3. That of "a good kidney" with a normal urogram. The patient stands a 40 per cent chance of cure and a 30 per cent chance of death within five years. This picture emphasizes that even when the urogram is normal, acid-fast organisms may be coming from the kidney. 4. That of a kidney in which caseous necrosis, ulceration and a pyogenic reaction are taking place at the renal papilla, allowing the excretion of pus. With or without surgery the prognosis is poor."

Comment: A most praise worthy investigation which was badly needed to determine actually what our operative results produced in surgical renal tuberculosis. I was particularly happy to see that bilateral renal bacilluria is no contradiction to nephrectomy providing the good kidney presents no evidence of destructive changes. I have always been a bit hesitant in performing nephrectomy in the face of positive bacteriologic findings on the supposedly good side. This investigation shows that if we can rule out the good side so far as gross suppuration is concerned, nephrectomy for the "bad" side is the treatment of choice.

---o---

State Board of Medical Examiners

THE STATE BOARD OF MEDICAL EXAMINERS organized February 3, 1939, in Oklahoma City, electing the following members: President, Dr. Sam A. McKeel, Ada; Vice-President, Dr. C. E. Bradley, Tulsa; Secretary, Dr. Jas. D. Osborn, Jr., Frederick, re-elected. The appointment by the governor of Drs. McKeel and Newman of Shattuck as new regular members of the Board, meets with the unanimous approval of the medical profession of Oklahoma, as these are outstanding men in their profession and will well and gracefully accept the responsibility.

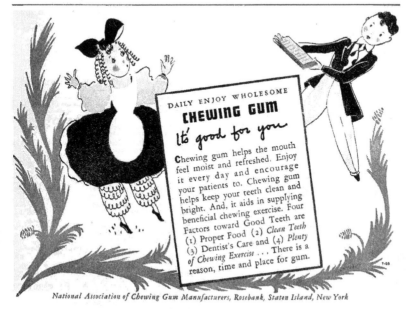

OFFICERS OKLAHOMA STATE MEDICAL ASSOCIATION

President, Dr. H. K. Speed, Sayre.

President-Elect, Dr. W. A. Howard, Chelsea.

Secretary-Treasurer-Editor, Dr. L. S. Willour, McAlester.

Executive Secretary, Mr. R. H. Graham, McAlester.

Speaker, House of Delegates, Dr. J. D. Osborn, Jr., Frederick.

Vice Speaker, House of Delegates, Dr. P. P. Nesbitt, Medical Arts Building, Tulsa.

Delegates to the A. M. A., Dr. W. Albert Cook, Medical Arts Building, Tulsa, 1938-39; Dr. McLain Rogers, Clinton, 1937-1938.

Meeting Place, Oklahoma City, May 1, 2, 3, 1939.

SPECIAL COMMITTEES 1938-39

Annual Meeting: Dr. H. K. Speed, Sayre; Dr. W. A. Howard, Chelsea; Dr. L. S. Willour, McAlester.

Conservation of Hearing: Dr. H. F. Vandever, Chairman, Enid; Dr. J. B. Hollis, Mangum; Dr. Chester McHenry, Oklahoma City.

Conservation of Vision: Dr. W. M. Gallaher, Chairman, Shawnee; Dr. Frank R. Vieregg, Clinton; Dr. Pauline Barker, Guthrie.

Crippled Children: Dr. Earl McBride, Chairman, Oklahoma City; Dr. Roy L. Fisher, Frederick; Dr. M. B. Glismann, Okmulgee.

Industrial Service and Traumatic Surgery: Dr. Cyril C. Clymer, Medical Arts Bldg., Oklahoma City; Dr. J. Wm. Finch, Hobart; Dr. J. A. Rutledge, Ada.

Maternity and Infancy: Dr. George R. Osborn, Chairman, Tulsa; Dr. P. J. DeVanney, Sayre; Dr. Leila E. Andrews, Oklahoma City.

Necrology: Dr. G. H. Stagner, Chairman, Erick; Dr. James L. Shuler, Durant; Dr. S. D. Neely, Muskogee.

Post Graduate Medical Teaching: Dr. Henry H. Turner, Chairman, Oklahoma City; Dr. H. C. Weber, Bartlesville; Dr. Ned R. Smith, Tulsa.

Study and Control of Cancer: Dr. Wendell Long, Chairman, Oklahoma City; Dr. Paul B. Champlin, Enid; Dr. Ralph McGill, Tulsa.

Study and Control of Tuberculosis: Dr. Carl Puckett, Chairman, Oklahoma City; Dr. W. C. Tisdal, Clinton; Dr. F. P. Baker, Talihina.

Study and Control of Venereal Disease: Dr. Robert H. Akin, Chairman, Medical Arts Bldg., Oklahoma City; Dr. Shade D. Neely, Muskogee; Dr. D. V. Hudson, Medical Arts Bldg., Tulsa.

ADVISORY COUNCIL FOR AUXILIARY

Dr. H. K. Speed, Chairman ....Sayre
Dr. C. J. Fishman..Oklahoma City
Dr. W. S. Larrabee..Tulsa
Dr. J. M. Watson..Enid
Dr. T. H. McCarley..McAlester

STANDING COMMITTEES 1938-39

Medical Defense: Dr. O. E. Templin, Chairman, Alva; Dr. L. C. Kuyrkendall, McAlester; Dr. E. Albert Aisenstadt, Picher.

Medical Economics: Dr. C. B. Sullivan, Cordell, Chairman; Dr. J. L. Patterson, Duncan; Dr. W. M. Browning, Waurika.

Medical Education and Hospital: Dr. V. C. Tisdal, Chairman, Elk City; Dr. Robert U. Patterson, Oklahoma City; Dr. H. M. McClure, Chickasha.

Public Policy and Legislation: Dr. Finis W. Ewing, Surety Bldg., Chairman, Muskogee; Dr. Tom Lowry, 1200 North Walker, Oklahoma City; Dr. O. C. Newman, Shattuck; Dr. R. O. Early, Medical Arts Bldg., Oklahoma City.
(The above committee co-ordinated by the following, selected from each councilor district.)

District No. 1.—Arthur E. Hale, Alva.
District No. 2.—McLain Rogers, Clinton.
District No. 3.—Thomas McElroy, Ponca City.
District No. 4.—L. H. Ritzhaupt, Guthrie.
District No. 5.—P. V. Annadown, Sulphur.
District No. 6.—R. M. Shepard, Tulsa.
District No. 7.—Sam A. McKeel, Ada.
District No. 8.—J. A. Morrow, Sallisaw.
District No. 9.—W. A. Tolleson, Eufaula.
District No. 10.—J. L. Holland, Madill.

Scientific Exhibits: Dr. E. Rankin Denny, Chairman, Tulsa; Dr. Robert H. Akin, Oklahoma City; Dr. R. C. Pigford, Tulsa.

Scientific Work: Dr. W. G. Husband, Chairman, Hollis; Dr. J. S. Rollins, Prague; Dr. J. L. Day, Supply.

Public Health:

Chairman—Dr. G. S. Baxter, Shawnee.
District No. 1.—C. W. Tedrowe, Woodward.
District No. 2.—E. W. Mabry, Altus.
District No. 3.—L. A. Mitchell, Stillwater.
District No. 4.—J. J. Gable, Norman.
District No. 5.—Geo. S. Barber, Lawton.
District No. 6.—C. E. Bradley, Tulsa.
District No. 7.—G. S. Baxter, Shawnee.
District No. 8.—M. M. De Arman, Miami.
District No. 9.—T. H. McCarley, McAlester.
District No. 10.—J. B. Clark, Coalgate.

SCIENTIFIC SECTIONS

General Surgery: Dr. F. L. Flack, Chairman, Nat'l Bank of Tulsa Bldg., Tulsa; Dr. John E. McDonald, Vice-Chairman, Medical Arts Bldg., Tulsa; Dr. John F. Burton, Secretary, Osler Building, Oklahoma City.

General Medicine: Dr. Frank Nelson, Chairman, 603 Medical Arts Bldg., Tulsa; Dr. E. R. Musick, Vice-Chairman, Medical Arts Bldg., Oklahoma City; Dr. Milam McKinney, Medical Arts Bldg., Oklahoma City.

Eye, Ear, Nose & Throat: Dr. E. H. Coachman, Chairman, Manhattan Bldg., Muskogee; Dr. F. M. Cooper, Vice-President, Medical Arts Bldg., Oklahoma City; Dr. James R. Reed, Secretary, Medical Arts Bldg., Oklahoma City.

Obstetrics and Pediatrics: Dr. C. W. Arrendell, Chairman, Ponca City; Dr. Carl F. Simpson, Vice-Chairman, Medical Arts Bldg., Tulsa; Dr. Ben H. Nicholson, Secretary, 300 West Twelfth Street, Oklahoma City.

Genito-Urinary Diseases and Syphilology: Dr. Elijah Sullivan, Chairman, Medical Arts Bldg., Oklahoma City; Dr. Henry Browne, Vice-Chairman, Medical Arts Bldg., Tulsa; Dr. Robert Akin, Secretary, 400 West Tenth, Oklahoma City.

Dermatology and Radiology: Dr. W. A. Showman, Chairman, Medical Arts Bldg., Tulsa; Dr. E. D. Greenberger, Vice-Chairman, McAlester; Dr. Hervey A. Foerster, Secretary, Medical Arts Bldg., Oklahoma City.

STATE BOARD OF MEDICAL EXAMINERS

Dr. Sam A. McKeel, Ada, President; Dr. C. E. Bradley, Tulsa, Vice-President; Dr. J. D. Osborn, Jr., Frederick, Secretary; Dr. O. C. Newman, Shattuck; Dr. L. E. Emanuel, Chickasha; Dr. S. D. Leslie, Okmulgee; Dr. G. H. Stagner, Erick.

STATE COMMISSIONER OF HEALTH

Dr. Grady F. Mathews, Oklahoma City.

COUNCILORS AND THEIR COUNTIES

District No. 1: Texas, Beaver, Cimarron, Harper, Ellis, Woods, Woodward, Alfalfa, Major, Dewey—Dr. O. E. Templin, Alva. (Term expires 1940.)

District No. 2: Roger Mills, Beckham, Greer, Harmon, Washita, Kiowa, Custer, Jackson, Tillman—Dr. V. C. Tisdal, Elk City. (Term expires 1939.)

District No. 3: Grant, Kay, Garfield, Noble, Payne, Pawnee—Dr. A. S. Risser, Blackwell. (Term expires 1941.)

District No. 4: Blaine, Kingfisher, Canadian, Logan, Oklahoma, Cleveland—Dr. Philip M. McNeill, Oklahoma City. (Term expires 1941.)

District No. 5: Caddo, Comanche, Cotton, Grady, Love, Stephens, Jefferson, Carter, Murray—Dr. Walter Hardy, Ardmore. (Term expires 1941.)

District No. 6: Osage, Creek, Washington, Nowata, Rogers, Tulsa—Dr. James Stevenson, Medical Arts Bldg., Tulsa. (Term expires 1941.)

District No. 7: Lincoln, Pontotoc, Pottawatomie, Okfuskee, Seminole, McClain, Garvin, Hughes—Dr. J. A. Walker, Shawnee. (Term expires 1939.)

District No. 8: Craig, Ottawa, Mayes, Delaware, Wagoner, Adair, Cherokee, Sequoyah, Okmulgee, Muskogee—Dr. E. A. Aisenstadt, Picher. (Term expires 1939.)

District No. 9: Pittsburg, Haskell, Latimer, LeFlore, McIntosh—Dr. L. C. Kuyrkendall, McAlester. (Term expires 1939.)

District No. 10: Johnson, Marshall, Coal, Atoka, Bryan, Choctaw, Pushmataha, McCurtain—Dr. J. S. Fulton, Atoka. (Term expires 1939.)

THE JOURNAL
OF THE
OKLAHOMA STATE MEDICAL ASSOCIATION

| VOLUME XXXII | McALESTER, OKLAHOMA, MARCH, 1939 | Number 3 |

Adrenal Cortex in Surgery

L. C. NORTHRUP, M.D.
TULSA, OKLAHOMA

A great deal of research work has been done on the function of the adrenal gland as a whole. Adrenalin, the secretion of the medulla, has been known and u s e d for years. The function of the cortical portion has remained a mystery. However, we do know a few important facts about the cortex. We know that life in the higher forms cannot exist more than a few hours without the adrenal cortex. It is known that Addisons disease is due to a progressive destruction of the adrenal gland. Research on Adrenalectomized animals has shown definite chemical changes in the b l o o d. There is a lowering of sodium and chlorides and an increase in non-protein nitrogen. This disproportion increases as death nears. Dr. A. Scott Worthim, in his autopsy reports of patients dying from shock, always brought out the fact that there was a state of exhaustion present in the adrenal glands.

Many investigators h a v e maintained adrenalectomized dogs in apparently normal physiologic condition by daily administration of sufficient amounts of extract of adrenal cortex. The symptoms, following the removal of the adrenal glands, are asthenia, falling blood pressure, edema, failing kidney function, anorexia, nausea and vomiting, g r e a t physical weakness, profuse cold perspiration, coma and death. The frequency that some of these symptoms are seen following operations has prompted the experimental use of adrenal cortex extracts to prevent shock in surgery and then later to make convalescence more smooth and more rapid.

In 1931, Zwemer reported on the use of adrenal cortex in the treatment of severe intestinal intoxication in babies. The improvement was very marked and almost instantaneous. Wilson, in 1936, reported on the use of adrenal cortex in the treatment of s e v e r e burns. Reed has been using adrenal cortex since 1932 in non-surgical patients. He first started using it in surgery in 1936. Since then, he has reported on a large number of cases in which he has used the extract to advantage. Several of his cases were almost moribund, in the last stages of exhaustion from peritonitis. The sudden change in the condition of the patient upon the administration of adrenal cortex extract was very remarkable; they all made a rapid recovery. At the present time, he is using it routinely pre-operatively to p r e v e n t shock and to prevent many of the post-operative symptoms, such as vomiting and weakness. My own experience with the extract, covers the past two years. I have used it only on the serious cases where they were obviously in for a stormy time.

In general, the following conditions have been noted when the extract was used:

1. Heart action has been stabilized.

2. It has a very stimulating effect on the kidneys. In several cases the urine has become f r e e of albumin and casts that were present before.

3. No change in the blood chemistry, as long as the extract was given.

4. Blood pressure levels maintained.

5. Pulse rates showed very little change during and after operation.

6. Absence of profuse diaphoresis even to the absence of the u s u a l post-operative period of sweating during the reaction from the anaesthetic.

7. No dehydration.

8. Almost entire absence of nausea and vomiting post-operatively.

9. There has been only one case of ileus in all of my cases.

10. Fluids and solids have been retained earlier and there has been a quick return to the normal appetite.

11. There has been a noticeable feeling of well being. No cases of extreme exhaustion.

12. Wounds have healed more rapidly and there has been a marked notice-able d e c r e a s e in pain and a less amount of narcotics have been required.

13. There is a definite increase of re-sistance to infection.

CASE REPORTS

Mr. H. had two operations for perforated ulcer of the stomach, two and one-half years apart. He had a spinal anaesthetic with each operation. With the first opera-tion, he did not have adrenal cortex ex-tract, with the second operation he did. Both operations were performed approxi-mately the same length of time after onset of symptoms. His temperature, following the first operation, reached 103, 24 hours post-operative, and did not reach normal until the seventh post-operative day. With the second operation, the highest tempera-ture was 100.8, and came to normal in 48 hours. The high pulse the first time was 120, which came down to 70 on the eleventh day. The second time, his pulse was 112, and came to 70 in 24 hours. Nausea and vomiting with distension was troublesome the first time. He was unable to retain any s o l i d food until the twelfth post-operative day, while the second operation, he did not vomit once, was not nauseated, and was able to eat solid food on the fourth day. He had his first bowel movement, following the first operation, on the sev-enth post-operative day, while after the second operation, his bowels moved on the third post-operative day. He was in the h o s p i t a l 14 days the first time, and 8 days the second time. Following the first operation, he had 27 doses of morphine, $\frac{1}{4}$ grains, 3,000 c.c. saline, 2,000 c.c. glu-cose, but after the second operation, he had only 10 doses of morphine, 4,000 c.c. of saline and no glucose. He received 11 doses of adrenal cortex extract. He was given 1 c.c. every six hours after the op-eration.

My procedure is to give 1 c.c. 12 hours before the operation, 1 c.c. one hour before the operation, and 1 c.c. or 2 c.c. every six hours after the operation until the patient is out of danger.

The preparation I have used, for the past two years, is made by Parke Davis Company, and is marketed under the trade name of Eschatin.

REFERENCES

Zwemer, R. L., and Sullivan, Endocrinology, 18:97, 1934.
Zwemer, R. L., Endocrinology, 15:382, 1931.
Reed, R. R., American Journal Surgery, XL:514, 1938.

————————0————————

The Complications of Gonorrhea*

ALLEN R. RUSSELL, M.D.
McALESTER, OKLAHOMA

The complications of gonorrhea are va-riable and many, and as a rule, these com-plications are not given the serious consid-eration which they deserve, but instead, it

*Read before the Section on Urology, Annual Meeting, Oklahoma State Medical Association, Muskogee, Oklahoma, May, 1938.

has been the custom to accept many of these appearances as unavoidable features of the disease itself, as the patient's mis-fortune, and no one's f a u l t, whereas in reality, a thorough understanding of the disease, and a little time spent with the patient at the beginning, e x p l a i n i n g the seriousness of this d i s e a s e, could have well prevented a great many of these complications. Many of these complications are disastrous and far-reaching and for that reason, any steps toward their prevention are well-worth the most painstaking investigation and study in the beginning. It is considered today that more than 50 per cent of the complications of gonorrhea are avoidable conditions, and that gonorrhea on the whole, is the most poorly treated of diseases.

Considering the complications of gonorrhea, we can divide our patients practically into three groups. The first group are those patients whose conduct is above reproach throughout the attack, and who receives oral treatment, a prescription, and syringe, and turned loose to treat themselves. In this group you see most of those complications that are as a rule, not the serious type, but rather either continue with recurrence, or finally become chronic.

In group number two, are patients having extremely mild and local treatment absolutely free from trauma, and of exemplary conduct. Among this group you have those patients who are under the best conditions of treatment, and therefore, where you see the smallest number of complications.

Group number three, are patients receiving strenuous treatment such as passage of catheters, sounds, high-pressure irrigations, injections, solutions being too strong, large doses of gonococcus vaccine, and various types of unwarranted treatment, and also whose conduct is generally bad. In this group you may see any, or all, of the complications expected in this condition, and the variable stages or extent of these same complications. Of course, even in this group itself, some of the complications are a result of the disease itself, as a result of continuity of surface, but by far the greater percentage, are the direct result of what the patient, or the physician, does, and as such are usually preventable.

I shall attempt to take these complications up one at a time, and discuss them as such.

Chronic Gonorrhea: In a consideration of chronic gonorrhea, one must make some very close distinctions, for it is often the custom to i n c l u d e under this condition, what is not really gonorrhea, but instead, conditions that have lingered long after the disappearance of the gonococcus, which may or may not be due to secondary infection, occurring upon the soil previously prepared for their invasion. Chronic gonorrhea should never be classified as such until the gonococcus has been present for more than six months, also, it might be said here that it is very seldom that the chronic gonorrhea is seen in those cases, whose treatment has been exemplary, and whose conduct has been satisfactory.

Gonorrheal Epididymitis: In s o m e groups of treated cases, this complication ranges as high as 30 per cent or more, and since it often renders from 25 to 50 per cent of these patients permanently sterile, it is well worth serious consideration as to its prevention. In the past there has been much discussion and differences of opinion as to the causative factor of epididymitis. Now, it is generally agreed that the usual cause is as follows: That when the bladder is full of urine, or partially distended, a small amount of the urine escapes through the relaxation of the internal sphincter into the posterior urethra, ejaculatory duct, or seminal vesicle, and u n d e r physical exertion or lifting, the lower abdominal muscles are brought into action producing an increased bladder pressure, which forces a s m a l l amount of urine down the vas deferens, and it eventually reaches the epididymal tube. This is the reason that the history of these complications brings out the fact that within 24 to 48 hours preceding the epididymal complication, that they have indulged in coitus, sexual excitement, or some form of strenuous exercise, with a full bladder. Or that some form of injurious treatment was carried out, which r a i s e d the intraurethral or intravesicle pressure, resulting in the infected urine being forced into the vas deferens, and on to the epididymal tube.

Seminal Vesiculitis: There are m a n y conditions wherein this diagnosis is made erroneously, because of the belief that a diseased seminal v e s i c l e is always palpable, and a palpable one is always diseased. To make a definite diagnosis of acute or sub-acute seminal vesiculitis is rather difficult, however on the other hand, to deny that some degree of infection of the seminal vesicles exists in any case of gonorrhea, is like saying that you have a pyelitis without a kidney infection. Clinically speaking, in those cases where there is a prolonged urethral discharge in patients receiving the proper treatment and having followed the proper conduct, gonorrheal seminal vesiculitis often results in a constant feeding source. With such a condition in the seminal vesicles, with accumulation of purulent material, in the face of a poorly draining organ, especially where there is a certain amount of flare-up from the urethra, w i t h an increased amount of discharge, it is easily seen that the seminal vesicles could be the source of such an infectious condition. Pain in the rectum and along the vas deferens when present, together with a mild grade of fever in the absence of evidence of a prostatic abscess, especially, also, if there is bloody seminal emission, is strongly suggestive of an acute seminal vesiculitis.

Gonorrheal Cowperitis: This condition is f a i r l y well limited to those patients who have had instrumentation of the urethra during the acute or sub-acute stage, and especially in those cases where strictures are present. In other words, this condition is rarely seen in those patients who have had proper treatment, unless there is a stricture formation, or s m a l l urethral meatus, or some other condition resulting in an increased back-pressure in the urethra. When present the infection usually breaks through the gland capsule and points towards the perineum, resulting in an abscess formation, which may destroy in whole, or part, Cowper's g l a n d. When such occurs, there is very good possibility of the additional complications of urinary extravasation. In those rare cases where gonorrheal cowperitis does develop without the formation of an abscess, there results a very chronic condition because of the poor drainage facilities and the prolonged gonorrheal infection that remains.

One of the best methods to diagnose this condition is by placing the gloved finger into the rectum and pressing into the fossa the thumb externally to the corresponding side of the bulb, and rolling the tissue between the thumb and finger. The enlarged glands can readily be palpated.

Gonorrheal Arthritis: Gonorrheal arthritis rarely occurs in the absence of some form of t r a u m a to the infected mucous membranes. Its appearance may be made after meatotomy, passage of a sound, opening of an infected gland, or any other procedure that may serve to introduce the gonococcus into the blood stream. On the other hand, those poorly behaved individuals who subject themselves to traumatic influences in the presence of an active infection of the urethra, tend to support this theory. This is perhaps the most damaging of all complications of gonorrhea, occurring in about two to five per cent of all cases, and is extremely resistant to treatment. It may present itself at any time during the attack, more frequently however, during the acute or sub-acute s t a g e s. The pathology is variable and in m a n y instances it may confine itself to one joint, more frequently being polyarticular, which may often offer a differential diagnosis from the commoner forms of rheumatic fever. It is, also, to be remembered that the degree of fever is not in proportion to the intensity of the local involvement. The disease is often periarticular, and extends along the tendon sheaths. This form is probably the least common, and thought by some authorities to be due to the gonorrheal t o x i n s, rather than the actual presence of the organism at the site. A simple effusion in the joint is sometimes noted, and in the absence of the gonococci, rarely becomes purulent. The most severe forms are those in which the actual presence of the organism are in the joints, with exudate and pus formation involving and destroying the synovial membrane of the articular surfaces and eventually ending in ankylosis. We have seen the clinical courses characterized by the great variability of the condition, and its obstinacy to therapeutic measures. In some cases the involvement is transitory, in others ending in variable degrees of ankylosis. Concerning the treatment of this obstinate condition, of course, the force of the attack should be the focus of infection, the same with urethral, prostatic and seminal vesicular gonorrhea.

Periurethritis or Spongyitis: Here there is a varying degree of infiltration of the corpus spongiosum, g r e a t l y limiting its distensibility. B e c a u s e of this, there is great pain on erection, and in the presence of extreme infiltration, there is a definite downward curve of the organ, which is commonly referred to as cordee. Along with this condition, you have the development of periurethreal abscesses, which if allowed to go untreated, may r u p t u r e either externally or internally, the former of which often results in sinuses which may harbor the gonococci almost indefinitely, and be an important etiological factor in the production of chronic gonorrhea.

Lymphangitis: This condition is characterized by the presence of small indurated cords, which may be felt running longitudinally in the subcutanious tissue of the p e n i s. There is generally an associated edema of the distal areolar tissue. It seldom causes any great amount of trouble, if the original infection is treated properly. The disection of these indurated cords has been suggested by some authors, but it is well to state that unless you have had some experience or are prepared as to what the possibilities may be, difficulties may be encountered, because of the fact that these cords sometimes run deep into the perineum.

Follicular Abscess: W h e n infiltrations around the urethral follicles undergo suppuration, they show a decided tendency to point towards the skin surface. It is well to incise these fairly early instead of waiting until they reach the skin to point, as such reduction may be avoided and possibility of sinus formation prevented. Also, f o l l o w i n g the incision of these abscesses, all active treatment should be discontinued otherwise it will greatly enhance formation of a permanent urethral sinus.

Suppurative Tysonitis: Infection of the paraphrenal glands results in this condition, which often go on to abscess formation. As soon as these form, they should immediately be incised and drained, and if possible, every effort made to keep up the drainage until healing. Otherwise, a mucous channel will be left, which will harbor the gonococci for m a n y months, which will result in numerous recurrences, and probably, chronic gonorrhea. After drainage has ceased, fulgaration of these glands is suggested by some authors, in o r d e r to more completely destroy any gonococci that may be left.

Prostatic Abscess: Infection of some degree in the prostate is c e r t a i n to occur whenever the posterior urethra is involved. The prostate may have become infected unknown to both patient and doctor even though its condition has been continually looked for throughout the course of the case. Differentiation between acute prostatitis and prostatic abscess of gonorrheal origin often is very difficult, particularly in the early stages. Urinary discomfort, frequency, and urgency, terminal hematuria, difficulty, even complete retention may occur with either. They may run a febrile or afebrile course and usually both show some degree of leukocystosis. In each, the prostate may be swollen, hot and tender on palpation but as a rule the diagnostic feature of prostatic abscess is the a r e a of fluctuation together with high temperature and sudden onset of chills. Also, the intense rectal pain is more common with gonorrheal abscesses. The acute prostatic abscess complicating gonorrhea is entirely different from the more common sub-acute or chronic pyogenic abscess. This differentiation is usually brought out by the findings of complete examination and history.

———o———

Removal of Spleen Controls Purpura

Blood transfusions and snake venom are temporarily helpful, and the removal of the spleen controls most cases of chronic thrombopenic purpura (tendency to easy bleeding due to the decrease in number of certain type of blood cell), Nathan Rosenthal, M.D., New York, states in The Journal of the American Medical Association for January 14.

There are many causes of purpura, some of which are measles, scarlet fever, chickenpox, infections of the respiratory tract and drug idiosyncrasy. However, in most cases the causative factor cannot be determined.

The condition is either acute or chronic, and the symptoms may be mild or severe in either type. Recovery is often spontaneous in the acute cases.

Some of the means suggested for the treatment of purpura include vitamin C, sesame oil, liver extract, parathyroid extract, X-ray radiation and ligation of the artery of the spleen.

———o———

Famed German Professor Retires

Having reached the age of 65, Prof. Otfried Forster has retired from the chair of neurology and psychiatry at Breslau University, the regular Berlin correspondent of The Journal of the American Medical Association reports in the January 14 issue. Through his basic research in anatomy and physiology as well as in the pathology of the nervous system, Forster has gained for himself an illustrious name. Neurosurgery likewise is much in his debt. The intradural resection of the dorsal nerve roots, for abolishment of spastic paralysis and tabetic crises, is known as Forster's operation; it was done by him as early as 1909. In 1935 Forster was awarded a British prize, the Jackson gold medal.

Diagnosis and Treatment of Gall Bladder Disease*

J. Hobson Veazey, M.D.
ARDMORE, OKLAHOMA

The gall bladder is an organ which has been generally poorly understood. Many s y m p t o m complexes related to the gall bladder still persist after a removal of the gall bladder.

In presenting this paper a study of the physiology of the gall bladder is a help in giving a clearer concept in the treatment and prognosis of gall bladder disease. The gall b l a d d e r is controlled through the vagus nerve and the sympathetic nervous system. These nerves also s u p p l y the sphincter of Odii at the duodenum. The sphincter of Odii is supplied also by the Auerbach plexus. Hence, an irritation in the duodenum can cause a reflex action in the gall bladder. The common duct and pancreatic duct empty into the duodenum in its second part at the Ampulla of Vater.

DIAGNOSTIC MEASURES

I. Cholecystogram:

Since the advent of the gall bladder dye administration, we have g a i n e d much knowledge about the gall bladder. The following terms are used in describing or interpreting the cholecystogram.

1. Normal emptying.
2. Faint visualization.
3. Delayed visualization.
4. No visualization.
5. No emptying.

II. Biliary tract drainage:

The non-surgical drainage of the gall bladder is a diagnostic measure of value. The tube should be taken in the morning following a 12-hour fast. The tube should be passed in the sitting position. Water should not be given to pass the tube in the stomach. To determine if tube is in the duodenum or stomach: (1) Stomach contents will be turbid, duodenal contents will be clear, homogenous. (2) Blow air into tube by small syringe. If it returns immediately the tube is in the duodenum. (3)

*Read before the Southern Oklahoma Medical Association Meeting, at Ardmore, December, 1936.

Fluoroscope. (4) Congo red reaction. The acid reaction of gastric contents (turns red to blue) disappears after entering the duodenum.

After the tube has passed into the duodenum usually one to two ounces of golden yellow bile is obtained. After the bile flow has ceased, one ounce of $MgSO4$ (25 per cent solution) is injected and allowed to remain two minutes. After which the $MgSO4$ solution is siphoned off and the returning $MgSO4$ is discarded. The $MgSO4$ may be repeated for two more injections. If no concentrated dark brown or olive green bile is obtained, one ounce of warm olive oil is injected and allowed to remain 10 minutes and the returning oil discarded.

The gross findings of biliary drainage:

1. Concentrated bile.
2. Absence of dark green bile usually indication of non - functioning g a l l bladder.
3. Bile sediments.

The microscopical findings of the biliary drainage:

1. Cholesterol crystals are thin ˙plates colorless with nick in one corner.
   (a) Usually indicates stones.
2. Calcium bilirubinate c r y s t a l s are lumps of heavy plates with yellow, orange, or red color.
   (a) Nearly 100 per cent diagnostic of stones.
3. Calcium crystals, are irregular, colorless and transparent.
   (a) Of no significance.

III. Chemical tests of blood. The most used tests are:

1. Cholesterol — Normal, 150-180 mgs per 100 c.c.
   (a) Elevation of blood Cholesterol; Hypercholesterolemia is usually associated with stones.
2. Cholesterol Esters — Normal, 80-120 mgs per 100 c.c. usually 50 per cent

of cholesterol. Drops to 5 to 10 per cent in liver damage.

3. Icterus Index — Normal value, 4-8. Reading 8-10 suggests g a l l bladder disease.

4. Van Den Berg.
   (a) Direct reaction, positive of common duct obstruction as 200 mgs per 100 c.c.
   (b) Indirect reaction, indicates hemolytic type of jaundice.

5. Bromsulphthalein.
   (a) Positive without jaundice, indicates p o r t a l Cirrhosis, cancer metastasis, or chronic p a s s i v e congestion.
   (b) Positive with jaundice indicates either obstruction or catarrhal jaundice.

CLASSIFICATION OF GALL BLADDER DISEASES
ACCORDING TO SYMPTOMS

I-II. Indefinite abdominal symptoms. Indigestion, distention, belching of gas, nausea, discomfort after meals, constipation with no acute attacks of pain.

III - III-A. One or more acute attacks of upper right quadrant pain such as colic, with typical radiation at times requiring hypodermics with or without nausea, vomiting or fever.

Types of Gall Bladders:

I. These patients have symptoms of gall bladder disease without a history of colic and without stones. The symptoms namely are epigastric distress, flatulence, nausea, tenderness over gall bladder.

Clinical findings: X-ray shows:

A. Faint visualization or delayed emptying or failure to empty.
B. Duodenal drainage shows crystalline sediment.
   1. Concentrated bile in which crystals of calcium, cholesterol or calcium bilirubinate are present.
C. Negative X-ray and examination of other parts of abdominal cavity.

Treatment:

A. Duodenal drainage.
B. Antispasmodics.
C. Bromides.
D. Hydrochloric acid or alkalies.
E. Saline cathartics or olive oil.

II. These patients have symptoms of gall bladder disease without a history of colic but with a stone. The symptoms are as mentioned in Type I.

This type due to stasis of bile in the gall bladder. There is a normal sphincter tone but a deficient r e s p o n s e to stimulation, h e n c e, atony and dilitation of the gall bladder. The stasis of bile c a u s e s the stone. The stone forms gradually and there is only one stone. The other types with stones will have numerous families because of numerous attacks. This type will eventually contract down. This type of gall bladder you will find in fair, fat and 40. There is no history of colic.

Clinical findings:

A. Gastric hypochlohydria.
B. X-ray shows:
   1. Dilated gall bladder with faint visualization.
   2. Incomplete emptying of gall bladder.
   3. Gall b l a d d e r does or does not show stone.
C. Icterus Index normal.
D. Cholesterol crystals in biliary sediment.

Treatment:

1. Dilute HCL.
2. Bland diet to promote emptying of gall bladder.
3. Olive oil before meals for drainage of gall bladder.
4. Strychnine is given to increase muscle tone.
5. Removal of the gall bladder is advocated because of mechanical menace of stone.

III. These patients give a history of right upper quadrant pain such as colic with typical radiation at times with or without nausea, vomiting and fever. There are two subdivisions under this type.

A. The hyptertonic individual with hyperacidity. This type is found at middle age. In women it disappears at the climateric. This gall bladder disturbance is caused by local duodenal irritation as duodenitis. The spasm p r o d u c e s a spasm of the sphincter of Odii. Diagnosis is made of duodenitis.— (1) X-ray, (2) Will have trouble getting tube in duodenum, (3) MgSO4 injected into tube will b r i n g no drainage, (4) O l i v e oil will promote drainage. This type will not get relief after gall bladder removal because pain is not due to stone but to acute duodenitis.

Clinical findings:

1. Duodenal drainage shows dark bile with cholesterol crystals because bile is stagnant.
2. Gastric hyperacidity.
3. Enlarged gall bladder shadow at X-ray.
4. Delayed emptying of gall bladder at X-ray.
5. Gall bladder may not visualize.
6. R e s p o n s e to olive oil but not to MgSO4 at biliary drainage.
7. Periodic increase of the Icterus Index.

Treatment:

1. Bland ulcer diet as Sippy.
2. Antispasmodics as t i n c t u r e Belladonna.
3. Alkalies are indicated to combat the gastric hyperacidity.
4. Olive oil is given before meals.
5. Duodenal drainage will give relief.
6. If stones are present operate because of the mechanical menace from stones.

III-A. Hypertonic t y p e without hyperacidity.

This type of gall bladder is due to reflex disturbances. A stimulation of the Vagus as neurosis, worry, nervousness, chronic appendicitis, colitis, infected tubes, etc., can cause reflex stimulation. There will be violent contractions of the gall bladder giving periodic attacks of colic or indigestion. The mechanism is produced by an increased tone of the sphincter of Odii, by a reflex of stimulation from the C.N.S.

Clinical findings:

1. Gastric acidity is normal.
2. There is no duodenitis.
3. X-ray shows normal emptying gall bladder.
4. X-ray may or may not show stones depending upon stage of formation.
5. Drainage response to b o t h MgSO4 and olive oil.

6. There is stasis in gall bladder as noted by crystalline biliary sediment.
7. Icterus index normal.

Treatment:

1. Removal of exciting cause as foci of infection.
2. Bromides or some sedative for nervous factor.
3. Antispasmodics.
4. Bland diet.
5. R e s p o n d to duodenal drainage or saline cathartics.
6. Removal of gall bladder if stones are present.

MANAGEMENT OF GALL BLADDER DISEASE

I. Avoid biliary stasis.
  A. General hygenic measures.
    1. Regularity of meals.
    2. Rest after meals.
    3. Outdoor exercise, deep breathing.
    4. Avoidance of constipation.
    5. Eliminate w o r r y and nervousness.

II. Prevention and treatment of inflammation:
  1. Bed rest.
  2. Bland diet.
  3. Remove foci of infection.

III. Dietary regulation:
  1. Bland type of diet.
  2. Frequent small meals for gall bladder drainage.
  3. Control of weight.
  4. Low cholesterol diet when Hypercholesterolemia is present.
  5. High cholesterol diet for stimulating gall bladder emptying, when not contraindicated.

IV. Medications:
  1. Sedatives such as bromides, etc.
  2. Antispasmodics as t i n c t u r e Belladonna.
  3. Hydrochloric acid or alkalies.
  4. Saline cathartics.
  5. Cholagogues.
  6. Duodenal drainage.

BIBLIOGRAPHY

Lectures—R. Franklin Carter and Associates New York Post Graduate Medical School April 1 to June 30, 1935.
Manual—"Diagnosis and Treatment of Diseases of Liver and Biliary Tract." New York Post Graduate Medical School.

Think of It First*
Some Comments on the Diagnosis of Tuberculosis

RICHARD M. BURKE, M.D.
SULPHUR, OKLAHOMA

In the years to come there shall probably be less ado over the diagnosis of tuberculosis. With the declining morbidity, our diagnostic approach is assuming a more aggressive character. We now attempt to d e t e c t tuberculosis in the pre-clinical stage. This means diagnosing the disease by the case finding method. This is being done by s u r v e y s in this state, most of which has been done by the State Tuberculosis Association under Dr. Puckett. The State Health Department's new mobile X-ray unit is extending this survey work. Incidentally, Oklahoma ranks high as regards the v o l u m e of tuberculin testing done, thanks to Dr. Puckett. Not long ago we were content to pick the disease up by physical examination and an occasional X-ray film. Today our aim is to diligently search out the positive reactors and then protect them, if possible, from further infection. If clinical tuberculosis is found, then active treatment is instituted. The time will probably come when all positive reactors will be registered and their infection followed from childhood. When such a day does come, the diagnosis of the few cases of tuberculosis then encountered will not be such a problem. For the present, however, we still must be on our toes to avoid overlooking clinical tuberculosis.

Let us consider somewhat informally some of the occasions when tuberculosis should be before our mind when examining the patient. While taking the history, always consider the possibility of tuberculosis when a story of exposure is given, especially family contact. Also, don't overlook coughing r e l a t i v e s with so-called bronchitis. Always think of it first when a patient gives a history of repeated or protracted colds or recurrent attacks of the "flu." Keep it in mind when the patient tells of exposure to irritant dust. A very

high percentage of silicotics develop tuberculosis. We might also recall that patients who shop around nursing an old diagnosis of tuberculosis rarely have clinical tuberculosis.

As to symptoms, think of it first when your patient complains of fatigue. This tiredness recalls the ill localized malaise of the early hypertensive. Pain and cough are seldom mentioned. Your patient complaining of persistent chest pain, unless it is a typical pleurisy pain, often has arthritis. The patient, with cough as a prominent symptom, rarely has early tuberculosis. Of course, there are some doctors who carry this idea a little too far. One sees patients coughing their heads off with advanced tuberculosis who have been diagnosed typhoid fever. Don't neglect the patient who seems genuinely fatigued and probably has lost a little weight. A slight temperature elevation is, of course, always suggestive.

Keep in mind, though, that the so-called fevers of unknown origin are rarely due to pulmonary tuberculosis. Here it is important to use your agglutination tests. Think of it first in patients with pleurisy or shoulder ache in the absence of acute respiratory infection. When a pleural effusion is present, treat as tuberculosis.

Likewise, a patient spitting blood is to be considered guilty until proven otherwise. Don't be guilty yourself of glibly assigning such bleeding to the upper respiratory tract as so often is done. Hemorrhage from this region is quite rare except for nose bleeds which usually can be easily spotted. Blood from the stomach is ordinarily in large clots. Blood from the lungs is mixed with mucus and 90 per cent of the time it is due to tuberculosis. The most common causes of streaking are bronchiectasis and bronchitis. Blood spitting of obscure origin, especially in young individuals, always demands prolonged ob-

*Presented before the Post Graduate Course on Tuberculosis in Oklahoma City, October 13, 1937.

servation. The hemoptysis occurring in mitral stenosis is not infrequently ascribed to tuberculosis. Patients are inclined to exaggerate when telling about the amount of blood raised. Quiz them carefully. The typical hemoptysis ("tossing the ruby"), of tuberculosis is about one ounce or more followed by blood streaked sputum for several days.

In physical examination, think of it when you encounter a chest exhibiting asymmetry such as a slight lag on one side or a slight wasting on one side. Tuberculosis is a disease which produces asymmetry. Unfortunately, t h e stethoscope plays a very minor role in diagnosing the early lesion. Of course, think of it first when moderately coarse post cough rales are heard above the third rib and fourth dorsal spine—the so-called zone of alarm. On the other hand, r a l e s in the lower lobes may be considered as non-tuberculous until proven otherwise. Rhonchi almost always indicate a non - tuberculous lung condition, such as asthmatic bronchitis. However, remember that tuberculosis co-exists with other diseases. When sputum is raised, always have it examined for tubercle bacilli. Club fingers usually point away from tuberculosis to o t h e r forms of chronic lung suppuration. Always think of it when anal fistula is encountered. Old scars of tuberculous adenitis are significant.

Next we come to laboratory aids. Repeated negative sputum examinations in the presence of a purulent sputum usually serves to rule out tuberculosis. Often we see relatives and doctors who are reluctant to give up a diagnosis of tuberculosis in the presence of a chronic productive cough such as occurs in bronchiectasis. Tuberculosis is no longer a universal disease, so use the tuberculin test on adults as well as children. Think of it whether the test is four plus or one plus. The fluoroscope is a fine routine but use it cautiously. An early lesion can be easily overlooked. Always take a chest film when any doubt exists. I feel that the fluoroscope is adequate in children under 12 years. We are inclined to over interpret the X-ray, i.e., see things that are not really present. Our chief concern s h o u l d be the outer and upper third of the lung fields. Fine and

moderately coarse mottling in this region means to think of it first. Chronic upper respiratory tract infection causes thickening about the hilus and along the descending bronchial trunks, which is confused with tuberculosis. Don't get too excited about healed primary complexes in persons over 30. When in doubt as to activity, always insist on serial films. Bronchoscopy and lipiodol mapping of the lung fields are important diagnostic aids. Use them especially in obscure lower lobe disease.

The pulmonary conditions which I have found most frequently misdiagnosed as tuberculosis have been bronchitis (usually with emphysema), bronchiectasis and lung abscess. The extra pulmonary conditions so diagnosed have been heart disease, malaria, syphilis and hyperthyroidism. I have not found disease of the paranasal sinuses per se quite as frequently misdiagnosed as others report. A difficult task sometimes is to tell whether or not a case of pneumoconiosis has an associated tuberculosis. Repeated sputum examinations help. The bronchomycoses are difficult to diagnose but fortunately, they are rare. Primary cancer of the lung is on the increase and it seems that errors in its diagnosis are also on the increase. An X-ray diagnosis is very hazardous. Bronchoscope your patient. If a pleural effusion develops, do a guinea pig even though the fluid is hemorrhagic.

Keep in mind that many of the things I have mentioned are merely diagnostic aids and not dogma or infallible truths. In concluding, let me remind you that to "Think of It First" is an excellent habit. By so doing you are bound to pick up an occasional early case of tuberculosis, which is still considered somewhat of a minor triumph in medicine.

—————————o—————————

Further Study of Lobar Pneumonia in the Tulsa Area

SAMUEL GOODMAN, M.D.

TULSA, OKLAHOMA

A statistical study of the pneumonias relative to the incidence of lobar pneumonia in the Tulsa area during the period from 1930 to 1937 revealed some interesting data. The results of this study in a series of 721 pneumonias was given in two previous papers, one read before the Tulsa Clinical Society in June of 1936, and one read before the Oklahoma State Medical Association in May, 1937. This s t u d y showed that prior to 1935 the incidence of lobar pneumonia was rather low. In the period from 1930 to 1935, it constituted but 10.6 per cent of the total number of pneumonias. In the period from January, 1935, to May, 1936, it constituted 25.5 per cent of the total number. From May 1, 1936, to May 1, 1937, it constituted a maximum of 46.8 per cent of the total number of pneumonias. The latter was based on a survey of 109 cases of pneumonia admitted into St. John's Hospital in that year.

Thus, it is seen that in the period from 1930 to 1937 there had been a decided increase in the incidence of lobar pneumonia.

From May, 1937, to May, 1938, there was a decided fall in the total number of pneumonias and a slight decrease in the inci-

dence of lobar and atypical pneumococcus pneumonia admitted into the hospital. The number of pneumococcus pneumonia cases made up 45.3 per cent of the total.

The importance of the pneumonia problem, both from a public health and economic standpoint can be appreciated from the fact that among the infectious diseases, pneumonia out-ranks all others as a cause of death. In 1936 the death rate in the United States was 69.8 per 100,000 population as compared to 54.2 per 100,000 due to tuberculosis. The mortality rate has increased at a rather disturbing rate since 1932.

According to the United States Bureau of Vital Statistics, the death rate per 100,-000 population in Oklahoma, from pneumonias other than broncho-pneumonia, increased from 38 in 1932 to 55.9 in 1936. The broncho - pneumonia mortality increased from 25.8 in 1932 to 35.6 in 1936 per 100,000 population. The total pneumonia mortality rate in Oklahoma during the year of 1936 was 91.5 per 100,000 population and was second only to heart disease among all other diseases as cause of death.

TABLE No. I

Survey of 569 Pneumonia Cases From January 1, 1935, to May 1, 1938						
January 1, 1935 to May 1, 1936				May 1, 1936 to May 1, 1938		
Morningside Hospital and St. John's Hospital				St. John's Hospital		
	Cases	%	Mortality	Cases	%	Mortality
Lobar & Atypical Pneumococcus Pneumonia	136	34.4	26.5	81	46.8	29.6%
Broncho Pneumonia	260	65.6	25.9	92	53.2	32.6%
Combined Total	396		25.6	173		31.2%

Average days ill before entering hospital—4.5

TABLE No. II

Analysis of 81 Lobar and Atypical Pneumococcus Pneumonia Admitted to St. John's Hospital From May 1, 1936, to May 1, 1938

AGE GROUP		MONTHS	
Less than 1 year	4	January	11
1 to 4 years	5	February	23
5 to 9 years	8	March	10
10 to 19 years	9	April	3
20 to 29 years	11	May	7
30 to 39 years	11	June	3
40 to 49 years	10	July	1
50 to 59 years	9	August	2
60 to 69 years	4	September	0
70 to — years	10	October	6
		November	4
SEX		December	11
Male	49		
Female	32		

Onset preceded by upper respiratory infection	50
Onset not preceded by upper respiratory infection	20
Unknown	11

Onset sudden	51
Onset gradual	22
Unknown	8

While it may seem fundamental to review the various phases of lobar pneumonia, I believe it is of the utmost importance that certain aspects of the disease be clearly understood in order to obtain the best results, particularly with specific treatment. In this connection it is significant that 96 per cent of lobar pneumonias and about 50 per cent of broncho-pneumonias in adults are caused by one of the various t y p e s of pneumococci. Of these, Types Nos. I, II, III, IV, V, VI, VII, VIII, XIV cause 89 per cent of the pneumococcus pneumonias. At the p r e s e n t time specific sera are commercially available for all the above individual types. In view of the above statements, it is clearly evident that we should be concerned more with the necessity of making a bacteriological diagnosis rather than an anatomical one.

In this series of cases the age group, sex, and seasonal incidence coincide with those found in various other localities. The role of the common cold as a predisposing factor in lobar pneumonia should not be overlooked. It is to be noted that 61 per cent were preceded by acute respiratory infections. Since at the present time no satisfactory protective antigen against pneu-

TABLE No. III

Symptoms and Physical Findings

Previous Attacks	9
No Previous Attacks	28
Unknown	44

SYMPTOMS		PHYSICAL FINDINGS	
Fever	73	Rales	60
Cough	68	Dullness	48
Pain in chest	55	Broncho-vesicular breathing	54
Chill	38	Limited expansion	32
Blood streaked sputum	26	Increased fremitus	13
Dyspnea	21	Cyanosis	7
Aching	6	Distant breath sounds	6
Nausea	8	Right side	44
Vomiting	8	Left side	17
Anorexia	5	Both sides	13
Abdominal pain	4	No record as to side	4
No record	1	Friction rub	3
		No record of physical examination	3

monia has been developed, it becomes our duty as physicians not to minimize the common cold and to consider all acute respiratory infections as potential pneumonias.

The diagnosis of lobar pneumonia with a typical explosive onset, most often seen with Type I and II is usually not difficult. However, an early diagnosis in an atypical case with inconspicuous onset, variable presenting symptoms, and physical signs may be rather difficult. It is with this group that diagnosis is often deferred, resulting in an unfavorable condition and a doubtful outcome of the disease. Since early and adequate specific treatment is the important factor in a given case of pneumococcus pneumonia regardless of its seeming mildness, it is necessary that we employ all available facilities to make an early diagnosis. Aside from the clinical findings these consist of laboratory aids such as sputum typing, blood culture, leucocyte, and differential count, and roentgenograms of the chest.

The symptoms of chill or chilliness, fever, cough, pain in the chest, accelerated respiration, with expectoration of blood tinged sputum, without clinical evidence of consolidation are sufficient to make a tentative diagnosis of pneumococcus pneumonia.

In cases with an atypical onset, acceleration of the respiration with a change in the respiration to pulse rate ratio may furnish valuable information of an underlying pneumonic process. A change in the normal pulse to respiratory rate ratio of 4 to 1 to a rate of 3 or 2 to 1 is one of the most common findings early in the course of a pneumonia. Other early physical signs such as slight cyanosis, intensification of the whispered voice sounds, suppressed breath sounds, limited respiratory excursion, and occasional crepitant rales over a localized area may be present and are of considerable diagnostic importance. Evidence of consolidation, which may not be elicited until the third or fifth day, particularly in centrally located lesions, is not necessary for the diagnosis of lobar pneumonia. Much valuable time may be lost in waiting until consolidation is manifested. In this connection it has been our routine to have roentgenograms made on every patient who enters the hospital with suggestive acute respiratory symptoms. X-ray evidence of consolidation is often superior to p h y s i c a l findings in detecting early lesions. These lesions may be visualized within the first 24 hours.

Typing of the sputum should be done as early as possible in order to determine the

TABLE No. IV

Laboratory Findings

WHITE BLOOD COUNT		PER CENT NEUTROPHILS	
5-10	8	50-59	1
11-15	20	60-70	0
16-20	30	71-80	9
21-30	14	81-90	38
31-40	5	91-100	30
41-50	1	Unknown	3
Unknown	3		

SPUTUM EXAMINATION			
Sputum examined	62	Group B	4
Sputum not examined	19	Group C	2
Sputum negative	4	Group D	6
Type I	14	Group E	3
Type II	7	Group F	1
Type V	4	Group G	2
Type VII	8	Group H	1
		Other pneumonia Morphology	6

ROENTGENOLOGICAL EXAMINATION	
Bronchial Pneumonia	13
Lobar Pneumonia	26
Influenzal Pneumonia	3
Pleuritis	11
Abscess	2
Fluid	10
Not X-rayed	32

etiological organism. Rapid pneumococcus typing by the Neufeld reaction as advocated by Sabin is a simple and very accurate procedure. It depends on the fact that a swelling of the pneumococcus capsule o c c u r s when the pneumococcus is mixed with a homologous type of rabbit antiserum. It is definitely type specific.

Since the pneumococci of the h i g h e r types are f r e q u e n t l y found in normal mouths, the question, as to their etiological relationship to the e x i s t i n g pneumonia might be raised. In a small percentage of cases there may be no relationship. Bullowa, however, has shown in a large series of cases that in a pneumonia patient the type of organism found in the patient's sputum corresponded in 93 per cent of the instances to the type found in the lungs.

It has been our custom to have the sputum retyped when members of the higher types are reported in the initial sputum examinations.

That physicians have become "type conscious" is evident from the fact that in 1935 less than 50 per cent of the sputums were examined or typed; that from May 1, 1936, to May 1, 1937, 76 per cent were typed. From May 1, 1937, to May 1, 1938, 76.5 per cent were examined or typed. These figures were taken from the records of pneumonia patients in St. John's Hospital.

Leucocytosis with an increase in the percentage of the neutrophils is almost always a constant finding in l o b a r pneumonia. Counts up to 40,000 per cubic millimeter with the neutrophils composing from 80 to 90 per cent of the total number of cells is not infrequent. Counts below 10,000 indicate a poor p r o g n o s i s. I wish to again stress the value of routine blood culture. Despite the significance of bacteremia as the factor in recovery, and as a guide to adequate serum dosage, it is regrettable that so few requests for blood culture have been made. The incidence of bacteremia apparently increased with age and also increases the mortality rate from three to five-fold. Even with serum treatment the mortality rate is high. In a series of bacteremic cases of the Massachusetts Study the mortality rate in Type I, treated with serum within the first four days, was 28.6 per cent as compared to a mortality rate of 8.2 per cent in the non-bacteremic cases. In Type II the mortality rate in the bacteremic cases treated with serum was 46.8 per cent as compared to a mortality rate of 15 per cent in the non-bacteremic cases. Bacteremia occurs in about one-fourth of Type I cases and in about one-third of Type II. Cases with positive blood cultures demand maximum serum dosage.

The vast amount of evidence which has been accumulated relative to the efficacy of specific serum leaves no doubt as to its therapeutic value in pneumococcus pneumonia. The results of serum treatment in a large series of cases gathered from the literature show that the mortality rate in Type I has been reduced from about 25 per cent in the non-serum treated cases to less than 10 per cent. In Type II the mortality rate has been decreased from about 43 per cent in the non-serum treated cases to about 22.5 per cent in the serum treated cases. Available data, as to the efficacy of rabbit antiserum in Type III pneumonias, which have a mortality rate of about 50 per cent is insufficient to draw any definite conclusion. The results obtained in Types V, VII, VIII, XIV treated with serum parallels the r e s u l t s obtained in serum treated Type I cases.

As shown by various investigators the importance of early serum treatment cannot be over emphasized. The results obtained depend upon a definite time relationship to the onset of the disease. According to Cole in a series of 462 patients with Type I pneumonia treated with serum within the first three days the mortality rate was 4.8 per cent, on the fourth day it was 8.2 per cent, on the fifth day it was 8.6 per cent, and after the fifth day it was 19.5 per cent. Bullowa reported a mortality rate of 8.8 per cent in a series of cases treated with serum before the fifth day. Cecil reported a mortality rate of five per cent in the cases which were treated with serum on the first day. Horsfall and his co-workers have recently treated a number of pneumococcus pneumonia with rabbit antisera. The results have been remarkable in that their mortality rate was but 3.7 per cent. The advantages of rabbit serum over horse serum are that the small molecule to w h i c h the antibody is attached is much less likely to produce dangerous reactions; that in the rabbit the antibody is more easily and rapidly developed to a much higher titer; that the cost is considerable less due to the fact that concentration of the serum is not required.

Before serum is administered it is necessary to test the patient for sensitivity. It is obvious that patients who are sensitive to horse serum or who develop asthma or vasomotor rhinitis w h e n exposed to horse emanations should not receive horse serum even by testing. In the cases of using horse serum the conjunctival and intradermal tests with d i l u t e d normal horse serum are performed.

Since practically all persons show a positive skin reaction to rabbit serum, Horsfall adopted the method of blood pressure and heart rate variations to determine sensitivity. If, within a period of five minutes after an intravenous injection of .01 c.c. to .05 c.c. of normal rabbit serum diluted with 5 c.c. of physiological salt solution, there is a fall in the blood pressure of 15 millimeters or more and there is an increase in the cardiac rate of 15 or more, it denotes that the patient is sensitive.

Serum should always be given slowly intravenously and in divided doses. The initial dosage of serum according to the Massachusetts program is from 60,000 to 100,000 units. This initial dosage is doubled, if: (1) Treatment is begun after the third day of the disease. (2) The p a t i e n t is over 40 years of age. (3) The patient is pregnant or in the first week of the puerperium. (4) There is involvement of more than one lobe. (5) Bacteremia is present. Additional doses of 40,000 to 60,000 units at intervals of three or four hours are recommended, if, in any case: (1) The temperature does not fall below 102 degrees by rectum within 18 hours after beginning serum treatment. (2) If the temperature rises again after having fallen below 102 degrees Fahrenheit by rectum. (3) Bacteremia is demonstrated by blood culture regardless of the clinical course. (4) There is evidence of a spreading lesion.

CONCLUSIONS

1. The importance of pneumonia with particular reference to the pneumococcic group as an economic and public health problem is emphasized.

2. An analytical study of 81 cases of pneumococcic pneumonia from May, 1936, to the present date, showing age, sex, seasonal incidences, symptoms, physical signs, laboratory findings, and mortality rate is presented.

3. The necessity of early diagnosis from the standpoint of symptoms and laboratory aids such as sputum typing, blood culture, blood counts, roentgenograms of the chest; and the importance of an etiological rather than an anatomical diagnosis are stressed.

4. The results of specific serum treatment in the various types of pneumococcic pneumonia in a large series of cases gathered from the literature are given. Initial serum dosage and the outline of serum treatment are set forth as advocated by the Massachusetts Pneumonia Study.

REFERENCES

1. Cole: Annals of Internal Medicine: 10:1, July, 1936.
2. Cecil: J.A.M.A.; 108:869; February, 1937.
3. Horsfall: J.A.M.A.; 108:1483; May, 1937.
4. Lord & Heffron: Pneumonia & Serum Therapy; pp. 57.
5. Lord & Heffron: Pneumonia & Serum Therapy; Treated Bacteremic and Non-Bacteremic Cases; Massachusetts Series; pages 116 and 117.
6. Bullowa: Etiological Agent By Lung Puncture; Management of the Pneumonias.

Functional Hearing Test

C. A. PAVY, M.D.
TULSA, OKLAHOMA

Of all the special senses, I am sure we will agree that sight is the most important, hearing second. Partial loss of the sense of hearing in the child, especially of school age, is unfortunate. Practically all education is acquired either by seeing or by hearing. The child who is unable to hear all that is said to him is frequently looked upon by the teacher, pupils, and even the parents as being mentally deficient. The adult with partial or complete loss of the sense of hearing is put to great disadvantage in his business and social activities, much more so than in years past. The age we are now living in is highly competitive, requiring all our facilities to meet this competition.

We as Otologists haven't much to boast about, for there are entirely too m a n y people, both children and adults, deficient in their ability to hear. This fact places a great responsibility upon us. What can be done about it? If there is any branch of m e d i c i n e that should be preventive rather than curative, it is Otology. We all know too well that permanent loss of hearing is m u c h more common than a loss which can be relieved. We, like the Oculists who prescribe glasses, may prescribe hearing aids; but the Occulist's patient will wear glasses with ease and comfort, while our patient will object seriously to wearing a hearing instrument, and, in many cases, rightly so. Not until we know just the instrument to prescribe and can write a prescription for it to be filled by a recognized institution, will we have gone far in this direction. At present, these instruments are sold m a i n l y on a commercial basis.

If we are to accomplish much, it seems that it must be through education. When I say education, I do not mean education for the public alone, but for the medical profession as well.

Before the depression, the public was becoming more and more educated to the necessity of periodic examinations. Many of them came in regularly, either annually or semi-annually, for these examinations. But what about the ears? Were they examined by a competent man? The examiner was often an internist, a pediatrician, or a general practitioner whose equipment u s u a l l y consisted of an otoscope and a watch. He would make a superficial examination, not sufficient to detect beginning deafness which might be corrected with little effort. But it was not detected, and the condition gradually grew worse until the subject was advised by his family or business associates that he was becoming deaf. Then he consulted the otologist with an advanced case of deafness, when there was little that could be done.

In recent years the public has paid less attention to these periodic examinations, and must be re-educated as to their value.

They must also be taught that these checkups are not only a saving of physical facilities, but a saving of m o n e y — not a scheme advanced by the medical profession for financial gain. We are not free from blame, for frequently we do not find this beginning deafness, the reason often being the fact that we do not follow a definite routine of examination. This is the one point which I wish to stress in this paper, "Functional Hearing Test."

I shall of necessity discuss t e s t s used which you all know, but, if I may insist upon your a d o p t i o n of a step-by-step method of examination, I shall feel that my time has been well spent. Before beginning an examination, one should have a complete history—that of the family, past history and present condition of the patient, with the beginning and progress of the complaint. One should also have a general physical examination. An otologist can no more practice within himself than a part of a machine can operate without its companion parts. We must have the cooperation of the m e d i c a l men in order to learn much which we cannot know without their help.

The examination of the ear should be made in a noiseless room. This is almost impossible in the city where t r a f f i c is heavy. Most of us do not have a soundproof room, but must compromise by using the quietest room we have for hearing examinations.

The equipment used in these examinations may i n c l u d e all the instruments known. It makes very little difference. One may make a very accurate estimation of hearing with his voice and two or three tuning forks, while another may have all the instruments at his command and make a very poor estimation. Thorough knowledge of the test used and its interpretation is necessary. What is normal hearing? Unfortunately we have no standard. The pulse, blood pressure, metabolic rate, etc., have no different standards, but are considered normal when found within certain limits. So we may take our own ear, if it is good, and be almost as definite as we could be with standards.

The object of the hearing tests is to find whether the ear is normal. If not, how much loss of hearing there is; and which parts are causing the loss must be determined. Deafness is divided into two types, depending upon the part responsible for such loss; namely, conductive and perceptive. Conductive deafness is caused by some interference with the parts which conduct the waves of vibration to the inner ear. These parts are the external canal, tympanic membrane, ossicles, middle ear, and eustachian tube. Perceptive deafness is caused by some disease or condition interfering with the receiving of vibrations to the cochlea, organ of Corti, the eighth nerve, or the center within the brain.

The instruments used in t e s t i n g the hearing function are the watch, the voice (both conversational and whispering), several tuning forks and the audiometer. I am not including a few of the instruments commonly used. One of the oldest tests is the watch test. It has been used since the beginning of the 16th century. In years gone by the watch had a more uniform tick than the modern watch, which has a wide variation in pitch and volume. For use as an office record this is still a very good test, but, in comparison with other examinations, it is of little value. In making the test, one must know his watch; that is, how many inches it can be heard from the ear. Each ear should be tested separately, holding the watch farther away from the ear than it can normally be heard and approaching the ear until the patient indicates that he hears the first tick. Although this is a very good test, the watch with its one high frequency is of little importance if used alone.

The voice tests are very important, for in most cases, a conversational range is the thing we are m o s t interested in. One should have a space of 30 feet between patient and examiner. Few of our offices have this much space, so the test is done at 15 feet with the proximal ear closed tightly, not by the patient, but by the doctor's assistant to make sure that the ear is really closed. One may use names of cities, objects, etc., but in my own work I use the simple numerals between one and ten. Many use double numerals, but it seems to me that the single numerals are more e-a-s-i-l-y handled at a definite frequency. These numerals should be spoken in an ordinary conversational tone. Much practice is required to become proficient. If the patient hears these numerals and can

repeat them after the examiner, we say that his hearing is normal; but, if he should not hear the numerals, he should be approached slowly until he is able to repeat them. The number of feet multiplied by two should be your numerator, 30 the denominator. The whispered voice test is done in the same way e x c e p t six feet is the distance used from the patient to the examiner. The examiner stands back of or by the side of the patient, again using numerals. If the patient repeats these numerals, we should consider his hearing normal. For the whispering voice, if you do not approach the patient as before, note the number of feet from which he can detect your whispering voice. The result will be a repetition of the spoken voice test except that the denominator will be six.

Now we have done three tests: the watch with a high frequency, the conversational voice, and the whispered v o i c e with a medium frequency. We now have a fair idea of the patient's ability to hear, but we have not found whether we are dealing w i t h a conductive or a perceptive deafness. The following tests are made for this purpose.

The selection of tuning forks is very important. First, the size should be neither too large nor too small. If too large, they are awkward to use; and, if too small, they are also inconvenient. I should say that the size should be from eight to ten inches at most. Medium forks should be weighted in order that we may produce a true tone. The number depends upon your other equipment. If you are going to use the forks in conjunction with an audiometer, one or two forks are sufficient; but, if you are going to d e p e n d upon forks alone, you should have at least five (a 64, 256, 512, 1048, and a 2096). These forks will take in all the range that is ordinarily used. In exciting the forks, all kinds of methods have been suggested. It makes little difference which method you use as long as you use the same method every time and become fairly accurate in doing so. One will never get an accurate test if one strikes the fork against anything which is most handy. If you use a pleximeter all well and good; but use it every time in exactly the same way. I let the tine of the fork fall from a perpendicular to a horizontal position, striking my wrist. I use this method every time. My 64 fork has a 22 vibrating time, my 128 fork has a 28 vibrating time, and so on, each fork having a definite vibrating time. By using these five forks and knowing their vibrating time, one may make a log similar to the one used with the audiometer and make a very accurate test even to percentages.

The fork tests as used by most men are three in number; namely, the Schwabach, the Weber, and the Rinne. These tests are not used to determine ability to hear, but to locate the part or parts involved if there is deafness present. Even with these tests, one can determine the groups of parts responsible; that is, they indicate whether we are dealing with a conductive deafness or a perceptive deafness. We cannot tell by giving tests whether the trouble is due to a tympanic membrane, eustachian tube, or any other particular part. The same is true of conductive deafness.

The Schwabach test is used in many ways, but I think one of the most common methods of testing is the use of a 128 or 256 fork set in vibration. The handle is placed to the forehead vortex or over the mastoid, the patient indicating when he or she no longer hears the tone. Then the fork is placed on the examiner's head, the same location being used. If the patient hears the vibration longer than the examiner, we say that the patient has a prolonged bone conduction, and, if a shorter time, that he has a bone conduction of short duration. The former indicates a conductive deafness; the latter shows a perceptive deafness.

The Weber test is a lateralization test. One must be very careful in interpreting this procedure as most patients think the vibrations should be heard more loudly in the good ear. The test is performed by setting a 256 fork into vibration and placing it on the forehead, the patient indicating the ear by which the vibrations are heard most distinctly. If the vibrations are heard louder in the good ear, perceptive deafness of the opposite ear is shown; but, if heard louder in the bad ear, conductive deafness is probably present. This is not universally true. If the patient says that the vibrations are louder in the bad ear, there must be some obstruction in the mid-

dle ear, the tympanic membrane, or the external canal to deflect the vibrations toward the inner ear. Therefore, in interpreting the findings, one must keep this fact in mind.

The Rinne test is a comparison of bone conduction and air conduction. Air conduction is about twice as long as bone conduction. The same fork or forks are used as are used in the other tests. The handle of the fork is placed over the mastoid process, and the patient tells the examiner when he can no longer hear the vibrations. The tines are then brought before the ear, and the patient makes known the point at which the vibrations are no longer heard. As I have said before, the ratio should be two to one. If there is a long bone conduction, conductive deafness is s h o w n. Should there be a short bone conduction as compared to air conduction, perceptive deafness is present. When one has done these tests and has properly interpreted them, a fairly accurate diagnosis may be made as to the type of deafness one is dealing with.

Some years ago, an instrument was perfected to measure rather accurately the ability to hear. This instrument, called the audiometer, has a frequency starting as low as 32 and reaching a height of 20,000 vibrations per second. In former years, the audiometer, because of its price, was almost prohibitive for the average otologist. In the last few years, the price has been reduced until it is within the range of every man doing ear work. This instrument is not a diagnostic instrument, but is used to determine the amount of hearing. It is especially useful in determining whether progress is being made, and, if so, how much. In compensation w o r k where a patient may claim loss of hearing as a result of accident, it is possible to measure accurately the actual loss and to have the findings compare favorably with those of other men using like instruments.

After compiling the results of all these tests, and having a complete history and physical examination, one may arrive at a very accurate diagnosis. However, let me again insist upon the importance of using a systematic routine of making examinations.

THE JOURNAL
OF THE
Oklahoma State Medical Association

Issued Monthly at McAlester, Oklahoma, under direction of
the Council.

Copyright, 1939, by Oklahoma State Medical Association,
McAlester, Oklahoma.

Vol. XXXII	MARCH	Number 3

DR. L. S. WILLOUR......................................Editor-in-Chief
McAlester, Oklahoma

DR. T. H. McCARLEY..............................Associate Editor
McAlester, Oklahoma

Entered at the Post Office at McAlester, Oklahoma, as
second-class matter under the act of March 3rd, 1879.

This is the official Journal of the Oklahoma State Medical Association. All communications should be addressed to The Journal of the Oklahoma State Medical Association, McAlester Clinic, McAlester, Oklahoma. $4.00 per year; 40c per copy.

The editorial department is not responsible for the opinions expressed in the original articles of contributors.

Reprints of original articles will be supplied at actual cost provided request for them is attached to manuscripts or made in sufficient time before publication.

Articles sent this Journal for publication and all those read at the annual meetings of the State Association are the sole property of this Journal. The Journal relies on each individual contributor's strict adherence to this well-known rule of medical journalism. In the event an article sent this Journal for publication is published before appearance in The Journal the manuscript will be returned to the writer.

Failure to receive The Journal should call for immediate notification of the Editor, McAlester Clinic, McAlester, Oklahoma.

Local news of possible interest to the medical profession, notes on removals, changes of addresses, births, deaths and weddings will be gratefully received.

Advertising of articles, drugs or compounds unapproved by the Council on Pharmacy of the A. M. A., will not be accepted.

Advertising rates will be supplied on application.

It is suggested that wherever possible members of the State Association should patronize our advertisers in preference to others as a matter of fair reciprocity.

Printed by News-Capital Company, McAlester.

EDITORIAL

ANNUAL MEETING

Arrangements are practically complete for the Annual Meeting, to be held at the Skirvin Hotel, Oklahoma City, May 1, 2, 3. The various local Chairmen have been appointed by Dr. L. J. Starry, and are properly functioning. Three of our Guest Speakers have already accepted an invitation to be present and are Doctors Wayne Babcock of Philadelphia; J. F. Hamilton, Campbell's Clinic, Memphis; and Edw. N. Smith, Oklahoma City, Instructor in Post Graduate work in Obstetrics. We also expect there will be a representative from the American Medical Association headquarters; however, as yet we do not know who this will be.

With the new assembly rooms that have been completed at the Skirvin Hotel we will have ample and commodious space for all Sections; the spaces for technical exhibits has practically all been taken.

The Oklahoma City physicians and surgeons are arranging for Clinics on Monday, May 1, at the various hospitals. The program of these Clinics will be published in the next issue of the Journal along with the entire program of the Annual Meeting.

We are looking forward to the usual good presentations in the Section meetings and all in all the prospects bid fair to be one of the best meetings in the history of the Association.

MEMBERSHIP DUES

The Roster of members of the State Association must be completed before the Annual Meeting, to be held May 1, 2, 3, as a membership card is necessary for registration.

It is also important that the dues be paid promptly in order that certification of membership may be made to the American Medical Association as membership in the A.M.A. will not be accepted until such certification. As the National meeting is to be held May 15th it is important that the dues be paid so that those desiring may obtain their Fellowship card before the meeting.

We wish to call attention to the fact that the payment of dues has been very slow this year and if the program, as outlined by the House of Delegates at their last meeting, is to be carried out it will be necessary that the funds be supplied and they are only supplied by the payment of dues.

Your prompt attention to this matter of paying dues is very important.

REVISION OF CONSTITUTION AND BY-LAWS

The House of Delegates at the Annual Meeting in 1937 appointed a Committee for the revision of the Constitution and By-Laws, composed of Drs. L. H. Ritzhaupt, Guthrie, C. P. Bondurant, Medical Arts Bldg., Oklahoma City, and E. Albert Aisenstadt, Picher Hospital, Picher, Oklahoma. This Committee is now busy making this revision and they ask that members who have suggestions to offer communicate with them immediately as they are desirous of receiving from all members interested, information, guidance, and recommendations so that the revised Constitution, when submitted for final passage, will represent the ultimate desire of a cross section of the largest majority of our membership, and will thereby assure passage without unnecessary controversy at the next annual meeting.

You may address any suggestions to any one of the above named Committee.

--------o--------

THE ANNUAL EARLY DIAGNOSTIC CAMPAIGN

Ordinarily, finding disease early is up to the p h y s i c i a n s. But in tuberculosis there is a difference, for the patient has it in an active, transmissable stage, months to years before he has any symptoms that suggest going to his doctor. Queries and Minor Notes of the Journal of the American Medical Association say that in the average case diagnosis may be made two and one-half years before the patient feels any symptoms whatever. For this reason the efforts of physicians must largely be linked with that of other citizens in making people tuberculosis conscious, so they will do their part to find out their own condition as a routine, or at least be alert when the possibility of tuberculosis occurs.

The National Tuberculosis Association has published and is distributing the April issue of "Tuberculosis Abstracts," preliminary to the annual nationwide Early Diagnosis Campaign conducted in April each year. The slogan this year is in the nature of an appeal to all the citizenship, "Help Find Early Tuberculosis."

A second catch phrase of this campaign is: "Eight out of Ten Who Come to the Sanatorium are ADVANCED Cases." The thoughtless might blame this situation on the medical profession. But the fact that most cases are advanced before they go to their doctors takes most of the blame away, if there be any. However, the medical profession should not be content to do nothing about it. Certainly an alibi is not what physicians usually seek. It is a part of the creed to meet public responsibilities. In doing so with tuberculosis a great service is rendered in solution of a problem of society. Of course we may be disposed to ease up on public service since the medical profession has been kicked around a good deal of late. But the best answer to that is obvious service, and nothing can be more impressive than a definite reduction in tuberculosis.

We suggest that you read this "Tuberculosis Abstract." County medical societies should join in observance of the Early Diagnosis Campaign by having a paper or discussion on tuberculosis. The Oklahoma Tuberculosis and Health Association, 22 N.W. 6th St., Oklahoma City, will furnish material helpful in preparation of papers. The new Diagnostic Standards is available on request of any physician in the state. The National Tuberculosis Association has an excellent sound moving picture for physicians called "Diagnostic Procedures." The State Association can obtain this in 16 mm. for a rental of $1.00, plus return postage. If your medical society can arrange for a picture machine a showing of this picture, 20 minutes, will make a fine addition to your program.

We urge physicians to be alert to the possibility of tuberculosis, both for the sake of their patients and to speed up·the eradication of this disease; for it will be conquered as a part of the onward progress of medical science.

--------o--------

DEAN UNIVERSITY OF TEXAS SCHOOL OF MEDICINE

Dr. John W. Spies, for the past three years director of the Tata Memorial Hospital in Bombay, India, and an internationally known authority on the study and treatment of cancer, has been appointed dean of the University of Texas School of Medicine, located at Galveston. His appointment was effective November 10. He replaces as dean Dr. W. S. Carter, retired. Dr. Spies will also serve as professor of preventive medicine and hygiene.

A native Texan and an academic graduate of the University of Texas, Dr. Spies has spent the last 20 years studying, practicing and teaching medicine in this country and in Belgium, Germany, China and India. He graduated in medicine at Harvard University in 1924. He received the degree of master of science from Yale University in 1930. Dr. Spies served as interne at St. Luke's hospital in New York City, which was followed by a residency and clinical fellowship at the Memorial Hospital in New York City. He has twice held fellowships under the a u s p i c e s of the American-Belgian Foundation at the University of Louvain.

During the academic years of 1929-1931 he was instructor in surgery and pathology at the Yale University School of Medicine and in the summer of 1930 he served as surgical assistant in the University of Berlin. From 1931 to 1935 he held the position of associate professor of surgery and head of the tumor clinic in the Peking Union Medical College which was established and is maintained in China by the Rockefeller Foundation. From 1935 to 1938 he was director of the Tata Memorial Hospital which was founded in Bombay, India, by the Sir Dorabji Tata Foundation to promote the study and treatment of cancer.

Dr. Spies is a member of the American Board of Radiology, the American Association of Pathologists and Bacteriologists, the American Radium Society, the American Association for Cancer Research, the Chinese Medical Association, the Indian Surgical Association, the Royal College of Surgeons and Physicians in England, and Sigma Xi, honorary scientific fraternity. He is holder of the certificate of the National Board of Medical Examiners of the United States, which is the only organization in this country affiliated with similar European Boards and which entitles the holder to practice in practically all of the States of the Union.

Dr. Spies has had an unusually extensive experience in first-hand visits to important educational institutions in North America, Europe, and the Orient. He has published numerous articles pertaining to investigations in various fields of medicine.

His brother, Dr. Tom D. Spies, is professor of medicine at the University of Cincinnati and has recently done very important work in connection with pellagra.

---o---

For the fifth consecutive year, the psychiatric staff of the Menninger Clinic, Topeka, Kansas, will offer a week's postgraduate course in Neuropsychiatry in General Practice, April 17-22. This practical presentation of dynamic psychiatry through lectures and case presentations has been attended by physicians from 19 states in the past four years. Enrollment is limited to 30. Address inquiries to Dr. Robert P. Knight, Chairman.

Editorial Notes—Personal and General

DR. and MRS NED BURLESON and sons of Prague, are spending the winter in New Orleans, where Dr. Burleson is taking postgraduate work at Tulane University.

DR. W. H. NEWLIN, Sallisaw, has been appointed as County Health Superintendent of Sequoyah County.

DR. D. E. LITTLE, Eufaula, has been appointed County Health Superintendent of McIntosh County.

DR. J. W. FRANCIS, Perry, has been appointed County Health Superintendent of Noble County.

---o---

News of the County Medical Societies

PITTSBURG County Medical Society met February 17th with Doctors A. R. Sugg and E. M. Gullatt, of Ada, as their guest speakers. Their subjects were "Perinephretic Pathology" and "Empyema" respectively.

MUSKOGEE County Medical Society met February 6, with Dr. A. Ray Wiley, Tulsa, and Dr. V. K. Allen, Oklahoma City, as their guests. They spoke on "The Relation of Endocrines to Neoplasma of the Breast" and "Individual Technique, in Ano-Rectal Surgery," respectively.

---o---

OBITUARIES

DOCTOR JOHN M. WELLS

Dr. John M. Wells (Dec. 14, 1875-Jan. 25, 1939) was born in Livingston, Tenn., December 14, 1875. He was married in 1905 to Miss Jeanette McNabb at Aurora, Mo. Was graduated from Vanderbilt University at Nashville in 1909. Doctor Wells had Post Graduate work from Northwestern University, Chicago, Tulane University, New Orleans and Vanderbilt University. After graduation he moved to Newby community south of Bristow, Okla., where he engaged in private practice until 1915 when he moved to Bristow and had lived there ever since. He became associated in 1926 with the Bristow Clinic and was a member of the staff until March, 1936, when he resumed private practice. Dr. Wells was a member of the Masonic and Odd Fellows lodges, of the Creek County Medical Association and the Presbyterian Church. He was a past president of the local Rotary Club.

He is survived by the widow, two sons, one daughter and four grandchildren. Milton K. Wells, U. S. Vice Consul, Lima, Peru, Raymond P. Wells, Jefferson City, Mo., and Mrs. Jack Carman, Bristow, Okla. He also leaves one brother, Dr. M. H. Wells, Watertown, Tenn.

Dr. Wells died of pneumonia and a heart ailment. Burial was in Oak Crest Memorial Park, Bristow, Okla.

DR. CHARLES B. BARKER

Born in Niobe, New York, February 27, 1884.

Graduated from Loyola University Medical College, Chicago, Ill., 1912. Internship at Illinois Charitable Eye and Ear Infirmary, Chicago.

Came to Guthrie, 1913.

Married to Dr. Pauline Quillin, 1914, with whom he operated eye, ear, nose and throat clinic.

In 1925 took as their associate Dr. Wm. C. Miller.

Took courses in ophthalmology and otolaryngology in Vienna, 1927, and Egypt, 1932.

Member American Medical Association, Oklahoma State Medical Society, Logan County Medical Society, Kansas City Society of Ophthalmology and Otolaryngology. In 1923 passed American Board of Otolaryngology. In 1930 received Fellowship in American College of Surgeons.

Died February 12, 1939, at St. Anthony Hospital, Oklahoma City, of streptococcus septicemia.

DOCTOR ARTHUR E. HALE

RESOLUTION:

At a recent meeting of the Woods-Alfalfa County Medical Society the following resolution was enacted:

WHEREAS, our fellow member and esteemed co-worker, Dr. Arthur E. Hale, has been called by the Great Physician, and

WHEREAS, for many years he was a prominent and active member of our Society and our profession, and

WHEREAS, his professional achievements as a specialist in eye, ear, nose and throat work has made him recognized by the doctors of these counties and his state, as one of the most beloved members of the medical profession,

THEREFORE Be It Resolved by the Woods-Alfalfa County Medical Society that we record our sadness, and in his untimely going we hold in memory his splendid skill and wonderful personality as a professional man, one who was always generous in his services to the poor, an active civic leader, a prominent Boy Scout worker and above all a gentleman of the first rank, and

BE IT FURTHER RESOLVED that a copy of these resolutions be made a part of the minutes of this meeting, and a copy be sent to the members of the family and that a copy be published in the Journal of the Oklahoma State Medical Association and local newspapers.

Signed: Woods-Alfalfa Medical Society,
C. A. Traverse,
L. T. Lancaster, Committee.

RECENT DEATHS
(Insufficient Data for Obituaries)

Dr. Chas. B. Barker, Guthrie, January, 1939.
Dr. J. P. Bartley, Duncan, February, 1939.
Dr. Ross D. Long, Oklahoma City, January, 1939.
Dr. S. M. Meredith, Vinita, January, 1939.
Dr. J. P. Nelson, Beggs, February, 1939.
Dr. A. G. Wainright, Tulsa, January, 1939.
Dr. J. M. Wells, Bristow, January, 1939.

Foundation Prize

The American Association of Obstetricians, Gynecologists and Abdominal Surgeons announces that the annual Foundation Prize for this year will be $100.00. Those eligible include only (1) interns, residents, or graduate students in Obstetrics, Gynecology and Abdominal Surgery, and (2) physicians (M.D. degree) who are actually practicing or teaching Obstetrics, Gynecology or Abdominal Surgery.

Competing manuscripts must (1) be presented in triplicate under a nom-de-plume to the Secretary of the Association before June 1st, (2) be limited to 5,000 words and such illustrations as are necessary for a clear exposition of the thesis, and (3) be typewritten (double-spaced) on one side of the sheets, with ample margins.

The successful thesis must be presented at the next annual (September) meeting of the Association, without expense to the Association and in conformity with its regulations.

For further details, address Dr. James R. Bloss, Secretary, 418 11th Street, Huntington, W. Va.

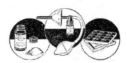
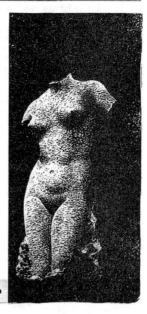

ABSTRACTS : REVIEWS : COMMENTS
and CORRESPONDENCE

SURGERY AND GYNECOLOGY
Abstracts, Reviews and Comments from
LeRoy Long Clinic
714 Medical Arts Building, Oklahoma City

Surgery for Ulcerative Colitis: Fred W. Rankin, M.D., Sc.D., F.A.C.S.; Surgery, Gynecology and Obstetrics; February 15, 1939; Vol. 68, No. 2A, page 306.

This disease of the large bowel is characterized pathologically by ulcerations, abscesses, and scars, and clinically by a syndrome associated with diarrhea, blood and pus in the stool, violent febrile reaction, prostration and weakness followed by periods of remission and with a proneness to multiple complications. Many names have been given to this ailment. It seems probable that American surgeons have been discussing a different pathological entity from continental surgeons when they speak of "chronic ulcerative colitis." This probably explains the divergent opinions on the etiology, pathology, and particularly the treatment of this not uncommon disease.

The typical clinical course, along with sigmoidoscopic and roentgenographic evidence, accurately establishes the diagnosis.

Medical management of chronic ulcerative colitis, which consists of a dietary regime, administration of vitamin C, elimination of focal infection, and the use of vaccines and serum, is effectual in most of the cases to a certain degree. Intractability to medical treatment with resulting damage of considerable extent to the colon, from which follows its loss of function and under which conditions the colon becomes filled with pus and detritus and is a source of absorption, is the principal indication for surgery.

In the author's opinion, surgery for chronic ulcerative colitis (as for duodenal ulcer) is indicated only for the complications which occur in about 15 per cent of the cases. These complications, except for hemorrhage and perforation, occur mostly in the chronic, intractable stages of the disease and fall readily into several classifications: (1) perforation, abscess formation, and hemorrhage usually occurring during the acute stages; (2) polyposis; (3) cancer developing on polyposis; (4) visceral degenerative changes; (5) unique complications such as erythemia nodosum, pyodermia gangrenosa, liver abscess, gastro-jejunocolic fistula, etc.; (6) evidences of focal infection, the lead-pipe colon filled with pus furnishing the source, as in arthritis; and (7) rectal complications such as stricture, fissure, peri-anal abscess, etc.

These complications, depending upon their distribution, the extension of the disease, and the acuteness or chronicity of the disease in each individual case, are indications for surgery of various types. The distribution is of particular importance because in 80 per cent of chronic ulcerative colitis cases as diagnoses by X-ray, the involvement of the large bowel is very extensive, being beyond the rectosigmoid juncture. In the experience of the author regional or segmental ulcerative colitis occurs very infrequently, the usual experience being that the disease has involved a major portion of the large bowel.

The operative procedures usually employed are: (1) colostomy; (2) ileostomy; (3) segmental resection by exteriorization; (4) subtotal colectomy following ileosigmoidostomy; and (5) subtotal or total colectomy following ileostomy.

Dr. Rankin's conclusions are as follows:

"1. Surgery in ulcerative colitis is indicated only for complications. These complications occur, first, as rectal or perirectal lesions, or second, usually affect the entire colon from rectosigmoid to cecum. The removal of part or all of the large bowel for chronic ulcerative colitis is definitely desirable when the colon has lost its function and becomes a focus of absorption.

"2. Surgery in the acute, fulminating or hemorrhagic forms of ulcerative colitis have few, if any, advantages. In this type of condition, ileostomy which completely by-passes the fecal current may be done under local anesthesia and occasionally appears to accomplish something.

"3. Operations for colectomy, total or subtotal, should be carried out in multiple stages. Multiple stage operations increase the margin of safety enormously and sufficient time after performance of ileostomy should be allowed to elapse before resection is undertaken, to replace fluid loss, balance the blood chemistry, and increase body weight and strength.

"4. Mortality statistics, following colectomy, parallel statistics for surgery of other major lesions of the colon.

"5. The treatment of chronic ulcerative colitis is predominantly medical and no operation should be attempted until all other efforts have proved futile. But when surgery is undertaken, it should be only after adequate and prolonged preoperative preparation and rehabilitation."

LeRoy D. Long.

Urologic Complications Following Complete and Supravaginal Hysterectomy: A. J. Murphy; American Journal of Obstetrics and Gynecology; February, 1939, Vol. 37, No. 2, page 201.

This is a study of the urologic complications following complete and supravaginal hysterectomy at the Woman's Hospital in New York City during the past eight years. It was undertaken largely because of the increasing number of advocates of routine complete hysterectomy and because of the fact that during the last eight years there had been 438 complete hysterectomies, whereas in a period of the same duration from 1922 to 1929 there were only 223 such operations in the Woman's Hospital.

During the last eight years at the Woman's Hospital there were performed 1,229 supravaginal operations while during the same time 438 complete hysterectomies were done. Forty-seven of the supravaginal operations were complicated by an acute postoperative pyelonephritis and 47 of the complete hysterectomies had a similar complication or three times as many as in the supravaginal series.

In the supravaginal group of 1,229 operations,

there were only three ureteral traumatic complications and the bladder was accidentally opened while separating it from the anterior surface of the uterus in two patients. In all of these the injury was recognized and repaired with no additional trouble.

In the series of complete or total hysterectomies, numbering 438, the bladder was accidentally opened twice and there were ten serious urological complications. Of these, four patients had left ureterovaginal fistula resulting in one death, one nephrectomy, destruction of function of one kidney by radiotherapy and one patient unable to be traced but probably requiring nephrectomy in order to be cured.

The right ureter was divided in three patients. In these three, repair was made at once and they had an uneventful postoperative recovery.

There were three vesicovaginal fistulas. The three were operated upon within four months and cured of their fistulas.

Three patients were readmitted to the hospital with an acute pyelonephritis.

It was, therefore, shown in this study that acute postoperative pyelonephritis was three times more frequent following complete hysterectomy. However, it was noted in their cases that such infections were not as serious after complete hysterectomy as those which developed after the supravaginal operation.

"In this series of cases ureteral and bladder injury was ten times more frequent following complete hysterectomy." "The seriousness of unrecognized ureteral injury with late renal complications cannot be minimized."

The author concludes that routine complete hysterectomy is not advisable because of the greater frequency of urinary infection and ureteral and bladder injury.

Comment: This study is an important one principally from the standpoint of demonstrating the fact that serious urinary tract infections and injuries occur more frequently with total or complete hysterectomies than with the supravaginal operation.

Despite the arguments of the advocates for routine total or complete hysterectomy, it is the general feeling among gynecologists that supravaginal hysterectomies will meet the requirement for operative procedure in the greatest number of patients needing hysterectomy. The choice of the complete or total hysterectomy over the supravaginal procedure rests entirely in the condition of the cervix, the general health of the patient as an operative risk, and the experience of the individual operator in the two procedures. In other words, the election of complete hyserectomy in preference to the supravaginal procedure is an individual matter with each patient and each surgeon.

Upon the basis of this report and the experience of most pelvic surgeons there can be little doubt that the urinary complications are more frequent and serious after complete hysterectomy. This does not mean that complete hysterectomies should not be elected in spite of this additional risk when the cervix is in such condition that the risk of subsequent malignancy is probably far greater than the operative risk incurred.

Wendell Long.

Bartholinitis and Skeneitis Due to Trichomonas Vaginalis; H. A. Shelanski and Saul P. Savitz; American Journal of Obstetrics and Gynecology; February, 1939, Vol. 37, No. 2, page 294.

These authors discovered that fresh smears taken from the glandular secretions of Bartholin's and Skene's glands in patients who had recurrent attacks of trichomonas vaginalis vaginitis were positive for vaginal trichomoniasis.

"The clinical picture is typical and in most cases resembles gonorrheal bartholinitis or skeneitis. However, some of the cases show only a slight swelling of the labia and are not quite as inflamed or edematous as are the gonorrheal cases."

Their recurrent cases demonstrating trichomona infestation of Bartholin's and Skene's glands were treated by injecting the glands with one cc. of one per cent aqueous solution of silver picrate. They found that two injections in seven patients and that one patient required four injections while another required the maximum of five injections. The injection of the glands was followed by the silver picrate treatment for vaginal trichomoniasis.

In two patients the Bartholin glands were excised. Each patient was observed for a period of four months after the last treatment and at the end of that time all were found to be negative.

The discussion and conclusions of the authors are quoted below because of their importance in the proper recognition and treatment of the resistant recurring instances of trichomonas vaginalis vaginitis.

"One of the outstanding obstacles in treating trichomonas infestations in the vaginal tract is reinfestation, for which several explanations have been suggested such as:

"1. Reinfestation from the male.

"2. Recurrence due to the organisms in the cervical plug of mucus.

"3. Infestation of the glands of Bartholin and Skene.

"4. Contaminated plumbing fixtures on which organisms will remain viable for as long as 24 hours if kept moist.

"5. Reinfestation from the bladder or urethra.

"Silver picrate has been used in the treatment of trichomonas vaginalis and has been shown to be highly germicidal to this organism in vitro. Thus its use in trichomonas bartholinitis and skeneitis is an extension of these former investigations."

Conclusions:

"Trichomonas vaginalis has been demonstrated in Bartholin and Skene's glands, and is a specific factor in producing bartholinitis and skeneitis.

"2. The presence of trichomonas vaginalis in these glands demonstrates that they act as foci of infestation. These glands, therefore, are one source of constant reinfestation in recurrent cases of trichomonas vaginalis vaginitis.

"3. Injection of the glands with one per cent solution of silver picrate has been found to be a satisfactory treatment for this infestation."

Comment: I have seen several patients who had an infestation of Skene's and Bartholin's glands which apparently caused reinfestation of the vagina with recurrence of the symptoms. These patients responded well when the infested areas were properly treated. This article also bears upon the very practical subject of both non-specific Bartholinitis and Skeneitis as well as a cause for reinfestation in some of the persistent recurring instances of trichomonas vaginalis vaginitis.

It has been our practice for a number of years to use the pentavalent arsenicals rather than silver picrate in the treatment of this disease.

This method has been satisfactory and silver picrate has, therefore, not been employed extensively by us.

Wendell Long.

Selective Surgery in Operable Rectal Cancer: George E. Binkley; The American Journal of Surgery; January, 1939, page 51.

There is no one operative procedure that is suitable for routine employment in all cases. Two factors, one the variation in the extent of disease at the time patients are referred for treatment, and two the variation in the ability of patients to withstand radical resection, make selective surgery preferable to the routine use of any one method.

The two types of operation that have proven of greatest value and appear worthy of consideration in selecting treatment for operable diseases are: (1) abdomino-perineal resections completed in one or two stages; and (2) perineal resections with or without preliminary colostomy. Each of the above procedures has a field of usefulness in the surgical treatment of this disease. Most appropriate selection can be made from the knowledge of the comparative advantages and limitations of each procedure, the pathologic factors of the disease presented, and the general physical condition and the psychology of the patient.

If it were possible to obtain patients for operation in the early incipient stages, treatment would be greatly simplified and excellent results obtained by the majority of the above methods of procedure. Unfortunately, many operable lesions are well established and extensive at the time patients come under observation. The extent of the disease has a marked bearing upon the prognosis. The ability of patients to withstand operation must be very carefully considered. Combined abdomino-perineal resection is accompanied by greater degree of shock and more severe complications than perineal resection. In the treatment of cancer of the rectum, it is advisable to employ the most radical dissection that the patient appears able to withstand, since one is never positive of the extent of the disease.

The problem of selecting treatment is a comparatively simple one when dealing with patients in good physical condition. Unfortunately, rectal cancer usually occurs in patients of mature and old age. Many of these patients are also victims of heart, lung, kidney, metabolic, or other chronic diseases, factors which greatly increase the hazards of successful resection. It is impossible to treat rectal cancer adequately without a certain percentage of operable fatalities. The latter, however, may be held at a reasonably low figure by attempting to keep the treatment within the tolerance of the patient and at the same time to afford him the benefit of the most radical resection that he is able to withstand. In recent years operable mortality, following all types of resections, has been lessened by more careful preoperative preparation, by liberal employment of blood transfusions, better surgery and more detailed after treatment.

Abdomino-perineal resection is considered the ideal surgical method of approach in eradicating rectal and rectosigmoidal cancers. Unfortunately, it must be reserved for good surgical risks. Making this procedure a two-stage affair allows one to accept for operation patients who are not in quite as good shape. Nevertheless, even for a two-stage type of abdomino-perineal resection the general condition of the patient must necessarily be fairly good. It is this fact (which the author does not mention) which has caused me to become less enthusiastic about abdomino-perineal resections. Also it has been repeatedly demonstrated (particularly by Lockhart-Mummery) that a large amount of gland-bearing tissue can be removed with perineal excision. Lockhart-Mummery's cases of perineal resection compare favorably with cases of abdomino-perineal resection by Miles and others. The operative mortality in any surgeon's hands is at least 50 per cent less with perineal excision than with combined abdomino-perineal excision. (Dr. Binkley gives an operative immediate mortality of 12.5 per cent for abdomino-perineal whereas he has a mortality of five per cent for perineal excision.)

However, it must be admitted that from the standpoint of obtaining clinical cure that perineal resections are best suited for cancer within the lower half of the rectum in which the disease is well localized.

Selective surgery in operable rectal cancer is advisable because of variations in (1) the location of lesions, (2) the extent of the disease, and (3) the physical condition of the patient. If the patient is a good surgical risk, abdomino-perineal resection, completed in one or two stages, probably affords the widest form of dissection, and is to be preferred for that reason.

Perineal resections, with or without preliminary colostomy (preferably with preliminary colostomy), are best suited for tumors situated in the lower two-thirds of the rectum in patients classified as only fair or poor surgical risks.

Resections which attempt continuity of bowel and sphincter control have not proved to be very satisfactory in the treatment of rectal cancer. Perineal anus is less satisfactory than permanent abdominal colostomy. Procedures such as local excision, perineal resections with preservation of the anal sphincter, and abdominal resections with anastomosis, are employed in an effort to avoid a permanent artificial anus. Any of these procedures is probably unsatisfactory in most cases and it certainly lends to increase in recurrences because they may result in incomplete removal of the cancer.

LeRoy D. Long.

EYE, EAR, NOSE AND THROAT

Edited by Marvin D. Henley, M.D.
911 Medical Arts Building, Tulsa

The Fluid Equilibrium of the Body and Its Relation to the Eye. J. Douglas Robertson, M.D., London. The British Journal of Ophthalmology, February, 1939.

There is a discussion and definition of the vascular and lymphatic systems and the tissue spaces. The interchange between these systems include a passage of gases, water, inorganic salts, organic crystalloids, and in certain tissues colloids.

Factors which normally play a part in the distribution of fluid throughout the body are:

1. Hydrostatic pressure in the capillaries.
2. Colloid osmotic pressure of the plasma.
3. The pressure of fluid in the tissues.

Methods of upsetting the fluid equilibrium of the body are discussed. Experiments are given and "the conclusions drawn are that the eyes does not share in the water-logging common to other tissues of the body. The equilibrium level of the intra-ocular pressure is not maintained by the hydrostatic pressure in the capillaries minus the difference in osmotic pressure between the aqueous humour and the blood."

Further experiments proved that the eye does not behave as a simple fluid depot as do connective tissue spaces, and the aqueous humour does not appear to be formed by the same process as the tissue fluid.

Evidence that the aqueous humour does circulate is supported by observations of Priestley Smith, Friedenwald and Pierce and three pertinent examples are given.

Discussion is given as to the site of formation of the aqueous humour and also the site of removal of the aqueous humour.

This appears to be a very valuable contribution to ophthalmological research and must have entailed an incalculable amount of work.

The author's own conclusions are:

1. The formation of the aqueous humour is not

governed by the same simple laws that govern the lymph, pleural and peritoneal fluids and other dialysates. Dialysis is therefore not a satisfactory explanation of the production of the aqueous humour.

2. When the osmotic equilibrium in the body is disturbed in various ways the fluid formed in the stomach and the eye are disturbed rather similarly. This suggests that a secretory process in the eye may play some part in controlling the intra-ocular pressure.

3. Ample evidence is available that the aqueous humour circulates from the posterior to the anterior chamber.

4. Evidence seems to point to the site of formation of the aqueous humour being in the ciliary process.

5. The aqueous humour leaves the eye at the angle of the anterior chamber into Schlemm's canal by some process which is not osmosis, and no fluid can leave the eye normally by the posterior chamber.

Late Results in Retinal-Detachment Operations. Dohrmann K. Pischel, M.D., San Francisco. American Journal of Ophthalmology, February, 1939.

The article is opened with a discussion of Weve's results in his operations at the Utrecht Eye Clinic. F. Ramach's results at Linder's Clinic in Vienna are also discussed. These reports do not give the findings at the end of a certain period as found on re-examination post-operatively.

The author's thought was what late results followed such a radical surgical insult as the eyeball suffered during a diathermy operation. He lists seven possible untoward late results: reappearance of the retinal detachment, degeneration of the macula, atrophy of parts of the retina, optic atrophy, scleral ectasia, troublesome hyperphoria and most important of all development of cataract.

Sixty-three patients are reported who had been operated at least a year. Of these 37 or 58 per cent were considered successful. Only 32 of these could be found for examination.

The safer method of multiple diathermy puncture was used in all cases. Patients were kept in bed for two weeks after operation. The earlier cases operated had only one line of pins inserted; later cases had double rows and transcleral treatment or application of bident electrode. Stenopeic spectacles were worn for two months.

In regard to the reappearance of the detachment he shows four cases in which the detachment recurred within three months of operation; the second operation was successful in all four cases. Another patient was operated three times before a cure was effected. In the author's opinion if a case remains cured three months, there is no danger of further relapse.

There was not any late degeneration of the macula found; no late atrophy of the retina was noted; there was no ectasia of the sclera noted.

Troublesome hyperphoria is reviewed in 16 cases where there was a complete tenotomy of a vertical rectus. He says this condition "never develops as a result of a complete tenotomy of a vertical rectus (with muscle resutured to insertion), when only one operation is undertaken. A slight hyperphoria may develop without tenotomy, due to the formation of scar tissue."

Considered the most important late development of all is cataract. The author's analysis showed only one case of cataract which developed in previously uninjured lenses; three cases of traumatic complicated cataract showed an increase in density of the lens opacity, as did one of complicated cataract.

Ruling out cataracts, vision was retained, when regained.

The time element on these cases showed: Four cases of more than four years' standing; five of more than three years' standing; six of more than two years' standing and 18 of more than a years' standing.

Incidence of Malignant Tumors of the Head and Neck. Noah D. Fabricant, M.D., Chicago. Archives of Otolaryngology, January, 1939.

This is a statistical survey of malignant tumors (confirmed microscopically) of the head and neck which occurred in the Department of Otology, Rhinology, and Laryngology of the University of Illinois College of Medicine during a period of seven years from July 1, 1930, to July 1, 1937. These were gleaned from 1,103 biopsies. Undoubtedly there were more malignancies than this during the stated interval since there are approximately 2,500 patients admitted per annum but only proven cases are reported.

The youngest patient was a boy of 17 years; the oldest was a man of 85 years. A total of 87.37 per cent occurred in men; 12.63 per cent occurred in women (seven times as frequent in men as in women). This ratio the author thinks is of significance, since an analysis of 250 malignant tumors in Cook County Hospital showed 88.4 per cent in men and 11.6 per cent in women.

Most investigators show the incidence to be greatest in the fifth decade with the fourth and sixth decades in the second place. This survey shows most malignancies occurring during the fifth decade, then the sixth and fourth decades, respectively.

The survey shows a two-page chart of the anatomic site and type of tumor. This shows the majority of malignancies occur in the larynx; next in numerical significance is the nose and paranasal sinuses; respectively then follows the esophagus, tongue, bronchi and tonsils.

Seventy per cent of the total number (249) were squamous cell; 8.7 per cent were basal cell carcinomas; 2.7 per cent were transitional cell carcinomas; 2.7 were undifferentiated tumors and 2 per cent were adeno-carcinomas.

"The heavy predominance of squamous cell carcinoma is manifested by the fact that 95 per cent of the tumors invading the larynx, almost 97 per cent of those invading the esophagus, 100 per cent of those invading the bronchi and the tongue, 55 per cent of those invading the bronchi and the neck and 90 per cent of those invading the tonsils were of this type."

Bronchoscopic and esophagoscopic examinations are necessary.

The Treatment of Acute Nasal Accessory Disease. A. C. Furstenberg, M.D., Ann Arbor, Michigan. Annals of Otology, Rhinology and Laryngology, December, 1938.

"The only generalization, which seems accurate about the treatment of acute nasal accessory sinus disease is that an inordinate variety of methods are in practice and that no specific cure, either medicinal, surgical or biological, has yet been discovered."

This is a confusing subject to the medical student as well as to the one who has been graduated many years. Furstenberg aptly sums it up in the above paragraph. Eminent authorities differ to an extreme degree on the method of treatment. Furstenberg admits the lack of knowledge on the subject by discussing in particular the negative phases of the disease and the things not to do.

In the Department of Otolaryngology, University of Michigan, there is no bone work done during the course of any acute infection. Condemned is the use of irritating solutions, such as silver salts, colloidal preparations, mercurochrome, etc., suction, tamponade or surgical intervention. Conservative methods are employed such as might be used in any infection. These include: rest, promotion of drainage (steam inhalations, unmedicated, and three per cent aqueous solution of ephederine sprayed in nose or dropped in nasal cavity according to the Proetz method), relief of pain (morphine and codeine), hydration and nutritional support of the patient. The argument given against irrigation is that frequently there is a pansinusitis and irrigation of, say a single antrum, is a futile gesture. Hot and cold applications are thought by Furstenberg to be of doubtful value.

In the "mine-run" of complications that appear in this clinic are osteomyelitis, orbital cellulitis, blood stream infections, etc. It was noted that the one who had such a complication gave a history of some surgical manipulation at some recent date before appearing at the clinic. Patients hospitalized by the clinic early in an acute sinusitis and treated conservatively as outlined did not develop such sequellae.

A series of 300 cases were observed. History, clinical examination and radiographic study showed them to be acute nasal accessory sinus infections. The conservative treatment was used. They were hospitalized for a period of one week, the first five days of which were spent in bed. Six months to two years later check-ups were done on this group; 296 were asymptomatic; four showed a chronic maxillary sinusitis, but gave history of an exacerbation with surgical intervention since they had left the hospital.

There is an account given of the experiments of the effect of mucin. Furstenberg thinks that when bacteria are suspended in a menstruum of mucin, they become most destructive invaders of the animal host.

Furstenberg says: "After taking into account the possibilities of error in diagnosis, the vagaries and fallacies of statistical computations, not to mention the whims and prejudices of observers, we are still forced to the conclusion that utmost conservatism as the treatment of acute nasal accessory sinusitis is worthy of avowed recommendation by members of our profession."

---o---

INTERNAL MEDICINE
Edited by Hugh Jeter, M.D., 1200 North Walker, Oklahoma City

Studies on Trichinosis—XII The Preparation and Use of An Improved Trichina Antigen; by John Bozicevich. From the Public Health Reports, Vol. 53, No. 48, December 2, 1938, pg. 2130-2138.

In connection with a series of studies carried on in the Division of Zoology, the National Institute of Health, of the United States Public Health Service on various aspects of trichinosis, an attempt was made to effect improvements in the preparation of trichina antigen in order that more reliable results might be obtained in the diagnosis of trichinosis by the precipitin and intradermal tests.

The author describes various methods for the recovery of trichina larvae with a minimum of debris, and for the preparation of trichina antigen by extraction with a neutral 0.85 per cent solution of sodium chloride without the use of preservatives. Such antigen may be put up in hermetically sealed vials and stored at room temperature until needed for use.

A convenient method for measuring intradermal

reactions is described. The progressive development of the reaction is followed by means of cellophane tracings which can afterwards be measured by means of a planimeter. By this method a progressive graphic picture of the reaction may be preserved for further reference.

The author concludes that the saline extracted antigen is superior as a diagnostic agent to other types of antigen.

Studies on Trichinosis—VII. The Past and Present Status of Trichinosis in the United States, and the Indicated Control Measures; by Maurice C. Hall, Chief, Division of Zoology, National Institute of Health, United States Public Health Service. Public Health Reports, Vol. 53, No. 33, August 19, 1938, pages 1472-1486.

Since 1936 the Division of Zoology, National Institute of Health, United States Public Health Service, has undertaken a study of trichinosis in the United States. On the basis of this study the author has arrived at some definite conclusions. They are:

1. Abundant evidence indicates quite clearly that trichinosis is probably a greater problem in the United States than in any other country in the world.

2. Human trichinosis rests primarily on the basis of swine trichinosis.

3. Swine trichinosis rests primarily on a basis of uncooked or inadequately cooked pork scraps fed to swine in garbage, table scraps, swill and similar material.

4. The indicated control of trichinosis in the United States is primarily a matter of keeping such uncooked pork scraps out of the feed of swine and either cooking such feed as garbage or refraining from feeding any food containing pork scraps.

5. Rats appear to have a very minor roll in the production of porcine trichinosis.

6. The incidence of trichinosis in man has not been lowered during the past 50 years.

7. Prompt action looking towards the control of trichinosis is imperative for the protection of the public health on the one hand and the protection and improvement of the swine industry and the packing industry on the other hand.

The author discusses the prevalence of trichinosis in the United States 50 years ago and has compared it to the incidence of trichinosis today. In addition he presents the incidence of trichinosis in European countries as compared to that of the United States. In this discussion the author states that the lowest of the recent figures for the United States is higher than all but one of the European figures cited.

Further, the author discusses the effectiveness of previous control measures, the prevention of trichinosis in swine and outlines the organization of a program for the control of human trichinosis.

---o---

PLASTIC SURGERY
Edited by
GEO. H. KIMBALL, M.D., F.A.C.S.
404 Medical Arts Building, Oklahoma City

Plastic Surgery in Children. The Medical and Psychological Aspects of Deformity. Claire L. Straith, M.D., and E. Hoyt De Kleine, M.D., Detroit. Journal of American Medical Association, December 24, 1938, Vol. 3.

The past two decades have brought forth intenseive campaigns in behalf of crippled and otherwise physically handicapped children of this country. Equally serious, but less widely publicized, are the childhood handicaps that are the results of deformity. By "deformity" we refer to those visible abnormalities which handicap their victims because of a peculiar appearance.

As examples of this group, the authors cite, harelip and cleft palate, facial birthmarks, saddle nose, hunchback, webbed fingers, crossed eyes, ptosis of the eyelid, disfiguring scars, lop ears, crooked teeth and contractures resulting from burns. Many of these congenital deformities and others are acquired during childhood. Of the acquired deformities, many might have been minimized at their onset or might have been prevented. In addition to efforts at prevention, the greatest service to such children is the work being done in the correction of such defects by plastic surgery. Plastic surgeons must of course give due credit to the achievements of orthopedists, dentists, ophthalmogoligists, and dermatologists, whose efforts have made many other deformities amenable to treatment.

Although the effects of deformity are largely psychologic, the ultimate responsibility for their management generally falls on the shoulders of some physician. It is for these physicians that we present this summary of the pertinent facts relating to childhood deformities. Let it be said at the outset that we are not professional psycologists. We are primarily surgeons interested in the correction of these deformities and our discussion on psychology is derived from personal experience in the management of such cases.

The authors list three psychologic effects of deformity:

1. Inferiority and Shame: Children are notoriously observant of the unusual. A great deal of undue attention is invariably directed at any cosmetic abnormality possessed by a playmate. They do not attempt to refrain from remarking about the afflicted companion. Sometimes he is nicknamed to suit the deformity. It is no wonder then that the majority of children quickly develop a feeling of inferiority and shame. As the child matures he becomes increasingly more sensitive.

2. Modifications of Self Expression: Lowery tells us that personality depends on two fundamental drives. The one is for self-expression and the other for conformance with accepted social standards. When this is applied to the deformed child, the result is obvious. The deformed child may have every mental and physical faculty for self-expression possessed by other children but because of his deformity he is either restrained by others or avoids the personal contacts necessary for such expression. Activities are either shunned or altered.

3. Anti-social Tendencies: Before a handicapped child can gain recognition of the group he must first overcome the tendency of other children to maintain the natural impression of abnormality and undesirability. Many unfortunates are inclined to give in to these difficulties and to make no effort to become one of the group. Others become resentful, blame is placed on all manner of circumstances and people. These children may develop objectionable social behavior, may resort to criminal tendencies and activities, etc.

The rarely spontaneous reaction occurs when the handicapped child sets out to make himself popular regardless of obstacles. This is a goal toward which mental therapy should be aimed when dealing with handicapped children.

Surgical Care of Deformities

1. Prevention: Very little is known about the prevention of congenital deformities. Acquired deformities on the other hand are largely preventable through safety measures. However, once an injury capable of producing a deformity has been inflicted, the preventive measures employed are entirely dependent on the resources of the physician responsible for its care.

Accidental injuries to the face lead the list of acquired deformities. The authors relate the necessary management of such cases.

2. Earliest Possible Correction: When a deformity of any type of severity is present the most important single item in the avoidance of undesirable personality changes is the most complete surgical restoration possible at the earliest date that is feasible. This is a hard and fast rule with no exceptions of which we are aware.

It is of particular importance to have deformities corrected if possible before the child enters school.

3. Management of Common Deformities: Among the congenital deformities there is a group which allows correction immediately after birth. Most conspicuous of these are the harelips. In the absence of specific contraindications to surgery, harelip should be corrected during the first week of life. With paregoric for premedication this repair can be safely and efficiently performed with a simple nerve block anesthesia. We have performed such surgery within 24 hours after birth, often with the child sleeping through the operation.

Cleft palates, we feel, should not be operated before the child is from 18 to 21 months of age, the authors state. Earlier than that the palatal tissue is too flimsy to permit adequate repair without tearing. Prevention of speech defects is the paramount aim, and, since most children begin to talk at about two years of age, this is the age choice for surgery of the cleft palate. Even after a satisfactory anatomic repair, speech training with hours of patient practice is required to insure a satisfactory speaking voice. In certain cases in which there is difficulty due to shortness of the palate, the Dorrance "push-back" operation may be performed to give the palate its needed length.

Plastic surgery involving the legs or abdomen must usually be delayed until the child passes the diaper age because of the danger of infection. This includes the use of skin or fascial grafts taken from the lower part of the abdomen and the upper part of the thighs.

The authors list a number of very common and very annoying deformities and use some very fine illustrations of each type. The authors are to be commended on the results shown by their procedure. Some of those listed and explained are, lop ears, nasal deformities, cleft palates, harelips, saddle nose, hump of nose, automobile injury to face, web fingers, contracture of axilla from burns, etc.

Development of Sound Mental Health

Surgical correction in early childhood is the most valuable method of preventing undesirable personality traits. Unfortunately early correction of the deformity in some instances is impossible; in others it is impossible to obtain a perfect cosmetic result. Theraphy, therefore, must often be supplemented by special training to prepare the child for his handicap. This so-called "special" training is really not special in any sense of the word. It is the same training that might be recommended for any normal child, with emphasis on certain aspects which are most important to the deformed child.

First, the deformed child must learn to "face the facts." He must learn to anticipate difficulties and to be self-reliant.

Second, the handicapped child is most likely to be deprived of many things commonly sought after for their supposed value; for example, money, friends, esteem, beauty, amusements and romance. Parents of such children should make every effort to help them readjust their sense of values. Above all, the children must learn that true friendship exists only in those who like them in spite of the deformities and irrespective of their possessions or ability to do something to buy their favor.

Thirdly, compensatory education and importance of speech training for children with cleft palate is almost as important as the surgical repair. Physical therapy and gymnastics are important for children with orthopedic deformities, and contractures from burns, after correction, frequently require muscular rehabilitation. It is known that crossed eyes are greatly improved by exercises to develop the use of extra-ocular muscles.

Summary:

1. Deformities in children are serious and have failed to attract adequate attention within the medical profession. The seriousness lies in the severe mental reactions and alterations of personality which result.

2. Many of the acquired deformities are preventable and the technical information regarding this phase of preventive medicine should be more widely publicized among medical schools and medical organizations.

3. Wherever possible childhood deformities should be corrected before the child reaches school age, and a few are best corrected within the first week of life.

4. Many childhood deformities have b e c o m e amenable to plastic surgery with the development of that specialty which has taken place since the World War.

5. In addition to surgical care, deformed children require more than ordinary "bringing up" at home and at school. They must be prepared to face greater hardships than normal persons and should be given special training to compensate for altered facilities for self-expression.

Comment: Dr. Straith is to be congratulated on a very comprehensive article pointing out the complexes which may develop in some of the congenital anomalies. Men doing plastic surgery encounter these complexes often.

It is remarkable how they can be completely relieved by operation. The illustrations show that Dr. Straith is doing outstanding work in this field.

UROLOGY

Edited by D. W. Branham, M.D.
514 Medical Arts Building, Oklahoma City

The Influence of Sulfanilamide on Gonococci and Gonococcal Infections. Russell D. Herrold, M.D., and Edward Palmer, M.D., Chicago, Illinois. Reprinted from American J o u r n a l of Syphilis, Gonorrhea and Venereal Diseases, November, 1938.

This report presented by a careful observer seems to present an accurate picture of the present day status of sulfanilamide therapy of gonorrhea. Unlike the majority of papers presented the past year on this remarkable drug the authors have not had the 84 per cent average of successful cures reported by other investigators. However, their standards of evaluation have been more strict than those who have previously reported on the drug.

They are of the opinion that if the drug produces eradication of the gonococci under a period of 30 days, a successful result has been obtained. If complications are presented and are promptly controlled, even though benefit is not gained within a short period of time, it should be considered partially satisfactory. In a total of 89 cases a satisfactory result was obtained in approximately one-third and a partially satisfactory result in another one-third. No results or poor results were obtained in the remaining one-third of cases studied.

Other observations made on this form of therapy were; patients who previously had the disease showed better result than those with initial infections—also better results were obtained the earlier the drug was used in the course of the disease. In a substantial percentage of patients a latent or carrier state has been found to exist for long periods of time. Local treatment of the infected urethral and glandular structures is a valuable therapeutic adjunct and will aid in expediting cure.

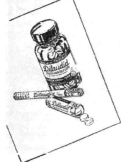
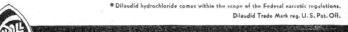

OFFICERS OKLAHOMA STATE MEDICAL ASSOCIATION

President, Dr. H. K. Speed, Sayre.

President-Elect, Dr. W. A. Howard, Chelsea.

Secretary-Treasurer-Editor, Dr. L. S. Willour, McAlester.

Executive Secretary, Mr. R. H. Graham, McAlester.

Speaker, House of Delegates, Dr. J. D. Osborn, Jr., Frederick.

Vice Speaker, House of Delegates, Dr. P. P. Nesbitt, Medical Arts Building, Tulsa.

Delegates to the A. M. A., Dr. W. Albert Cook, Medical Arts Building, Tulsa, 1938-39; Dr. McLain Rogers, Clinton, 1937-1938.

Meeting Place, Oklahoma City, May 1, 2, 3, 1939.

SPECIAL COMMITTEES 1938-39

Annual Meeting: Dr. H. K. Speed, Sayre; Dr. W. A. Howard, Chelsea; Dr. L. S. Willour, McAlester.

Conservation of Hearing: Dr. H. F. Vandever, Chairman, Enid; Dr. J. B. Hollis, Mangum; Dr. Chester McHenry, Oklahoma City.

Conservation of Vision: Dr. W. M. Gallaher, Chairman, Shawnee; Dr. Frank R. Vieregg, Clinton; Dr. Pauline Barker, Guthrie.

Crippled Children: Dr. Earl McBride, Chairman, Oklahoma City; Dr. Roy L. Fisher, Frederick; Dr. M. B. Glismann, Okmulgee.

Industrial Service and Traumatic Surgery: Dr. Cyril U. Clymer, Medical Arts Bldg., Oklahoma City; Dr. J. Wm. Finch, Hobart; Dr. J. A. Rutledge, Ada.

Maternity and Infancy: Dr. George R. Osborn, Chairman, Tulsa; Dr. P. J. DeVanney, Sayre; Dr. Leila E. Andrews, Oklahoma City.

Necrology: Dr. G. H. Stagner, Chairman, Erick; Dr. James L. Shuler, Durant; Dr. S. D. Neely, Muskogee.

Post Graduate Medical Teaching: Dr. Henry H. Turner, Chairman, Oklahoma City; Dr. H. C. Weber, Bartlesville; Dr. Ned R. Smith, Tulsa.

Study and Control of Cancer: Dr. Wendell Long, Chairman, Oklahoma City; Dr. Paul B. Champlin, Enid; Dr. Ralph McGill, Tulsa.

Study and Control of Tuberculosis: Dr. Carl Puckett, Chairman, Oklahoma City; Dr. W. C. Tisdal, Clinton; Dr. F. P. Baker, Talihina.

Study and Control of Venereal Disease: Dr. Robert H. Akin, Chairman, Medical Arts Bldg., Oklahoma City; Dr. Shade D. Neely, Muskogee; Dr. D. V. Hudson, Medical Arts Bldg., Tulsa.

ADVISORY COUNCIL FOR AUXILIARY

Dr. H. K. Speed, Chairman..................................Sayre

Dr. C. J. Fishman..................................Oklahoma City

Dr. W. S. Larrabee..................................Tulsa

Dr. J. M. Watson..................................Enid

Dr. T. H. McCarley..................................McAlester

STANDING COMMITTEES 1938-39

Medical Defense: Dr. O. E. Templin, Chairman, Alva; Dr. L. C. Kuyrkendall, McAlester; Dr. E. Albert Aisenstadt, Picher.

Medical Economics: Dr. C. B. Sullivan, Cordell, Chairman; Dr. J. L. Patterson, Duncan; Dr. W. M. Browning, Waurika.

Medical Education and Hospital: Dr. V. C. Tisdal, Chairman, Elk City; Dr. Robert U. Patterson, Oklahoma City; Dr. H. M. McClure, Chickasha.

Public Policy and Legislation: Dr. Finis W. Ewing, Surety Bldg., Chairman, Muskogee; Dr. Tom Lowry, 1200 North Walker, Oklahoma City; Dr. O. C. Newman, Shattuck; Dr. R. O. Early, Medical Arts Bldg., Oklahoma City.

(The above committee co-ordinated by the following, selected from each councilor district.)

District No. 1.—Arthur E. Hale, Alva.

District No. 2.—McLain Rogers, Clinton.

District No. 3.—Thomas McElroy, Ponca City.

District No. 4.—L. H. Ritzhaupt, Guthrie.

District No. 5.—P. V. Annadown, Sulphur.

District No. 6.—R. M. Shepard, Tulsa.

District No. 7.—Sam A. McKeel, Ada.

District No. 8.—J. A. Morrow, Sallisaw.

District No. 9.—W. A. Tolleson, Eufaula.

District No. 10.—J. L. Holland, Madill.

Scientific Exhibits: Dr. E. Rankin Denny, Chairman, Tulsa; Dr. Robert H. Akin, Oklahoma City; Dr. R. C. Pigford, Tulsa.

Scientific Work: Dr. W. G. Husband, Chairman, Hollis; Dr. J. S. Rollins, Prague; Dr. J. L. Day, Supply.

Hospital Insurance Board—Dr. H. D. Collins, Oklahoma City; Dr. W. P. Neilson, Enid; Dr. R. L. Fisher, Frederick; Dr. W. A. Howard, Chelsea; Dr. P. M. McNeill, Oklahoma City.

Public Health:

Chairman—Dr. G. S. Baxter, Shawnee.

District No. 1.—C. W. Tedrowe, Woodward.

District No. 2.—E. W. Mabry, Altus.

District No. 3.—L. A. Mitchell, Stillwater.

District No. 4.—J. J. Gable, Norman.

District No. 5.—Geo. S. Barber, Lawton.

District No. 6.—C. E. Bradley, Tulsa.

District No. 7.—G. S. Baxter, Shawnee.

District No. 8.—M. M. De Arman, Miami.

District No. 9.—T. H. McCarley, McAlester.

District No. 10.—J. B. Clark, Coalgate.

SCIENTIFIC SECTIONS

General Surgery: Dr. F. L. Flack, Chairman, Nat'l Bank of Tulsa Bldg., Tulsa; Dr. John E. McDonald, Vice-Chairman, Medical Arts Bldg., Tulsa; Dr. John F. Burton, Secretary, Osler Building, Oklahoma City.

General Medicine: Dr. Frank Nelson, Chairman, 603 Medical Arts Bldg., Tulsa; Dr. E. R. Musick, Vice-Chairman, Medical Arts Bldg., Oklahoma City; Dr. Milam McKinney, Medical Arts Bldg., Oklahoma City.

Eye, Ear, Nose & Throat: Dr. E. H. Coachman, Chairman, Manhattan Bldg., Muskogee; Dr. F. M. Cooper, Vice-President, Medical Arts Bldg., Oklahoma City; Dr. James R. Reed, Secretary, Medical Arts Bldg., Oklahoma City.

Obstetrics and Pediatrics: Dr. C. W. Arrendell, Chairman, Ponca City; Dr. Carl F. Simpson, Vice-Chairman, Medical Arts Bldg., Tulsa; Dr. Ben H. Nicholson, Secretary, 300 West Twelfth Street, Oklahoma City.

Genito-Urinary Diseases and Syphilology: Dr. Elijah Sullivan, Chairman, Medical Arts Bldg., Oklahoma City; Dr. Henry Browne, Vice-Chairman, Medical Arts Bldg., Tulsa; Dr. Robert Akin, Secretary, 400 West Tenth, Oklahoma City.

Dermatology and Radiology: Dr. W. A. Showman, Chairman, Medical Arts Bldg., Tulsa; Dr. E. D. Greenberger, Vice-Chairman, McAlester; Dr. Hervey A. Foerster, Secretary, Medical Arts Bldg., Oklahoma City.

STATE BOARD OF MEDICAL EXAMINERS

Dr. Sam A. McKeel, Ada, President; Dr. C. E. Bradley, Tulsa, Vice-President; Dr. J. D. Osborn, Jr., Frederick, Secretary; Dr. O. C. Newman, Shattuck; Dr. L. E. Emanuel, Chickasha; Dr. S. D. Leslie, Okmulgee; Dr. G. H. Stagner, Erick.

STATE COMMISSIONER OF HEALTH

Dr. Grady F. Mathews, Oklahoma City.

COUNCILORS AND THEIR COUNTIES

District No. 1: Texas, Beaver, Cimarron, Harper, Ellis, Woods, Woodward, Alfalfa, Major, Dewey—Dr. O. E. Templin, Alva. (Term expires 1940.)

District No. 2: Roger Mills, Beckham, Greer, Harmon, Washita, Kiowa, Custer, Jackson, Tillman—Dr. V. C. Tisdal, Elk City. (Term expires 1939.)

District No. 3: Grant, Kay, Garfield, Noble, Payne, Pawnee—Dr. A. S. Risser, Blackwell. (Term expires 1941.)

District No. 4: Blaine, Kingfisher, Canadian, Logan, Oklahoma, Cleveland—Dr. Philip M. McNeill, Oklahoma City. (Term expires 1941.)

District No. 5: Caddo, Comanche, Cotton, Grady, Love, Stephens, Jefferson, Carter, Murray—Dr. Walter Hardy, Ardmore. (Term expires 1941.)

District No. 6: Osage, Creek, Washington, Nowata, Rogers, Tulsa—Dr. James Stevenson, Medical Arts Bldg., Tulsa. (Term expires 1941.)

District No. 7: Lincoln, Pontotoc, Pottawatomie, Okfuskee, Seminole, McClain, Garvin, Hughes—Dr. J. A. Walker, Shawnee. (Term expires 1939.)

District No. 8: Craig, Ottawa, Mayes, Delaware, Wagoner, Adair, Cherokee, Sequoyah, Okmulgee, Muskogee—Dr. E. A. Aisenstadt, Picher. (Term expires 1939.)

District No. 9: Pittsburg, Haskell, Latimer, LeFlore, McIntosh—Dr. L. C. Kuyrkendall, McAlester. (Term expires 1939.)

District No. 10: Johnson, Marshall, Coal, Atoka, Bryan, Choctaw, Pushmataha, McCurtain—Dr. J. S. Fulton, Atoka. (Term expires 1939.)

THE JOURNAL
OF THE
OKLAHOMA STATE MEDICAL ASSOCIATION

VOLUME XXXII	McALESTER, OKLAHOMA, APRIL, 1939	Number 4

Internal Derangements of the Knee

D. H. O'Donoghue, M.D., F.A.C.S.
OKLAHOMA CITY, OKLAHOMA

ANATOMY OF THE KNEE

The knee joint is potentially one of the weakest j o i n t s of the body, from the standpoint of bony structure. The articular facets of the upper end of the tibia are mere shallow depressions, deepened somewhat by the semi-lunar cartilages, which form but a poor receptacle for the lower tuberosities of the femur. This is in sharp contrast to the other large joints of the lower extremity, namely the hip and ankle, the one a deep ball and socket joint, the other a well constructed mortise and tenon. To compensate for this potential weakness, the knee is stabilized and fortified by a complete envelopment of extremely dense ligaments, which serve capably to maintain the integrity of the joint under all ordinary stress.

For purposes of discussion, these ligaments may be divided into several more or less distinct groups: 1. Internal lateral ligament. This structure encompasses the entire mesial aspect of the joint, being attached above to the margin of the mesial condyle of the femur, below to the margin of the upper end of the tibia. It is intimately connected to the capsule of the joint, and indistinguishable from it. It is also closely attached to the internal semi-lunar cartilage. 2. External lateral ligament. This structure is a definite ligamentous band in two sections, the anterior and posterior, and p a s s e s from the external condyle of the femur to the head of the fibula. It is distinct from and but loosely attached to the capsule of the joint, and thus has no connection with the ex-

ternal semi-lunar cartilage. 3. Posterior ligament. This structure is a fascial and capsular thickening, with interdigitating fibers strongly supporting the joint posteriorly. 4. Anterior c r u c i a l ligament. This structure is intra-articular, running from the front of the spine of the tibia as a pencil-sized band, backward, upward and outward, to insert in the mesial side of the lateral condyle of the femur posteriorly. It effectively c h e c k s forward displacement of the tibia on the femur, and is taut on complete extension of the knee. 5. Posterior crucial ligament. This is a thick, short ligament, running from the posterior part of the spine of the tibia obliquely upward, forward and inward, to attach to the outer side of the medial condyle of the femur. It serves to check posterior displacement of the tibia on the femur, and is most taut on flexion. These two ligaments acting together tend to limit rotation of the tibia on the femur. 6. Internal and external semi-lunar cartilages. These are crescentic slips of cartilage, thick on the outer border, and thinning toward the joint, and closely attached to the margin of the articular surface of the tibia and the capsule of the joint. Thus the internal meniscus is fixed to the internal lateral ligament, while the lateral is more freely movable, being attached only to the capsule of the joint. They serve to prevent lateral motion of the joint by their wedge action, and also deepen slightly the articular facets of the tibia. Altogether these structures serve to stabilize the joint, and prevent undue rotation and lateral motion, while allowing flexion and extension.

INJURIES

With this brief consideration of the anatomy of the more important structures of the knee, let us correlate injury and anatomy in a rational discussion of traumatic internal derangements of the knee joint.

Although there are a multitude of various injuries to the mechanism of the knee, many of these are so infrequent as to be negligible in a brief discussion of this sort. Investigation of case series reveals that about 75 per cent of the injuries to the knee consist of injury to the internal or external lateral ligament or its corresponding cartilage. This leaves a comparatively small percentage to include injury to the crucial ligaments, fracture of the tibial spines, loose bodies, injured fat pads and major fractures. For this reason the major portion of this discussion will be confined to the more common injuries, namely, lateral ligament and cartilage injuries, with only a brief description of the more uncommon ones.

I.—Injury to the internal lateral ligament.
  A. Etiology.
      The mechanism of production of an injury to this structure is a forced abduction of the leg at the knee, and external rotation of the leg on the thigh, with the knee slightly flexed. Usually the foot is fixed, and the knee is forced mesially, with the thigh and body rotating inward.
  B. Pathology.
      Partial or complete severance of the fibers of the ligament at either insertion or of the body of the ligament itself. A continuation of the force will dislocate or rupture the internal semi-lunar cartilage, and a further continuation will injure the crucial ligaments.
  C. Symptoms and diagnosis.
      1. History of the type of injury.
      2. Severe pain over the ligament, with a sensation of the knee "giving away."
      3. Effusion into the joint, which de-

pends upon the severity of the injury to the ligament.
      4. Local tenderness over the site of rupture.
      5. Pain on external rotation of the tibia, with the knee flexed.
      6. Pain on passive abduction of the leg at the knee.
      7. Increase in lateral motion if the ligament is entirely ruptured.
  D. Complications.
      1. Dislocation of the internal semi-lunar cartilage, with symptoms of cartilage injury.
      2. Avulsion of the tibial spine.
      3. Injury to the crucial ligaments.
      4. Fracture of the tibia or femur.
  E. Treatment.
      The treatment of injury to the internal lateral ligament depends to a large extent upon the severity of the injury and the presence of complications. It is unfortunately true that the major portion of these injuries are very inadequately treated. A great number of knee injuries which result in instability of the knee, with a so-called "game knee," can be prevented by adequate treatment, instituted early. In too large a proportion of cases the doctor is not consulted until permanent damage has been done. In many other cases, however, the doctor tends to minimize the injury, encouraging early weight bearing and active and passive motion, to the marked detriment of the injured structures. The rational of the treatment depends entirely upon the pathology. In the presence of a ruptured ligament, it is obvious that complete rest should be maintained until union is complete, if we are to prevent a relaxed, redundant ligament, with resulting instability. If the patient is seen early, the treatment consists of:
      1. Absolute bed rest.
      2. Application of alternate heat and cold to the knee.
      3. Snug bandage to prevent effusion.
      4. Aspiration of effusion into knee

as frequently as is necessary to prevent u n d u e tension. Strict asepsis is imperative.

5. After the effusion is under control a plaster cast should be applied from the toes to the groin. In about 10 days the cast may be b i v a l v e d for the institution of heat and massage, but *not* motion. This immobilization should be continued for from three to six weeks, depending upon the severity of the injury. The patient may t h e n be allowed up with a snugly fitting e l a s t i c bandage to the knee, and the inner side of the sole and heel of the shoe raised ¼ inch, in order to relieve the strain on the internal lateral ligament.

II.—Injury to the external lateral ligament.

Injury to the external lateral ligament is much less common than injury to the internal lateral ligament. The method of production is practically the reverse of that causing injury to the internal lateral ligament, and the injury is such that the leg is *internally* rotated on the t h i g h, and *adducted* at the knee joint, while the knee is in slight flexion. It can readily be seen that this is a much less common type of injury than the former. The symptoms of this injury are practically the same as those of injury to the internal lateral ligament, except localizing signs are over the external lateral ligament.

A. History of the type of injury.

B. Severe pain over the external lateral ligament.

C. No effusion into the joint, unless the injury is very severe, since the ligament and capsule of the joint are separate.

D. Local tenderness over the site of injury.

E. P a i n on passive *adduction* at the knee.

F. Pain on *internal rotation* of leg.

G. Possibly increased lateral motion of the knee if the injury is severe.

Treatment is identical to that of treatment of internal lateral ligament, except that when weight bearing is permitted the *external* portion of the sole and heel of the shoe is raised, rather than the internal.

III.—Injuries to the internal semi-lunar cartilage.

Injuries to the internal semi-lunar cartilage are much more common than injuries to the external, the proportion being about nine to one. This is due to the fact that the internal lateral ligament is integral with the capsule of the joint, and the internal semi-lunar cartilage is in turn attached to the capsule, while on the outer side of the knee there is no connection between cartilage and ligament.

A. Etiology.

The m e c h a n i s m of production is identical with that of injury to the internal lateral ligament, t h a t is, with the knee slightly flexed the foot is fixed and the body weight is thrown inward and rotated inward, throwing a strain directly on the internal lateral ligament. This procedure rotates the anterior portion of the cartilage backward and inward, and the posterior part of the cartilage backward and outward.

B. Pathology.

This may do one of several things to the cartilage:

1. The cartilage may be torn loose at its front attachment.

2. The cartilage may be ruptured in the central portion.

3. The cartilage may be split longitudinally, "bucket handle" type.

4. The posterior s e g m e n t of the cartilage may be caught in the articulation when the j o i n t is straightened, thus rupturing the cartilage.

Any one of these injuries may permit the cartilage to slide into the joint, and thus lock the knee on attempted extension.

C. Symptoms.

1. Following the acute injury.

a. History of the type of injury.

b. Pain on attempted extension of leg.

c. Inability completely to extend the knee without first manipulating the leg.

d. Pain o v e r the anterior attachment of the semi-lunar cartilage.

e. Swelling and effusion of the knee joint.

2. Diagnosis of an old cartilage injury.

   a. History of acute onset.
   b. Synovitis of the knee.
   c. Pain over the detached cartilage, especially anteriorly.
   d. Locking of the joint repeatedly.
   e. Pain on abduction at the knee.
   f. Pain on external rotation of the leg on the thigh, with the knee flexed.
   g. Pain on forced extension of the knee.
   h. Recurrent effusion following each successive locking.

D. Treatment.

There is a good deal of debate as to the proper procedure in a recent case of injury to the semi-lunar cartilage. There should be no question, however, but that following the first attack the treatment should be conservative.

1. Conservative treatment.

   a. Complete reduction of the displacement. With or without an anesthetic the knee is completely flexed. Then abduct the leg at the knee and externally rotate the leg, while rapidly extending the leg on the thigh. If the patient is not under an anesthetic, he should be required to kick down at the time of this extension. If reduction is complete, the leg can be easily and painlessly e x t e n d e d to an equal degree with the opposite leg.

   b. After reduction, complete immobilization of the knee for from four to six weeks, preferably by a plaster cast running f r o m the toes to the groin.

   c. Elastic support following removal of the cast, or a brace to protect knee.

   d. Elevate the inner side of the heel and sole of the s h o e about $\frac{1}{4}$ inch.

2. Surgical treatment.

If the patient gives a history of repeated attacks, it is advisable to remove the cartilage. This requires the strictest asepsis, and most careful technique. There seems to be no particular handicap to the k n e e following removal of the semi-lunar cartilage. Cases that have been re-operated for some other involvement of the knee reveal that the cartilage is replaced with a formation of fibrous tissue, which seems to satisfactorily fulfill the function of the internal semi-lunar cartilage.

IV.—Injuries to the external semi-lunar cartilage.

This condition is much less common than injuries to the internal semi-lunar cartilage, the exact mechanism of production being rather indefinite. A great many cases of injury to the internal semi-lunar cartilage may have symptoms referable to the outside of the knee. For this reason one must be particularly careful in making a diagnosis of injury to the external semi-lunar cartilage alone. The conservative management of the two conditions is identical, so the exact diagnosis of course is not essential. Should the case go to operation, however, it is inadvisable to approach the external cartilage through a small incision, but is essential to use an approach which will permit exploration of both cartilages, in order to assure removal of the site of the trouble.

V.—Injuries to the anterior crucial ligament.

We have seen that the principal function of the crucial ligaments is to stabilize the knee antero-posteriorly, the anterior crucial ligament c h e c k i n g anterior displacement of the tibia on the femur, the posterior checking posterior displacement of the tibia on the femur. The anterior crucial ligament, however, also serves to check abduction at the knee and internal rotation of the leg on the knee.

A. Etiology.

1. Forcible hyper-extension at the knee.

2. Forced hyper-abduction at the knee.

3. Forced internal rotation of the tibia on the femur.

It can be seen that the anterior crucial ligament is likely to be injured only after severance of the internal lateral ligament, and displacement of the internal semi-lunar cartilage. A continuance of the force then either ruptures the anterior crucial ligament or fractures the tibial spine.

B. Pathology.

1. Rupture of the ligament proper.

2. Avulsion of the tibial spine.

3. Tearing loose of the ligament from the femoral attachment.

C. Symptoms.

We have the symptoms of a severe injury to the knee joint, with all the findings referable to injury to the internal lateral ligament. In addition, there is definite lateral instability of the knee, and also instability in the antero-posterior plane. That is, with the knee extended, the tibia may be displaced somewhat anteriorly upon the femur.

D. Treatment.

This condition requires prolonged immobilization of the joint. Following an acute injury it may be advisable to institute some preliminary treatment in the way of reducing the swelling and effusion, prior to immobilization. This can be accomplished by hot and cold applications and aspiration of the joint while the patient is at bed rest. Following this the knee should be completely immobilized in a plaster of paris cast, preferably from the toes to the groin, with the knee at about 30 degrees flexion. After about two months in the cast, it is sometimes permissible to apply a cast from the ankle to the groin in the same position, and allow weight bearing. Immobilization should be complete for about six months. Following this a brace should be worn, which limits extension at the knee to about 160 degrees. This should be worn for another two to six months, during which time physiotherapy should be instituted, consisting of heat, massage, and active and passive motion. Operative treatment is gaining popularity and is indispensable in any but the most acute cases. It will often shorten the period of convalescence.

VI.—Rupture to the posterior crucial ligament.

A. Etiology.

1. Forcible backward displacement of the tibia on the femur. This is an unusual type of injury, and occurs with the knee flexed. It requires very serious injury to rupture the posterior crucial ligament.

B. Pathology.

1. Rupture of the fibers of the crucial ligament.

2. Fracture of the tibial spine.

3. Tearing loose of the attachment of the ligament to the femur.

C. Symptoms.

In a case of this kind, we have the symptoms of a very serious injury to the knee, with swelling, effusion, dysfunction and severe pain. The cardinal sign of rupture of the posterior crucial ligament is the ability to displace the tibia posteriorly on the femur, with the knee flexed. In the majority of cases many other structures of the knee are injured as well, diagnosis being based entirely on antero-posterior instability.

D. Treatment.

The treatment is identical with that of injury to the anterior ligament. Care must be taken in the application of the cast that the tibia is well forward on the femur. The prognosis in primary injuries to the crucial ligaments is at best doubtful. In many cases there will be a resulting instability at the knee joint. It is unquestionably true, however, that a large proportion of this disability can be minimized by early adequate treatment. Since the operative treatment is unsatisfactory, it renders the initial period of treatment much more important, since there is little or no recourse if the liagament is allowed to heal with increased length, resulting in instability.

VII.—Fracture of the tibial spine.

This condition is probably much more common than has been suspected. Careful X-ray of the knee will oftimes reveal a f r a c t u r e of the tibial spine, in cases where ligament i n j u r y only has been suspected.

A. Etiology.

The mechanism of production of this injury is identical with that of rupture of the anterior c r u c i a l ligament. There are of course many cases of major fractures around the knee in which the tibial spine is involved, but these cases are beyond the realm of this discussion.

B. Symptoms.

The symptoms are the same as those of rupture of the crucial ligaments. In some cases, however, there is not increased mobility, since the spine is not completely torn loose. In certain other cases there is sufficient displacement of the spine to cause actual locking of the knee, and this is in the nature of a bony block, rather than the cartilaginous locking incident to injury to the semilunar cartilage. All severe injuries to the knee joint should have careful X-ray study, and this will reveal fractures of the tibial spine.

C. Treatment.

1. If there is bony block, this must be eliminated by manipulation of the knee under an anesthetic. If this fails, the knee must be opened and the bony block removed in toto.

2. Preliminary period, during which time the swelling and effusion of the knee is reduced.

3. Complete immobilization of the knee by a plaster cast from the toes to the groin, with the knee slightly flexed. It is not usually necessary to immobilize the knee over so prolonged a period in fracture of the tibial spine as in rupture of the crucial ligaments, six to eight weeks probably being sufficient.

CONCLUSION

In conclusion, then, let me make a plea for early and adequate treatment of injuries about the knee. In all of these injuries there is a tremendous advantage in early care. Many times satisfactory treatment cannot be instituted late with any degree of success. With careful examination, prompt, accurate diagnosis, and immediate adequate care the percentage of disability resulting from intrinsic injuries to the knee can be sharply reduced.

The Management of Pulmonary Tuberculosis

C. A. THOMAS, M.D.   S. C. DAVIS, M.D.   R. A. WILSON, M.D.
TUCSON, ARIZONA

In dealing with the management of pulmonary tuberculosis, the time-worn subject of early diagnosis is of too great importance to pass without mentioning. The present high death rate in tuberculosis is largely dependent upon two factors; first, failure to make the correct diagnosis while the condition still has a favorable prognosis; and second, failure to use the methods of treatment which will, when used properly, offer the best chance for cure and at the same time markedly shorten the length of convalescence.

Failure to make a diagnosis early is not necessarily incompetence on the part of the attending physician.

Often the patient does not consult a doctor until this stage is passed. Sometimes the internist sees only infrequent cases of tuberculosis and consequently is not always tuberculosis-minded.

Then, too, there are moderately advanced cases with indefinite symptoms and obscure physical signs in which the X-ray film alone will tell the true story. It is conceded by all phthisiologists that the X-ray is today the greatest single guide in the detection and management of cases of pulmonary tuberculosis.

The physician should always and forever be looking for early tuberculous lesions, and without exception any and every patient presenting himself with either a history or physical signs, or both, that suggest in any way tuberculosis should have an X-ray of the lungs.

It is not within the scope of this paper to go into the signs and symptoms of tuberculosis; however, we want to invite your attention to this fact: all tuberculosis does not begin insiduously and progress as a chronic disease.

Not infrequently, the disease begins with symptoms of an acute illness, and often is mistaken for lobar-pneumonia.

In fact, it may be a tuberculous pneumonia, and have all the signs and symptoms of a pneumococcic or streptococcic disease.

If it be a tuberculous process, however, it will not clear up so rapidly nor so completely as a pneumococcic pneumonia; therefore, every patient having a slowly resolving pneumonia with a continued productive cough and a low grade temperature after the acute sypmtoms have subsided should have not one, but many, sputum examinations for tubercle bacilli, and an X-ray of the chest.

More frequently than this, there is a type of tuberculosis which begins acutely but less dramatically and is erroneously called influenza, cold in the chest, or bronchitis. Here, also, it is our conviction that every patient with these symptoms which fail to clear up as readily as we are justified in expecting, should also have the same careful examination.

If these procedures are followed, a large number of patients will be spared much

suffering; and often unnecessary deaths will be prevented.

Furthermore, a patient who has had a pulmonary hemorrhage and, after a few days rest in bed, is returned to work without an X-ray of the chest has been grossly mistreated. Yet such a gross omission as this is no greater than relying on bed rest over an indefinite period of time without consideration as to the need of local rest; by local rest we mean some form of collapse therapy.

The clinical material which serves as a basis for this paper is drawn from a private group practice of many years in a community which is a mecca for tuberculous patients and from the Southern Pacific Tuberculosis Sanatorium, a 100 bed institution located in Tucson. In this institution and in our private practice, strictest bed rest is enforced, but it is not relied upon solely.

In this Sanatorium we have an average of 70-80 per cent of our patients under some form of collapse therapy, and at intervals that percentage has risen above 80 per cent. It is often attempted in those patients who appear hopeless at the start, and we have frequently benefitted and sometimes even secured an arrested disease in patients whose outcome, without such help, would be fatal.

Collapse therapy in all types of pulmonary tuberculosis is the greatest boon that has come to the tuberculous patient since the principles of bed rest and good food were generally accepted as fundamental in the treatment of this disease.

It is our serious conviction that in certain cases of pulmonary tuberculosis, particularly those with cavities, collapse therapy is just as much indicated as surgery is in acute appendicitis; because without this, their hope of ultimate cure is greatly lessened.

The absence of acute symptoms and the tragic demise of the patient makes us none the less responsible than if we were to permit a patient with an acute appendicitis to go without surgery.

There are many beautiful stories of early recoveries from bed rest alone. We have all seen them. No one is more convinced than we are that complete bed rest is the fundamental and the most essential principle in the treatment of this disease. Our purpose is to show that it should not be depended upon solely.

Very little has been said by the advocates of bed rest without collapse therapy of those patients who have extensions in the same and in the contralateral lung, as well as in other organs, while the patient is at rest in bed. Neither do they write about those who have cavities to form and those who have hemorrhages from these cavities; we hear no one taking credit for the case with an open cavity who, because of a continued positive sputum, is a menace to every one with whom he is in contact.

We hear little of the patient who, by waiting for bed rest to cure him, has had pleural adhesions to form and has, therefore, lost forever his opportunity for a successful pneumothorax.

Different forms of collapse therapy will be enumerated in the order of the frequency of their use: (1st) pneumothorax, (2nd) phrenic interruption (temporary and permanent), (3rd) intrapleural pneumonolysis, (4th) extrapleural pneumonolysis, (5th) scalenotomy, (6th) oleothorax, (7th) intercostal neurectomy, (8th) thoracoplasty (partial and complete).

This group of procedures can be used separately, collectively, or successively; and we want here to advocate and emphasize the principle of using them as successive steps until cavities have been collapsed, and the patient has been rendered free of sputum and bacilli.

In other words we feel that the only way that the best interest of the patient can be served is to start the use of collapse therapy with one object in view — placing the disease process at rest even if all of these procedures are required.

If the first procedure is not successful in accomplishing this, then an additional one or more of these methods is to be used in conjunction with or as a subsequent procedure until absolute collapse with arrest of the disease has occurred.

We feel that the use of surgery early in the disease is often overlooked. Many men are coming more and more to look upon collapse as a valuable adjunct in the treatment of tuberculosis, but too often they use it as a last resort. So often the

waiting is the one thing that changes a patient from a hopeful to a hopeless case.

One should always have in mind those dangers of delay which have been pointed out earlier in this paper.

Our methods of procedure of studying and handling patients can best be illustrated by following a patient into the Southern Pacific Sanatorium. When a patient enters this institution and when his history, physical examination, laboratory studies, and X-ray films are completed, his case is presented before the Staff.

Depending upon the duration of the disease, the amount of involvement, the location of the lesions, the amount of previous rest he has had, and how he has reacted to it, the decision is made as to what therapeutic measures will be instituted at this time. If the disease is of short duration, minimal in character, and he has had no previous rest, he may be put on complete bed rest for a period of 30 to 60 days, when he is studied again. Then if there is not ample evidence that there is a retrogression of the lesion, immediately help is given him by some form of collapse therapy.

On the other hand, if the disease is more advanced, if he has had a previous period of bed rest with evidence of a progressing disease process, especially if he has open cavity, then we immediately begin to supplement his bed rest with collapse therapy. We consider an open cavity is always a menace to the patient, and the patient who has a cavity remaining open is always regarded as being in jeopardy. Consequently in cavity cases collapse in some form is always undertaken at once.

PNEUMOTHORAX

Pneumothorax is usually the first thought in collapse therapy and is indicated wherever the disease is sufficiently advanced to justify collapse therapy. The selective, or more properly, ideal pneumothorax is that which collapses the diseased area only and allows the healthy lung to continue to function; in early cases, it is the one which is most desirable.

At the present time there are ample figures to prove that in collapse by pneumothorax, for instance, the cures are in direct proportion to the amount of collapse the patient receives.

Therefore, where, on account of adhesions, a complete collapse is impossible, a Jacobeus operation or some other method should be used to cut the adhesions; if this is impractical a phrenic interruption may be effective.

It is a deplorable fact that many cases of unilateral pneumothorax with a good contralateral lung, where only partial collapse has been obtained, have been and are being kept up without any other procedures being instituted, while the patient with his open cavity progresses gradually until death. This is also true of phrenic interruption.

Pneumothorax has the advantages that it can be continued either unilaterally or bilaterally, or discontinued on one or both sides when the symptoms indicate the necessity.

Contrary to the once popular opinion, the use of pneumothorax in bilateral tuberculosis does not necessarily aggravate the condition in the contralateral l u n g. More often a good collapse of the lung with the more advanced lesion, by a diminution in the general toxicity and probably a transference of pressure t h r o u g h the mediastinum, allows the opposite lung to improve. This is so commonly seen that we do not feel that bilateral lesions constitute a contra-indication to pneumothorax, but rather an added indication.

Furthermore, in cases with bilateral disease when the better lung fails to improve, while its opposite has been collapsed by pneumothorax, we have no hesitancy in instituting pneumothorax bilaterally, or a phrenic interruption on the side with the better lung.

Vital capacity studies are important in such cases.

Pneumothorax, when it accomplishes complete collapse is successful in producing a cure in about 80 per cent of the c a s e s of unilateral involvement, and a smaller percentage in bilateral disease.

A difficult problem for decision is the length of time pneumothorax should be continued.

Usually the patient is loath to give up the thing which he feels has saved his life —the attending physician is usually in accord with him. The decision is made by consideration of the pathology that was present when the pneumothorax was instituted and the present X-ray appearance of the lung. In general, we may assume that a successful pneumothorax will have accomplished its purpose in two to two and one-half years, if cavity were present at time of its induction, and sooner if there were no cavity. Furthermore the compressed lung is capable of expanding and resuming its function in most cases, which are not collapsed for longer periods.

COMPLICATIONS

There are two serious complications to pneumothorax; (1) spontaneous collapse, and (2) development of an effusion which may l a t e r become purulent. The spontaneous collapse is always looked upon as serious. Some may survive without any interference—we had one patient who had three separate spontaneous collapses. It never became necessary to interfere on any occasion, and he is well today. This is the exception. More often the air must be aspirated, and if this is not sufficient, a small catheter is introduced over the outer end of which is fastened a condom with a small slit in the end—this acts as a valve, allowing air to escape but not return.

Fluid develops frequently—more often when a complete collapse is prevented by adhesions and when positive intrapleural pressures are used. It is our practice to aspirate the fluid when it forms. We feel that the risk to the patient is greater by leaving it in than by withdrawing it.

PHRENIC NERVE INTERRUPTION

Recently there has been considerable unfavorable criticism of phrenic nerve interruption. This criticism grew out of the fact that all of the original operations caused permanent paralysis of the diaphragm. We agree with these objections.

However, we avoid the unfavorable results of a permanent paralysis by doing a temporary nerve interruption. In doing a phrenic operation we use the method devised by Goetz, advocated and popularized in this country by Dr. John Alexander. The paralysis of the hemidiaphragm, when the operation is performed in this manner, persists four to nine months, when the function gradually returns. When the diaphragm begins to function again, and if the patient still needs the benefit of its paralysis, a second similar operation may be performed easily. In some patients we have repeated it the third time and have a diaphragm which is capable of resuming its function.

We find the use of phrenic nerve interruption as important in conjunction with other measures as it is when used independently. Many unsatisfactory collapses by pneumothorax can be converted into a satisfactory measure by the use of this minor operation. This is especially true in those cases with adhesions to the diaphragm. The relaxation obtained w i l l often allow a cavity to be collapsed by the pneumothorax which, before the paralysis of the diaphragm, was continuously pulled open by every cough and r e s p i r a t o r y movement.

It is a matter of frequent observation that by the use of a combination of these methods, additional beneficial results may be accomplished amounting to 25-35 per cent of the heretofore unsuccessful cases.

Temporary phrenic interruption is used routinely on a patient who has had a successful pneumothorax long enough and the lung is going to be permitted to re-expand. Thus the once diseased lung is protected from full function for several m o n t h s longer. Phrenic interruption has another important function as preliminary to complete thoracoplasty—its use here is to test the contralateral lung and, too, a high rise of the diaphragm may make it unnecessary to remove as many ribs as would otherwise be necessary.

OLEOTHORAX

Oleothorax is a valuable supplement to pneumothorax, and has a distinct place in collapse therapy. It is not uncommon to note that often with the continued use of pneumothorax, particularly where o n l y partial collapse has been obtained, as a result of adhesive pleuritis, the pneumothorax space becomes reduced. This indicates that the collapse is soon to be lost through this process. The collapse can frequently be maintained for an indefinite period of time by displacing the air with oil.

This procedure is only adapted to those cases having the lower part of the lung adherent to the chest wall and diaphragm;

this prevents the oil from resting upon the diaphragm. The preparation with which we have had the greatest success is ordinary Wesson oil. This causes but little, if any, reaction, and prevents by its weight further reduction of the pleural space. Our experience with Gomenal or other antiseptic oils has been most unsatisfactory.

SCALENOTOMY

Scalenotomy is used in moderately advanced apical tuberculosis, usually in conjunction with phrenic interruption with the hope of effecting a cure by this minor procedure and avoiding the more formidable procedures. It adds additional rest to the apex by relaxation and also affords some restriction of motion of the upper three ribs. This procedure probably has not been as widely used as it should have been, especially in the earlier cases. Our experience with this procedure has been most satisfactory.

EXTERNAL PNEUMONOLYSIS

External pneumonolysis, while not as popular as the other procedure, certainly has its place, particularly in the very sick patients who have not yielded to the less drastic measures and where there are specific contradictions to thoracoplasty. In this type of cases, it is indicated (1st) in a single, small, apical cavity with a good contralateral lung, (2nd) with involved contralateral lung, or bilateral, apical cavities, (3rd) in some cases of posterior thoracoplasty where the cavity has not been successfully closed. Materials used in this procedure are muscle, fat, gauze, rubber dam, and paraffin.

Complications to be considered in this procedure are (1st) rupture of external cavity wall during operation, with infection of pleural space and resultant empyema, (2nd) interference with c a r d i a c function due to e x c e s s pressure, (3rd) where paraffin is used, perforation of wax through cavity wall into a bronchus with extrusion of wax.

INTERCOSTAL NEURECTOMY

Intercostal neurectomy has more limited use in collapse therapy than other measures. Its field of greatest usefulness is in those patients in whom the other minor procedures have failed to effect an arrest and whose present physical condition contraindicates thoracoplasty. It is used with the hope of the patient's improving to the point that he may be a suitable risk for thoracoplasty.

THORACOPLASTY

If all other measures fail to accomplish the desired result, or if the case is such that it is obvious that other procedures can but cause a waste of time, we resort to an extrapleural thoracoplasty, either partial or complete, or one that is bilateral and partial. The details of this procedure will be omitted. Suffice it to say, many cures have been effected by virtue of thoracoplasty which would, with anything less radical, certainly, surely and fairly rapidly have resulted in death.

The attitude of patients regarding these measures is significant. Very frequently we have patients who ask when they will get their collapse procedure started and even get impatient because it is not done immediately. This is especially true in the Southern Pacific Sanatorium where there is always a large percentage of patients under collapse therapy. Further-more, even though looked upon as radical by many, it is not uncommon to have patients come to us of their own volition to ask if they are suited for thoracoplasty.

In closing, I want to emphasize again the opening thoughts — two factors are largely responsible for tuberculosis being of such tremendous importance—first, failure to make the correct diagnosis while the prognosis is good, and while cure may be effected with a minimal morbidity; second, failure to use the methods of treatment which will offer the best, the surest, and the quickest prospects for a cure.

SUMMARY

1. The importance of early diagnosis of pulmonary tuberculosis is discussed.

2. The necessity of collapse therapy in addition to routine bed rest is emphasized.

3. The importance of using the methods of collapse individually, collectively, and successively, is stressed.

4. The various surgical methods used with their indication, contra-indications, and complications, are discussed.

---o---

Rupture of Tendo Achilles
Report of a Case

ROBERT L. NOELL, M.D.
Instructor in Orthopaedic Surgery,
University of Oklahoma School of Medicine
OKLAHOMA CITY, OKLAHOMA

This rather rare injury has been briefly described by Whitman, and J o n e s and Lovett. Very little has appeared in the literature in regard to end results in this lesion.

Two types of injuries have been described by Jones and Lovett: "(1), A rupture of the fibers in the transverse plane. This injury usually occurs at about one-half inch above the attachment to the os calcis or slightly higher at its narrow portion, or at the musculotendinous junction. (2), Sliding tears, the tendon bundles being dragged apart in a coronal plane."

The case reported is of the second type.

CASE REPORT

J. L., white, male, aged 41, came to my office on August 3, 1936, complaining of an injury to the right foot and leg. The injury occurred on June 5, 1936, eight weeks prior to my first examination. He gave a history of having injured the right leg while p l a y i n g volley ball. While standing on his toes ready to receive the ball he noticed a severe pain in the right leg in the region of the tendo Achilles.

The only treatment given was an adhesive strapping which was applied the day following the injury. The patient removed the adhesive in about one week.

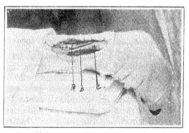

FIG. 1

Photograph of the ruptured tendon taken immediately after the incision was made. (a) Proximal portion of ruptured tendon. (b) Plantaris tendon intact. (c) Distal portion of the ruptured tendon.

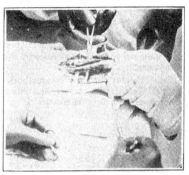

FIG. 2

Shows the ruptured proximal portion of the tendon being dissected from the underlying structures.

Examination was negative except for the injured right tendo Achilles. He walked with a limp characteristic of a loss of function of the gastrocnemius and soleus muscles. A calcaneous deformity of the right foot was being developed.

Examination of the tendo Achilles revealed a definite defect in the tendon about one and one-half inches proximal to its attachment to the os calcis. There was very little function exercised through the combined action of the gastrocnemius and soleus muscles. A diagnosis of a ruptured tendo Achilles was made, and open repair advised. The operative procedure was done on August 12, 1936. The condition of the ruptured tendon may be seen in the photographs taken after a complete exposure was made (figures 1 and 2). The

proximal portion of the ruptured tendon was completely detached from the distal portion and was adherent to the underlying structures. The plantaris tendon was intact and may be seen in the photographs. There was evidence of considerable hemorrhage, having occurred at the point of injury. The tendon sheath was incorporated in the m a s s of adhesions. This was a sliding type of rupture.

The adherent portion of the tendon was carefully dissected from the underlying structures. After freshening the opposing edges they were sutured with black silk to the distal portion of the tendon. After closing the incision a plaster casing was applied from the mid-thigh to the toes, with the knee flexed about 30 degrees and the foot in a moderate equinus position. This was changed in three weeks, and the foot brought up to about a 110 degree angle with the leg. He was allowed to walk at the end of eight weeks, with a short leg brace, which limited dorsiflexion of the foot to 90 degrees, the heel of the shoe being raised three-eighths of an inch. This was worn for three months.

E x a m i n a t i o n when last seen, eight months after operation, revealed an excellent return of function of the t e n d o Achilles. He w a l k e d without a limp. There was no evidence of a calcaneous deformity of the foot, and there was a normal range of active motion in the ankle joint.

CONCLUSION

This rather rare injury, of a sliding type of rupture involving the tendo Achilles should be treated by open operation. Early operative repair is desirable, but as demonstrated in this case a good result may be obtained when repair is done s e v e r a l weeks after the injury.

REFERENCES

Whitman: Orthopaedic Surgery, Ninth Edition Revised, 1937, Lea and Febiger, Philadelphia, Pa.

Jones and Lovett: Second Edition Revised, William Wood & Co., Baltimore.

Handbook of Orthopaedic Surgery: by Alfred Rivers Shand, Jr., the C. D. Mosby Co., 1937.

Orthopaedic Surgery: by T. P. McMurray, 1937, William Wood & Co., Baltimore.

————o————

State Dues will not be accepted at the Registration Desk, Annual Meeting, except through C o u n t y Secretaries.

TYPHOID FEVER

CARLTON E. SMITH, M.D.
HENRYETTA, OKLAHOMA

A general infection caused by baccillus typhosus characterized by hyperplasia and ulceration of intestinal lymphatics, swelling of mesentive glands and spleen.

History: In 1829 Louis gave the disease the name of typhoid fever. Gerhard of Philadelphia gave the first satisfactory description of the disease in 1837.

ETIOLOGY

Typhoid is a disease of filth and is an index of the sanitary conditions of a community. It is most prevalent in the autumn. The disease is more common in the male than female.

The typhoid bacillus is a short, thick, flagellated motile bacillus with round ends, about 3 u. in length and .6 u. in width. Early in the disease its bacilli are probably circulating in the blood. They are probably always present in the rose spots.

Fingers, food and flies are means of propagation. Infected water supply has been the source of numerous large epidemics. Typhoid carriers are always a source of danger. The organism may be present in the urine, bile or intestine. Flies as a means of spreading the disease are important in camps or where large groups of people are closely segregated.

Typhoid is a disease of youth and young adult life. The ages of 336 cases examined ranged from eight months to 60 years of age, about 90 per cent being between the ages of 5 and 30. The greater number for any one year was 20, at the age of 11.

MORBID ANATOMY

There is a catarrhal condition throughout the small and large bowel. There is hyperplasia of Pyers patches, the follicles are swollen, grayish white and the patches project. The solitary glands are swollen and project. Later there is a great increase in cells of the lymph tissue which may infiltrate the surrounding mucosa. When the hyperplasia is very severe the lymph follicle can no longer return to normal and is followed by necroses and sloughing. The ulcerations due to sloughing, if extensive, results in hemorrhages which may be extensive, frequently leading to death. The thin ulcerated areas may perforate at any time. After the sloughs have separated healing begins and regardless of the extent of the slough, stricture never results.

The mesenteric glands show hyperemia and become greatly swollen. Occasionally these may rupture causing hemorrhage or peritonitis.

The spleen is invariably enlarged. The tissue is soft and occasionally rupture occurs.

SYMPTOMS

Three hundred and thirty-six cases were received extending over a period of four years. One hundred and seventeen gave history of positive exposure, having been out of town on fishing trips, drinking of well or spring water, or contact with typhoid patient.

The most constant symptom was fever, practically 100 per cent showing an elevation of temperature. Fifty per cent of the patients complained of headache, 132 had diarrhea, 34 complained of constipation, 136 complained of abdominal pain, 119 complained of generalized ill feeling and muscular aching, 52 complained of vomiting and 43 had epistaxis. The patients usually began to complain of general ill feeling, slight fever followed in a few days by the increase in the above symptoms, sometimes accompanied by vomiting, diarrhea or more or less indefinite abdominal distress. The fever becomes more intense, being higher in the afternoon, a rash may be noted, the patient is forced to bed and a definite diagnosis can usually be made. The fever usually takes about one week to reach its' height, then remaining of the plateau stage for one week to ten days and then begins to fluctuate more widely as the fever subsides.

A large number of patients complain of abdominal pain, this varies from mild discomfort to sharp pain. One patient was operated for appendicitis and many complain so bitterly that perforation must be considered. In case of perforation the pain usually comes on suddenly, is i n t e n s e, sometimes cramping in character, usually accompanied by v o m i t i n g, abdominal rigidity, loss of liver dullness, and X-ray may show layer of air u n d e r the diaphragm. In practically every case of perforation the layer of air was demonstrable.

COMPLICATIONS AND SEQUALAE

	Year 1928 1929	Year 1929 1930	Year 1930 1931	Year 1931 1932	Year 1932 1933	Total	%
Number of Cases	65	39	88	46	98	336	
Broncho Pneumonia	4	3	8	5	21	41	12.2
Lobar Pneumonia	0	0	1	1	2	4	1.19
Distension	23	18	23	12	19	95	28.2
Furunculosis	3	1	4	5	10	23	6.9
Intestinal Hemorrhage	10	13	16	7	12	58	16.2
Perforation	3	0	4	1	2	10	2.9
Psychosis	2	1	5	1	5	14	4.1
Convulsions	2	0	1	2	1	6	1.79
Thrombophlebitis { Left	1	1			9	12	3.58
Thrombophlebitis { Right					6	6	1.79
Acute Otitis Media	1	1	5		5	12	3.58
Acute Myocarditis	4	1			5	10	2.9
Chronic Myocarditis	0			2	1	3	.9
Pregnant	2	1	1			4	1.19
Miscarriage		1	1			2	.6
Cholecystitis				1	1	2	.6
Cholecystotomy					2	2	.6
Empyema					2	2	.6
Peripheral Neuritis					2	2	.6
Nephritis					1	1	.3
Orchitis				1	1	2	.6
Paronychia		1		2		3	.9
Periostitis				1		1	.3
Pericardial Effusion				1		1	.3
Parotitis					1	1	.3
Uremia				1		1	.3
Stomatitis			1		1	2	.6
Pressure Sores				2	2	4	1.19
Cellulitis			2	1		3	.9
Pleural Effusion					3	3	.9
Fecal Impaction		2		1	1	4	1.19
Ishiorectal Abscess				1		1	.3
Mastoiditis			1		1	2	.6
Stricture of Rectum		1				1	.3
Cystitis	1					1	.3
Pyelitis	2		3		1	6	1.79
Operated for Appendicitis	1		1			2	.6
Mortality	14	7	15	2	6	44	13.1
Average Stay In Hospital	35.3	39.6	41.6	39.1	33.7	37.4	

INCIDENCE ACCORDING TO AGE

Age in Years	Number of Cases
1	3
2	3
3	3
4	3
5	7
6	15
7	7
8	9
9	12
10	11
11	8
12	20
13	13
14	10
15	8
16	8
17	9
18	14
19	15
20	9
21	8
22	13
23	12
24	11
25	10
26	7
27	9
28	2
29	11
30	3
31	13
32	6
33	4
34	4
35	2
36	4
37	0
38	1
39	2
40	5
41	0
42	1
43	2
44	1
45	2
46	2
47	1
48	3
49	1
50	1
51	2
52	1
53	0
54	1
55	1
56	0
57	0
58	2
59	1
60	1
61	0

PHYSICAL FINDINGS

The patient is usually drowsy and has washed out appearance. Face is frequently flushed, temperature is high and the pulse is relatively slow in adults, children may fail to show the slow pulse. The tongue is heavily coated, furred, and dry. The abdomen is moderately to markedly distended and has a somewhat doughy feel. Of the 336 cases examined 37 showed a dicratic pulse, 131 had rose spots and 130 had palpable spleen, 85 were irrational and 95 showed marked distention. Rose spots usually appear over the upper abdomen and chest, in the form of a moderately sized macular rash, about ⅛ inch in diameter, they fade on pressure, are pink in color and the typhoid organism may be cultured from these lesions.

The spleen is usually enlarged and palpable at some time during the disease, the consistency is rather soft and mushy.

Distension has been a rather troublesome symptom, but has been greatly relieved by improvement in the typhoid diet in which the fermentable sugars were replaced by other sugars. Dextrose has largely taken the place of succrose in the diet at the St. Louis Isolation Hospital. Lactose has been used by some.

DIAGNOSIS

Patient takes sick with high persistent fever, slow pulse, drowsy, sometimes irrational, abdominal distress, vomiting or diarrhea. Rose spots, dicratic pulse, palpable spleen may be noted. The patients entering isolation had admission blood culture, stool and urine ran and three discharge urine and stools. There were 27 patients with positive urine, 24 with positive stools and 76 with positive blood culture. The Widal was the most reliable positive finding, being positive in 289 cases.

Severe typhoid cases may be mistaken for meningitis, the patient is irrational or unconscious, muscles may show considerable spasticity, both have high fever and slow pulse. In meningitis the rash if present, is petecheal in character, does not fade on pressure and the spine is stiff, Kernig positive, neck stiff and spinal fluid shows cloudy fluid, with increased pressure and cell count, the gram negative diplococcus may be found.

Miliary tuberculosis may be mistaken for typhoid, exhibiting chills, fever, malaise. The finding in chest of consolidation, rales, increase in voice and breath sound. X-ray will confirm the diagnosis. Undulant fever may cause some difficulty in diagnosis, there is remittent fever, absence of signs of typhoid, and positive agglutination tests for bacillus brucella abertus.

Generalized pyemia may simulate typhoid, findings of infection elsewhere, absence of signs of typhoid and increased white blood count aid in the differential diagnosis. The white blood count is usually low in typhoid, five cases observed had white blood count below 3,000, a count of 2,000 was the lowest, 34 per cent showed white blood count of 3,000 to 6,000, 35 per cent of 6,000 to 8,000 and remainder above 8,000. There was quite a shift to the left, many young cells being present at the expense of a reduction in segmented cells, the lymphatic count being practically normal.

COMPLICATIONS AND SEQUELAE

The most frequent complication was intestinal hemorrhage being present in 58 cases or 17.2 per cent. These varied from a small amount of blood in stool to severe hemorrhage in which the patient was found lying in a pool of blood. The greater number were of the moderately severe type. The pulse became rapid, weak, blood pressure dropped if the hemorrhage was severe. Red blood count showed considerable anemia. These were watched closely, pulse and blood pressure checked at frequent intervals.

Second in incidence was broncho-pneumonia which was present in 41 cases or 12.3 per cent. Patients had cough, moderate impairment of resonance, rapid breathing and rales over both sides of chest. There were four cases of lobar pneumonia in the series of 336 cases examined. There were three cases of pleural effusion following broncho-pneumonia.

Toxic psychosis developed in 14 cases or 4.2 per cent, these patients were disoriented, had various delusions, often of persecution, some would mutter to themselves while a few were very loud and noisy, screaming at the top of their voice and disturbing everyone in the hospital. These usually cleared up after the patient had recovered from the typhoid, some requiring several weeks after the temperature was normal.

There were 16 cases of thrombophlebitis, nine occurring in the left lower extremity and six of the right with one bilateral. There was pain and swelling over the femoral vein with elevation of fever and local heat. Acute purulent otitis media was present in 12 cases or 3.6 per cent.

Acute toxic myocarditis was present in 10 cases or 3.3 per cent. The pulse was rapid, weak, heart tones were very distant, liver was enlarged and some edema of ankles were shown. There were three cases of chronic myocarditis which had been present for some time. One case of pericardial effusion developed.

Because of the long confinement to bed furunculosis is frequent, being present in 23 cases or 6.9 per cent. The skin must be kept clean, alcohol rub daily and patient should change position frequently. Four cases of rather extensive pressure sores developed.

Intestinal perforation is the complication most dreaded. The patient has sharp pain in his abdomen, sometimes cramping in nature, usually vomits, the abdomen becomes rigid, white blood count is elevated, liver dullness obliterated and X-ray shows layer of air under the diaphragm. There may be drop in temperature and elevation of pulse. Perforation occurred in 2.9 per cent (10 cases) of the cases, all being present in male patients, the youngest being five years of age. Of these eight died and 2 recovered. The patients were operated immediately, but practically all had a more or less diffuse peritonitis.

Six patients had a pyelitis, as shown by chills, fever and white blood cells in urine.

Four of the patients were pregnant at the time they developed typhoid fever, two of these miscarried, while the other two seemed to suffer no ill effects.

Because of abdominal pain two patients had been operated for appendicitis at the time they entered the hospital.

One patient had a periostitis of the rib which had developed about 15 years following his typhoid. A thoractomy was done and because of persistent positive cultures from duodeonal drainage his gall bladder was removed. Patient eventually recovered.

There were two cases of cholecytitis, one of which had cholecystotomy done on two occasions. In spite of the routine enema given every morning four cases of fecal impaction developed.

Other less frequent complications were, empyemia (2), peripheral neuritis (3), convulsions were present in six cases, orchitis (2), mastoiditis (2), nephritis (1), stomatitis (2) cellulitis (3), external otitis (1), ischo-rectal abscess (1), stricture of rectum (1) and cystitis (1).

A number of patients had more than one disease. Twenty-two patients had positive Wasserman reaction, three had measles, three patients were dementia praecox, two had scarlet fever and varicella, malaria (1), impetigo (1), pulmonary tuberculosis (1), scabies (1), diphtheria (2), influenza (1), and one diphtheria carrier.

IMMUNITY

Typhoid fever usually confers an active immunity that lasts for life. Of the patients examined only three gave history of previous typhoid, one was 12 years previous, and another 33 years previous. The time elapsed in third case was unknown.

Typhoid vaccine has been very effective in the prevention of the disease. Three patients had received the vaccine, one had the shots four days previous to onset so an immunity had not had time to develop. The other two had their series of shots three years and four years previous. If the typhoid vaccine had been repeated every three years the immunity would probably be practically 100 per cent.

The Widal is of little value in diagnosis if the patient had previously had typhoid vaccine. Widals were run on 13 people who had previously had typhoid vaccine, of these five were negative, while eight gave a positive Widal reaction which varied from the lowest which was 1:20 to the highest which was 1:1280.

PROGNOSIS

The prognosis is fairly good in uncomplicated cases, however there will be a few deaths among the extremely toxic cases. In the 336 cases examined there were 44 deaths or 13.1 per cent. Of the cases dying there were 18 cases of intestinal hemorrhage (40.9 per cent), 14 cases of broncho-pneumonia (31.8 per cent), two cases of lobar pneumonia (4.5 per cent) and eight cases of perforation (18.1 per cent). Others were complicated by myo-carditis, pleural effusion, pericardial effusion and less common complications.

The youngest patient to die and also to contract the disease was eight months old while the oldest to die was 58 years of age. Only four patients below 10 years of age died, 30.9 per cent of the deaths were between the ages of 10 and 20, and 35.7 per cent between the ages of 20 and 30 years.

TREATMENT

The treatment is chiefly dietary and good nursing care. Patient is in bed at absolute bed rest, being fed liquids until their temperature has been down for one week. They are given a high caloric liquid diet with feedings every two hours. The diet is made up largely of milk, cream, gruels, fruit juices and custards. For the past few years the successe sugar has been largely replaced by dextrose which seems to have lessened the amount of distension.

The fever is treated by ice bags, sponge baths, alcohol fans and in extreme cases by cephalic douche.

The patient routinely receives an enema every morning. Distension may develop which is treated by reduction in the feedings to ¼ or ½ the amount usually given, rectal tube and occasionally hot turpentine stoops.

Intestinal hemorrhage is treated by sedation to keep the patient quiet, all food by mouth is stopped, ice bag is placed to the abdomen, subcutaneous fluids administered, calcium in large doses intra-muscular or by mouth may be given. The ceanothyn and other hemo stiptics may be given but their value is rather questionable. Intra-muscular blood may reduce the coagulation time. Transfusions and intra-venous fluids are given only in extreme cases at the time of the hemorrhage. After the bleeding stops small transfusions are given slowly to make up for the blood lost. Pulse and blood pressure are checked frequently.

Perforations have been treated by immediate operation. The course is always very stormy as the patients are extremely sick before perforation occurs. Fluids and transfusions are given to help keep up the patient's strength.

Transfusions have been given rather frequently to acutely ill typhoid patients always being given small amounts, 250 to 300 cc. at a time, and given very slowly. The patients are "pepped up" considerably in most cases. There were 31 transfusions given with average drop in temperature of .78 degrees in 24 hours and .93 degrees in 48 hours after being administered, besides general improvement in their appearance.

In acute myo-carditis the patient is digitalized, stimulants such as strychnine and small doses of adrenalin may be given.

Acute cholecystitis is treated conservatively by ice bag to upper abdomen, and sedation, in cases where the symptoms are marked cholecystotomy should be done.

After the temperature has been normal for seven days the diet is gradually increased, the increases coming every other day until the patient is on a soft diet. At this time the patient is allowed to sit up in bed. When patient is placed on a soft diet he is allowed out of bed. After temperature has been normal for 10 days, three urine and stool cultures are taken on successive days. Provided these are negative the patient may be discharged. If stool or urine returns positive the patient should be isolated until negative. Sometimes the patient becomes a chronic carrier after the disease has subsided. Large doses of hexamethalamine are given in hope it will clear up the urine and stool culture.

Of the cases examined seven were admitted as carriers without any clinical symptoms of typhoid fever. One patient ran away after being in the hospital nine days, one was discharged after 57 days in hospital still with positive stool cultures, the other four obtained negative cultures, one remaining in hospital 88 days before the negative cultures were obtained. One patient had repeatedly positive culture from Lyon's drainage of the gall bladder, this patient had his gall bladder removed and was discharged with negative cultures at the end of 40 days in the hospital. The carriers are treated by large d o s e s of hexamenthalamine, and vaccination with typhoid vaccine, which sometimes helps.

An antogenous vaccine w o r k s in some cases. The average stay in the hospital for all the typhoid cases treated was 37.4 days.

————————o————————

The Autonomic Nervous System

C. J. ROBERTS, M.D.
ENID, OKLAHOMA

The autonomic nervous system differs from the cerebrospinal nervous system in that the former supplies smooth or involuntary muscle while the latter supplies striated or voluntary muscle.

The autonomic system is composed of two main parts (1) the sympathetic or thoraco-lumbar division and (2) the parasympathetic or craniosacral division. The sympathetic division is composed of two chains of ganglia situated on either side of the vertebral column extending from the superior cervical ganglion, in the head, down to the upper sacral segments, in the pelvis. All the viscera of the thorax and abdomen and some organs in the head, as the ciliary muscle of the eye and the salivary glands have a reciprocal innervation, i.e. they are supplied with both sympathetic and parasympathetic fibers. The parasympathetic division is composed of fibers in the III, VII, IX, X cranial nerves and the pelvic or nerve irigens from the first three sacral segments of the cord.

The efferent fibers of both divisions of the autonomic system consist of pre- and postganglionic fibers. Most of the preganglionic efferent sympathetic fibers are comparatively short, passing from the cord out the anterior spinal nerve root and through the ramus communicans to the sympathetic ganglion lying close to the vertebral c o l u m n. The preganglionic f i b e r s passing to the superior cervical ganglion are long, however, as they emerge from the thoracic region of the cord and must pass up the sympathetic chain to the superior cervical ganglion b e f o r e they form synaptic connections with the postganglionic fibers. The preganglionic efferent fibers of the parasympathetic division are long, especially those of the vagus. They pass from the brain or sacral portion of the cord to ganglia on or very near the organ to be innervated before they form synaptic connections with the postganglionic fibers. The postganglionic fibers of the sympathetic division are consequently long and those of the parasympathetic division are short. The autonomic nervous system is essentially an efferent system, but afferent fibers are concerned in some of the visceral reflex acts.

It has been quite conclusively proved that the efferent fibers only are concerned in the production of pain, whether referred or visceral and that the afferent autonomic fibers play no part. For instance, pain referred to the shoulder tip from irritation of the central portion of the diaphragm. The impulse passes up the phrenic nerve to the cord, an adjustor neuron then carries the impulse to a synapse with the sympathetic efferent preganglionic fiber, thence to the sympathetic ganglion where the postganglionic fiber takes the impulse to the shoulder tip to the posterior column of the cord, to the lateral spinothalamic tract of the opposite side and thus up the cord to the cortical center in the postcentral gyrus.

There are certain tests for function of the autonomic system. Vasomotor function is determined by measurements of the skin temperature, and heat elimination by the extremities. Blood pressure response to standard forms of stimulation and posture, and response of the cardiac rate to standard exercise tests are also used. Measurement of vasoconstriction is made by determining the temperature response of the digits, hands and feet to fever. Blood pressure response to cold and inhalation of CO2 (10%) are measured. Responses of the blood pressure and pulse to standard exercise tolerance tests, as 15 trips up and down a set of two stairs 1½ feet high, are also measured. The vasodilatation tests are useful in differentiating organic and vasomotor disturbances of the extremities, and in the selection of patients who have occlusive arterial diseases for sympathetic ganglionectomy. Sweating tests are used (1) to assist in diagnosis of diseases affecting the function of sweating and, (2) to demonstrate whether or not complete denervation of the sympathetic f i b e r s to the hands or feet is present after cervicothoracic or lumbar sympathetic ganglionectomy. T e s t s of vasomotor reactability are valuable in determining the presence or absence of the disposition to essential hypertension. Test of the response of the heart to standard exercise tests are important in diagnosing cardiac neuroses, such as effort syndrome and neurocirculatory asthenia.

Of the 350,000 organic drugs known, practically all of them act to some extent upon the autonomic nervous system. A few of them act solely on the autonomics. Of these few, some act on the parasympathetics and s o m e on the sympathetics. Pilocarpine, physostigmine, muscarine and arecoline stimulate parasympathetic nerve ends; atropine, hyoscine and homatropine p a r a l y z e the parasympathetic endings. Adrenaline, tyramine, ergotoxine (in small doses) and ephedrine stimulate sympathetic nerve ends; while ergotoxine (in large doses) paralyzes them. Some of the drugs acting on the autonomic ganglia are nicotine, lobeline, methylhordenine and coniine which c a u s e s marked primary stimulation followed by depression if the dose is large enough; curare is purely depressent on the ganglia. Recently two terms have been coined to differentiate the function of the two types of autonomic fibers, "cholinergic" and "adrenergic," depending upon whether the fibers liberate acetycholine or adrenalin at their terminations. Thus, the postganglionic parasympathetic fibers will liberate acetylcholine at their terminations, this liberation being inhibited by atropine and augmented by physostigmine. The sympathetic f i b e r s

are considered to liberate adrenaline at t h e i r terminations. Cocaine potentiates this "adrenergic" action. In some instances fibers that belong anatomically to the true sympathetic system are cholinergic in action; e.g. the nerves to the sweat glands, and apparently some to the blood vessels, for in a normal animal acetylcholine dilates the arteriols, while after atropine it no longer has this effect. Experimental evidence has been obtained to the effect that the passage of impulses from the endings of pregangliomic fibers over to the ganglion cells of the postganglinic fibers is accomplished by the liberation of acetylcholine, probably in all instances, including both the true sympathetics and the parasympathetics.

Surgery of the autonomics is instituted in the severe cases or in the mild and moderately s e v e r e cases in which medical treatment has failed. Raynaud's diseases and the frequently associated scleroderma yield strikingly to sympathectomy in the suitable cases. Essential hyperhidorosis immediately and permanently responds to sympathectomy. Sympathetic ganglionectomy in carefully s e l e c t e d cases of thromboangitis obliterans has yielded as striking results as in Raynaud's diseases. Spastic and trophic lesions such as osteoporosis, poliomyelitis, t r o p h i c ulcers, causalgia and painful stumps have been treated successfully in some cases by sympathetic ramisectomy. Resection of the splanchnic nerves has had some success in lowering essential hypertension in selected cases of young people less than 40 who had a history of short duration and of slow progression of the diseases. Hirschsprung's diseases or congenital megacolon has responded to resection of the superior hypogastric plexus, as has also cord bladder.

--------------------o--------------------

Notice For Interns and Residents

Mr. Tom Testerman, Morrison, Oklahoma, advises there is an excellent opportunity for a young physician to practice in that vicinity. Anyone interested should get in touch with Mr. Testerman.

--------------------o--------------------

State Dues will not be accepted at the Registration Desk, Annual Meeting, except through C o u n t y Secretaries.

THE JOURNAL
OF THE
Oklahoma State Medical Association
Issued Monthly at McAlester, Oklahoma, under direction of
the Council.
Copyright, 1939, by Oklahoma State Medical Association,
McAlester, Oklahoma.

| Vol. XXXII | APRIL | Number 4 |

DR. L. S. WILLOUR...............................Editor-in-Chief
McAlester, Oklahoma

DR. T. H. McCARLEY...............................Associate Editor
McAlester, Oklahoma

Entered at the Post Office at McAlester, Oklahoma, as
second-class matter under the act of March 3rd, 1879.

This is the official Journal of the Oklahoma State Medical Association. All communications should be addressed to
The Journal of the Oklahoma State Medical Association,
McAlester Clinic, McAlester, Oklahoma. $4.00 per year; 40c
per copy.

The editorial department is not responsible for the opinions expressed in the original articles of contributors.

Reprints of original articles will be supplied at actual
cost provided request for them is attached to manuscripts
or made in sufficient time before publication.

Articles sent this Journal for publication and all those
read at the annual meetings of the State Association are
the sole property of this Journal. The Journal relies on
each individual contributor's strict adherence to this well-
known rule of medical journalism. In the event an article
sent this Journal for publication is published before appearance in The Journal the manuscript will be returned to
the writer.

Failure to receive The Journal should call for immediate
notification of the Editor, McAlester Clinic, McAlester,
Oklahoma.

Local news of possible interest to the medical profession,
notes on removals, changes of addresses, births, deaths and
weddings will be gratefully received.

Advertising of articles, drugs or compounds unapproved
by the Council on Pharmacy of the A. M. A., will not be
accepted.

Advertising rates will be supplied on application.

It is suggested that wherever possible members of the
State Association should patronize our advertisers in preference to others as a matter of fair reciprocity.

Printed by News-Capital Company, McAlester.

EDITORIAL

STATE DUES WILL NOT BE ACCEPTED AT THE REGISTRATION DESK, ANNUAL MEETING, EXCEPT THROUGH COUNTY SECRETARIES!

State Dues will not be accepted at the Registration Desk, Annual Meeting, except through County Secretaries.

The reason for this is that we do not know the amount of the County dues, and whether or not the Applicant has been acted upon favorably by the membership of his County Society. It has never been the policy of the State Association to accept dues direct; they must come through the Secretary of the component County Medical Society.

ANNUAL MEETING

You will note in this issue of the Journal the complete program of the State Meeting and you will agree that there will be presented some of the leading authorities of the country, with subjects that will be of vital and universal interest. You will note that the meetings of the House of Delegates have been arranged so that the Delegates will have the opportunity to attend the General Sessions on Tuesday and Wednesday mornings.

The Section programs are of unusual interest this year and the very best State talent will be presented on these programs.

The Skirvin Hotel has every facility for a meeting of this kind both as to hotel accommodations and accommodations for the various Section Meetings. It is particularly fine to have all of the functions under one roof; the only exception to this is the President's Reception and Dance which will be held in the beautiful Silver Glade Room in the Skirvin Tower. An excellent orchestra and floor show has been engaged for this social gathering.

With the Clinics which will be held throughout the day, Monday, May 1st, at the various Hospitals in Oklahoma City you can expect three days of edification and entertainment.

———o———

February 11, 1939

Dr. L. S. Willour, Secretary
Oklahoma State Medical Association
McAlester, Oklahoma

Dear Doctor:

At the suggestion and advice of a number of Councilors, it is requested that a prominent notice be published in the next issue of the Journal inviting the attention of officers and members of our Association to the fact that their committee on the revision and amendment of the Constitution and By-Laws is desirous of receiving from all members interested, information, guidance, and recommendations, so that the revised Constitution when submitted for final passage will represent the ultimate desire of a cross section of the largest majority of our membership and will thereby assure of passage without unnecessary controversy at the next annual meeting.

Communications relative to this matter may be addressed through the Councilors of the respective districts, or directly to a member of the committee composed of Dr. Ritzhaupt of Guthrie, Oklahoma; Dr. C. P. Bondurant, Medical Arts Building, Oklahoma City; and Dr. E. Albert Aisenstadt, American Hospital, Picher, Oklahoma.

Thanking you for giving this matter your early attention, I am

Very truly yours,

E. ALBERT AISENSTADT.

CC:—Dr. H. K. Speed
Dr. J. D. Osborn, Jr.

——————o——————

CONSTITUTION

Article 1. Name of Association

The name of this organization is the Oklahoma State Medical Association.

Article 2. Purpose

The object for which this Association is formed is to promote the science and art of medicine.

Article 3. Component Societies

The membership of this Association shall be organized into county medical societies or district medical societies as circumstances may dictate and the Association may determine. The functions of each such society and its relations to the Association shall be defined in a charter issued by the Association subject to amendment and revocation by the Association in accordance with such terms as may be prescribed by the By-Laws.

Article 4. Membership

The membership of this Association shall comprise all members in good standing of its component societies as indicated by the membership records of the Association.

Article 5. House of Delegates

Section 1. The House of Delegates shall be composed of (1) Delegates elected by the component county and district societies of the Association. (2) The officers of the Association enumerated in Article 8, Section 1, of this Constitution.

Section 2. All legislative powers of the Association reside in the House of Delegates which alone shall have authority to determine the policies of the Association. The House of Delegates shall transact all business of the Association, directly or through agencies created by it, the transaction of which is not vested by this Constitution in any other agency. The House of Delegates shall elect the general officers of the Association.

Section 3. The House of Delegates may provide for a division of the scientific work of the Association into such sections as in the judgment of the House will best promote the scientific and professional activities of the Association, or may delegate the Council to do so.

Section 4. The House of Delegates may provide for the organization of such Councilor District Societies as in its judgment will promote the best interests of the profession, but the membership of any such society shall be limited to members of the component county societies of which it is made up.

Article 6. Council

Section 1. The Council shall be composed of (1) Councilors elected by the House of Delegates from one or more nominations submitted by the component county and district societies of the Association grouped as Councilor Districts and provided for in the By-Laws, and (2) Officers of the Association enumerated in Article 8, Section 1, of this Constitution.

Section 2. The Council shall be the Executive or governing Board of this Association and shall carry out the mandates and policies of the Association which are determined by the House of Delegates. Between sessions of the House of Delegates the Council may initiate emergency legislation, but in no case may such legislation conflict in policy or mandates of the House of Delegates or be in conflict with this Constitution or By-Laws, and such legislation to be valid subsequent to the next annual meeting, shall be approved by the House of Delegates. The Council shall have supervision and control of the finances and particularly the expenditures of the Association, the investment of its funds, and the direction and control of its property.

Section 3. The Council shall meet at least once during the annual session, and on call by the President between annual sessions of the Association on his own initiative or by petition to the President by at least one-third of the members of the Council.

Article 7. Sessions and Meetings

Section 1. The Association shall hold an annual session. The time and place for holding each annual session may be fixed by the House of Delegates or, by authority of the House, by the Council.

Section 2. During the annual session there shall be at least one general meeting open to all registered members and guests; at least one meeting of the House of Delegates, either immediately preceding, during the session, or immediately following; and at least one meeting of the Council.

Section 3. Time and place fixed for an annual session, whether by the House of Delegates or the Council may be changed for cause by a two-thirds vote of the full membership of the Council.

Section 4. Special meetings of the Association or of the House of Delegates may be called by a two-thirds vote of the full membership of the Council, and shall be called upon petition to the Council by 30 or more delegates of the Association. At such a meeting only such business may be transacted as is specified in the call.

Article 8. Officers

Section 1. Officers of this Association shall be a President, a President Elect, a Secretary-Treasurer-Editor, a Speaker of the House of Delegates, a Vice-Speaker of the House of Delegates, and ten Councilors.

Section 2. The President shall be elected for a term of one year; the Secretary-Treasurer-Editor, the Speaker of the House of Delegates, the Vice Speaker of the House of Delegates and the Councilors, for three years; the Council being divided into classes, a portion will retire each year.

Section 3. The President shall assume office at the time of his inauguration, during the Annual Session. Delegates to the American Medical Association shall assume office at the close of the Annual Session. Speaker and Vice Speaker of the House of Delegates, Secretary-Treasurer-Editor and the Councilors shall assume their duties on January 1st, following their election.

Section 4. Vacancies created by the death, resignation, or removal of the above named officers shall be filled by temporary appointment by the Council, such appointment being effective until the next annual meeting of the House of Delegates, which shall elect a successor to complete the un-expired term, if any.

Article 9. Finance

Section 1. Funds for meeting the expenses of the Association may be arranged for by the House of Delegates by an equal per capita assessment upon each component county or district society. The amount of such assessment shall be fixed by the House of Delegates. Funds may also be ap-propriated by voluntary contributions requested by resolution of the House of Delegates, and in any other manner approved by the House of Delegates.

Section 2. Request for expenditure of funds may be voted by the House of Delegates but all appro-priations must be authorized for expenditure by the Council.

Section 3. The Council shall submit an annual budget for approval by the House of Delegates, detailing its financial needs for the ensuing year, and the House of Delegates is authorized to accept, reject, or amend the budget submitted.

Article 10. Referendum

Section 1. At any session of the House of Dele-gates, the House may by two-thirds vote of its registered members submit any question to the membership of the Association for its vote. A ma-jority vote of all the members of the Association shall determine the question.

Section 2. The Council shall be in charge of the referendum and may designate an officer of the Association or a Committee to canvass the vote and announce the results.

Article 11. Seal

The Association shall have a common seal. The power to change or renew the seal shall rest with the House of Delegates.

Article 12. Ethics

Principles of Medical Ethics of the American Medical Association in force at the time of the adoption of this Constitution, and as they may from time to time be thereafter amended by the American Medical Association, shall be accepted as the Principles of Medical Ethics of the Oklahoma State Medical Association and is binding on its members and component county and district so-cieties.

Article 13. Amendments

The House of Delegates may amend any article of this Constitution or any section or part thereof by a two-thirds vote of the delegates registered at any annual session, provided that such amendment shall have been presented in writing in open meet-ing of the House of Delegates at the previous an-nual session and that it shall have been published at least once during the year, in the Journal or a bulletin of the Association.

Article 14

Upon the adoption of this Constitution all pre-vious Constitutions are thereby repealed, and all By-Laws and enactments in conflict with this Constitution are declared as of no effect.

———o———

Editorial Notes—Personal and General

DR. H. L. RAINS, Okmulgee, has been appointed County Health Superintendent of Okmulgee County.

DR. WALDO B. NEWELL, JR., Enid, has been appointed County Health Superintendent of Gar-field County.

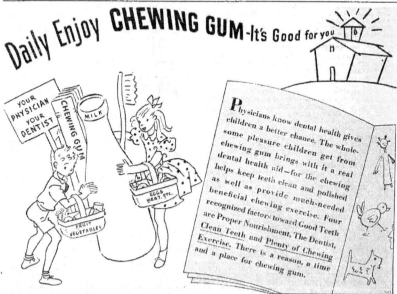

DR. and MRS. WALTER HARDY, Ardmore, have returned from Rochester, Minn., where they spent two weeks in March.

DR. CARROLL M. POUNDERS, Oklahoma City, professor of pediatrics at the University of Oklahoma, was speaker on the program of the Dallas Southern Clinical Conference in Dallas, March 13th.

○

Southeastern Oklahoma

The Southeastern Oklahoma Medical Association held a meeting at Durant, Wednesday, April 12th, which was well attended. All sessions were held at the Bryant hotel, commencing at 10:30 a.m., with noon-day luncheon, and closing late in the afternoon. Dr. W. K. Haynie is president and Dr. John A. Haynie, secretary-treasurer. Following is the program:

Scientific program:

"Endocrinology in General Practice," Dr. T. H. Briggs, Atoka. Subject unannounced, Dr. E. H. Shuller, McAlester. "Sub-Acute Bacterial Endo-Carditis," Dr. B. B. Coker, Durant.

Afternoon program:

Invocation, Rev. W. T. White, pastor, Nazarene church, Durant. Welcome address, Dr. A. J. Wells, Calera. Response, Dr. L. S. Willour, McAlester. President's annual address, Dr. W. K. Haynie, Durant. "History, Progress, and Needs of the University of Oklahoma School of Medicine," Dr. Robert U. Patterson, Dean, Oklahoma City. "Progressive and Organized Medicine," Dr. W. A. Howard, president-elect, Oklahoma State Medical Asso-

ciation, Chelsea. "Some Aspects of Pathology and Surgery of Gall Bladder," Dr. John Munal, Holdenville. "Activities of the Present Session of the Legislature," Mr. R. H. Graham, executive secretary, Oklahoma State Medical Association, McAlester.

Officers were elected as follows: president, Dr. W. L. Shippey, Poteau; vice-president, Dr. J. S. Fulton, Atoka; Dr. John A. Haynie, Durant, succeeded himself as secretary-treasurer.

○

OBITUARIES

J. P. NELSON, M.D.

Dr. J. P. Nelson, of Beggs, Past President of the Okmulgee County Medical Society, was called from his labors February 18, 1939, due to a short illness from streptococcic infection which gained entrance through the throat. Dr. Nelson graduated from the Chicago University, School of Medicine, in 1903. He established his first practice in Piatt, Ill., moving to McAlester, Oklahoma, in 1908. He moved to Okmulgee County in 1915.

The 68-year-old doctor was a member of the Okmulgee County Medical Society, the Oklahoma State Medical Association, and the American Medical Association.

In the death of Dr. Nelson, Okmulgee County has lost an honorable public spirited citizen and gentleman of the highest type in our profession. During his long career as a physician, he always placed his own comfort secondary to the comfort of those he

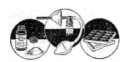
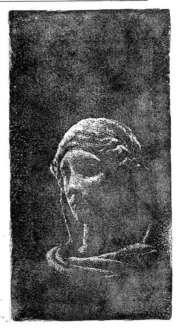

served. It is tragic that the career of a gentleman so genial and a friend so true should end so suddenly, but for those who mourn him there is a solace that his was a happy life. He was a devoted husband, indulgent father, and truly a "friend to man."

His affability, beaming smile, and spontaneous good fellowship characterized him as one of the most lovable members of our society.

It is not easy to say farewell to such a man, nor to relinquish his genial smile and fine companionship, but pleasant memories will endure after time has eased the hurt of parting; and there is the consolation for us, his friends, and for those who loved him most, that there has been less suffering and more sunshine because he lived among us.

Now be it resolved by the Okmulgee County Medical Society that a copy of the foregoing written expression of our esteem be placed in the minutes of the County Society and a copy mailed to the office of the State Medical Association Journal and a copy be sent to the widow of the deceased.

Adopted unanimously.

> J. C. Matheney,
> S. D. Leslie,
> O. M. Uling, Committee.

RECENT DEATHS
(Insufficient Data for Obituaries)
Dr. W. W. Gill, Enid, March, 1939.

New Books

CANCER, ITS DIAGNOSIS AND TREATMENT, By Max Cutler, M.D., Associate in Surgery, Northwestern University Medical School; Chairman, Scientific Committee, Chicago Tumor Institute; Consultant Tumor Clinic and Director Cancer Research, U. S. Veterans Administration, Hines, Illinois. AND Franz Buschke, M.D., Assistant Roentgenologist, Chicago Tumor Institute; Late Assistant Roentgen Institute University of Zurich; ASSISTED by Simeon T. Cantril, M.D., Director Tumor Institute, Swedish Hospital, Seattle; Late Assistant, Chicago Tumor Institute.

The purpose of this text, according to the authors in this preface, is to present the essential known clinical facts of cancer in diagnosis and therapy; to separate the second or proven evidence on cancer from this huge mass of controversial and confusing literature that has been produced since the advent of X-ray and radium irradiation.

Doctors Cutler and Buschke have accomplished their purpose admirably in this text, and are to be commended. The common types of cancer are presented under different chapters. The manner of presentation makes one feel he is reading some well planned lectures of the authors. The signs and symptoms of early and late cancer are discussed from the clinical aspect, chiefly as observed by the authors from their huge clinical

material. Voluminous quotations on theory, physics and experimentation are conspicuous by their absence. Pathology and histology are discussed in their importance to proper therapy. The value of surgery, X-ray and radium therapy are carefully evaluated by the authors, and the preferential therapy is clearly stated in most instances. The details of therapy and the confusing details as used by different authorities are omitted.

The book is to be commended for its practicability.

Pneumococcic Meningitis

Four recoveries out of seven cases of pneumococcic meningitis treated with sulfanilamide are reported by Barbara A. Hewell, M.D., and A. Graeme Mitchell, M.D., Cincinnati, in The Journal of the American Medical Association for March 18.

This disease is an infection of the meninges, or membrane coverings of the brain and spinal cord, by a pneumococcic organism.

A review of the literature up to 1927 shows 150 authentic recoveries from this disease, the authors say. Approximately 30 additional recoveries have occurred during the years 1927 to 1937. Most of these have been attributed to spinal drainage and the administration of antipneumococcus serum or the drug, ethylhydrocupreine, but in general results with these treatment measures have been unsuccessful.

The authors point out that "in the ten years preceding 1937 there were in the Children's Hospital of Cincinnati and in the pediatric service of the Cincinnati General Hospital 23 children suffering from pneumococcic meningitis, the mortality in this group being 100 per cent. Since the use of sulfanilamide four of seven patients with the condition have recovered."

Stating that there are at least 30 cases of recovery from the disease, including four observed by them, in which part of the treatment consisted in the use of sulfanilamide or related compounds, the authors say that "it appears reasonable to conclude that sulfanilamide was responsible for these recoveries, since the mortality rate was so high with other forms of treatment. Recovery occurred with the use of different compounds, such as prontosil, sulfanilamide and sulfapyradine; that is to say, the data now available do not permit conclusions concerning the relative merit of these different compounds in the treatment of pneumococcic meningitis.

"There are at least eight cases of pneumococcic meningitis, including three observed by us, in which sulfanilamide was given and in which recovery did not follow.

"Of the patients receiving sulfanilamide who recovered, only one showed pneumococci in the blood culture. Of the eight patients receiving sulfanilamide who died, the blood cultures were positive for seven. This indicates that even with the use of sulfanilamide a blood stream infection with pneumococci is a factor in mortality and perhaps also that with such infection large doses of sulfanilamide should be tried."

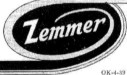

PROGRAM

Forty-Seventh Annual Session of the Oklahoma State Medical Association at Oklahoma City, May 1, 2, 3, 1939

General Information

Headquarters—Skirvin Hotel.

Registration and Commercial Exhibits— Fourteenth Floor, Skirvin Hotel. All physicians, except those outside the State and visiting guests, must hold membership receipt for the year 1939 before registering. Please attend to this at once, if you are not in good standing, by seeing your County Secretary.

Woman's Auxiliary — Annual Meeting, Tuesday, May 2nd, 10:00 A.M., Y. W. C. A. Luncheon, Tuesday, May 2nd, 1:00 P.M., Y.W.C.A. All other information will be given to visitors at the Registration Desk at the time of the Convention.

Guest Speakers—Dr. W. Wayne Babcock, Professor of Surgery, Temple University, Philadelphia; Dr. J. F. Hamilton, Willis C. Campbell Clinic, Memphis; Dr. Austin A. Hayden, Secretary, Board of Trustees, American Medical Association, and Chairman, Department of Oto-Laryngology and Ophthalmology, St. Joseph Hospital, Chicago; Dr. Edw. N. Smith, Instructor Orthopedics, State Medical Association Post Graduate Course, Oklahoma City.

Council—The Council will meet at 3:00 P.M., Monday, May 1st, Wilson Room, Mezzanine Floor, Skirvin Hotel, for the transaction of business affairs, and thereafter on call of the President.

House of Delegates—The House of Delegates will meet at 8:00 P.M., Monday, May 1st, Second Floor, Skirvin Tower, and at 8:00 A.M. Tuesday and Wednesday, May 2nd and 3rd, in the same place.

Resolutions—Any resolutions that you may desire to submit to the House of Delegates should be prepared and presented at the first meeting of the House of Delegates.

General Sessions—Will be held, beginning at 10:00 A.M., Tuesday, May 2nd, and 10:00 A.M., Wednesday, May 3rd, Venetian Room, Fourteenth Floor, Skirvin Hotel.

Public Health Meeting—Will be held at 1:30 P.M., May 1st, Empire Room, Skirvin Hotel. Program on page 140.

Oklahoma Pediatric Society—Meetings at Children's Hospital and Skirvin Hotel. See Program, page 140, for details.

Golf Tournament—The Oklahoma State Medical Association Golf tournament will be held on Monday, May 1st, at the Oklahoma City Golf and Country Club Course. The fee will be Two Dollars per player and the tournament round may be played any time Monday. If players would enjoy playing more golf than this, arrangements can be made by contacting Dr. Everett B. Neff, Chairman of the Golf Committee.

The tournament awards are unusually attractive and are donated by the following concerns in Oklahoma City: Prichard Oil Company; Caviness Surgical Company; Veazey Drug Company, and the Osler Drug Shoppe.

We are anticipating a large turnout and would like to make a request that all players who wish to play in the Handicap tournament bring with them their individual handicap scores, endorsed by their local professional. Locker room facilities are available free of charge to all players, members of the Association.

Clinics—Medical and Surgical Clinics are to be held by the Oklahoma City profession, Monday, May 1st. Program on pages 138, 139, 140, this issue.

Fraternity Dinners — Arrangements for these dinners will be made with the Committee of which Dr. Tom Wainright is Chairman.

Medical Reserve Officers—Dinner will be held Tuesday, 6 P.M., May 2nd, Parlor G, Skirvin Hotel. Reservations may be made through Dr. George Borecky, Chairman.

Women Physicians —

Tuesday May 2, at 7 P.M., in the Young Woman's Christian Association Building, there will be a dinner for all women m e m b e r s of the State Medical Association.

Reservations made through Dr. Ruth S. Reichmann, Chairman.

―――――o―――――

Committees In Charge

L. J. STARRY, General Chairman

Advisory Committee — Arthur W h i t e, Chairman; C. E. Clymer, LeRoy D. Long, R. M. Howard, Horace Reed, J. C. MacDonald, Chas. E. Barker, Henry H. Turner, C. J. Fishman.

Program Committee—N. P. Eley, Chairman; R. Q. Goodwin, D. W. Branham.

Scientific Exhibits—Robert H. Akin, Chairman; Basil Hayes, Elias Margo.

Commercial Exhibits—S. R. Fryer, Chairman; John H. Lamb, Hervey A. Foerster.

Finance—Ralph Bowen, Chairman; Hervey A. Foerster, Wm. H. Bailey.

Entertainment — Dick Lowry, Chairman; Henry C. Morrison, J. J. Caviness.

Stationery and Badges—Frank Harbison, Chairman; Jess Herrmann, J. H. Huggins.

Hotels—C. W. Lemon, Chairman; Floyd Moorman, O. G. Hazel.

Women Physicians — Ruth S. Reichmann, Chairman; Grace Hassler, Mary V. S. Sheppard.

Auxiliary—Mrs. L. C. McHenry, Chairman; Mrs. N. Price Eley, Mrs. J. F. Kuhn, Jr., Mrs. Lea A. Riely, Mrs. Nesbitt Miller, Mrs. W. K. Ishmael, Mrs. D. H. O'Donoghue, Mrs. Joe H. Coley.

Golf—Everett B. Neff, Chairman; W. J. Thompson, Robt. U. Patterson.

Reserve Officers — Dr. Geo. B o r e c k y, Chairman; Leo Cailey, W. F. Keller.

•

Fraternity Dinners — T o m Wainright, Chairman; O. A. Watson, W. W. Rucks, Jr.

Section Hosts — J. P. Wolff, Chairman; Gerald West, O. A. Watson.

―――――o―――――

SECTIONS

All Sections will meet at 1:30 P.M., Tuesday, May 2nd, and at the same hour on Wednesday, May 3rd. Meeting places will be as follows:

Surgery — Venetian R o o m, Fourteenth Floor, Skirvin Hotel.

Medicine—Second Floor, Skirvin Tower.

Eye, Ear, Nose & Throat—Crystal Room, Mezzanine Floor, Skirvin Hotel.

Obstetrics & Pediatrics — Wilson Room, Mezzanine Floor, Skirvin Hotel.

Genito-Urinary & Syphilology—Room 1005, Skirvin Hotel.

Dermatology & Radiology — Room 1006, Skirvin Hotel.

―――――o―――――

CLINICS

Committee in Charge of Surgical Clinics (All Hospitals)

DR. W. K. WEST, Chairman (St. Anthony Hospital).

DR. J. C. McDONALD (Wesley Hospital).

DR. OSCAR WHITE (University Hospital).

DR. R. L. NOELL, (Crippled Children's Hospital).

Operative Clinic
St. Anthony Hospital
South Surgery
May 1, 1939

Room 1—9:00-10:30, Dr. H o r a c e Reed, General Surgery.

10:30-12:00, Dr. L. J. Starry, General Surgery.

Room 2—9:00-10:30, Dr. J. F. Kuhn and Dr. J. F. Kuhn, Jr., Gynecology.

10:30-12:00, Dr. Curt Von Wedel, Plastic Surgery.

Room 3—9:00-12:00, Dr. Leroy Long, General Surgery; Dr. LeRoy D. Long, General Surgery; Dr. Wendell Long, Gynecology.

Room 4—9:00-10:30, Dr. Harry Wilkins, Neuro-Surgery; Dr. J. D. Herrmann, Neuro-Surgery.

10:30-12:00, Dr. T. O. C o s t o n, Eye Clinic.

North Surgery

Room 2—9:00-12:00, Symposium on Injuries to the Upper Extremity. Dr. H. Dale Collins, General Surgery; Dr. Geo. Kimball, General Surgery; Dr. D. H. O'Donoghue, Orthopedic Surgery; Dr. W. K. W e s t, Orthopedic Surgery.

Room 5—9:00-10:30, Dr. R. H. Akin, Urology.

Obst. Dept.—9:00-10:30, Dr. E. P. Allen, Obstetrics.

10:30-12:00, Dr. J. B. Eskridge, Jr., Obstetrics.

Surgical Clinics
May 1, 1939
University Hospital

Room 1 — 9:00-10:30, Dr. C. E. Clymer, General Surgery.

10:30-12:00, Dr. F. M. Lingenfelter, General Surgery.

Room 2 — 9:00-10:30, Dr. Joseph Kelso, Gynecology.

10:30-12:00, Dr. Grider Penick, Gynecology.

Room 3—9:00-10:30, Dr. L. M. Westfall, Eye Surgery.

10:30-12:00, Dr. W. L. Bonham, Ear, Nose and Throat Clinic.

Room 4 — 9:00-10:30, Dr. Rex B o l e n d, Urology.

10:30-12:00, Dr. R. L. Murdoch, Proctology.

Obst. Dept.—9:00-10:30, Dr. W. W. Wells, Obstetrics.

10:30-12:00, Dr. Dick Lowry, Obstetrics.

Crippled Children's Hospital

Room 1—9:00-10:30, Dr. L. C. McHenry, Bronchoscopy.

10:30-12:00, Dr. John F. Burton, Plastic Surgery.

Room 2—9:00-10:00, Dr. E. Gordon Ferguson, Eye Clinic.

10:00-11:00, Dr. Paul C. Colonna, Orthopedic Surgery.

11:00-12:00, Dr. C. R. Rountree, Orthopedic Surgery.

Bone and Joint Hospital and McBride Clinic

9:00 to 12:00—Drs. Earl D. McBride, Elias Margo and Howard B. Shorbe, Orthopedic Surgery.

---o---

Wesley Hospital

General Surgery—Dr. J. H. Robinson, Dr. A. H. Bell.

General Surgery—Dr. Louis H. Ritzhaupt.

Nose and Throat—Dr. J. C. McDonald, Dr. Ed D. McKay.

Urological—Dr. Basil A. Hayes.

Gynecology—Dr. LeRoy H. Sadler.

---o---

Medical Clinics
May 1, 1939
Wesley Hospital

2:00 P.M.—Dr. D. D. Paulus, Gallbladder disease.

2:30 P.M.—Dr. W. W. Rucks, Jr., Heart disease.

3:00 P.M.—Dr. Walker Morledge, Diseases of the Chest.

3:30 P.M.—Dr. R. Q. Goodwin, Pneumonia.

4:00 P.M.—Round Table Discussion.

St. Anthony's Hospital

1:30 P.M.—Dr. Ray M. Balyeat, Allergic Clinic.

2:00 P.M.—Dr. Lea Riely, Blood Dyscrasia.

2:30 P.M.—Dr. Louis J. Moorman, Nontuberculous pulmonary infections.

3:00 P.M.—Dr. John A. Roddy, Physical (mechanical) Treatment of Decompensated Cardio-Vascular Diseases.

3:30 P.M.—Dr. Price Eley, Gastro Intestinal Diseases.

4:00 P.M.—Round table discussion.

University Hospital

1:30 P.M.—Dr. A. W. White, Gastro Intestinal Diseases.

2:00 P.M.—Dr. C. J. Fishman, Neurological Clinic.

2:30 P.M.—Dr. Henry H. Turner, Endocrinology.

3:30 P.M.—Dr. Wann Langston, Cardiac Clinic.

3:30 P.M.—Dr. Phil McNeill, Chest Clinic.

4:00 P.M.—Round table discussion.

Oklahoma Pediatric Society
Monday, May 1, 1939

President, A. L. Solomon, Oklahoma City.

President-Elect, Hugh Graham, Tulsa.

Secretary, Ben H. Nicholson, Oklahoma City.

9:30 A.M.—Children's Hospital.
Presentation of C a s e s and Clinical Program by the Pediatric Staff.

2:00 P.M.—Crystal Room, Mezzanine Floor, Skirvin Hotel.

"Nutrition of the Infant and Child."

The afternoon will be devoted to a discussion of this subject by Dr. P. C. Jeans, Professor of Pediatrics, University of Iowa. All members of the State Medical Association who are interested are invited to attend.

6:00 P.M.—Crystal Room, Skirvin Hotel. Dinner in honor of Dr. Jeans.

Council Meeting—3:00 P.M., Wilson Room, Mezzanine Floor, Skirvin Hotel.

Public Health Department Program
Monday, May 1, 1939

1:30 P.M., Empire Room, Skirvin Hotel

G. F. Mathews, State Health Commissioner, Presiding.

"Contact Examination in Syphilis Control —Methods and Results," Mack I. Shanholtz, Wewoka.

"A Backslider Testifies," Ned R. Smith, Tulsa.

"Management of A Maternity Service With Nurse Attendance At Delivery In A Rural Area—A Preliminary Report," Isadore Dyer, Tahlequah.

Election of Officers.

House of Delegates
Monday, May 1, 1939

8:00 P.M., Empire Room, Mezzanine Floor, Skirvin Hotel.

Tuesday, May 2, 1939

8:00 A.M. — House of Delegates Meeting, Empire Room, Mezzanine Floor, Skirvin Hotel.

General Scientific Section
Tuesday, May 2, 1939

Venetian Room, 14th Floor, Skirvin Hotel

10:00 to 10:40 A.M.—"Toxemias of Late Pregnancy," Dr. Edw. N. Smith, Instructor Post Graduate Medical Teaching, Oklahoma City.

10:40 to 11:20 A.M.—"Peripheral Vascular Disease: Diagnosis and Treatment," Dr. J. F. Hamilton, Willis C. Campbell Clinic, Memphis, Tenn.

11:20 to 12:00 Noon—"Surgery of the General Practitioner," Dr. W. Wayne Babcock, Temple University, Philadelphia.

Section on General Surgery
Tuesday, May 2, 1939

Charles M. O'Leary, Sponsor

Venetian Room, 14th Floor, Skirvin Hotel

Chairman—F. L. Flack, Tulsa.

Vice-Chairman—John E. McDonald, Tulsa.

Secretary — John F. Burton, Oklahoma City.

1:30 P.M.

"Injuries of the Brain and Spinal Cord"— Chairman's Address, F. L. Flack, Tulsa.

"The Anatomy of Operative Incisions"— E. Eugene Rice, Shawnee. Discussion: Oscar White, Oklahoma City.

"Septicemia"—Geo. A. LaMotte, Oklahoma City. Discussion: R. M. H o w a r d, Oklahoma City.

"Diagnosis and Treatment of Infection and Gangrene in Extremities of Diabetics" W. D. Hoover, Tulsa. Discussion: Fred Watson, Okmulgee.

"Abdominal Decompression with Discussion of Means and Measures to Obtain Same"—A. S. Risser, Blackwell. Discussion: Cyril E. Clymer, Oklahoma City.

"Gall Bladder Surgery"—F. A. Hudson, Enid. Discussion: A. Ray W i l e y, Tulsa.

(All papers presented before the Sections are property of the Association, for publication in the J o u r n a l and should be presented to the Secretary of the Section when read.)

————————o————————

Section on General Medicine

Tuesday, May 2, 1939

George J. Seibold, Sponsor

Second Floor, Skirvin Tower.

Chairman—Frank Nelson, Tulsa.

Vice-Chairman—E. R. Musick, Oklahoma City.

Secretary — Milam McKinney, Oklahoma City.

1:30 P.M.

"Presentable Data on Mercurial Diuresis" —Frederic G. Dorwart, Muskogee.

"Therapeutics in Allergy (Lantern Slides)" —E. Rankin Denny, Tulsa.

"Enemas: Their Uses and Abuses" — S. Charlton Shepard, Tulsa.

"The Use of Autohemotherapy Re-Inforced With Artificial Fever in the Treatment of Rheumatic Disease"—Wm. K. Ishmael, Oklahoma City.

"The Clinical Significance of S y s t o l i c Murmurs"—Fred C. Rewerts, Bartlesville.

(All papers presented before the Sections are property of the Association, for publication in the J o u r n a l and should be presented to the Secretary of the Section when read.)

Section on Eye, Ear, Nose and Throat

Tuesday, May 2, 1939

Lee R. Emenhiser, Sponsor

Crystal Room, Mezzanine Floor, Skirvin Hotel.

Chairman—E. H. Coachman, Muskogee.

Vice-Chairman—F. M. Cooper, Oklahoma City.

Secretary—James R. Reed, Oklahoma City.

1:45 P.M.

"Diphtheria Carriers"—E. H. Coachman, Muskogee.

"Tendon Transplantation in Ocular Muscle Paralysis"—Harvey O. Randel, Oklahoma City. Discussion: C. H. Haralson, Tulsa.

"Tempero-Mandibular Syndrome (Costen's Syndrome)"—Lee K. Emenhiser, Oklahoma City. Discussion: L. Chester McHenry, Oklahoma City.

"Remarks on Treatment of Dacryocystitis" —D. L. Edwards, Tulsa. Discussion: J. P. McGee, Oklahoma City.

"Postoperative Management of Tonsillectomies" — G. E. Haslam, Anadarko. Discussion: Paul J. Craden, El Reno.

"Removal of Non-Magnetic Foreign Bodies from Vitreous"—J. J. Caviness, Oklahoma City. Discussion: E. G o r d o n Ferguson, Oklahoma City.

(All papers presented before the Sections are property of the Association, for publication in the J o u r n a l and should be presented to the Secretary

————————o————————

Section on Obstetrics and Pediatrics

Tuesday, May 2, 1939

Gerald Rogers, Sponsor

Wilson Room, Mezzanine Floor, Skirvin Hotel.

Chairman—C. W. Arrendell, Ponca City.

Vice-Chairman—Carl F. Simpson, Tulsa.

Secretary — Ben H. Nicholson, Oklahoma City.

1:30 P.M.

"Some Observations on the Diagnosis and Treatment of Pneumonias of E a r l y

Childhood"—C. W. Arrendell, Ponca City.

"Further Observations on the Relationship of Vitamin A Deficiency in Pregnancy to Congenital Malformations"—G. R. Russell, Tulsa. Discussion: Clark Hall, Oklahoma City, and P. C. Jeans, Iowa City, Iowa.

"Convulsions in Childhood"—Jess D. Herrman, Oklahoma City. Discussion: C. E. Bradley, Tulsa, and C a r r o l l M. Pounders, Oklahoma City.

"Anaesthesia and Analgesia in Obstetrics and Its Relation to Asphyxia Neonatorum"—H. J. Reichert, Moore. Discussion: Chas. Ed White, Muskogee, and Roy Emanuel, Chickasha.

"Laryngotracheo Bronchitis"—Geo. Felts, Oklahoma City. Discussion: L. Chester McHenry, Oklahoma City.

(All papers presented before the Sections are property of the Association, for publication in the J o u r n a l and should be presented to the Secretary of the Section when read.)

───────o───────

Section on Genito-Urinary Diseases and Syphilology

Tuesday, May 2, 1939
Basil A. Hayes, Sponsor
Room 1005, Skirvin Hotel
1:30 P.M.

Chairman—Elijah S. Sullivan, Oklahoma City.
Vice-Chairman—Henry S. Browne, Tulsa.
Secretary — Robert H. Akin, Oklahoma City.

1:30 P.M.

"Bilharziasis" — Chairman's Address, Elijah S. Sullivan, Oklahoma City.

"Preliminary Report on the Use of Histidine in the Treatment of Hunner's Ulcer"—K. F. Swanson, Tulsa.

"Bladder Infections in the Female"—D. W. Branham, Oklahoma City.

"Urethral Strictures"—J. W. Rogers, Tulsa.

"Bladder Diverticuli" — J. Holland Howe, Ponca City.

"Hypernephroma, With Case R e p o r t" — Allen R. Russell, McAlester.

(All papers presented before the Sections are property of the Association, for publication in the J o u r n a l and should be presented to the Secretary of the Section when read.)

───────o───────

Section on Dermatology and Radiology

Tuesday, May 2, 1939
Onis George Hazel, Sponsor
Room 1006, Skirvin Hotel

Chairman—W. A. Showman, Tulsa.
Vice-Chairman—E. D. Greenberger, McAlester.
Secretary—Hervey A. Foerster, Oklahoma City.

1:30 P.M.

Election of Officers

"The Common Skin Diseases of the Lower Extremities," Chairman's Address — Winfred A. Showman, T u l s a. Discussion: M. M. Wickham, Norman.

"Intestinal Perforations Roentgen Aspects" — Edw. D. Greenberger, McAlester. Discussion: Ralph E. Myers, Oklahoma City.

"Interstitial Radium Treatment of Cancer of Lower Hip"—L. K. Chont, Resident in Radiology, University Hospital, Oklahoma City. Discussion: Wm. Eastland, Oklahoma City.

"Atrophy of the Subcutaneous Fat—Case Report"—Onis G. Hazel, and John H. L a m b, Oklahoma City. Discussion: Chas. P. Bondurant, Oklahoma City.

"Common Lesions of the Oral Cavity, Local in Origin"—E. S. Lain, Oklahoma City. Discussion: Harry Green, Tulsa.

(All papers presented before the Sections are property of the Association for publication in the J o u r n a l and should be presented to the Secretary of the Section when read.)

───────o───────

PROGRAM GENERAL MEETING

Tuesday, May 2, 1939
8:00 P.M.
Second Floor, Skirvin Tower
L. J. STARRY, General Chairman, Presiding

Invocation—Rev. Frederick W. Beckerle, Oklahoma City.

Vocal Solo — "Morning" (Oley Speaks) Miss Mary Newman (Mary Lou of Showboat fame).

Introduction of Guests—L. J. Starry, Oklahoma City.

Address of Welcome—Carroll. M. Pounders, President of Oklahoma C o u n t y Medical Society.

Response—W. Pat Fite, Muskogee.

Vocal Solo — "On The Beautiful B l u e Danube" (Strauss), Miss Mary New- man.

Introduction of President-Elect — H. K. Speed, Sayre, Retiring President.

President's Address—W. A. Howard, Chelsea.

9: 30 P.M.

PRESIDENT'S RECEPTION AND DANCE

Silver Glade Room, Skirvin Tower

———o———

House of Delegates

Wednesday, May 3, 1939

8: 00 A.M.—Meeting of the House of Delegates, Second Floor, Skirvin Tower.

———o———

General Scientific Section

Wednesday, May 3, 1939
Venetian Room, Fourteenth Floor
Skirvin Hotel

10:00 to 10:40 A.M.—*"Pseudomycotic Leg Ulcers"*—J. F. Hamilton, Memphis.

10:40 to 11:20 A.M. — *"Intestinal Malignancy"* — W. Wayne Babcock, Philadelphia.

11:20 to 12:00 Noon—*"The Democracy of American Medicine"*—Austin A. Hayden, Secretary of Trustees, American M e d i c a l Association, and Chairman Department of Oto-Laryngology and Ophthalmology, St. Joseph Hospital, Chicago.

Section on General Surgery

Wednesday, May 3, 1939
Charles M. O'Leary, Sponsor
Venetian Room, Fourteenth Floor,
Skirvin Hotel
1: 30 P.M.

Election of Officers.

"Use of Vitallium Metal in Treatment of Fractures"—Frank A. Stuart, Tulsa. Discussion: D. H. O'Donoghue, Oklahoma City.

"The New Extra Pleural Pneumothorax Treatment" — Paul B. Lingenfelter, C l i n t o n. Discussion: F. P. Baker, Talihina.

"Experiences with Internal Fixation in Fractures of the Hip"—Chas. R. Rountree, Oklahoma City. Discussion: John E. McDonald, Tulsa.

"Emergency Treatment of Hand Injuries" —Horton Hughes, Shawnee. Discussion: Ray Lindsay, Pauls Valley.

"Emergency Treatment of Airplane Injuries" — Roy L. Fisher, Frederick. Discussion: Clarence E. N o r t h c u t t, Ponca City.

(All papers presented before the Sections are property of the Association, for publication in the J o u r n a l and should be presented to the Secretary of the Section when read.)

———o———

Section on General Medicine

Wednesday, May 3, 1939
George J. Seibold, Sponsor
Second Floor, Skirvin Tower
1: 30 P.M.

Election of Officers.

"Gout: Its Systemic and Joint Manifestations"—E. Goldfain, Oklahoma City.

"Diaphragmatic Hernia" — E. G. Hyatt, Tulsa.

"Practical Management in Peripheral Vascular Disease" — B. E. Mulvey, Oklahoma City.

"Pancoast's Tumor: Case Report and Lantern Slides"—J. M. Byrum, Shawnee.

"The Private Practitioner and Vital Statistics"—Joe Rose, M.A., Oklahoma City.

(All papers presented before the Sections are property of the Association, for publication in the Journal and should be presented to the Secretary of the Section when read.)

Section on Eye, Ear, Nose and Throat

Wednesday, May 3, 1939
Lee R. Emenhiser, Sponsor
Crystal Room, Mezzanine Floor,
Skirvin Hotel
1:45 P.M.

Election of Officers.

"*Otomycosis of External Ear*" — Hugh Evans, Tulsa. Discussion: A. H. Davis, Tulsa.

"*Acute Glaucoma*"—Edw. D. McKay, Oklahoma City. Discussion: F. M. Cooper, Oklahoma City.

"*Nasal Plastic Operations*" — M. C. England, Woodward. Discussion: Lee K. Emenhiser, Oklahoma City.

"*Practical Technique of Office Refraction*" —H. F. Vandever, Enid. Discussion: Leo F. Cailey, Oklahoma City.

"*Heterophoria*" — C. H. Haralson, Tulsa. Discussion: F. M. Cooper, Oklahoma City.

"*Petrositis*" — Theodore G. Wails, Oklahoma City. Discussion: Wm. L. Bonham, Oklahoma City.

(All papers presented before the Sections are property of the Association, for publication in the Journal and should be presented to the Secretary of the Section when read.)

Section on Obstetrics and Pediatrics

Wednesday, May 3, 1939
Gerald Rogers, Sponsor
Wilson Room, Mezzanine Floor,
Skirvin Hotel

1:30 P.M.

Election of Officers.

"*Later Reaction of Children With Asphyxia at Birth*"—Chas. Ed. White, Muskogee.

"*Sterility*"—Dick Lowry, Oklahoma City.

"*Use of X-ray in Obstetrics*"—E. O. Johnson, Tulsa.

"*Report on Post Graduate Work in Oklahoma*"—Dr. Edward N. Smith, Oklahoma City.

(All papers presented before the Sections are property of the Association for publication in the Journal and should be presented to the Secretary of the Section when read.)

Section on Genito-Urinary Diseases and Syphilology

Wednesday, May 3, 1939
Basil A. Hayes, Sponsor
Room 1005, Skirvin Hotel
1:30 P.M.

Election of Officers.

"*Perinephritic Abscess*" — Chas. M. O'Leary, Oklahoma City.

"*Renal Emergencies*"—A. R. Sugg, Ada.

"*Toxic States Seen in Urology*"—Basil A. Hayes, Oklahoma City.

"*Lymphopathia eVnerea*" — Joseph Fulcher, Tulsa.

"*Some Problems of Syphilis Control in Oklahoma*"—David V. Hudson, Tulsa.

(All papers presented before the Sections are the property of the Association for publication in the Journal and should be presented to the Secretary of the Section when read.)

State Dues will not be accepted at the Registration Desk, Annual Meeting, except through County Secretaries.

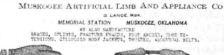

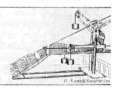

COMMITTEE REPORTS

These reports are made in compliance with provisions of the Constitution and By-Laws which call for publication of such matter in the issue of The Journal preceding the Annual Session.

Annual Report—Crippled Childrens Committee
Oklahoma State Medical Association

The Oklahoma Society for Crippled Children still operates as an independent organization. The Secretary of this organization is Mr. Joe N. Hamilton, 313 Franklin Building, Oklahoma City, Oklahoma.

Under provision of Senate Bill 15, each county has a crippled children's fund, through the appropriation of .1 mill ad valorem tax. In some counties the fund is ample, but in many counties it is used very quickly.

The State Crippled Children's Hospital, located in Oklahoma City, is a part of the University of Oklahoma School of Medicine and University Hospital system, and receives crippled children directed to it by the local county judge, but the county does not pay this hospital for services rendered. The Hospital is supported by state appropriation. The act provides for a Commission for Crippled Children, composed of five members, and for a Committee on Standardization of Hospitals. There are three types of hospitals:

1. Crippled Childrens.
2. General Hospitals.
3. Standard Hospitals.

1. Crippled Children's: Referring chiefly to the State Crippled Children's Hospital located in Oklahoma City. Included in this group are hospitals which are approved only for orthopedic and plastic work.

2. The general hospital is one that has been approved by the American College of Surgeons. The general hospital can accept committed cases including orthopedic and plastic cases, provided there are specialists approved for this work on the staff. When there is not an approved orthopedic or plastic surgeon on the staff, chronic deformities and plastic cases must be referred to a hospital where approved specialists' services can be obtained.

3. The second type is that of the standard hospital which meets the standards set up by the Committee on Standardization.

Any hospital that has on its staff a general surgeon and an internist or general practitioner and a specialist in eye, ear, nose and throat, and is willing to keep records according to the standards of the College of Surgeons and meet the ordinary requirements of such rules, can make application to the Committee on Standardization for approval. These hospitals may accept acute cases of injury or sickness in children under 21 years of age, but cannot accept orthopedic or plastic cases, or chronic bone disease or deformities. The counties from where the children are committed pay the rate of $17.50 per week for the entire care of a child. No fees can be collected by the doctor for services rendered.

The provision of the Department of Welfare, State of Oklahoma, through the State Assistance Fund, now provides for care of crippled children under certain regulations. When the county has run out of funds this organization may be able to provide for the crippled children in the county until funds are available.

The following statistics will indicate the scope of the crippled children's activities over the past year:

Total number diagnostic clinics.................. 38
Number children examined................... 1,258
Number counties in which clinics were held... 36
Number doctors participating in clinics........... 14

Number doctors approved for crippled children's work:

Orthopedic	14
Plastic	6
General	381

Hospitals approved:

Crippled Children	9
General	9
Standard	36
Total	54

Number children hospitalized:

Oklahoma Hospital for Crippled Children	2,400
Private	3,900
Total	6,300

Respectfully submitted,

Earl D. McBride, Chairman.

Copies:
Dr. Roy L. Fisher, Frederick.
Dr. M. B. Glisman, Okmulgee.

Report of Committee on Conservation of Hearing

Your Committee fells that the proper way to attack the problem of deafness is preventative. Certainly treatment of advanced hearing loss is unsatisfactory.

The Committee held a meeting in September with Mr. Baker Bonnell, State Supervisor of the program for the deficient of hearing, who works out of the office of the State Superintendent of Public Instruction. Mr. Bonnell is engaged and has been for some time in testing hearing of the children in our public schools and has collected a number of interesting statistics as to the number of hard of hearing children in the schools. He wished the Committee to endorse his work and to work out, if possible, a method of following up his work so that some definite benefit to the hard of hearing children might come about. His work is not a medical program and consists only of finding what individuals have deficient hearing among the groups tested. To result in any benefit to these hard of hearing individuals the work must be followed by medical examination and treatment when indicated.

With the cooperation of the chairman of this committee it was arranged for Mr. Bonnell to test the hearing of the children of the rural schools of Garfield County. A total of 1,707 children were examined. Three hundred and thirty-three of them, 13 per cent, showed a hearing loss of 15 or more sensation units. One hundred and eighty-three of these had a loss of 24 or more sensation units. Although the parents of each of these children found deficient in hearing were notified of the findings and were urged to seek medical attention, not one has so far reported to any of the five eye, ear, nose and throat specialists in the county seat for diagnosis or treatment.

This sort of result, or lack of result, is very discouraging. The apparent colossal indifference of the layman and perhaps of some physicians makes the committee doubt whether such a program is justified from an economic standpoint. If during the three months following the expenditure of so much effort and money we are not able to determine that any individual profited thereby we feel that there is some ground to be dubious as to the benefits of the program. However, the committee wishes to emphasize that this is a problem of education. No educational program brings results in a short period of time. The aim of the program must be first to make the public, including doctors, hearing conscious. We must first make it known that a large number of our children have deficient hearing. Of course in individual instances the parents and perhaps the teachers know that certain children do not hear well. By repeated and widespread group testing however, we can make people aware of the magnitude of the problem. The next step then is to let them know that at least some of these children can be benefited by trteatment. A large number may have hearing loss beyond repair already but even in these a great deal may be done to prevent further loss. If these children are all neglected, certainly many of them will become more greatly handicapped as the hearing loss progresses. Treatment of advanced hearing loss is discouraging at best but the earlier these cases are brought under treatment, the better the results that may be obtained.

Your committee recommends that each County Medical Association at some time during the year have someone outline before the Society the purposes and aims of a program for conservation of hearing. It must be stressed that this, of necessity, be at first a campaign of education. By means of group audiometric testing of hearing with individual re-examination of those found deficient it is first determined who are deficient in hearing. This should be then followed by medical examination of these individuals. As laymen and doctors become aware of such a program, the next step is to make them aware that benefits can only come from it by means of treatment of afflicted persons. In this way and only in this way can a great number of our school children who have already some loss of hearing be prevented from becoming more greatly handicapped as they grow older and enter the economic life of our state.

H. F. Vandever,
L. C. McHenry,
J. B. Hollis.

Report of the Committee on Public Policy and Legislation

Your committee has attempted with the limited funds available to do the things we thought the membership of the State Medical Association desired. We have with the invaluable aid of our Executive Secretary, Mr. R. H. Graham, attempted by bulletin to keep the membership advised as to what is going on in the state from a legislative and public policy standpoint. We have secured much and valuable information with reference to legislative matters. We have only promoted the passage of one act by this legislature. We have constantly attempted and have so far been successful in blocking the passage of numerous bills which have been introduced in the legislature, that in our minds would be harmful to the health of the citizens of Oklahoma, however at the time this report is submitted the legislature has not completed its session and numerous bills are pending that are in our minds harmful. We expect to continue our activities along the same lines. We would like to recommend that in the future a more liberal allowance be made to this committee to cover its activities, than has been this year.

The committee desires to thank the membership of the State Medical Association, the officers of the County Societies and the co-ordinating members of this committee for the invaluable aid they have rendered. The Committee desires also to thank the officers of this Association for their cooperation.

There will be at the state meeting a further report submitted to the House of Delegates.

Finis W. Ewing, Chairman
R. O. Early
Tom Lowry
O. C. Newman

ANNUAL REPORT
of the Secretary-Treasurer-Editor
April 1, 1938, to March 31, 1939

TO THE MEMBERSHIP OF THE
OKLAHOMA STATE MEDICAL ASSOCIATION:

In compliance with the Constitution and By-Laws the Secretary-Treasurer-Editor herewith submits his report to the House of Delegates as to the various activities of his office during the past year.

Detailed statements of all financial transactions, duplicate deposit certificates and other business matters have been submitted to the Council and the audit published with this report.

As to the membership of the organization I will say that we have had a decided decrease, the membership last year being 1,465 and up until this time we have received dues from 1,064 members. Undoubtedly the decrease is due to the increase in dues. With our present membership we will be able to certify two delegates to the American Medical Association.

We have lost by death about the usual number of members and the list of these departed ones will be published with the report of the Necrology Committee.

Medical Defense: The following cases have either been settled, dropped or disposed of in the following manner:

Settled:
Stephens County, No.........

Pending:
Caddo County, No. 9407.
Carter County, No. 16262.
Choctaw County, No. 8644.
Logan County, No. 1693.
Mayes County, No. ....
Pontotoc County, No. ....

In addition to the above the following cases are now pending, the progress of which is unknown as they are pending or dormant in the courts:

Blaine County, No. ....
Carter County, No. ....
Craig County, No.
Hughes County, No.
Payne County, No. ....
Pottawatomie County, No. ....

Advertising: During the year we have maintained practically all of the advertising contracts of the previous year. We have received the further support of the Cooperative Medical Advertising Bureau and as a result of this received a dividend check the first of the year for $490.82, which is one of the largest dividend checks we have ever received. Our advertising has maintained the high standard of previous years; we have accepted no advertising except of products approved by the various councils of the American Medical Association and the membership can always be sure that any advertised material, be it drug, apparatus or institution, has been thoroughly investigated and found to be of high ethical quality.

The Journal during the past year has not only maintained its usual size but several numbers have shown an increase in size and with our new contract with the publisher have been distributed at an approximate cost of 20½ cents per copy. This of course without the mailing expense.

The members of this Association are certainly indebted to our abstractors. These busy physicians and surgeons have given of their time to maintain the high standard of the abstract department. The very latest material being abstracted from the American Medical literature, and Dr. LeRoy Long very often has abstracted some of the outstanding French contributions. These contributions made by the physician at the head of the various abstract departments does much to maintain the high standard and is one of the most interesting departments of our publication.

You will note in the financial report that the Journal has shown a financial profit during the past year and the Secretary-Treasurer always feels that considerable has been accomplished when the Journal can pay its way.

Unfortunately we are able to publish but few of the Committee reports as they have not been submitted to the Journal, but will undoubtedly be submitted to the House of Delegates.

You will notice that our indebtedness to the First National Bank of McAlester has been reduced $2,000.00; we have contributed $2,000.00 to the support of the Post Graduate Course in Obstetrics; we have met the increased expense incurred by the employment of an Executive Secretary; some money has been appropriated by the Council for the work of the Legislative Committee; $750.00 has been authorized for the use of the Committee on the Study and Control of Cancer, and current bills have all been paid.

The Post Graduate department in Obstetrics has been carried on throughout the year under the direction of the Post Graduate Medical Teaching Committee and the work of the Instructor, Dr. Edw. N. Smith, has been very acceptable and we have received many very complimentary letters as to his very efficient work.

AUDIT REPORT

Oklahoma State Medical Association
Dr. L. S. Willour, Secretary-Treasurer
McAlester, Oklahoma

For Period from April 1, 1938, to March 31, 1939
By J. K. Pemberton, McAlester, Oklahoma

April 5th, 1939

Dr. H. K. Speed, President,
Oklahoma State Medical Association,
Sayre, Oklahoma.

Dear Dr. Speed:

Upon request, I have audited the books of account, records and investments of

Dr. L. S. Willour, Secretary-Treasurer,
Oklahoma State Medical Association,
McAlester, Oklahoma.

for the period beginning April 1st, 1938, and ending March 31st, 1939, and submit the following schedules, together with comments and supporting exhibits.

Cash receipts were traced into the bank through a detailed check of the items received, against deposit tickets as shown by the files of the bank. Cash expenditures and disbursements were c h e c k e d against bank records, all vouchers and checks were examined and compared with original entries; endorsements scrutinized and found to be in order.

In company with Dr. L. S. Willour, Secretary-Treasurer, I have examined the following investments which are kept in a safety deposit box in the First National Bank, McAlester, Oklahoma, which box is registered in the name of the Oklahoma State Medical Association; except at this date the bonds are held by the bank as collateral to a loan totaling $5,000.00 executed by the Oklahoma Medical Association:

GENERAL FUND:
3¼% U. S. Treasury Bonds of 1944-46—

Bond Number	Par Value	
94180L	$ 500.00	
94181A	500.00	
95099K	1,000.00	$2,000.00

MEDICAL DEFENSE FUND:
3¼% U. S. Treasury Bonds of 1943-45—

Bond Number	Par Value	
878J	$1,000.00	
879K	1,000.00	
880L	1,000.00	$3,000.00

April 15th, 1939, coupons were attached to the bonds together with all subsequent coupons.

I find upon examination the following Notes Payable owing by the Association:

NOTES PAYABLE:

To The First National Bank, McAlester, Oklahoma (Secured by $5,000.00 par 3¼% U. S. Treasury bonds as described above) $5,000.00

I further find that proper resolutions were passed authorizing said loan, and said loan therefore is a valid and binding obligation of the Oklahoma State Medical Association.

I respectfully submit the following Audit and Report for your information.

J. K. PEMBERTON, Auditor.

* * * *

The above and foregoing statement and following Audit is submitted as my report for the period beginning April 1st, 1938, and ending March 31st, 1939.

L. S. WILLOUR, Secretary-Treasurer,
Oklahoma State Medical Association.

THE FIRST NATIONAL BANK
McAlester, Oklahoma
April 5th, 1939

Dr. L. S. Willour, Secretary-Treasurer,
Oklahoma State Medical Association,
McAlester, Oklahoma.

Dear Dr. Willour:

This is to certify that according to our records at the close of business on March 31st, 1939, the following accounts reflected a credit balance, subject to check, as follows:

Oklahoma State Medical Association:
General Fund $9,696.93
Medical Defense Fund 895.50

It is further certified that the following direct obligations of the Oklahoma State Medical were owing to the First National Bank, McAlester, Oklahoma, at the close of business on March 31st, 1939, as follows:

Date of Note	Description of Collateral	Date Due	Amount
2-10-37	3¼% U. S. Treasury Bond of 1944-46 No. 95099K $1,000.00 par.	4-10-39	$1,000.00
2-18-37	3¼% U. S. Treasury Bonds of 1944-46 Nos. 94180L, 94191A, 2 @ $500.00 each; & 3¼% U. S. Treasury Bonds of 1943-45 Nos. 878J, 879K, 880L being 3 @ $1,000 each Total	4-10-39	$4,000.00

Yours very truly,
J. K. PEMBERTON,
Vice-President and Cashier.

Oklahoma State Medical Association
Dr. L. S. Willour, Secretary-Treasurer
McAlester, Oklahoma
March 31st, 1939

BALANCE SHEET

ASSETS

CURRENT ASSETS:

First National Bank, McAlester, Oklahoma:
General Fund $8,740.76
Medical Defense Fund 895.50 $9,636.26

INVESTMENTS—U. S. GOVERNMENT BONDS:
General Fund (Par Value) 2,000.00
Medical Defense
Fund (Par Value) 3,000.00   5,000.00

TOTAL $14,636.26

LIABILITIES

EXCESS OF ASSETS OVER LIABILITIES:
Balance March 31st, 1938 ......$8,736.37
Less: Post Graduate Fund 2,630.08 $6,106.29

Add:
Excess of Income over Expenditures:
General Funds 3,476.54
Medical Defense Fund 1,197.50
Legislative Fund 1,144.07 $9,636.26

NOTES PAYABLE:
To First National Bank,
McAlester, Oklahoma, (Secured) 5,000.00

TOTAL $14,636.26

Oklahoma State Medical Association
Dr. L. S. Willour, Secretary-Treasurer
McAlester, Oklahoma
April 1, 1938, to March 31, 1939

CASH RECEIPTS AND DISBURSEMENTS

GENERAL FUND:

Balance March 31st, 1938 ...... $ 5,764.22

RECEIPTS:
Advertising ....$ 5,631.57
Exhibits 81.00
Memberships 12,296.00
U. S. Bond Interest 227.50
Repayment of Advance 28.72
Rebate Interest 6.20
Transfer from Medical De-
fense Fund 1,500.00
Transfers from Special
Fund (Balance) 660.00

Total Receipts 20,430.99

Total Cash to Account For $26,195.21

DISBURSEMENTS:

Dr. L. S. Willour, Sec.-Treas.
Salary to 4-1-39 ....$ 2,400.00
Oltha Shelton: Ass't. Sec.
Salary to 4-1-39 .... 1,500.00
R. H. Graham, Executive Sec.
Salary 850.00
Nigel Gilbreath, Ass't. Ex. Sec.
Salary 135.00
Other Office Salaries 25.00
Traveling Expense Ex. Sec.... 84.06

Social Security Tax 62.18
Rent 300.00
Telephone & Telegraph 112.14
Postage 354.44
Stationery and Printing 235.76
Treasurers Bond & Audit 75.00
Printing Journal 5,069.18
Press Clipping Service 36.00
Expense Annual Meeting 645.74
Expense Executive Council
and Delegates 554.44
Expense—Legislative 274.50
Insurance 8.52
Office Expense—Executive
Secretary 77.05
Interest Paid on Borrowed
Money 75.00
Office Repairs & Equipment 19.67
Sundry Expense 27.62
Payment on Note 2,000.00
Advance to Public Policy &
Public Relations Committee 375.00
Payment to Post Graduate
Fund 2,158.15

Total Disbursements 17,454.45

Balance on Hand March 31, 1939 ...... $ 8,740.76

MEDICAL DEFENSE FUND:

Balance March 31, 1938 .... $ 1,198.00

RECEIPTS:
Fees Collected ....$ 1,200.00
U. S. Bond Interest 97.50   1,297.50

Total Cash to Account For .... $ 2,495.50

DISBURSEMENTS:
Transfer to General Account $ 1,500.00
Medical Defense of Members   100.00

Total Disbursements 1,600.00

Balance on Hand March 31, 1939 ...... $ 895.50

CASH ON DEPOSIT
Oklahoma State Medical Association
Dr. L. S. Willour, Secretary-Treasurer
McAlester, Oklahoma
March 31, 1939

FIRST NATIONAL BANK,
McAlester, Oklahoma.

GENERAL FUND:
Balance as per Records .... $ 8,740.76
ADD:

Outstanding Checks:	No.	Amt.	
	3617	4.00	
	3574	1.00	
	4115	4.00	
	4663	6.50	
	4677	6.50	
	4701	6.50	
	4878	3.70	
	4879	60.00	
	4880	272.88	
	4882	26.15	
	4885	550.94	
	4886	3.00	
	4887	11.00	956.17

Balance as per Bank Statement
and Verification Letter .... $ 9,696.93

MEDICAL DEFENSE FUND:

Balance as per Records	$ 895.50
Outstanding Checks:	None
Balance as per Bank Statement and Verification Letter	$ 895.50

INCOME AND EXPENDITURES

Oklahoma State Medical Association
Dr. L. S. Willour, Secretary-Treasurer
McAlester, Oklahoma
For Period from April 1, 1938, to March 31, 1939

GENERAL FUND:

INCOME:

Advertising	$ 5,631.57
Exhibits	81.00
Memberships	12,296.00
U. S. Bond Interest	227.50
Repayment of Advance	28.72
Rebate Interest	6.20
Received from Special Fund (Balance)	660.00
Total Income	$18,930.99

EXPENDITURES:

Salary Secretary-Treasurer	2,400.00
Salary Ass't. Secretary	1,500.00
Salary Executive Secretary	850.00
Salary, Ass't. Ex. Sec.	135.00
Other Office Salaries	25.00
Traveling Expense Executive Secretary	84.06
Social Security Tax	62.18
Rent	300.00
Telephone & Telegraph	112.14
Postage	354.44
Stationery and Printing	235.76
Treasurers Bond and Audit	75.00
Printing Journal	5,069.18
Press Clipping Service	36.00
Expense Annual Meeting	645.74
Expense Executive Council and Delegates	554.44
Expense—Legislative	274.50
Insurance	8.52
Office Expense—Executive Secretary	77.05
Interest Paid on Borrowed Money	75.00
Office Repairs & Equipment	19.67
Sundry Expense	27.62
Advance to Public Policy and Public Relations Committee	375.00
Payment to Post Graduate Fund	2,158.15
Total Expenditures	15,454.45
Balance—Net Excess of Income over Expenditures	$ 3,476.54

MEDICAL DEFENSE FUND:

INCOME:

Fees collected	$ 1,200.00	
U. S. Bond Interest	97.50	$ 1,297.50
Total Income		$ 1,297.50

EXPENDITURES:

Medical Defense of Members	100.000	100.00
Balance—Net Income Over Expenditures		$ 1,197.50

Influx of Refugee Physicians Focuses Attention on Citizenship Question

The influx of refugee physicians has focused attention on the question of citizenship in the granting of licenses to practice medicine.

J. E. McIntyre, M.D., Lansing, Mich., secretary of the Michigan State Board of Registration in Medicine, in The Journal of the American Medical Association for March 18 says:

"It is interesting to note that most states have already required either United States citizenship or first papers as a condition precedent to taking the state board examinations. Only the following states require neither citizenship nor first papers at the present time: California, Illinois, Massachusetts, New Hampshire, New Mexico, New York, Ohio, Texas, Utah and the District of Columbia. Either by state law or by a ruling of the state boards of registration in medicine, the following states now require full United States citizenship: Alabama, Arkansas, Delaware, Florida, Georgia, Indiana, Kansas, Kentucky, Michigan, Missouri, Montana, Nevada, Nebraska, North Carolina, North Dakota, Oklahoma, South Carolina, South Dakota, West Virginia, Wyoming and, except in the case of Canadians, Arizona, Iowa and Minnesota.

"States now requiring that first papers for United States citizenship must be taken out are Colorado, Connecticut, Idaho, Louisiana, Maine, Mississippi, New Jersey, Pennsylvania, Rhode Island, Virginia, Washington and Maryland except in the case of Canadians. In addition to these requirements there is a great variety of other restrictions.

"In some states, such as South Carolina and Wyoming, foreign graduates are not accepted under any circumstances. In some other states there is a requirement of a senior year's work in an approved United States medical school and a one year rotating internship in a United States hospital approved for internship training. Still others require that the candidates pass the National Board examination and apparently there is no uniformity whatever as to these special requirements."

Place of Sulfanilamide in Pneumonia Treatment Not Yet Established

The future specific treatment of pneumonia probably will be with a combination of sulfanilamide and pneumococcus serum, especially in those cases caused by types II and III pneumococci, Alvin E. Price, M.D., and Gordon B. Myers, M.D., state in The Journal of the American Medical Association for March 18.

Although the results obtained from using the drug in the treatment of pneumonia are encouraging, the two men point out, the place of sulfanilamide in the treatment of the disease is not yet definitely established.

Their paper in The Journal is a preliminary report, based on 115 cases of pneumococcic pneumonia treated with uniform doses of sulfanilamide, 40 cases with Felton serum and 94 controls with no specific treatment.

The death rate was 15.7 per cent for the group of patients treated with sulfanilamide and 30.8 per cent for the controls. The death rate for 57 patients with types I, II, V, VII and VIII pneumonia treated with sulfanilamide was 10.5 per cent, whereas it was 27.5 per cent for the 40 patients with the same types of pneumonia treated with serum.

Of 21 patients with pneumococci in the blood

stream treated with sulfanilamide seven died, of 12 treated with serum six died and of 15 controls 13 died.

Some adverse reactions due to sulfanilamide treatment occurred. In 5.2 per cent of the patients treated with sulfanilamide a severe anemia developed and in an additional 18.2 per cent moderate secondary anemia, influenced by the infection, developed.

---o---

DRUG TREATMENT IN CORONARY DISEASE

Drugs have practically no value as a speific treatment for coronary disease if the patient is free of symptoms, Harry Gold, M.D., New York, declares in The Journal of the American Medical Association for Jan. 7. The one exception is syphilis involving the blood vessels of the heart.

At the present time there are no drugs that definitely influence the course of disease of the muscles and blood vessels of the heart. However, when pain exists certain drugs are beneficial.

The nitrites are the preferred drugs in the treatment of effort angina (pain on effort). The nitrites do not impair awareness of pain but abolish the mechanism that causes it.

The nitrites are not entirely free of disagreeable effects. They may bring about such minor symptoms as flushing of the face, headache, a sensation of throbbing and tension in the head, palpitation and, in excessive doses, collapse. Sometimes these symptoms can be averted by reducing the dose without losing the effect of the drug.

The dose should be taken at the first suggestion of the oncoming pain. Some patients, guided by a mistaken notion that danger of inquiry or the development of habit is involved in frequent use of the nitrites, wait for the full development of pain.

The frequent use of the nitrites will neither lead to dependence on them nor reduce their efficacy.

Of the numerous other drugs used in heart disease, the xanthine compounds exert no action that is useful for the routine treatment of heart pain.

The purine bases are extremely valuable in promoting the secretion of urine in congestive heart failure.

In a typical case of coronary thrombosis in which there is agonizing pain, anguish and terror of impending death, morphine is the preferred drug. It not only relieves pain but also abolishes the desire to move about and in many instances gives rise to a sense of well-being which is quite apart from its analgesic effects.

By reducing nervous excitability the barbiturates decrease the number and severity of the attacks of effort angina. By means of the barbiturates fear, anxiety and restlessness in acute coronary thrombosis may be controlled.

Digitalis is useful in heart failure and in certain disorders of heart rhythm.

The indications for drugs promoting the secretion of urine include in part those for digitalis. These drugs are useful for the control of congestive heart failure and attacks of recurrent labored breathing.

While in many instances great suffering is spared and a life is saved through the judicious use of these many drugs, the major part in the control of this disease lies not in drugs, but in expert guidance in making the mental and physical adjustments which will enable these patients to carry on within their capacity without symptoms of heart disease.

---o---

State Dues will not be accepted at the Registration Desk, Annual Meeting, except through C o u n t y Secretaries.

Animal Experimentation and Scientific Medicine Endorsed By Voters

The voters of California and Colorado, November 8, by overwhelming majorities emphatically rejected proposals made in those states to undermine the structure of scientific medicine, The Journal of the American Medical Association for November 19 says. In California an initiative humane pound law, so called, proposing to cripple scientific research by hampering animal experimentation, was decisively defeated. In Colorado an initiative measure proposed by a group of chiropractors, to debase the quality of medical care in the state by repealing the basic science act and by destroying other safeguards that have been erected to assure adequate and scientific medical service, was met by an avalanche of negative votes, running as high as ten to one in some counties.

In Oklahoma an initiative measure that would have sanctioned practices not conducive to public welfare failed to get on the ballot, because of court action instituted by the medical profession. In Ohio a chiropractic initiative somewhat similar to the Colorado initiative ded abornng, the cultist sponsors apparently becoming disheartened shortly after the proposal was submitted to the attorney general for the approval as to form. Petitions in Ohio were not circulated and the proposed initiative measure was not submitted to the people for a vote.

The medical associations in the states named assumed the lead in thwarting the selfish interests behind these proposals, interests that would subordinate the public welfare to their own private ends. In California and Colorado the state medical associations, aided by many lay and other professional groups and by public spirited citizens, informed the people fully of the dangers implicit in the proposals. To bring these dangers to the attention of the voters necessitated great sacrifices of time and money, but the results show that such sacrifices were well worth while and indicate that an informed electorate will support scientific medical care under proper legal and ethical safeguards.

Radio Short Waves Now Used in Giving Fever Treatment

The use of radio short waves to produce artificial fever for the treatment of disease is a striking demonstration of the relationship of progress in various fields of knowledge, Richard Kovacs, M.D., New York, declares in the May issue of Hygeia, The Health Magazine.

Such disease as gonorrhea, St. Vitus's dance, some forms of arthritis and of bronchial asthma, sinus disease and neuritis are being successfully combated by short wave treatment, the author points out.

Describing the method employed, Dr. Kovacs explains that local heating of any part of the human body is produced by placing it in the energy field of a short wave radio set.

This method is known as short wave treatment or short wave diathermy. An older method of diathermy involves the placing of plates in direct contact to the body or an extremity and the passing of a high frequency electric current through the afflicted part. The newer form of diathermy has the advantage that it can be applied to pratically any surface or part of the body and its heat is more uniform.

"Fever treatment must be combined with other recognized forms of treatment, by diet and if necessary by surgery," the author observes. "Experienced medical advice and skilled nursing care are more important in administering artificial fever than the best apparatus in unskilled hands.

"The large majority of medical men agree that it is the well directed and well controlled deep heating effect of radio waves on the human body which brings about relief. The idea that certain wave lengths exert special effects on certain diseases is untenable or at least not proved."

For the man listening to his radio, Dr. Kovacs admits, the use of radio waves for medical treatment is sometimes anything but a blessing. "When some of the apparatus used for treatment is improperly constructed," he explains, "it may become a nuisance not only for every radio set which derives electricity from.the same power line, but for those within several miles.

"Steps are under way to abate such nuisance by cooperation of the medical profession and reliable manufacturers of medical equipment. All apparatus may be properly screened to minimize interference, or a special wavelength may be allocated for treatment purposes.

"Induced fever," says the author, "has proved especially effective in disease caused by so-called 'parasitic' germs. Some germs, such as those of gonorrhea, have become so completely used to living in the human body at its normal temperature that an increase of temperature by a few degrees affects them.

"Artificial fever maintained for some hours either directly destroys the germs of gonorrhea or sufficiently stimulates the natural defensive forces of the body to stop the further growth of germs.

"In joint inflammation or arthritis caused by gonorrhea, almost dramatic relief from pain and swelling can be accomplished by artificial fever. Similar results have been accomplished in gonorrhea inflammation of the eye and in stubborn infections of the pelvic organs in both women and men.

"Fever treatment is also effective in the disease of children known as St. Vitus's dance, as well as

in certain forms of bronchial asthma resisting all other forms of treatment.

"Short wave diathermy is employed by physicians for treating inflammatory conditions of inner organs and of joints. These include some forms of arthritis, sinus disease and rheumatic conditions such as neuritis. Repeated treatment by diathermy brings about an increased flow of blood, which speeds up the return of normal function; it also relieves pain due to nerve irritation."

Explains Means of Preventing the Reactions From Vein Feedings

Means of preventing the fever and chills which may follow intravenous or vien feedings are explained by Charles M. Nelson, M. D., Richmond, Va., in The Journal of the American Medical Association for April 8.

Although these reactions have been commonly attributed to various causes, Dr. Nelson says that experiments show the real factor is bacterial contamination of the distilled water used in the solutions for these feedings.

Boiling the water to be used for six hours will destroy the fever-producing agent. Autoclaving (sterilization under steam pressure) for three or four hours will also destroy it. The usual sterilization period tends to enhance its growth.

Even when sterilized by the usual method, the tubing and flasks used in giving intravenous feedings may sometimes cause fevers, as the fever-producing factor may have lodged in them previously while a solution (not autoclaved) was passing through the apparatus.

Dr. Nelson points out that "any organism that is capable of elaborating a fever-producing substance, which thrives at room temperature and which is a common contaminant may be the offender. No organism will ever be the offender if the distilled water is taken directly from the still—most storage tanks are contaminated by backflow of air when the still cools—and autoclaved immediately."

Gastroscopy Aids Diagnosis

The diagnosis of cancer, ulcer and hemorrhage of the stomach and chronic gastritis is aided by gastroscopy (the direct visualization of the stomach), Elmer B. Freeman, M.D., Baltimore, reports in The Journal of the American Medical Association for January 21.

Before use of the gastroscope (a flexible illuminated tube) will give its utmost in results the physician must be familiar with the appearance of the normal stomach.

Gastroscopy is also of value in determining the results of treatment. The author declares that there no longer need be any doubt as to whether a gastric ulcer is healing under medical care, as this can be definitely determined gastroscopically. Gastroscopic observations have proved beyond a question of doubt that gastric ulcer may be completely healed under appropriate medical treatment.

The author believes that cancer of the stomach can be diagnosed by gastroscopic study before it can be determined by X-rays, thereby permitting early operation when complete cure is generally impossible.

State Dues will not be accepted at the Registration Desk, Annual Meeting, except through C o u n t y Secretaries.

ABSTRACTS : REVIEWS : COMMENTS
and CORRESPONDENCE

SURGERY AND GYNECOLOGY
Abstracts, Reviews and Comments from
LeRoy Long Clinic
714 Medical Arts Building, Oklahoma City

Painful Lumbo-Sacral Syndrome (Syndrome Douloureux Lombo-Sacre): J.-Ed. Samson, Chirurgien de l'hopital du Sacre-Coeur, Montreal; L'Union Medicale du Canada; December, 1938, Vol. 67, No. 12, page 1267.

This is a very practical contribution upon an extremely important subject. The author insists upon a careful examination of persons who have pain in the lumbo-sacral region because he believes that pain in that region is due very often to demonstrable pathology, provided a careful examination is made.

In reviewing the anatomy, the author calls attention to a combination of diarthrodial and amphiarthrodial articulations of the sacrum with the ilia, while there is a true amphiarthrodial articulation between fifth lumbar and sacrum. Taking into consideration the types of articulations, together with the contiguous nerve filaments, ligaments and interoseus cartilages, one has the ground work of the anatomy of this important region.

In the standing position all these things begin to complicate themselves, in connection with the multiple movements of the different articulations. In studying this situation, one must realize that he has before him the principal connections between the trunk and the pelvis.

Each of these articular surfaces is subject to organic disturbance with concomitant hyperostosis, congenital malformation, defective position, inflammatory lesions, traumatic or infectious. Practically all these conditions are accompanied by pain, but the pain may be due to variable causes. The author remarks, "We are, you will see, far away from the time when one classified, without frowning, this immense chapter in three words: rheumatism, lumbago, and Pott's disease." (Nous sommes, vous le voyez, bien loin du temps ou l'on reduisait, sans sourciller, ce chapitre immense en trois mots: rhumatisme, lumbago, mal de Pott.)

Today one speaks frequently in the surgical literature about sacralization, lombalisation, spondylosis, spina-bifida-occulta, spondylolisthesis, fasciitis, myositis, hernia of the intervertebral disc, chronic arthritis involving the lumbo-sacral joint, etc.

In connection with the congenital malformations the author indicates that it is important not to conclude that every congenital malformation causes lumbo-sacral pain. At the same time, it is his conclusion that the presence of congenital defects, or acquired defects, such as osteoarthritis, may enhance difficulties that might follow trauma.

Particular attention is directed to the careful taking of a history. He quotes Leriche as saying, "Many times the striking point in connection with the history of the patient escapes us because we do not know how to listen, or because we listen to the history with preconceived ideas." This is a very free translation. The original is as follows:

"Bien des fois, nous ratons notre coup aupres d'un malade, parce que nous ne savons pas l'ecouter, ou que nous ecoutons son histoire avec des idees preconceues." In other words, we miss fire in our efforts. He quotes another author, Mathieu Weil, who says, "We group all the patients whose histories we do not understand and whose suffering we are not able to demonstrate in the class of pithiatics." (Pithiatism is a term that was suggested by Babinski as the equivalent of hysteria.)

The sex of the patient, the condition of life, and the age are important. In a group of 109 collected by the author there were 65 females and 44 males. In connection with the condition of life, 61 were laborers and 44 were of sedentary habits. In connection with the age, 20 were under 20 years of age, 65 between 20 and 50 years, and 24 from 50 to 70 years of age.

In middle life it has been found, according to Weil, quoted by the author, that the lumbo-sacral syndrome is frequently found about the menopause in women, and in the case of men of like age the syndrome is more frequently in connection with traumatic or infectious disease—most often in connection with trauma because of the exposure of the male at that age to trauma.

It is preferred that the examination of the patient be made, if possible, during the stage when there are no very acute symptoms. As a rule, the patient presents himself with a distinctly lumbo-sacral syndrome in the acute stage, characterized by symptomatic sciatica; or he presents himself during the chronic stage of the lumbo-sacral syndrome. In the latter case, the diagnosis may be a little more difficult but, after all, the data secured by a systematic clinical examination will be of more value. One must determine whether the pains are severe, persistent, continued or intermittent. He ought to ascertain, if possible, whether the patient suffers more because of the duration of the pain than because of the intensity of it. He ought to try to secure information from the patient as to the exact site of the pain, the patient designating the areas where pain is pronounced, and he ought to ascertain some information as to whether the pain is relieved by position; whether it is more persistent at night; whether it becomes necessary for the patient to get up and move about at night in order to be relieved of the pain.

In the physical examination, the patient is examined without clothing. The first part of the examination is inspection of the front of the patient as he stands, of the side of the patient and of the posterior portion of the body and extremities as he stands. In this way one notes the general aspect of the trunk and of the muscular groups. He notes whether there are distortions or deformities. He notes the general contour of the lumbar spine—whether it is flat or whether the lumbar curve is more pronounced; whether the back appears short in this region, and whether there are evidences in the lumbar spine or in the adjoining dorsal spine of angulation. When such data are secured by careful inspection, combined with the other methods of physical examination, important information is secured. For example, the lumbar spine appears short, with a saddleback appearance. In the angle between the lumbar spine and the buttocks the finger may be introduced into a very marked depression. Altogether, the trunk appears to be short when compared to the length of the legs. In addition to that, there are cutaneous folds, rather pronounced, just above the buttocks, and the lower portion of the abdomen is very prominent. As the author remarks, there is a falling of the abdomen upon the thighs, and he winds it all up by saying, "And you have there before your eyes the trunk of the patient who has a spondylolisthesis." (Et vous avez la, sous vos yeux, le tronc du spondylolisthesique.)

In connection with a lumbar segment that is short, flat, movable in all directions, there is a suggestion of sacralisation. In chronic arthritis of the lumbo-sacral region, the lumbar spine may be short and flat, but the movements are distinctly limited.

The author calls attention to a sign of considerable importance in connection with spina-bifida-occulta, but it is very often overlooked—that is, a tuft of hair in the lumbar region.

Attention is directed to the various other procedures in connection with the physical examination, such as the movement of the vertebral column, the hip, and of the lumbo-sacral region in particular. In order to make a differentiation between ordinary sciatica, the sign of Lasegue is employed. (In the employment of the sign of Lasegue, there is no pain on flexion of the thigh upon the abdomen, provided the leg is flexed at the knee, in the presence of ordinary sciatica not associated with pathology of the bones or joints.)

An X-ray examination of the spine is usually important. The author indicates that there ought to be an anteroposterior view, an oblique view, and a side-to-side view.

The anteroposterior view will show the number of vertebrae, their form, their architecture, their histological structure. It will show, also, the changes that may have taken place in connection with the inter-vertebral spaces to a certain extent. It will show spina-bifida-occulta, the general orientation of the pelvis, the position of the sacrum, and such abnormalities as sacralisation of the fifth lumbar vertebra.

A side-to-side X-ray negative is important because in that way one is able to determine many conditions, such as angulation, differences in the thickness of the inter-vertebral cartilages, structure of the cartilage with the extrusion of the nucleous pulposus, the difference in the density and the regularity of the bodies of the vertebrae, etc. Again, a good side-to-side X-ray negative will give distinct evidences of such abnormalities as spondylolisthesis.

Finally the author says, "When one suspects a diminution of the calibre of the medullary canal by a herniated nucleus pulposus or by any other mechanical object, one is justified in making an inspection of the canal after the injection of some opaque material, like lipiodol, the progress of which is followed by a fluoroscopic examination. One may thus determine the site and the degree of obstruction of the medullary cavity."

The following is the conclusion of the author: "Painful lumbo-sacral syndrome is more frequent than is usually believed. This frequency is accounted for, in part, by a complete examination, both clinical and radiologic. An observation well made, in proper order, serves to differentiate pains that are due to visceral origin, such as calculosis, tuberculosis of the kidney, uterine affections, etc., from pains that are distinctly due to pathology of the bones or joints. Finally, an examination fairly establishes, once for all, that so-called idiopathic sciatica and lumbago are nearly always associated with pathology of the bones or joints, and that they very often require surgical treatment."

—LeRoy Long

Pulmonary Tuberculosis With Hyperthyroidism (Tuberculose Pulmonaire Avec Hyperthyroidie): J. A. Vidal, F.R.C.P., Chef de service a l'hopital du Sacre-Coeur, and Real Dore, Chirurgien a l'Hopital General de Verdun; Montreal L'Union Medicale du Canada, March, 1939, Vol. 68, No. 3, page 262.

Directing attention to the clinical observation that sometimes the differential diagnosis between a mild hyperthyroidism and incipient tuberculosis is not always made with facility, because of the presence of symptoms and signs, such as loss of weight, weakness, rapid pulse, etc. that might be found with either of these diseases singly, the authors report the case of a patient that is characteristically a good clinical picture when both pulmonary tuberculosis and hyperthyroidism exist at the same time.

A married woman, 39 years of age, came to hospital because she had cough, a small hemoptysis a few days before, fever in the afternoon, and with a history of having lost 40 pounds during the preceding two years, her actual weight at the time of admission being 97 pounds. There was increase in the rapidity of the pulse, with a relatively low blood pressure.

X-ray examination of the chest showed some density of the superior lobe on the right side, while on the left side there was a web-like opacity extending from the hilus to the costo-clavicular angle on each side.

The patient was given management, chiefly of a hygienic and dietetic character, from January 14, 1937, to May 12, 1937. During this time the radiographic findings had improved a good deal, and the weight had gone up to 111½ pounds. The appetite was better, but pulse remained rapid, being from 115 to 125 per minute. When she entered hospital, tubercle bacilli were found in the sputum, and they were still present in the sputum after the management indicated above.

About this time there was some family disturbance, the patient became excessively nervous, lost appetite for food, and found it difficult to sleep. At the same time there was some tremor of the hands and fingers, and a rapid pulse rate that was increased on exertion. There was progressive loss of weight. In connection with these symptoms and signs, enlargement of the thyroid gland was demonstrable, and there was some exophthalmus.

Repeated examinations showed that the pulmonary lesions were apparently stationary, but evidences of hyperthyroidism increased rapidly. The basal metabolism was plus 45. The pulse from 120 to 130, the patient lost weight, and there was nervousness and insomnia. It appeared to be pretty clear that there was a coexistence of pulmonary tuberculosis and a rather pronounced hyperthyroidism. Repeated examinations showed that the B.M.R. varied from plus 33 to plus 69.

Reasoning that a continuation of the hyperthyroidism would greatly interfere with the proper and successful management of the pulmonary tuberculosis, it was decided to do a thyroidectomy in two stages. The first operation was on August 24, 1937, the second September 17, 1937.

In support of the decision to perform a thyroidectomy in the presence of a stationary tuberculosis, reports by Lahey, of Boston, and Crile, of Cleveland, are quoted.

The operations were done under local anesthesia, combined with general superficial anesthesia produced by nitrogen oxide gas in whiffs (anesthesie generale superficielle au protoxyde d'azote, par bouffees).

The histological examination disclosed an interlobular hyperplasia, with masses of lymphoid cells. In addition, there was at one point a tuberculous granuloma.

The patient was discharged September 30, 1937. At that time the weight was 102 pounds, the pulse varied from 94 to 100, the temperature was sometimes irregular, and there was still cough and raising of material.

The management for pulmonary tuberculosis was continued. By the middle of December, 1937, the weight was 126 pounds, pulse 88 to 92. The expectoration was greatly reduced. At the end of January, 1938, there was an absence of suspicious expectoration, the weight 132 pounds, the pulse 84 to 88.

On March 29, 1938, radiographic examination showed that there was much improvement in connection with lung shadows. The weight was 136 pounds, pulse 84 to 90. The patient was seen again in the latter part of May, 1938, at which time she was feeling well.

In conclusion, the authors indicate that when there is an active hyperthyroidism which interferes with the management of a pulmonary tuberculosis there ought to be a thyroidectomy.

—LeRoy Long.

The Diffuse Colloid Goiter: C. A. Hellwig, M.D., F.A.C.S.; Surgery, Gynecology and Obstetrics; March, 1937, Vol. 64, No. 3, page 604.

McCarrison, one of the great authorities on goiter, has stated that there is little precise knowledge as to the geographic distribution, epidemiology, etiology, and biochemistry of the diffuse colloid goiter.

The study of this type of endemic goiter has been neglected. Few clinicians realize that in North America, about 90 per cent of the surgical goiters develop in this structure.

In regard to the function of the diffuse colloid goiter, most writers (Rienhoff, Plummer, Boothby) contend that it is hypo-active. Hellwig believes that adolescent goiter in this country is not associated with a low thyroid function. He points out that, although basal metabolic tests are valuable in adults, they are very unreliable in young individuals between the ages of 14 and 19 years. The author states that he has never seen a case of myxedema with diffuse colloid goiter.

He believes that diffuse colloid goiter during adolescence satisfies the increased demand of the organism for thyroid hormone. He also believes that in another period of physiological hypertrophy of the thyroid (pregnancy) diffuse colloid goiter often develops. It is again his opinion that this is a successful attempt of the thyroid to produce more secretion.

If the diffuse colloid goiter persists or develops after the twenty-fifth year, without pregnancy, then definite symptoms of hyperthyroidism are evident in the majority of cases (81 per cent).

He believes that there is a close histological relationship between the diffuse colloid goiter and exophthalmic goiter. He believes that these two conditions are related stages of thyroid activity and that one can change into the other.

He draws the conclusion that cretinism will never become a serious problem in our country as long as colloid goiter is the predominating type of endemic goiter.

If his conception is correct that the diffuse colloid goiter forms the anatomical basis for the development of exophthalmic goiter, it is reasonable to expect that a successful prevention of colloid goiter will lead ultimately to the disappearance of Grave's disease.

His conclusions in this article are set down as follows:

"1. The diffuse colloid goiter is the prevailing type of endemic goiter in level countries. In North America, about 90 per cent of the surgical goiters develop in this structure.

"2. The diffuse colloid goiter is not preceded, as a rule, by the parenchymatous, colloid-poor type of goiter, but it develops directly from the normal gland.

"3. During puberty and pregnancy, a small diffuse colloid goiter is physiological. It satisfies the increased demand of the organism for thyroxin during these periods.

"4. If the diffuse colloid goiter persists or develops after the twenty-fifth year of life and there is no pregnancy, symptoms of hyperthyroidism are very common.

"5. There is a close anatomical relationship between diffuse c o l l o i d goiter and exophthalmic goiter. This explains the fact that toxic goiter is much more common in level regions where colloid goiter is the prototype of endemic goiter.

"6. In white rats, diffuse colloid goiter can be produced by a diet containing a positive goitrogenic factor and a relatively large amount of iodine."

—LeRoy D. Long.

EYE, EAR, NOSE AND THROAT
Edited by Marvin D. Henley, M.D.
911 Medical Arts Building, Tulsa

The History of Cancer of the Larynx. Sir StClair Thomson, London. The Journal of Laryngology and Otology, February, 1939.

This is an extremely interesting article about 25 to 30 pages in length. The rapid increase in the death rate of cancer is compared with the steady, though slower, diminution of tuberculosis. Tubercular death rate has decreased 30.01 per cent in 12 years; cancer death rate has increased 27.75 per cent. Cancer of the larynx, is relatively to its occurrence in other regions, a rare manifestation. In every 100 cases of cancer only 1.8 are in the larynx. Investigation of the past 20 years shows cancer of the larynx to be on the increase more, relatively speaking, than elsewhere in the body.

Since 1855 it has been possible to observe more accurately cancer of the larynx. Literature shows reference to this disease as far back as 100 A.D. by Aretaeus and 200 A.D. by Galen. Garcia demonstrated auto-laryngoscopy in 1854 but the frequency of the disease was not well recognized before 1883, when Butlin spoke of intrinsic and extrinsic cancer and stated that the vocal cords were the most common site of the lesion.

The diagnosis of cancer of the larynx has made its most rapid strides in the last 20 years. Excluding tuberculosis and syphilis, in a patient at or over middle age (particularly a man), a limited neoplasm, located within the larynx and especially on the vocal cord, should be regarded as possibly malignant, a diagnosis on clinical appearances proved correct in 61 of 63 cases. Recent advance in pathology indicate a biopsy when a proper specimen can be obtained for examination. "Intrinsic cancer, from the view point of early diagnosis, offers the great advantage of causing the symptom of persistent hoarseness. In the extrinsic form this warning signal is lacking."

Intrinsic cancer, on a vocal cord, diagnosed and operated early gives a favorable prognosis (80 per cent). Extrinsic cancer is seldom arrested or cured by operation. It is hard to diagnose early. Aetiology is unknown. Predisposing factors mentioned are heredity, chronic irritation, excessive use of the voice, abuse of alcohol and tobacco and syphilis. Sex is an important factor. Intrinsic cancer is nine to ten times more frequent in males than in females. The most common age for its occurrence is between the ages of 50 and 60.

Broders' four group classification pathologically suits the authors' views best.

Signs, symptoms and site are correlated as follows: 1. Intrinsic cancer is met with most frequently on the vocal cord. 2. The subglottic area is the next most frequent site. 3. It is rare in the ventricular band or in the sinus of Morgagni, almost unknown in the inter-arytenoid region. 4. Rarely originates in the posterior third of the cord or processus vocalis. 5. The central or anterior half of the cord is the favorite location. 6. The two extremities in the usual chordal cancer are generally quite free in early cases.

As early as 1886 it was noted that in many cases of intrinsic cancer, the movement of the affected cord was impaired or abolished. It was thought that this was an early symptom; it is now recognized as a symptom of advanced growth and depending on the degree of mobility aids greatly in the prognosis and method of treatment. Treatment is discussed in detail, relating failures as well as successes, after treatment and end results. It is discussed under the following headings: a. Removal by the laryngofissure route. b. Removal by laryngectomy. c. Removal by the lateral pharyngotomy route. d. The removal of glands. e. Treatment by radium and X-ray.

I will close with a paragraph from the author's conclusions:

"When we recall that 50 years ago Morell Mackenzie was obliged to say that, for cancer of the larynx, 'the only possible termination is death,' we may rejoice in realizing today that with laryngofissure we can effect lasting cures in over 80 per cent of cases, that there should be no operative mortality, that surgery (laryngofissure and laryngectomy) will cure practically all cases of intrinsic cancer and that, in skilled and careful hands, they are now well established as safe and justifiable procedures."

The Significance of Errors of Refraction in Chronic Blepharitis of Children. E. J. Somerset, London. The British Journal of Ophthalmology, March, 1939.

The purpose of the paper is to enquire into the significance of refractive errors as an aetiological factor in children suffering from chronic blepharitis or blepharo-conjunctivitis.

Ernest Clarke in 1894 examined 100 cases whose average age was 17 years, including 44 school children. Atropine was used as was with the author's cases in this present report. Clark found hypermetropia in 64, hypermetropic astigmatism in 96, mixed astigmatism in eight, myopia in five, myopic astigmatism in 26, and emmetropia in one. From his observations he concluded that asthenopia due to ametropia was invariably present and although there was an underlying tendency to eczema or struma, the important factor in treatment was the ordering of glasses to correct the ametropia which he defined as follows: Astigmatism of more than 0.25 D., myopia and hypermetropia of more than 1. D. The opinion today is that the new-born baby is almost a plus 4.0 D. (atropine); as the child grows older the hypermetropia diminishes until between the ages of four and eight years the most common findings are plus 1.50 to plus 3.50 D. (atropine). Maximum incidence plus 2.50 D.

The author's investigations showed:

1. There is no significant difference in the spherical refractive error in children suffering from blepharitis in comparison with the normal child.

2. The incidence of astigmatism is similar in blepharitis cases and normal children.

3. Uniocular cases do not show blepharitis more frequently in the eye with the greater ametropia.

4. Causes other than errors of refraction must be sought for in blepharitis of children.

The Diabetic Fundus. K. von Hofe, Koln, Germany. Digested from Graefe's Archiv. Ophth. (Germany), December, 1938. Published in Digest of Ophthalmology and Otolaryngology, March, 1939.

By examining the eyegrounds of 322 diabetics in the space of a few months, the author was able to formulate a definite opinion as to what constitutes the usual and what constitutes the exceptional diabetic fundus.

Retinitis in the strict sense of the word, i.e., white spots and hemorrhages in the retina, was found in 28 cases; 19 cases showed only punctate hemorrhages; and 16 cases showed choroidal changes.

There is nothing distinguishing or characteristic in the appearance of the retinitis as it was found in diabetics. The white spots represent the reaction of the retina to the disturbed nutrition caused on the one hand by a diseased vascular system and on the other hand by the faulty metabolism. They are by no means characteristic of diabetes. They are found in a multitude of retinal conditions where the metabolism of the retina is disturbed, especially where there are vascular changes.

Punctate hemorrhages were found to be the most characteristic lesions of the diabetic fundus. These lesions may lie in the superficial or in the deep layers of the retina, and are usually found in the neighborhood of the disc.

The third group shows an affection of the deeper layers of the retina and of the choroid. Yellowish spots that are sharply bounded are seen and only exceptionally are they accompanied by punctate hemorrhages. This type is not often seen except in diabetics.

Although most of the cases had a hypertension, there were enough exceptions to indicate that there were other factors more important in the causation of diabetic retinal pathology.

Some claim that vascular changes are of no importance in the diabetic fundus. Braun even goes so far as to state that the very lack of visible vascular changes is indeed characteristic. Of 47 cases 15 had no definite visible changes of the blood vessels. In the others it was not possible to decide whether the changes were caused by or merely coincidental with the diabetes. However the punctate hemorrhages can be nothing else but an expression of damaged blood vessels, and their very frequency makes vascular pathology an essential feature of the diabetic fundus.

The Retina in Septic and Chronic Endophthalmitis of Ectogenous Origin. Harvey D. Lamb, M.D., St. Louis. The American Journal of Ophthalmology, March, 1939.

E. Fuchs' definition of the term is "the ocular condition characterized by the exudation of pus cells into the vitreous from the ciliary body and retina following the deposit of toxins in the vitreous."

A table accompanies the report which tells the kind of injury or operation, interval between penetration and enucleation, anterior retina quantity of pus cells, posterior retina quantity of pus cells, anterior retina quantity of macrophages, posterior retina quantity of macrophages, anterior retina quantity of round cells, posterior retina quantity of round cells, degree of perivasculitis, presence of connective tissue on inner surface of retina. Microphotographs also accompany the report.

The author's own summary is as follows:

The principal retinal changes are tabulated in the case of 28 eyes with septic endophthalmitis and of seven eyes with chronic endophthalmitis. The 28 eyes with so-called complicated septic endophthalmitis were characterized by at least a small amount of small round-cell infiltration in the ciliary body and choroid together with the exudate of numerous pus cells and macrophages into mainly the anterior or the cyclitic portion of the vitreous. The term chronic endophthalmitis is introduced as a corollary to septic endophthalmitis for the clinical and pathologic diagnosis of eyes showing an exudate into the vitreous that is composed almost altogether of macrophages. The retinal change occurring first in endophthalmitis was perivasculitis. The latter was the source of all the inflammatory round cells that infiltrated the retina and migrated into the vitreous from the retina. In all the eyes tabulated, the macrophage was the predominant cell composing the perivasculitis. Perivasculitis in some degree was present in all but two of the 28 eyes with septic endophthalmitis and in all but two of the seven eyes with chronic endophthalmitis. The number of round cells infiltrating the retina entering the vitreous were generally fewer by far in chronic endophthalmitis than in complicated septic endophthalmitis. The retinal membrane on the inner surface of the retina like the cyclitic membrane was composed of connective tissue produced by fibroblasts that developed from the macrophages in the vitreous. This retinal membrane is more likely to occur in septic endophthalmitis than in chronic endophthalmitis because more macrophages develop in the former.

INTERNAL MEDICINE
Edited by Hugh Jeter, M.D., 1200 North Walker, Oklahoma City

Malignant Cells in Serous Effusions. John R. McDonald, M.D. and Albert C. Broders, M.D., Rochester, Minn. Archives of Pathology, January, 1939, Volume 27.

In this the authors review the reports on the subject dealing with cases in which malignant cells were demonstrated in effusions and discuss the criteria for diagnosis of malignant cells in serous effusions. In addition the authors present their results in microscopic examinations in which malignant cells were found and those in which malignant cells were not found.

The authors in a review of 30 cases in which malignant cells were found in the fluids were able to confirm the diagnosis in 12 cases by necropsy or biopsy and in the remaining 18 cases the clinical roentgenographical evidence was suggestive of malignancy in 12. In the six remaining cases there was no evidence that the diagnosis of malignancy was wrong, although definite proof was lacking. In an analysis of 41 cases in which malignant cells were not found in the effusion they found that 10 had carcinoma (proven by necropsy or biopsy), 17 had effusions due to lesions other than malignancies (tuberculosis, cirrhosis or inflammatory conditions), and in 11 cases it was impossible to arrive at a diagnosis.

The technique which was used in the examination of these specimens is presented and several excellent photomicrographs are shown.

The authors conclude that the examination of the sediment obtained from effusions is of definite value in cases in which malignant growths involving serous cavities are suspected and when malignant cells can be identified definitely in serous effusions, the diagnosis of malignant growth carries a high degree of accuracy.

Comment: In a critical analysis of the diagnoses based on the microscopic examination of 69 peritoneal and pleural fluids at the University Hospital the following results were obtained:

In 24 fluids (representing 23 patients) malignant cells were demonstrable. In 45 fluids (representing 31 patients) no tumor cells were demonstrable. In the 23 cases in which malignant cells were demonstrable the diagnosis was proven in 13 cases by necropsy or biopsy and in the 31 cases in which tumor cells were not demonstrable the diagnosis was proven in 18 cases. From this analysis the following conclusions were drawn:

1. When a diagnosis of malignancy is made from the cytological study of serous effusions, the diagnosis is accurate in approximately 75 to 85 per cent of the cases.

2. When tumor cells are not demonstrable, the diagnosis is accurate in but approximately 40 to 50 per cent of the cases.

3. A diagnosis of malignancy derived from the cytological examination of fluid from the pleural and peritoneal cavities carries a high degree of accuracy and warrants a routine examination for malignant cells.

PLASTIC SURGERY
Edited by
GEO. H. KIMBALL, M.D., F.A.C.S.
404 Medical Arts Building, Oklahoma City

The Fate of Living and Dead Cartilage Transplanted in Humans. Lindon A. Peer, M.D., F.A.C.S., Newark, N. J. S.G.&O., March, 1939, Vol. 68, Number 3.

The author has done original work to determine the fate of living and dead cartilage transplants in human beings. The following is an outline of the experiments:

"1. Six segments of cadaver cartilage preserved in alcohol were transplanted beneath the skin of six other humans (homografts) and removed for examination at intervals from six months to two years.

"2. Eight segments of living autogenous costal cartilage were buried beneath the skin of eight humans and removed for examination at intervals from six months to six years. All of these grafts were transplanted without perichondrium.

"Cadaver cartilage grafts. The use of cartilage preserved in alcohol to fill depressions of the nose, face and skull, like most surgical procedures, is not new. It was utilized rather extensively a generation ago and was discarded because of the belief that the grafts either suppurated or were absorbed and replaced by fibrous tissue. Recently there has been a revival of the method. Pierce and O'Conner, J. B. Brown, Claire Straith, C. R. Straatma, and I, among others have used cartilage preserved in alcohol to repair saddle nose and defects of the skull. Successful grafts examined by external palpation appear to retain their size and consistency to periods of over a year.

The advantage of this procedure is obvious, as fresh cartilage from cadavers is easily obtainable in almost any desired quantity, and a supply of this cartilage preserved in alcohol may be kept on hand in the hospital laboratory for use when needed. It goes without saying that the donor must be proved free from syphilis. The disadvantage of the method lies in the uncertainty as to the ultimate fate of the transplant.

Autogenous rib cartilage grafts. Koenig, in 1896, was the first to use the cartilage transplants in man, and since that time, living autogenous rib cartilage has been employed widely as a filling substance, and for the structural support of soft tissues. There is, however, a great difference of opinion concerning the fate of the autogenous cartilage graft following transplantation. A questionaire sent to 10 surgeons who frequently use the rib cartilage grafts, disclosed a variety of beliefs concerning the fate of the grafts. These opinions were based on clinical evidence and may be summarized as follows: 1. Cartilage tends to survive when transplanted. 2. Cartilage tends to degenerate when transplanted. 3. Cartilage survives when transplanted with its perichondrium, but tends to degenerate and disappear when transplanted without its perichondrium.

The author gives a comprehensive outline of the following experiments: Previous experimental work with living cartilage in animals. Previous experimental work with living cartilage in humans. Previous experimental work with the transplantation of dead cartilage in animals. Previous experimental work with the transplantation of dead cartilage in humans.

A detailed description of cadaver cartilage transplants after having buried and observed from six months to 24 months is told in a very enlightening manner.

Summary of findings in pickled cartilage grafts. The grafts remain, after transplantation as tolerated dead foreign bodies for about 9½ months. From this time on the surrounding host tissues invade the foreign cartilage, and very slowly absorb portions of the cartilage. This process, however, is very gradual and the bulk of the graft is still present two years after transplantation. The 14 month and two year specimens showed areas of calcification or early bone formation.

Description of living autogenous rib cartilage transplants: The five sections buried from six months to two years all appear as normal living cartilages. They are surrounded by a dense connective tissue capsule and there is no evidence of invasion or absorption of the cartilage by the surrounding host tissue.

The author gives magnified photographic illustrations of cartilagenous growth of cells of various stages and an interesting discussion of each.

Summary of findings in autogenous rib cartilage grafts:

The cartilage grafts buried from six months to two years showed no evidence of invasion by fibrous tissue or absorption. The graft buried 4½ years appeared in the form of a cylinder of living cartilage, with this bone formation at the core of the graft represents a degeneration of cartilage which failed to survive transplantation because of nutritional difficulties.

The segment buried six years appeared as normal living cartilage. The host connective tissue on one side of the graft slightly penetrated the edge of the cartilage and this may represent beginning invasion. The cartilage graft, however, was scraped with a scalpel before insertion in the nose, and I believe that the surrounding host tissue merely occupies the small depressions formed in the cartilage by the scraping.

Conclusions: The dead cartilage grafts buried from 9½ months to two years showed progressive invasion by fibrous tissue and partial absorption. In contrast to these findings autogenous rib cartilage grafts showed no invasion or absorption over the same period of time.

Two late autogenous rib cartilage grafts buried 4½ years and six years appeared as living cartilage.

From the evidence found in these sections one may conclude that autogenous rib cartilage survives after transplantation as living cartilage and, up to periods as long as six years, neither increases nor decreases in size.

Autogenous rib cartilage is better material for plastic repair than dead, pickled cartilage.

Comment: I have had satisfactory results with autogenous cartilage especially in reconstruction of the bony framework of the nose. I have not used the pickled cartilage because the ones that I had seen employed in this community in my judgement were not successful. Some of them showed softening and infection early.

I have not had the opportunity to examine by microscopic method any of the grafts that I have used. It is quite possible that the pickled cartilage in the hands of some men is quite satisfactory.

The author in this article has demonstrated what actually happens to both types of grafts, that is, living and dead grafts.

———————o———————

ORTHOPAEDIC SURGERY

Edited by Earl D. McBride, M.D., F.A.C.S.
717 North Robinson Street, Oklahoma City

"The Scalenus Anterior Muscle in Relation to Shoulder and Arm Pain," Joseph A. Freiberg, Jr. Bone & Joint Surg., Vol. XX, No. 4, October, 1938.

The author first reviews briefly the history of pain in nervous and vascular disturbances of the shoulder, citing first that J. B. Murphy in 1906 described the relation between the scalenus anterior muscle, but it was not until 1927 that definite relationship between the cervical ribs and the scalenus anterior muscle was really demonstrated. At this time it was pointed out by Adson and Coffey that division of the scalenus anterior muscle would relieve pain suspected due to cervical ribs.

The author briefly reviews the literature on the subject and then describes in some detail the anatomical position of the muscle, particularly in relation to the subclavian artery and the brachial plexus, in which there is rather extensive communication with the third, fourth, fifth, sixth, seventh and eighth cervical nerves. This spasm of the muscle or spasm associated with hypertrophy or contracture of the muscle may produce injury or lesions to the roots of the nerves themselves and be manifest as a simple nerve irritation with cutaneous or muscle pain in the areas supplied by the involved roots. There may be actual muscle weakness or paralysis. Vascular symptoms of coldness, swelling and patchy areas of subjective numbness may occur. The most common complaint is that of a dull ache in the hand and forearm, associated with a feeling of continual pressure as if someone were squeezing the extremity from without. It is easily seen that any lesion, traumatic or infectious, in which the cervical spine or the shoulder girdle is involved may be an initiating factor in causing the scalenus anterior syndrome. Even lesions of the shoulder girdle, such as a fractured clavicle or a painful shoulder associated with calcification of the supraspinatus tendon may initiate diffuse muscle spasm which accompanies the lesion.

The author describes 20 cases of scalenus anterior syndrome, associated with various lesions of the shoulder girdle and of the cervical spine. Six were associated with lesions of the supraspinatus or of the short rotator tendons of the shoulder; four, with arthritis of the shoulder, one case being bilateral; three, with the anatomical type initiated by strenuous exercise or a lesser trauma; three, with fracture of the clavicle; one, with an old traumatic arthritis of the cervical spine; one, with an infectious arthritis of the cervical spine; one, with an old unreduced dislocation of the shoulder; and one, with a traumatic subluxation of the third cervical vertebra on the fourth.

Therapy in these lesions has been directed first to the primary lesion and second to the syndrome. Frequently the annoying and distracting signs of the syndrome have disappeared with efficient management of the primary lesion. Traction in the line of deformity has been one method of therapy which relieved pain by overcoming the spasm of scalenus anterior.

The author feels that if time is of no importance traction is the method of choice. Tenotomy may always be resorted to if conservative therapy is unsuccessful.

The author feels that in the presence of a syndrome of three months' duration with definite muscle weakness and signs of vascular interference, scaleniotomy should probably be done. However, a trial of conservative treatment should be made first.

Note by abstractor: The scalenus anterior syndrome is not a rare condition, but one that is seen more frequently than was formerly supposed. Diagnostic points include vague, indiscriminate pain, numbness in the hand, forearm and shoulder, vascular disturbances and mild disturbances of sensation or some evidence of muscular weakness and atrophy. Once diagnosed the condition lends itself well to treatment following the methods suggested by Dr. Freiberg. After tried conservative therapy in the form of traction of the long axis of the arm, if no relief, a tenotomy of the scalenus anterior muscle should be undertaken. It is obvious that this is no simple procedure from the standpoint of the surgeon, although it is not dangerous to the patient if he is in the hands of one who knows anatomy of the cervical region. The post-operative course is usually uneventful. Pain is usually relieved immediately post-operatively.

———o———

UROLOGY
Edited by D. W. Branham, M.D.
514 Medical Arts Building, Oklahoma City

Precocious Hypertrophy of Prostate Following Persistent Treatment With Gonadotropic Hormone. Tracy O. Powell. Journal of Urology, February, 1939.

Experimentally the gonadotropic hormone stimulates the secondary sex organ when the gonads are intact. Prostatic hypertrophy may be easily produced by injecting suitable quantities of any type of gonadotropic hormone in the experimental animal such as the rat. In view of this information it is surprising that more reports of stimulation of the secondary sex organ such as the penis and prostate are not reported during the course of hormonal treatment of undescended testes.

Because no similar case has been reported the authors considered it of sufficient interest to report an instance of prostatic hypertrophy from hormonal treatment. The case reported was that of a 17-year-old boy who had been given hormonal therapy over a period of time and subsequently developed an enlargement of the prostate not unlike that seen in senile individuals. This enlargement was of sufficient size to produce obstructive symptoms so far as micturition was concerned. The treatment given was in addition to local measures the administration of a preparation of bull testes "contruin." On this treatment the patient's condition returned to an almost normal state with relief from the obstruction. The author warns that such a complication is possible and this should be remembered during the course of such hormonal treatment.

———

A New Operation For the Relief of Incontinence of Urine and Feces: Preliminary Report. Oswald S. Lowsley and Robert W. Hunt. The Journal of Urology. February, 1939.

The authors state that incontinence of urine and feces due to spina bifida or other causes is one of the cruelest developmental disorders of mankind. Any operation which may aid in relieving this distressing condition is most welcome. Accordingly he has discovered an operation by which through a single incision in the perineum using ribbon catgut he is able to plicate the bulbous portion of the urethra and the ventral portion of the rectum thereby narrowing the outlet of these structures.

Successful a n i m a l experimentation with this method induced him to try it on two young boys. The operation was performed with no difficulty and the end results were good. Both patients were able to control their urine and bowels when healing had taken place.

———

The Use of Testosterone Propionate in Prostatic Hypertrophy. Rex Bolend, B.S., M.D., Oklahoma City. Southern Medical Journal, February, 1939.

Twenty-three patients suffering from prostatic hypertrophy with urinary obstruction were given testosterone propionate in an attempt to evaluate its clinical effects on the disease. Seven of these cases were subjected to biopsies both before and after this course of treatment.

A total of 43.5 per cent of the patients in this series were dismissed from the hospital clinically well or symptom-free; 30.5 per cent were improved, and 26 per cent showed no improvement. Definite histological changes were noticed in the tissue removed from the gland, which undoubtedly resulted from the effects of the medication. These were: 1. Exaggeration of glandular hyperplasia. 2. A reduction in the inflammatory reaction. 3. A reduction or at least no increase in the stroma of the gland, however, no changes could be observed in the individual epithelial cells of the gland.

Comment: Apparently testosterone propionate does produce some beneficial effect at least on the symptomatology of this disease. Such a study as this adds something to our understanding of this most prevalent condition. Doubtless the improvement observed is due to a softening of the bladder neck, thereby allowing the vesical orifice to open more easily. The demonstration of a decrease in inflammatory reaction in the gland is significant as a considerable portion of the symptoms are often due to irritative factors which are produced by the complicating infection present. It seems to me that a profitable field of investigation would be a study to endeavor to find out if possibly testosterone propionate would be of value as an adjunct in the treatment of ordinary chronic prostatitis.

———o———

Warns Against Tying Off External Carotid Artery

Only the external carotid (the principal artery of the neck) should be tied off for otherwise uncontrollable profuse nasal hemorrhages, J. L. Fetterman, M.D., and W. H. Pritchard, M. D., Cleveland, warn in The Journal of the American Medical Association for April 8.

Their warning is based on a case in which not only the left external but also the left internal carotid artery was tied off. Following this ligation or tying off, convulsions, impairment of intelligence, defection in the understanding of the written or spoken word, numbness of the left side of the body, and one-sided paralysis resulted. Insufficient blood supply on the left side of the brain was the chief cause of these symptoms.

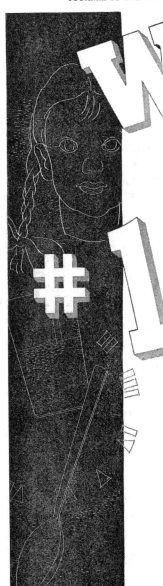

WHY

THE EMULSION...
Petrolagar
FOR CONSTIPATION

Petrolagar is more palatable. Easier to take by patients with aversion to plain oil— may be thinned by dilution.

2. Miscible in aqueous solutions. Mixes with gastrointestinal contents to form a homogeneous mass.

3. Does not coat intestinal mucosa. Petrolagar is an aqueous suspension of mineral oil — oil in water emulsion.

4. No accumulation of oil in folds of mucosa.

5. Will not coat the faeces with oily film.

6. Does not interfere with secretion or absorption.

7. Augments intestinal contents by supplying an unabsorbable fluid.

8. More even distribution and dissemination of oil with gastro-intestinal contents.

9. Assures a more normal fecal consistency.

10. Less likely to leak.

11. Provides comfortable bowel action.

12. Makes possible five types of Petrolagar to select from to meet the special needs of Bowel Management.

Petrolagar — Liquid petrolatum 65 cc. emulsified with 0.4 Gm. agar in a menstruum to make 100 cc.

Petrolagar

Petrolagar Laboratories, Inc. • 8134 McCormick Boulevard • Chicago, Illinois

OFFICERS OKLAHOMA STATE MEDICAL ASSOCIATION

President, Dr. H. K. Speed, Sayre.
President-Elect, Dr. W. A. Howard, Chelsea.
Secretary-Treasurer-Editor, Dr. L. S. Willour, McAlester.
Executive Secretary, Mr. R. H. Graham, McAlester.
Speaker, House of Delegates, Dr. J. D. Osborn, Jr., Frederick.
Vice Speaker, House of Delegates, Dr. P. P. Nesbitt, Medical Arts Building, Tulsa.
Delegates to the A. M. A., Dr. W. Albert Cook, Medical Arts Building, Tulsa, 1938-39,
Meeting Place, Oklahoma City, May 1, 2, 3, 1939.

SPECIAL COMMITTEES 1938-39

Annual Meeting: Dr. H. K. Speed, Sayre; Dr. W. A. Howard, Chelsea; Dr. L. S. Willour, McAlester.

Conservation of Hearing: Dr. H. F. Vandever, Chairman, Enid; Dr. J. B. Hollis, Mangum; Dr. Chester McHenry, Oklahoma City.

Conservation of Vision: Dr. W. M. Gallaher, Chairman, Shawnee; Dr. Frank R. Vieregg, Clinton; Dr. Pauline Barker, Guthrie.

Crippled Children: Dr. Earl McBride, Chairman, Oklahoma City; Dr. Roy L. Fisher, Frederick; Dr. M. B. Glismann, Okmulgee.

Industrial Service and Traumatic Surgery: Dr. Cyril C. Clymer, Medical Arts Bldg., Oklahoma City; Dr. J. Wm. Finch, Hobart; Dr. J. A. Rutledge, Ada.

Maternity and Infancy: Dr. George R. Osborn, Chairman, Tulsa; Dr. P. J. DeVanney, Sayre; Dr. Leila E. Andrews, Oklahoma City.

Necrology: Dr. G. H. Stagner, Chairman, Erick; Dr. James L. Shuler, Durant; Dr. S. D. Neely, Muskogee.

Post Graduate Medical Teaching: Dr. Henry H. Turner, Chairman, Oklahoma City; Dr. H. C. Weber, Bartlesville; Dr. Ned R. Smith, Tulsa.

Study and Control of Cancer: Dr. Wendell Long, Chairman, Oklahoma City; Dr. Paul B. Champlin, Enid; Dr. Ralph McGill, Tulsa.

Study and Control of Tuberculosis: Dr. Carl Puckett, Chairman, Oklahoma City; Dr. W. C. Tisdal, Clinton; Dr. F. P. Baker, Talihina.

Study and Control of Venereal Disease: Dr. Robert H. Akin, Chairman, Medical Arts Bldg., Oklahoma City; Dr. Shade D. Neely, Muskogee; Dr. D. V. Hudson, Medical Arts Bldg., Tulsa.

ADVISORY COUNCIL FOR AUXILIARY

Dr. H. K. Speed, Chairman...Sayre
Dr. C. J. Fishman..Oklahoma City
Dr. W. S. Larrabee...Tulsa
Dr. J. M. Watson..Enid
Dr. T. H. McCarley..McAlester

STANDING COMMITTEES 1938-39

Medical Defense: Dr. O. E. Templin, Chairman, Alva; Dr. L. C. Kuyrkendall, McAlester; Dr. E. Albert Aisenstadt, Picher.

Medical Economics: Dr. C. B. Sullivan, Cordell, Chairman; Dr. J. L. Patterson, Duncan; Dr. W. M. Browning, Waurika.

Medical Education and Hospital: Dr. V. C. Tisdal, Chairman, Elk City; Dr. Robert U. Patterson, Oklahoma City; Dr. H. M. McClure, Chickasha.

Public Policy and Legislation: Dr. Finis W. Ewing, Surety Bldg., Chairman, Muskogee; Dr. Tom Lowry, 1200 North Walker, Oklahoma City; Dr. O. C. Newman, Shattuck; Dr. R. O. Early, Medical Arts Bldg., Oklahoma City.
    (The above committee co-ordinated by the following, selected from each councilor district.)
District No. 1.—Arthur E. Hale, Alva.
District No. 2.—McLain Rogers, Clinton.
District No. 3.—Thomas McElroy, Ponca City.
District No. 4.—L. H. Ritshaupt, Guthrie.
District No. 5.—P. V. Annadown, Sulphur.
District No. 6.—R. M. Shepard, Tulsa.
District No. 7.—Sam A. McKeel, Ada.
District No. 8.—J. A. Morrow, Sallisaw.
District No. 9.—W. A. Tolleson, Eufaula.
District No. 10.—J. L. Holland, Madill.

Scientific Exhibits: Dr. E. Rankin Denny, Chairman, Tulsa; Dr. Robert H. Akin, Oklahoma City; Dr. R. C. Pigford, Tulsa.

Scientific Work: Dr. W. G. Husband, Chairman, Hollis; Dr. J. S. Rollins, Prague; Dr. J. L. Day, Supply.

Hospital Insurance Board—Dr. H. D. Collins, Oklahoma City; Dr. W. P. Neilson, Enid; Dr. R. L. Fisher, Frederick.

Public Health:
Chairman—Dr. G. S. Baxter, Shawnee.
District No. 1.—C. W. Tedrowe, Woodward.
District No. 2.—E. W. Mabry, Altus.
District No. 3.—L. A. Mitchell, Stillwater.
District No. 4.—J. J. Gable, Norman.
District No. 5.—Geo. S. Barber, Lawton.
District No. 6.—C. E. Bradley, Tulsa.
District No. 7.—G. S. Baxter, Shawnee.
District No. 8.—M. M. De Arman, Miami.
District No. 9.—T. H. McCarley, McAlester.
District No. 10.—J. B. Clark, Coalgate.

SCIENTIFIC SECTIONS

General Surgery: Dr. F. L. Flack, Chairman, Nat'l Bank of Tulsa Bldg., Tulsa; Dr. John E. McDonald, Vice-Chairman, Medical Arts Bldg., Tulsa; Dr. John F. Burton, Secretary, Osler Building, Oklahoma City.

General Medicine: Dr. Frank Nelson, Chairman, 603 Medical Arts Bldg., Tulsa; Dr. E. R. Musick, Vice-Chairman, Medical Arts Bldg., Oklahoma City; Dr. Milam McKinney, Medical Arts Bldg., Oklahoma City.

Eye, Ear, Nose & Throat: Dr. E. H. Coachman, Chairman, Manhattan Bldg., Muskogee; Dr. F. M. Cooper, Vice-President, Medical Arts Bldg., Oklahoma City; Dr. James R. Reed, Secretary, Medical Arts Bldg., Oklahoma City.

Obstetrics and Pediatrics: Dr. C. W. Arrendell, Chairman, Ponca City; Dr. Carl F. Simpson, Vice-Chairman, Medical Arts Bldg., Tulsa; Dr. Ben H. Nicholson, Secretary, 300 West Twelfth Street, Oklahoma City.

Genito-Urinary Diseases and Syphilology: Dr. Elijah Sullivan, Chairman, Medical Arts Bldg., Oklahoma City; Dr. Henry Browne, Vice-Chairman, Medical Arts Bldg., Tulsa; Dr. Robert Akin, Secretary, 400 West Tenth, Oklahoma City.

Dermatology and Radiology: Dr. W. A. Showman, Chairman, Medical Arts Bldg., Tulsa; Dr. E. D. Greenberger, Vice-Chairman, McAlester; Dr. Hervey A. Foerster, Secretary, Medical Arts Bldg., Oklahoma City.

STATE BOARD OF MEDICAL EXAMINERS

Dr. Sam A. McKeel, Ada, President; Dr. C. E. Bradley, Tulsa, Vice-President; Dr. J. D. Osborn, Jr., Frederick, Secretary; Dr. O. C. Newman, Shattuck; Dr. L. E. Emanuel, Chickasha; Dr. S. D. Leslie, Okmulgee; Dr. G. H. Stagner, Erick.

STATE COMMISSIONER OF HEALTH

Dr. Grady F. Mathews, Oklahoma City.

COUNCILORS AND THEIR COUNTIES

District No. 1: Texas, Beaver, Cimarron, Harper, Ellis, Woods, Woodward, Alfalfa, Major, Dewey—Dr. O. E. Templin, Alva. (Term expires 1940.)

District No. 2: Roger Mills, Beckham, Greer, Harmon, Washita, Kiowa, Custer, Jackson, Tillman—Dr. V. C. Tisdal, Elk City. (Term expires 1939.)

District No. 3: Grant, Kay, Garfield, Noble, Payne, Pawnee—Dr. A. S. Risser, Blackwell. (Term expires 1941.)

District No. 4: Blaine, Kingfisher, Canadian, Logan, Oklahoma, Cleveland—Dr. Philip M. McNeill, Oklahoma City. (Term expires 1941.)

District No. 5: Caddo, Comanche, Cotton, Grady, Love, Stephens, Jefferson, Carter, Murray—Dr. Walter Hardy, Ardmore. (Term expires 1941.)

District No. 6: Osage, Creek, Washington, Nowata, Rogers, Tulsa—Dr. James Stevenson, Medical Arts Bldg., Tulsa. (Term expires 1941.)

District No. 7: Lincoln, Pontotoc, Pottawatomie, Okfuskee, Seminole, McClain, Garvin, Hughes—Dr. J. A. Walker, Shawnee. (Term expires 1939.)

District No. 8: Craig, Ottawa, Mayes, Delaware, Wagoner, Adair, Cherokee, Sequoyah, Okmulgee, Muskogee—Dr. E. A. Aisenstadt, Picher. (Term expires 1939.)

District No. 9: Pittsburg, Haskell, Latimer, LeFlore, McIntosh—Dr. L. C. Kuyrkendall, McAlester. (Term expires 1939.)

District No. 10: Johnson, Marshall, Coal, Atoka, Bryan, Choctaw, Pushmataha, McCurtain—Dr. J. S. Fulton, Atoka. (Term expires 1939.)

THE JOURNAL
OF THE
OKLAHOMA STATE MEDICAL ASSOCIATION

VOLUME XXXII	McALESTER, OKLAHOMA, MAY, 1939	Number 5

MEDICAL OBJECTIVES*

W. A. HOWARD, M.D.
CHELSEA, OKLAHOMA

Within a little more than 300 years the land which we call the United States has become the home of the fourth largest national group in the world. China, of course, is first, India second, and Soviet Russia third.

When the United States was founded, republics were few and weak and Europe predicted a speedy end of the young nation. For a time the future did seem uncertain, but all the dangers were overcome until now in extent, stability, population, w e a l t h and power our republic ranks either first or among the first of the nations of the earth.

Daniel Webster said, "A m e r i c a has proved that it is practicable to elevate the mass of mankind—the laboring or lower class—to raise them to self-respect, to make them competent to act a part in the great right and the great duty of self government and she has proved that this may be done by education and the diffusion of knowledge."

Webster was right then and is today. Likewise, the words of another great patriot are as true now as when Emerson wrote them, "America is another name for opportunity. Our whole history appears like a last effort of divine Providence in behalf of the human race."

Opportunity is a word which, like so many others that are excellent, we get from the Romans. It means near port, close to haven. It is a favorable occasion, time or place for learning or saying or

*Presidents Address, Annual Meeting, Oklahoma State Medical Association, Oklahoma City, May, 1939.

doing a thing. It is an invitation to seek safety and refreshment, an appeal to make escape from what is low and vulgar and to take refuge in high thoughts and worthy deeds, from which flow increase of strength and joy.

Life is good and opportunities of becoming and doing good are always with us. Our house, our table, our tools, our books, our city, our country, our language, our business, our profession—the people who love us and those who hate, they who help and they who oppose, what is all this but opportunity?

Now we are ready to ask and answer, what are the "opportunities in the medical profession?"

1. The medical profession has the opportunity of furnishing an example of good citizenship. A good citizen is a man or woman who is doing something of service to the community. A good citizen is a workman who needeth not to be ashamed. There is no fitting place in society for the selfish and the greedy and you will see in time that only insofar as the range and circle of your duties may include others and help and bless them, will you find the true joy of living.

2. The medical profession has the opportunity of safeguarding the health of the community and the state.

3. The medical profession has an opportunity of setting an example of sympathy, charity and kindness.

   In each generation some of the best

minds have devoted themselves to the study of the healing art. This will always be so. There is an allure to the practice of medicine which keeps the conscientious physician struggling on for his patient in the face of any difficulty. I like to believe that it is an inherent love of human-kind, which makes life's ultimate goal the universal brotherhood of man.

4. The medical profession has the opportunity of an interesting future.

With the greater knowledge of the cause of disease which time will bring us, there will be put into the hands of the physicians of the future a weapon far more powerful than any we can wield today. We may reasonably look forward to the time when many of the e v i l s which afflict us now will be avoidable and as a result, the span of the life of man, which even in our own time has been materially increased, will be stretched several decades beyond the three score and ten, that at one time were allotted to man. Yet, to attain such results as these there will have to be cooperative efforts. On the willingness of the individual to accept the teaching of the science of those days, to obey the dictates of the medicine of the future, will depend the reward which science will then offer.

The practice of medicine had its origin in the far distant past. Primitive man, the ancient ancestor of the present generation, was a savage who roamed the earth, ignorant of the phenomena of his existence or of his surroundings. Fear of death was uppermost in his mind. He feared his fellow man, the wild beasts that inhabited the mighty forests and fled in terror from such natural phenomena as thunder and lightning. He attributed all his misfortunes, including disease, to evil spirits, that in his imagination inhabited the air about him. To protect himself from these evil spirits he invented good spirits, charms and mystic rites. In due time some one member of the clan or tribe appeared to be more successful than others in combating these evil influences. This man became the magician or medicine man of the clan. He was the progenitor of the physician.

About 400 years before the b i r t h of Christ, there lived in Greece a physician, whose name was Hippocrates. He became the greatest physician of his age. He was the first to recognize the error of mysticism, magic and religion in medicine. He taught that d i s e a s e was cured by the natural powers of the body. He practiced bedside observation of symptoms, examined the secretions of the body and investigated the digestibility of various foods. He established the practice of medicine on a rational basis. He also composed a code of ethics to govern the conduct of physicians. He declared that the true physician must be a man of honor, true to himself and honorable in his dealing with all men. This ancient code is the b a s i s for the present code of ethics that is in use today by the medical profession. In this date of many codes we of the medical profession can point with pride to this ancient code of ours that has been a lamp to guide the members of our profession throughout all the centuries of the past.

Gradually the science of medicine progressed until today we find not a finished product but a system that has reduced the incidence of disease to a point that is nothing short of miraculous. The death rate from disease has dropped to 9.6 per thousand and nearly 20 years has been added to man's age expectancy. The number of newborn infants that may reasonably expect to reach maturity has been vastly increased. Trench after trench of man's great enemy, "entrenched disease," has been taken in our war on that dread enemy of the human race. There remains much more to be done before disease will be entirely under control.

During all of these centuries past, the physician has never faltered in his endeavor to serve suffering humanity. Perhaps the most puzzling question a physician ever asks himself is "what do people expect from a doctor?" and that probably suggests another, "how do they make their choice when they decide to call a doctor?" The great majority of physicians have confessed an inability to get unqualified and uncolored answers to these questions.

The principal reasons for the selection of a particular physician may be grouped as follows:

1. Ability, which consists of economy,

willingness, reliability, honesty and quickness.

2. Personality, which means confidence, warmth of heart and sympathy. Universally there is a desire to find a physician in whom perfect trust can be placed.

The personal side of the practice of medicine, which has always played an important and comforting part, steps in at such times and renders a service which the people not only desire but demand. Sympathy, kindness, pity and cheerful hope— no amount of scientific efficiency can take the place_ of these in the dark hours of sorrow and trouble so common in the experience of all.

President Eliot of Harvard said, "In these intangible things are found the durable satisfactions of life; fame dies and honors perish, but loving kindness is immortal."

I would not belittle the importance of science in medicine — I bow in humble reverence before its beneficent power, nor would I magnify the personal element, yet many of us know from experience what comfort, hope and assurance the personality of a trusted physician may bring to the bedside of his patient.

The reaction of the public press to the indictment of the American Medical Association, its officers and permanent secretaries of the various councils, by the grand jury in Washington is most questionable as to a proper government procedure. This action has aroused tremendous resentment among the medical profession. The feeling that the profession has been treated most unfairly is not confined to its members. J u d g i n g from the editorials from the lay press it is obvious that there are many, many others in this country who feel that the indicting of these officials was an underhand act to prepare the way for socialized medicine. It is a distinct and direct effort to harm the medical profession and to weaken its stand against socialized medicine. There is no question but that this is the motivating purpose of the indictment. As an example of the reaction of the legal profession, the statement of a distinguished lawyer might be mentioned, he said that it is the first time lthat he ever knew or heard of an act which had to do with financial and business relations being called on to lash a noble

profession and to bring about a s o c i a l change which is unnecessary and undesirable.

Mr. Carter expresses well the feelings that the great majority of the profession have in regard to the underhand measures that have been taken by a few enthusiastic, misguided Washington officials to chastise medicine. He said:

"It is a remarkable commentary on our present day life that there should be held up to public scorn a profession such as that of medicine, which has always upheld the finest of traditions, which has labored day and night in the care of the sick, rich or poor, and which has alleviated sickness and death to such an extent that morbidity incidence and death rate have fallen to a degree which is astounding. In no other country in the world is there a comparable record of decreasing illness and diminishing death rate. That medicine should be punished and held up to public ridicule because it has been through the efforts of organized medicine, that quacks have been kept in restraint, that hospitals have the efficiency they have and that medical service is as excellent as it is, is utterly ridiculous. It is almost entirely through the efforts of the American Medical Association, through its policing p o w e r s, that medical ethics is where it is today, that quackery is on the decrease and that malp r a c t i c e is practically non-existent. It should be to the glory of organized medicine that such an honest, clean profession exists. Benighted reformers in Washington have done their best to destroy the ' faith of the American people in their physicians and doctors."

This is really most lamentable. American medicine needs no defense. One of the m o s t important officials of Washington has just pointed out that the death rate last year was lower than it had been in this country in many years. The health of the population, as a whole, is guarded most effectively by present day methods. The people of America receive better medical care than any country in the world. There is never a serious illness or epidemic which is not taken care of adequately. If the American man, woman or child is not getting medical care it is either because of their unwillingness to make use of the existing facilities or it is sure to be some minor condition which is of minimum moment. Did any one in Washington ever hear of an indigent patient with a broken leg, pneumonia or acute appendicitis who does not receive the same care, attention and skill that a person would receive who can afford to pay?

I have been following the quarrel between the group health association and the District of Columbia Medical Society.

How can any group of people who are capable of earning between $1,400.00 and $2,000.000 per year be so deluded by a plan that promises better medical care for $2.20 per year? G.H.A. boasts that it pays its physicians $6,000.00 per year. How many persons must join in order to pay one physician's salary? At least 2,713 persons. This does not include medical equipment, expendable supplies, office space, utilities and assistants. Hence the number will run well over 3,000 and these 3,000 will consult a physician many more times than they would if they were paying by the visit.

The present ratio is 300 patients per physician. Therefore the G.H.A. doctor will have to take care of 12 times as many people as the community physician now cares for. How can he give each patient the time and care he needs when good medical care and thorough diagnostic procedure is a long, drawn out process and cannot be done in a few minutes? At the present time, because the experiment is on trial, those physicians who have accepted such positions will do their utmost to satisfy all patients until it is on a running basis, in order to insure a salary they could not possibly equal otherwise.

Personally, I feel that patients get better care by going to a physician who can give them his time and personal attention, a man who is familiar with their family and history. One certainly gets what one pays for and one cannot expect much for $2.20 per year.

It has been argued that the middle class will now receive the care it needs but from personal experiences over a long period of time and knowing many physicians, I know that the community physician has always given such care, at a price commensurate with a patients' ability to pay. A woman who is employed by the H.O.L.C. was telling recently how good this plan would be for people in her circumstances; yet her

husband and three grown children are employed; they own a beautiful home in a nice section of the city and own a car. This is the type of person that group health will cater to.

The community physician does a great deal of charity. The G.H.A. doctor will do none, yet he throws the entire burden of charity on the community physician and at the same time robs him of part of his income. Perhaps this is the reason he accepted such a position in the first place. He stands to lose nothing and at the same time receives at regular intervals an adequate s a l a r y, something the community physician never has had. This type of doctor is not the type who would give his patients the best care and couldn't if he wished. And what will these members of group health, who are being intimidated into joining or going into it because it is a cheap way out, do in times of the year that are most conducive to illness or in times of epidemic? Perish like flies—because it is the cheap way out.

If the government could not administer medicine any better than it administers its various bureaus—if it indulged in the waste of medicine that it indulges in administering its various functions—if it had as little regard for ability in its physicians as it has in its servants, I fear that the health of America would be in serious jeopardy. Everyone knows or s h o u l d know that political appointments are often made for political expediency and not because of ability; and we have no reason to believe that it would be any different in federal medicine.

Some have pointed out that 430 doctors revolted against the American Medical Association in favor of federal medicine. A splitting off of 430 men from an organizatio nof 106,000 members cannot be called much of a revolt and especially not when we see that these men are not true family practitioners. Most of them are practicing on salaries in institutions and do not come in very personal contact with their patients; therefore they are not representative of the American family physician.

Under federal medicine, the doctor and patient relationship would exist no longer. "The doctor's duty would be to the state and not to the patient," and this astounding and un-American utterance is not my statement but the statement of one close to the administration. By serving each individual patient well the physician is performing a greater service to his country than by serving some bureau. The six per cent indigent are now being well attended by the various cities and towns. The 94 per cent of the population who are able to pay probably wish to choose their own physicians.

The agitators for federal medicine have not proved that there is any need for such legislation. Let them prove their case and not go off on a tangent, and then be compelled to beat a hasty and ignominious retreat.

The American people are a proud people and do not wish some political bureau to enter their home life, to administer their routine in illness, to invade their right of privacy. Federal medicine would be a tragedy for the American health record— the best in the world.

By means of a calm and dispassionate marshalling of facts let us redouble our efforts to convince the public that socialized medicine is "poorhouse medicine.".

Daily, one sees in the papers the work of m e d i c a l men, who have discovered something new, not only to lessen mortality but at the same time curtails the income of the physician and still there is propaganda fostered by the 19 other cults, who are poisoning the minds of the people against the only scientific body of men who are engaged in the healing art. There is not a regular physician in the state of Oklahoma who would not go, day or night, rain or shine, when he is called. The patient first and compensation last.

The medical units may be formed, they may flourish for minor ailments, but when they cannot pay their dues or death is imminent, the regular old doctor will be on the job. The future of public health must center around the family physician, who with his bag and office equipment still cares for 95 per cent of the nation's illness. The treatment of illness must remain a profession.

Now, what constitutes a profession? Personal service. It cannot be standardized. There is an intellectual character to this service, with considerable self-direction and individual responsibility. There can be but one master in the house of medicine and that is the physician himself.

State medicine cannot change human nature though it may alter relationships. Independence in medical practice is as essential to the happiness and prosperity of physicians and to the advance of scientific medicine as independence gained by prodigious expenditure of blood and treasure, should under all circumstances be sacredly preserved to the people of these United States.

In summarizing—I am opposed to state medicine for the following reasons:

First—Government subsidies mean government control of everything it subsidizes.

Second—Government subsidies to private institutions mean the appropriation of public funds — the tax money of the people.

Third—It means government paternalism.

Fourth.—It means the government entering into competition with private medical practice.

Fifth—It m e a n s the surrender of the sovereignty and independence of the people to government regimentation.

Sixth and lastly—It means the gradual reduction of the rights of citizens to the status of serfs and minors.

———o———

Injuries of the Brain and Spinal Cord*

F. L. FLACK, M.D., F.A.C.S.
TULSA, OKLAHOMA

There were 38,000 deaths due to automobile accidents in 1938. A large number of these were caused by injuries to the head and to the spinal column which involved the brain and spinal cord. It has been s t a t e d that approximately 35,000 deaths resulted in 1938 from accidental injuries involving the head and spine alone and it is reported that 112,000 c a s e s of fracture of the skull, from which recovery is made as far as immediate effects are concerned, occur annually in the United States, but we must realize that a considerable per cent of these are left with some disability and that probably 10 per cent are totally disabled. In medical centers, in hospitals with high grade neurological services and under the supervision of skilled neurological attendance these cases are well cared for today.

It m u s t be remembered that at the p r e s e n t time more than half of these cases happen on rural highways and must be treated by doctors who are in general practice. Such injured persons must not be moved long distances and it is a poor treatment to take them to the "big shots" in the larger towns and medical centers. However, we have all seen a sufficient number of such accidents and have read and studied methods which have given the big boys the most successful results that we can easily familiarize ourselves with the diagnosis and treatment in more than 90 per cent of these cases, and this treatment can be given practically any place. The treatment has been so well standardized that by far the greatest percentage can be well cared for by the doctor who sees the case at the scene of the accident.

Prior to 1920 the mortality rate for skull fractures varied from 28 to 40 per cent, even in the best equipped hospitals. In 1929, in Bellevue Hospital, New York, the m o r t a l i t y rate was 37.8 per cent.

Temple Fay's series of 7,000 cases during the last 15 years, treated with due consideration of cerebral hydrodynamics consisting of repeated spinal puncture, dehydrating measures and restriction of fluid intake showed an average mortality of 14.5 per cent. During the last two years Fay has shown a mortality of between nine and 11 per cent.

It seems like, with the standard method of treatment which can be carried out in any village and with a careful diagnostic survey, the discrepancy between the treatment which gives a mortality of 11 per cent and that which gives a mortality of 40 per cent should be corrected.

For this reason it seems proper to again review some of the high points in the diagnosis and treatment of these very common injuries.

We know that a fracture of the skull, whether of the vault or of the base, is of little significance as compared to the injury of the brain itself. We also realize that there is probably only one urgent emergency which requires operation and that is a rupture of the middle meningeal artery. All we can accomplish in operating on a case of acute head injury is to take something out and that something is an extra or sub-dural hemorrhage, depressed bone fragments or contused and lacerated cortical or sub-cortical b r a i n tissue.

A hemorrhage from the middle meningeal artery is an extra-dural hemorrhage and most cases put us on guard by the following diagnostic points. The patient may not have been unconscious immediately after the injury but usually is for a short period of time, then regains the conscious state and has a lucid interval and again gradually develops coma. Many descriptions have been given of the various findings or combinations of findings involving the p u l s e, the blood pressure, and the respiration, but the most characteristic and reliable sign of a middle meningeal hem-

*Chairman's Address, Section on General Surgery, Annual Meeting, Oklahoma State Medical Association, Oklahoma City, May, 1939.

orrhage is dilatation of the pupil upon the side of the hemorrhage. It should be remembered that bleeding from this artery may occur on the side opposite the skull injury. The coma may be slow in developing and, under such conditions, a careful neurological examination may reveal a weakness of the muscles on one side of the face, in one arm and in many cases in one leg. A constant watch should be kept on the facial muscles during emotional expression, the difference in the size of the palpebral fissures and the tendency of one upper extremity to be limp.

The treatment of a ruptured m i d d l e meningeal artery is, of course, to ligate the bleeding vessel. Someone skilled in this type of work must be called.

The clinical symptoms of head injuries change so rapidly that only the closest observation will enable us to make the diagnosis in time to be of the greatest help to the patient. Shock is present in the majority of cases and it should be emphasized that cerebral shock can be grafted on general shock. Marked restlessness, delirium, and persistent coma are signs indicating marked brain damage or increased intracranial pressure. When increased intracranial pressure comes on slowly, the pulse rate may be as low as 40 and this is a warning sign demanding relief before the medulla becomes compressed with a pulse changing to a rapid rate. The pulse and respiration should be taken at two hour intervals. Temperatures above 102 indicate compression of the medulla. The reflexes are variable. A dilated pupil on one side indicates a hemorrhage on the same side. It is to be remembered that in the brain there are three sets of circulation, the arterial, the venous and the brain and spinal fluid, and that in a head injury they all may be disturbed. Pupils which are widely dilated and do not contract are of serious import and significance. If the pupils are normal on admission and later become irregular or unequal or show variations to light, it is frequently helpful in determining the site of injury.

Without entering into a long discussion of matters that have been subject to controversy in the treatment of head injuries, the treatment which in general I have followed and the treatment which has been found successful by experts is about as fol-

lows: In the first place it certainly is not advisable to remove the patient to distant places or medical centers for care. The patient, whether unconscious or not, is as soon as possible put to bed and treated for shock. He is kept warm, a close record of his temperature, respiration and b l o o d pressure findings is kept. No effort is made to obtain an X-ray at this time. Formerly, patients showing any degree of shock were given a slow intravenous injection of 50 cc of 50 per cent glucose. However, it has been amply demonstrated that the administration of intravenous glucose is attended with a secondary rise in pressure. It also has been shown that this secondary rise is not experienced after sucrose has been used, although, to obtain the same effect of dehydration, about twice the amount of 50 per cent sucrose must be used because sucrose has only about one-half the osmotic pressure e f f e c t of glucose. One hundred c.c. of 50 per cent sucrose may be given by vein and may be repeated as indicated, depending largely upon the variations in clinical symptoms and cerebral spinal f l u i d pressure as determined by manometer r e a d i n g s. Fifty per cent sucrose does not cause phlebitis in the injected vein and the large amounts in the circulation are apparently non-toxic. It is also a marked diuretic. Caffeine sodium benzoate is a valuable drug in the treatment of these cases and it also has value as a dehydrating agent. It may be given in 0.5 gram doses every eight hours by hypodermic. Morphine is a medullary depressant and should not be used. Cheyne Stoke's respiration frequently disappears when morphine is stopped. Cardiac stimulants should not be used. Hot colonic irrigations are many times of help in maintaining the body temperature.

Lacerations of the scalp should have a sterile dressing applied and, when the patient has recovered from the shock, the wound should be thoroughly cleaned, devitalized tissue should be removed and a careful closure made.

In compound depressed fractures where the depression is of any consequence, (as soon as the patient has recovered from the stage of shock), the depression should be elevated and a debridement done.

In regard to lumbar punctures, I know that some good men say lumbar punctures should not be done. Equally as good men advocate their use. My practice has been to do repeated lumbar punctures as often as every six to eight hours under careful management and reduce the spinal pressure by one-half. If the pressure is elevated or if the fluid is bloody, this is a valuable procedure. The fluid intake should be limited to 1,500 c.c. a day.

The after treatment is of great importance. These c a s e s, with even m i l d cerebral symptoms, should remain in bed for two weeks and those with more severe head injuries, regardless of their wishes, should be kept in bed six to eight weeks.

SUBDURAL HAEMATOMA

Hemorrhage beneath the dura of sufficient extent to produce symptoms is more common than it was formerly thought to be and may occur soon after the injury or many months may elapse before such a hematoma may reach a size sufficient to cause findings. Subdural hematomata are not rare but because of the gradual onset of symptoms they are not easily diagnosed. Headaches are important. A careful neurological examination should be made for the detection of any slight difference in the muscular activity on the two sides of the body and this will frequently give a clew. The vital centers are at the base of the brain and are, of course, well protected by layers of white brain substance but just the same they are subject to oedema.

The treatment of subdural hematomata is a surgical procedure by someone who is skilled and experienced in this type of work and consists of removing the clot.

In general, the treatment of head injuries is to remove by every safe means fluid from the cranial cavity and thus reduce the pressure on the vital centers. It is, of course, a matter of everyday good judgment that patients who are unconscious should have their heads lowered in order that secretions will drain through the mouth and nose instead of being aspirated into the lungs where they are likely to produce serious complications. It is also to be remembered that these patients must not be starved and that dehydration can not be continued over an indefinite period of time.

INJURIES OF THE SPINAL CORD

Every practitioner of medicine, no matter how specialized or how generalized his field, has to treat, quite frequently, fractures and injuries involving the spinal column. Injuries to the spinal cord, like brain injuries, are serious and experience has taught doctors that they should be extremely cautious regarding the care given these cases. Because of the greater concentration of nerve fibers in a small area in the spinal cord for a given amount of tissue, destructive injuries are more serious and extensive. The frontal lobe of the brain may be destroyed by a tumor and the patient continue to carry on a normal existence but if an area the size of a pea is injured in the spinal cord, at a particular l e v e l, it may result in a permanent paralysis. The loss of f u n c t i o n of the spinal cord is probably more often the result of vessel damage due to thrombosis than due to actual l a c e r a t i o n of nerve tissues.

When the spinal cord is exposed for the removal of a tumor, a greater degree of compression of the cord is seen than is likely to be seen following a spinal fracture but the patient who has the compression of the spinal cord due to a slowly and progressively growing t u m o r frequently recovers following removal of the tumor and the patient with a compression due to an injury often will not recover his function although on gross examination the spinal cord may appear to be in a better condition. The reason that has been assigned for the cause of this is that trauma occurs suddenly and the blood vessels in the spinal cord are seriously damaged, lacerated or thrombosed, whereas the vessels in the spinal cord will withstand a slowly developing pressure from a progressively growing tumor. The vertebrae may be dislocated or, what is more common, there may be a fracture-dislocation involving fractures of the body and one or both articular processes.

The extent of injury of the spinal cord depends upon two factors, the amount of displacement anteroposteriorly and laterally and the rotation of the vertebrae. The outcome of the case d e p e n d s upon the amount of injury to the spinal cord, since fractures of the vertebrae will heal by bony union as well as fractures of other bones.

From the very first moment every attempt should be made to maintain immobilization of the back in order to protect the cord from damage. The patient should be placed flat on the floor or a stretcher until he can be moved to a place where more e l a b o r a t e facilities are available for his care. X-rays should be made with the least possible movement of the body and careful methods of support applied in the v a r i o u s necessary positions, keeping in mind that it is necessary to maintain the spinal column in its normal relations.

A complete physiological severance of the s p i n a l cord can not be determined from a complete anatomic section and unless one has inspected the cord there can not be sufficient reason for the assumption that the cord has been divided entirely and it should not be assumed that there is a contraindication to laminectomy. Both conditions are followed by a c o m p l e t e paralysis in the muscles supplied by nerves which originate below the level of the injury. In both conditions complete sensory loss results below the level of the injured segment and the bladder disturbance may be similar.

In complete transverse lesions there is, in most cases, first the stage of muscular flaccidity which is the period of spinal shock. The m u s c l e s are toneless and flabby. All reflexes are lost and sphincter disturbances occur. The second stage or stage of reflex activity begins with the first reflex response to an external stimulus, usually from the sole of the foot. The third stage is that of gradual failure of reflex functions. In complete lesions the posture of the lower limbs is one of flexion; in partial lesions, one of extension. In an incomplete lesion, an early Babinsky sign appears.

Of very great importance is the Queckenstedt test for intraspinal pressure. This, of course, consists of a compressing of the jugular veins and noting the prompt rise in the intraspinal fluid pressure and the prompt fall upon the release of the jugular compression which takes place in a normal individual. In other words, in a normal patient a change in the intracranial venous pressure is followed by a prompt change in intraspinal pressure. If there is an ob-

struction of the subarachnoid space above the l e v e l of the spinal puncture needle, compression of the jugular veins is not followed by a rise of the intraspinal fluid pressure. This is evidence of a complete subarachnoid space block. In the presence of a partial block, the fluid rises very slowly and either falls slowly or reaches a level beyond which it does not fall and which is higher than the original pressure.

X-Ray Findings

Very often the character of the dislocation or rotation of the fractured vertebrae as demonstrated upon the X-ray plates is in itself a sufficient indication for laminectomy. Symptoms of cord injury may sometimes be present in the absence of X-ray evidence of bone pathology. In such cases, one must depend entirely upon the presence or absence of block and it is justifiable to perform repeated Queckenstedt tests to follow the case.

The first demonstration of a compression of the spinal cord is the indication for a laminectomy and not alone the suspected extent of the spinal cord damage. One may, with justification, wait for several hours until the immediate effect of general shock has subsided before laminectomy is performed but this period should not be extended for the cessation of symptoms or improvement in the presence of a block. Of course, the amount of movement should be restricted. If laminectomy is to be performed on the patient, it is wise that it should be done under local block anaesthesia. Following laminectomy, spinal fixation is advisable. Splints which are properly selected should be used. An indwelling urethral c a t h e t e r should be placed. If there are no signs of improvement within three months of injury to the spinal cord, the chances of complete return of function are not considered to be good. Some of these individuals are seriously disabled but should be encouraged to study and develop their minds and take up some sort of work that can be accomplished sitting down.

Common s e n s e and good judgment,

which are acquired by observation and experience, of course, should be the guiding principles in the treatment of all head and spine injuries, the same as in any other field of medicine.

BIBLIOGRAPHY

1. Rawls, Julian L.: Treatment of Head Injuries; Journal Southern Medical Ass'n., Vol. XXV, No. 8.

2. Fay, Temple: Economic Readjustment Following Head Injuries. Surgery, Gynecology & Obstetrics, Vol. LIV, 362-370.

3. Sammons, W. P.: Head Injuries. West Virginia Medical Journal, Vol. XXXIV, No. 10.

————————o————————

Diphtheria Carriers*

E. H. COACHMAN, M.D.
MUSKOGEE, OKLAHOMA

Diphtheria carriers all show (1) positive culture, and (2) virulence test but (3) no membrane. It is the lack of this membrane which differentiates these from the a c u t e diphtheria. The diagnosis is made simply by the insertion of a sterile applicator into the eye, ear, nose or throat exudate. The cases included in this report are all from the general run of private practice and are listed in order of frequency found, viz.; nose, throat, ear and eye.

Nose: Ten c a s e s had been diagnosed "sinus trouble," treated for such, only to continue their headaches. The diphtheria headache parallels the amount of discharge, while the sinusitis headache is the reverse, and reaches its worst when the sinus becomes blocked. The quantity of nasal discharge in the carrier is always much less than that of the purulent sinusitis, and in addition more flaky and scabby in texture.

The temperature ranges normal to a rise of a degree while in acute sinusitis the elevation is usually several degrees.

Even after these carriers have been suffering for months and years they show clear sinuses to transillumination and X-ray, with no drainage present in the meatii, by nasoscopic examination. Instead there is a fluffy greyish to yellowish exudate scattered along the medial surface of the three turbinates, which usually are not engorged, and occasionally the adjoining portion of the nasal septum. Again there is no membrane and the m a t e r i a l when touched moves easily without leaving any eroded

*Chairman's Address, Section on Eye, Ear, Nose and Throat, Annual Meeting, Oklahoma State Medical Association, Oklahoma City, May, 1939.

or raw surface, and on culture yields the diphtheria organism. This in four of the ten cases has given positive virulence tests upon the guinea pig, and the diphtheria organisms again isolated from these lesions. The remaining cases have been positive on s m e a r and culture only, since financial reasons prevented the cycle completion, yet they have been relieved by the same therapy of X-ray deep irradiation, and alkaline nasal douches, as used in the virulent positive cases.

The one exception to the rule of clear sinuses in these carrier cases was in an adult female who had sustained several s i n u s operations bilaterally, turbinectomies, and a submucous resection elsewhere, only to continue with her nasal symptoms. Her nose showed a unilateral blockage with polyps drenched in pus, the culture of which was diphtheria positive, and relief followed X-ray therapy and nasal douching. Her previous history covered some 20 years of continual nasal complaint and headaches.

Throat: In these eight c a s e s the epipharynx was chronically inflamed and the adenoid area usually atrophic, but rose red in color, with scabbing and flaky exudate scattered over the posterior surface. The texture of the exudate varied from a sticky gelatinous to watery, serous consistency.

In one adult throat infection diphtheria was found accompanying a peritonsillar abscess. Several authors have previously stressed the probability of death following the abscess incision being due to diphtheria toxin absorption through the incision area. This patient was given 10,000 units of diphtheria antitoxin and the abscess incised, recovery was uneventful.

In a second case the father had continual sore throat, which showed scabbing over the posterior epipharyngeal wall. His tonsils and adenoid were moderately hypertrophied, and a mild anterior and posterior cervical adenitis were present. X-ray and nasal douching gave relief for a few weeks but symptoms and positive culture reappeared, so tonsilectomy and adenoidectomy were performed to eliminate the focus, following diphtheria antitoxin administration as a precautionary measure. Recovery was uneventful.

In a third throat case a purulent maxillary sinusitis had cleared but scabbing of the epipharynx and post nasal discharge continued. The culture was positive for diphtheria, and again X-ray and douching gave negative culture, but this case has not as yet entirely stopped the post nasal discharge.

Ear: The six discharging chronic otitis media cases had positive diphtheria smears and cultures, although not any of these have had a virulence test. They came in complaining, not of diphtheria, but of the discharging ear, which had persisted for months or years following original paracentesis for an acute condition. It was observed following X-ray therapy in these cases that the smears and cultures quickly became negative for diphtheria, w h i c h probably accounted for the improvement from the X-ray, although the streptococci and staphlococci persisted in the discharge, until healing occurred.

In addition to these chronic otitis media c a s e s there was one unusual external auditory c a n a l and concha eczematoid lesion, where the area involved was a typical crusting eczema of the left ear only. Eczema is usually a bilateral lesion. This site gave a positive diphtheria smear and culture which promptly healed with repeated applications of tincture of merthiolate. This case was in a young mother with a nursing child, but neither she nor her child had any other clinical symptoms of diphtheria.

Eye: The first eye case* was in a nurse suffering from c h r o n i c conjunctivitis,

*Diagnosed, treated, and permission for publication given by J. V. Roule, M.D., University of Georgia Eye, Ear, Nose and Throat Staff, Augusta, Ga.

which originally started while she was nursing in Philadelphia. The condition had persisted for a year, during which time she had consulted the specialist of that area, before she went South for the winter, where a chronic diphtheritic conjunctivitis was found, *without* any membrane being present. She, at first, gave a negative history for diphtheria exposure, but following positive smear, culture, and g u i n e a pig virulence test, recalled she had nursed a diphtheria case shortly before her symptoms began. Antitoxin administration cleared her condition. The second eye case was in a six-week-old baby with a unilateral purulent conjunctivitis since birth which cultured positive to diphtheria, no m e m b r a n e was ever present, and administration of antitoxin immediately cleared the condition.

CONCLUSIONS

1. There is nothing characteristic in the appearance, color or odor of the carrier d i s c h a r g e. Therefore the diagnosis is chiefly laboratory and requires merely the insertion of a sterile applicator to detect the organism at fault. The "mousy" odor of the acute diphtheria is never present.

2. Some authorities contend diphtheria carriers immunize themselves to their own infection by slow absorption of the toxin. In the eye cases both recovered following antitoxin administration, while a throat case developed no complications following antitoxin, and peritonsillar abscess incision, even in the presence of a positive culture.

3. Deep X-ray t h e r a p y coupled with mild alkaline nasal douches gave prompt relief in all nose cases, and these have remained culture free for one year.

4. In no instance was infection passed onto others, even where the mother (in one of the nose cases) had six children, nursed them all, while she had the same symptoms through all those years.

5. It appears that diphtheria is possessed of properties of chronicity, the same as tuberculosis and syphilis, and should be routinely searched for in eye, ear, nose and throat conditions.

6. Antiseptic medications help but little except where the infection is upon skin rather than mucous membrane.

BIBLIOGRAPHY

1. Neffson, A. H. and Brem, J.: Diphtheria simulating peritonsillar abscess: Danger of infection. Arch Oto. 25 :260-265. March, 1937.

2. Rudolf, G. deM. and Ashby, W .R.: Nasal diphtheria carriers. J. Hygiene 36 :129-139, June, 1936.

3. Mitman, M.: The problem of the diphtheria carrier. J. State Med. 45 :249-257, May, 1937.

4. Cummings, G. O.: Laryngeal diphtheria. Maine M. J. 27 :55-57, March, 1936.

5. Jackson, O and C. L.: Acute laryngotracheobronchitis; living pathologic conditions seen in acute respiratory diseases. J.A.M.A. 107 :929-933, September, 1936.

6. Francois, J.: Catarrhal diphtheria. British J. Opth. 19 :1-19, January, 1935.

7. McKee, S. H.: Two cases of diphtheria conjunctivitis. Canadian M.A.J. 35 :425-426, October, 1936.

---O---

Some Observations on the Diagnosis and Treatment of Pneumonias During Infancy and Childhood*

C. W. ARRENDELL, M.D.

PONCA CITY, OKLAHOMA

Eleven years ago I presented before this section a paper on the treatment of broncho-pneumonias during infancy and childhood in which methods to prevent anhydremia and to maintain optimum blood volume were advocated. Since that time the members of the staff of the Ponca City Hospital have more frequently used measures relating to the maintenance of normal blood chemistry in the treatment of pneumonias. Although the value of these measures has not been proved by the reduction of the mortality rate, observation tends to show that procedures designed to offset the effect of water and mineral salt loss and the low oxygen content of the blood and tissues are beneficial in carrying many pneumonia patients through a critical period. It is unfortunate that no record is kept of the total number of pneumonias in the Ponca City area, although it is estimated that 50 per cent are treated at the Ponca City Hospital. There is even a discrepancy in the records of the number of deaths from that disease. For example, the Oklahoma State Health Department in 1936 reports 21 pneumonia deaths from Ponca City, whereas records of the Ponca City Hospital alone show 26 deaths from primary and secondary pneumonias. In 1937 the State Department r e p o r t s 17 pneumonia deaths and the Hospital records 23. Thus a review of the pneumonia

experience in the Ponca City Hospital will not prove the value of any procedure, as far as mortality experience is concerned, but is made to show in a small way what is being done for this important medical problem.

Arbitrarily, the pneumonias from age one month to 16 years treated in the Ponca City Hospital during the years 1936-37-38 were chosen for this study. During these years there were 6,574 patients admitted, of whom 287, or 4.3 per cent, had pneumonia. A comparison made of the experience 10 years previously, 1926-27-28, shows a total of 4,523 patients, of whom 77, or 1.7 per c e n t, suffered with pneumonia. This may or may not indicate an increase in the total number of pneumonias in the community during recent years, though it is believed that the incidence has recently been higher and that the virulency has also increased.

As stated above, there were 287 pneumonia patients treated during the years 1936-37-38 of whom 75 died, a mortality of 26.1 per cent. Of these there were 128 pediatric pneumonias of whom 25 died, a 19.5 mortality. Of the 77 pneumonia patients treated during the years 1926-27-28, 13 died, a mortality of 16.9 per cent, and seven, or 15 per cent, of the 42 pediatric pneumonias treated during the p e r i o d failed to recover. Dividing the 128 pediatric pneumonias into three age groups, the first group of one month to two years,

*Chairman's Address, Section on Obstetrics and Pediatrics, Annual Meeting, Oklahoma State Medical Association, Oklahoma City, May, 1939.

inclusive, shows 60 patients with 17 deaths, a mortality of 28.3 per cent. The second group of three to five years, inclusive, has 33 patients with two deaths, a mortality of 6.06 per cent. The third group of six to 16 years, inclusive, shows 35 patients with six deaths, a mortality of 17.1 per cent. In comparison, during the years 1926-27-28, the first group shows 18 patients with four deaths, a mortality of 22.2 per cent; the second group has 15 patients with two deaths, a mortality of 13.3 per cent; and the third group shows nine patients with one death, a mortality of 11.1 per cent.

None of the 128 pediatric pneumonias were typed, and there was no indication otherwise of the bacteriology. Several of the adult group of 159 patients were typed. However, specific serum was used only a few times — not often enough to materially alter the mortality experience. It was noted that the mortality of the adult group was 31.4 per cent as compared to 19.5 per cent for the younger group. In 1926-27-28 the mortality of the adult group was 17.2 per cent as compared to 15 per cent for the pediatric group.

Clinically, all of the cases were classed in four groups: (1) lobar pneumonia, (2) broncho-pneumonia, (3) influenzal pneumonia, and (4) septicaemia. Of the first group there were 38 with six deaths; in the second group, 70 with 16 deaths; in the third group, nine with no deaths; and in the fourth group there were six with three deaths. There were five incomplete histories with no classification of any kind, and of these there were no deaths.

Further review indicated that 24 of the cases were classified as primary pneumonia with one death, and 98 were secondary, or complicating other diseases, with 21 deaths. Six were not classified, but of these there were three deaths.

Radiographs of 36 patients were taken, but of these, 11 did not show any evidence of pneumonia. However, in this group of 11, five died—one on the first day after admission, one on the second, one on the fifth, one on the sixth, and one on the eleventh day.

Of the 25 patients with positive X-ray findings, four died. This would leave 16 patients who died but did not have radiographs made.

It was also noted that of the 25 patients who died there were 15 deaths within three days after admission. This probably indicated that the disease process was highly virulent or had existed in the home before removal to the hospital long enough in advance that irreparable pathology had already developed. Often the primary disease overshadows the pneumonia itself —as indicated by five of the nine deaths in 1938 in children with violent pertussis and uncontrolled spasms of coughing which resulted in a severe anoxemia with cyanosis. White blood counts of patients who lived average 18,270 with 71.4 per cent polymorphonuclears, and the average count for those who died was 26,000 with 70.8 per cent polys. Unfortunately, the Schilling differential was not used.

In considering the treatment of this group of patients, it was noted that at least 20 did not receive any treatment or care that perhaps could not have been given in the average home. About half of the entire group were treated in a small ward which was often quite crowded; most of the others were in double rooms and a few in private rooms. Pneumonia jackets with camphorated oil chest rubs were used about three-fourths of the time. Orders to force fluids by mouth were invariably given, and depending on the age of the patient, simple foods were offered. Fifty-two patients had a varying number of hypodermic or intravenous infusions of saline, Ringer's or Hartman's solution, the latter being used over 90 per cent of the time. About half of this number had intravenous glucose infusions, and eight had one or more blood transfusions. Fifty-eight of the group had oxygen, the tent method being the usual choice. In practically all of these, the nurses' bedside notes contained comments relating to the presence of cyanosis. It was noted that only four out of the 25 deaths did not receive any oxygen. Codeine or morphine was apparently used rather infrequently in 22 patients, and a laxative or purgative was given to only 17 patients. However, enemas were given to practically all of the patients. In fact, both from the perusal of bedside notes, as well as from personal observation, especially in the more seriously ill patients, as many as four or five enemas were sometimes given in a 24-hour period. Apparently, enemas were given for the reduction of high temperature as well as the relief of abdominal tympanites. Hydrotherapy in the form of ice caps, tepid sponges, or cold packs was used more or less on all patients. Diathermy was used occasionally in the older children. The average duration of stay in the hospital for the whole group was 9.1 days, and the average duration of fever was 4.7 days.

As stated before, this review was made to gain some impression of the methods used in the diagnosis and treatment of pneumonias in the Ponca City community. Further observations coming out of this experience, together with the findings of investigators and other clinicians might be added to this review. It will be recalled that no attempt was made to type any of the pediatric pneumonias, and the chief reason for this was undoubtedly due to the difficulty in obtaining specimens of sputum. Furthermore, investigators have shown that a majority of the pediatric pneumonias fell i n t o the heterogenous group IV, for which there was no specific sera. R e c e n t developments, however, which have d i v i d e d this heterogenous group into 29 separate and distinct types and for which there has also been developed specific sera for each type, should cause a considerable increase in the interest toward the typing of pneumonias outside of the larger urban centers. Also in this connection more frequent use of blood cultures should be encouraged, particularly for their prognostic value. McKann reports that the majority of the pneumonias in infants and small children fall into groups XIV, V, and XIX, the frequency being in the order named. However, it is too early to know definitely if the results from use of specific sera in these types will produce satisfactory results.

In regard to the relation of lobar pneumonia, broncho - pneumonia, a n d septicaemia, the findings of Gaskell are most illuminating. He shows that invasion of the lungs by a pneumococcus of low virulency will cause a single small area of pneumonia to develop, while an organism of slightly higher virulency produces a larger single area involving one or more lobes as in lobar pneumonia, while an organism of still higher virulency sweeps through the whole lung or both lungs rapidly and produces a patchy pneumonia as in broncho-pneumonia, while an organism of even higher virulency produces a septicaemia.

Reports of investigators seem to agree that 96 per cent of the primary pneumonias are due to one or more types of pneumococcus; but in secondary pneumonias, that is, in those cases in which the pneumonia is secondary to a well-defined primary disease such as pertussis, measles, or influenza, or is secondary to some long illness, the bacteriologic picture is considerably changed. These secondary pneumonias usually present the picture of a patchy pneumonia, and their bacteriology is reported as being approximately 60 per cent to 70 per cent pneumococci and 30 per cent to 40 per cent streptococci, staphylococci, influenza bacilli, typhoid bacilli, and possibly other organisms. It has been said t h a t pneumonias due to pneumococcus, streptococcus, or influenza bacillus differ characteristically in their clinical manifestations. However, no particular characteristic sign or symptom has been noted in this study.

In further consideration of the treatment of pneumonias much emphasis must still be placed on the prevention of anhydremia and the maintenance of normal blood volume and also upon the value of oxygen administration. A valuable index to the relative anhydremia in any patient may be obtained by observing the amount and color of the urine output. As previously noted, Hartman's solution was most frequently used in those patients suffering from water and mineral salt loss. This solution is rather fool-proof in that it supplies chloride as needed; also sodium is balanced by the potassium and calcium, and sodium lactate is converted s l o w l y into sodium bicarbonate, which is retained in the tissues if needed and excreted if not. In other words, Hartman's solution quite effectively overcomes any tendency toward either acidosis or alkalosis and its use has made it possible to maintain a more normal circulation in many of these patients, thereby reducing the number of blood transfusions in recent years. However, blood transfusion still constitutes one of the most effective means of aiding in the establishment of immunity in infectious processes and is particularly advisable in t h o s e patients with diminished plasma protein.

Oxygen administration has become almost a necessity in the treatment of the more serious types of pneumonia. This is really one of the life-saving procedures that modern physiology has contributed to medicine. It is used to combat a condition of anoxemia or the lower oxygen content of the blood and tissues which may or may not be associated with c y a n o s i s. The symptoms of anoxemia will at least exaggerate, and oftentimes completely overshadow, the signs and symptoms of toxemia resulting from the pneumonic infection.

These signs and symptoms are hyperpnea, shallow breathing, rapid heart, nausea and vomiting, toxic ileus, and circulatory collapse. Of course, there are many quite mild types of pneumonias that do not need o x y g e n administration, but if possible oxygen should be given to all pneumonia patients whose breathing shows any embarrassment. It is important to note that a dangerous anoxemia can be present without cyanosis.

No paper on the subject of pneumonia would be complete without at least a word on sulfapyradine. Already reports indicate that the results in the treatment of pneumonias with this drug compare favorably with the results obtained in diphtheria or malaria with specific sero- and chemo-therapy. McKann reports 80 children under the age of two years treated with no deaths. Evans and Gainesford report a mortality of eight per cent as compared with 27 per cent under the control series. Tehin reports a mortality of f i v e per cent in his observations. Although this drug with its further development offers great promise for the future, its use alone will not solve the pneumonia problem. Much work, especially in the field of bacteriology, remains to be done, and, for the time being, therapeutic methods already developed will not be displaced. Keen discrimination at the bedside will ever r e m a i n the physician's greatest asset.

--------------------o--------------------

Bilharzia*

Report of a Case

ELIJAH S. SULLIVAN, M.D.
OKLAHOMA CITY, OKLAHOMA

Urinary bilharzias is a disease of man which often invades the urinary track due to the infusion of the trematode schistosoma hematobium, which was discovered by Bilharz at Cairo in 1851. The disease occurs chiefly in Southern Mediterranean Countries. It is endemic in Egypt, Greece, Turkey and South Africa. About 30 cases have been reported in the United States. One case was reported in a boy four years old that had never been out of the middle west. It is considered impossible for the disease to be transmitted because of the absence of appropriate snails to act as intermediate hosts.

Etiology and Pathogenesis. Schistosoma are unisexual flat worms that live in the smaller branches of the portal system. The larviae cercariae mature and mate in the larger branches of the portal system and then migrate to the smaller veins of the bladder, intestines and liver, according to the species of the fluke involved. The mature male of the schistosoma hematobium is broad, flat and of a whitish color, is about 15 mm. long and has gynecopharic groove on its ventral surface for accommodation of the female. The female is slender threadlike and of a brownish color, it is about 20 mm. long. After mating has occurred they migrate to the smaller veins in the m u c o s a and sub-mucosa of the

*Chairman's Address, Section on Genito-Urinary Diseases and Syphilology, Annual Meeting, Oklahoma State Medical Association, Oklahoma City, May, 1939.

bladder, but may take up lodgings in the veins of the intestines. There the female lays a number of eggs which set up an irritation and produce the characteristic disease. The ova pass through the mucosa and are discharged through urine or feces. On reaching water the ovum hatches in a few minutes and releases a c i l i a t e d larveun. The larveun cannot infect man, but die in 24 hours unless they reach the liver of certain species of the snail called genera bullinus. Within these snails the asexual stage occurs and a sporocyst is formed which is filled with smaller bifid-tail larvae called cercariae. The cercariae, expelled by the snail through pulmonary system, are then free to make their way toward the surface of the water, and are capable of e n t e r i n g the human body through the skin or mucous membrane[1].

The ova is an elongated oval, about 120 to 190 micron long and 50 to 73 micron b r o a d, yellowish in color, and slightly transparent. They possess no lid, such as characterizes the eggs of most of the trematodes, but are provided with a thorn-like spine which is placed at one end. Within is a ciliated embryo[2].

In Vesical Bilharzia, the predominating symptoms are pain in the bladder, terminal hematura, dysuria and a b d o m i n a l cramps. The bladder is thickened and congested, ulcerated or papillomatous. The cystoscopic p i c t u r e may be that of a chronic cystitis, but the ulcerated papillomatous is likely to suggest malignancy[3].

The treatment is intravenous administration of potassium antimony tartrate, (tartar emetic), beginning with ¾ grain and increasing to 1½ grains once a week for about 10 doses.

CASE REPORT

Mrs. G. L. E., white, age 39, weight 94, entered Polyclinic Hospital March 1, 1939. Complaint, hematuria. Family history, essentially negative. Personal history, usual childhood diseases without any complications or sequela. Tonsillectomy several years ago. Bilateral salpingectomy and uterine fixation 15 years ago. One normal pregnancy 20 years ago.

Present illness, 1935, patient began to have a frequency, urgency, nocturia, hematuria and severe pain in hypogastric region. Was sent to the hospital for a uro-

logical workout. Both kidneys were found to be of normal size and position, with normal kidney function. Urine from both kidneys was normal, no acid fast bacilli found. Examination of gross specimen, color red, specific gravity· 1.018, acid reaction, albumen 2 plus, sugar negative, acetone 1 plus, casts none, gross amount of RBC, few WBC.

Cystoscopic examination, bladder moderately contracted, capacity about 16 oz. There were multiple papillary reddened areas studded with whitish opaque nodules, around the posterior portion of trigone and along the left ureteral ridge. Some of these areas had broken down and were bleeding. They were all thoroughly electro-coagulated. A biopsy specimen was taken from one of the lesions, no evidence of malignancy was found. Hemorrhage was controlled for about two months. It was necessary to electrocoagulate the reoccuring papillomas at irregular intervals to control the excessive bleeding.

May, 1938, patient returned to hospital with severe hemorrhage of bladder, which necessitated a cystotomy to remove bladder full of blood clots. Excessive bleeding was controlled by ligation, and papillary area cauterized. Patient made an uneventful recovery and left the hospital in two weeks and continued well for about three months, at which time her usual bladder symptoms re-occurred. Frequency every hour of day and night, and passing about one to two ounces of urine at a time.

On March 2, 1939, cystoscopic examination, bladder wall very thick and contracted, with a c a p a c i t y of about four ounces. The usual papillary areas were observed. Catheterized u r i n e specimen, deep straw color, turbid appearance, acid reaction, albumen 4 plus, occult blood positive (macroscopic positive), sugar negative, acetone negative, mucus 2 plus, epithelium 4 plus, erythrocytes many, leucocytes per HPF., centrifugalized specimen too many to c o u n t, noncentrifugalized specimen many large and small clumps, bacteria 4 plus, bacilli coli predominating, ova of schistosoma hematobium.

Upon finding the ova, a diagnosis of bilharzia was made. Immediate administration of ¾ grain potassium antimony tartrate, intravenously, was begun and continued twice a week. At the end of four weeks, cystoscopic examination shows a great improvement, bladder capacity 12 ounces, with papillomatous areas disappeared, leaving a reddened area, with a few white streaks in the center. Patient is voiding seven to ten ounces of urine at a time, gets up two or three times at night, and has gained 10 pounds. However, treatment will be continued for about four or five weeks, or until cystoscopic examination reveals a negative bladder.

This patient is a native of Georgia, and lived in one of ·the sea port towns in Texas until 1934.

In quoting Dr. Vincent Vermooten of Johannesburg, South Africa, in a letter to the Urologists Letter Club, February, 1939:

One of the first diseases I had to learn about in South Africa was Bilharzia. It is so prevalent and so extensive in the Transvaal and in Natal, that, when a patient comes in complaining of attacks of renal colic and haematuria, one immediately suspects Bilharzia and is surprised when one finds a renal or ureteral calculus. The result is that, in bilharzial districts, p a t i e n t s with nephritis are frequently mistakenly treated with antimony injections and so too, are those with renal or vesical tumors.

The correct diagnosis by the urologist is easy, for the cystoscopic appearance is so characteristic. Patches about the size of a quarter, usually near the ureteral ori-

fices, are seen, giving the appearance of millions of tiny crystals, lying just under the epithelium. In Egypt they are known as "sandy patches" for they glitter like the sand on the banks of the Nile. Here on the Reef they remind us of "gold dust."

If no "gold dust" is visible, one frequently sees small raised nodules, quite white in appearance, about a millimeter in diameter and raised about one millimeter above the surface of the bladder mucosa. These nodules, either singly or in groups, resemble tubercles, but have no red ring around their bases. I have seen both these lesions disappear completely after an adequate amount of antimony has been administered.

Papillomata, ulcers or other bilharzial lesions are, in my experience, never seen without. one or both of the above lesions being present.

When therefore, we suspect bilharzia, we do not rely for diagnosis upon finding the ova in the urine, nor upon an eosinophilia, nor on a history of terminal haematuria. A cystoscopic examination will give us an immediate answer and it is also the only definite way of knowing when a patient is cured of the disease[4].

BIBLIOGRAPHY

1. L. W. Riba and F. Christensen, Urinary Bilharziasis, J. of Urol. (November) 1934.
2. J. C. Todd, Clinical Diagnosis.
3. F. C. Hinman, Principles and Practice of Urology.
4. Vincent Vermooten, Johannesburg, South Africa, Urologists Letter Club, (February) 1939.

————————O————————

The Common Skin Diseases of the Lower Extremities*

W. A. SHOWMAN, M.D.
TULSA, OKLAHOMA

Many of the more common skin diseases occurring on the lower extremities present rather bizarre lesions and even the most frequent eruption; those encountered

*Chairman's Address, Section on Dermatology and Radiology, Annual Meeting, Oklahoma State Medical Association, Oklahoma City, May, 1939.

routinely are often erroneously diagnosed, resulting in many instances in a misdirected treatment. A resume of these more common lesions with some of the newer methods to their successful management prompted me to discuss them.

The etiological factors are numerous but simplified when the normal and anatomical functions of the skin are remembered. The skin's natural thickness plays an important role, as well as man's upright position, which has been responsible for some of the more common eruptions on the lower extremities as stasis, or improperly fitted pedal coverings causing many hypertrophies. The endowed individual characteristics of the skin, whether it might be an altered sensitiveness or true allergic response, accounts for a certain number of the dermatoses. C o n t a c t substances must be remembered such as shoe leather, dyes, flax linings of shoes, hose, etc. A certain number of the diseases are merely expressions on the skin of constitutional disease (syphilis, pellagra, exanthemata, and other diseases). Others are p u r e l y cutaneous in origin, the entire process being limited to the skin (scabies, impetigo, pyogenic and mycotic infections).

The inflammations and hyperemias, particularly the eczemas, contact dermatitis, and stasis dermatitis still require considerable consideration. The complicated disease picture dermatomycosis r e q u i r e s much knowledge to accurately differentiate it from the eczemas and dermatitis. To assume, without confirmation, that all dermatitis occurring on the feet and lower extremities is caused by the many varieties of the mycoses only leads eventually to misdirected treatment. The disease eczema, if we still consider it a disease per se, and rightly should, as encountered on the lower extremities, presents the familiar picture, whether it is pustular, erythematous, papular, vesicular, squamous or the "Eczema Rubrum." Isolated nummular plaques are too frequently treated for a mycotic infection.

The dyshidrotic eruptions simula t i n g dermatitis-eczema processes, even psoriasis pustulosa, add to the already complicated picture, the latter being a most difficult diagnostic problem. Whether we admit dysidrosis as a disease e n t i t y, or as (1) Schuermann considers this process a syndrome of other processes and call them "Dyshidrotic Exanthems," must not be disregarded, since many persistent and recalcitrant vesicular processes will improve rapidly under dyshidrotic management. The stabilization of the sympa-thetic and parasympathetic nervous system with calcium therapy and high vitamin feeding, particularly the hypodermic injection of thiamin chloride in doses of 3,000 units or more daily, will often suffice to alleviate a troublesome dyshidrosis. The use of the follicular hormones, when indicated, likewise will be of value.

The invasion of the skin of the feet and lower extremities, including the appendages of the feet, by the large group of fungi is a prevalent disease. The sodden macerated interdigital lesions, the vesicobullous plantar eruptions, the associated streptococcus and staphlococcus infections, the desquamative and hyperkeratotic lesions, are familiar to those doing a specialty; yet how often do we fail because our assumption that it is mycotic rather than proven, leading us to reconsideration only to find a negative smear, culture, and dermatomycin test. The latter should not be considered diagnostic, if positive, but only an expression of sensitivity. The insistence upon routine smears can not be urged too strongly, since errors are in direct proportion to the inconsistency, or lack of preforming same, resulting in improper treatment. The steady stream of desirable patients could be redverted to their proper professional conferees if more diligence on the part of the physicians, as a whole, was expressed by an equivalent determined attitude. The most important single prerequisite for the successful management of these various mycotic lesions is individualization. No set rule of thumb treatment is applicable to a satisfactory end result. Overtreatment is equally undesirable as the mycotic infection and, at times, even more troublesome than the original infection. Proper attention to the secondary invaders s h o u l d concern us more immediately than the mycotic phase, since the latter in most instances responds to appropriate antifungicidal preparations. The approach by the intradermal desensitization, in my hands, has not proven to be the anticipated help which was hoped for after its standardization.

Contact dermatitis occurring on the lower extremities is o f t e n overlooked and treatment instituted for some other disease, more often a m y c o t i c infection. Many of the persistent lesions on the feet and legs are due to the contacting material;

for example, leather, dyes, hose, lining of shoes, rayon, foot powders, etc. The more acute onset which is characterized by an intolerable pruritis, absence of fungi in smear, positive patch test, lack of involvement of the interdigital spaces, predilection for the great toes and dorsa of the feet instead of the little toes and plantar surfaces of the feet in dermatomycosis with extension onto the ankles, leads to an early recognition. Appropriate therapy includes the removal of the offending agent with soothing or stimulating preparations as indicated.

The pyogenic invaders, especially the staphylococcus and streptococcus, producing a dyshidrotic pyodermia, complicate the picture. Occurrence of these lesions on the sides of the toes and the plantar surfaces with deep seated pools of pus on a more or less erythematous base; developing rapidly, especially with the streptococcus and its complicating lymphangitis; often quite painful and being rather poorly limited, presents a rather unique syndrome. The inspection of the hands will materially aid in the diagnosis since a number of these cases s h o w an associated dyshidroform eruption. Chronicity is the usual added feature; however, excellent results may be obtained by the judicious administration of staphylococcus toxoid or autogenous vaccine together with adequate local therapy.

Stasis in the lower extremities from the various pathological conditions, especially varicosities, thrombophlebitis or lymphatic obstruction, is one of the more common causes for a chronic dermatitis appearing on the legs, as well ulcers. These static conditions previously and incorrectly called "varicose dermatitis and ulcer" usually occur on the lower third. At times the ulcers appear over the internal malleolus. These ulcers with their characteristic features seldom give rise to any diagnostic problems; however, one must differentiate syphilis, erythema induratum, b r o k e n down tuberculids and cancer. The familiar solitarity, induration, indolence, arciform configuration, punched out appearance, central healing with an atrophic non-contracted scar, and peripheral hyperpigmentation is the usual appearance of the luetic ulcer.

Tuberculids are more frequently multi-

ple, occurring on the knees and elbows usually in crops. Erythema induratum is predominantly on the posterior a s p e c t, usually the lower portion of the leg, and begins with a bluish-red, firm nodule or plaque ultimately softening in the center to form an ulcer. Cancer, when present, is of the squamous variety. The correction of the underlying pathology in the stasis lesions by appropriate management is the most singular therapeutic requirement whether by sclerosing agents, application of f i x e d elastic bandages, semi-rigid plasters, or complete rest with elevation. The syphilitic ulcers require adequate anti-luetic therapy.

The soles are frequently the site for an early or late syphilid. The brownish-red, deep shotty, grouped papules with scant scales occurring symmetrically, s h o u l d arouse one's suspicion, and adequate search should be made for confirmation of the early syndrome. The late cutaneous lesions, other than ulcers previously described, in contrast to the early lesions, are more often unilateral. The keratoderma's with the thickened plantar surface, hyperkeratotic and verruciform lesions, are distinct in their expression. The dismissal of a mal-perforans as an "infected w a r t," callous or soft corn, is not uncommon. The examination of the pupils when encountering these lesions frequently pays dividends, since these individuals may be unaware of their syphilitic process.

Drugs taken internally, in many instances, produce various dermatological expressions on the lower extremities. These reactions, at times, involve actual deposition of the drug in the tissue, or a toxic expression such as a toxic dyshidrotic process. Again the process may be any of the many usual combinations. Arsenic, besides the a c u t e reactions, produces characteristic keratodermas on the soles, as well as the general cutaneous surfaces. The vegatative lesions produced by the bromides and iodides seldom give rise to any diagnostic difficulty; however, their identity should be established since appropriate treatment will depend upon their removal. Many of the newer drugs now being used are likely offenders, especially sulfanilamide, which may produce various type lesions. Confirmation of the suspected offender with p r o m p t removal and adequate specific therapy will result in satisfactory recovery.

Hyperhidrosis and bromidrosis are very annoying and unpleasant conditions. The excessive sweating, with the usual accompanying pungent odors, is often encountered among hyperactive individuals, or those individuals whose sympathetic nervous system responds to the slightest stimulation. The recalcitrant cases respond well to irradiation by the fractional method for immediate relief, but attention to the neurogenic element, for the final solution, is essential. Sedation, tonics, and vitamin therapy will materially aid these these individuals.

The most common hypertrophies occurring on the feet such as clavus, callosities, and verrucae, should demand a great deal more consideration by medical men. These lesions, to the average physician, seem so trivial that a casting glance is the only solace these patients receive. How often could these worthy individuals be properly directed if more consideration be given them. An orthopedic examination, for the correction or proper support, in conjunction with removal of the corns and callosities will not only materially alleviate the local process, but in addition, soothe many irritable, high strung neurotic women. The common plantar wart, verruca plantaris, whose presence demands immediate treatment to avoid additional lesions, as well, alleviation, and whose exploitation by the various individuals treating these lesions, in most instances for remunerations far in excess of the more satisfactory methods, will respond promptly to irradiation with less expense. A single treatment with unfiltered X-ray, in most instances, or an injection with a soluble (water) bismuth, as recently advocated, will produce excellent results.

Fortunately, the malignant lesions of the lower extremities are not common, but when they do occur their malignancy is of the highest order. Carcinoma or melano-carcinoma developing from a pre-existing lesion, such as moles or sarcoma, demand immediate and radical treatment. Surgery and irradiation offer the only methods to combat these highly malignant lesions and the end results, in most instances, are not any too good. Careful and adequate attention to the precancerosis of the skin is,

unquestionably, the better approach.

There are, in addition to the few more common diseases mentioned, many other diseases, s o m e of which are relatively common, and others rare. Time will not permit their discussion. The successful management of the more common lesions demand an accurate diagnosis with the institution of proper and early treatment.

BIBLIOGRAPHY

1. Dermat. Wchnschr. 106:461-471, April 23, 497-502, April 30, 1938.

---o---

CANCER

The following is taken from a bulletin and announcement cf the Division of Cancer Control, Department of Health, Commonwealth of Pennsylvania. This bulletin was edited by John J. Shaw, M.D., Secretary of Health, and issued from Harrisburg, April 26, 1939.

Cancer is now a reportable disease in Pennsylvania, but this in itself will not make possible the accumulation of sufficient data on which to base a rational program of progress in cancer control for the citizens of the state. For such a purpose it is necessary that many more facts be known and correlated.

There arc many questions of immediate practical importance w h i c h can be answered if only the proper data can be collected and correlated. S u c h important problems as the value of preoperative and postoperative irradiation in cancer of the breast, the value of irradiation of the lymph nodes of the neck when they are not clinically the seat of metastases from cancer of the lower lip, the general distribution of cancer by age and sex, and the extreme importance of delay time, all can be solved by the accumulation of proper data.

Recognition of these facts has been given by the Medical Society of the State of Pennsylvania. In the annual report of its Cancer Commission for 1938, the general principles were laid down showing how a fact-finding program could be organized for s u c h a program, and the provisions were ratified by the House of Delegates of the Society.

To this end, then, it is proposed to augment the simple reporting of cancer cases by collecting data for every tumor case in the State of Pennsylvania. The w o r d tumor is here defined as any neoplastic growth, benign or malignant, to include

Hodgkin's disease, the lymphomas, leukemias, proliferative c y s t s (this includes retention cysts), teratomas, etc. In addition, a microscopic slide preparation from all cases in which biopsy has been performed or specimens removed, and in some a block of tissue of the cancer, are to be sent to the State Department of Health Laboratory, 34th and Locust streets, Philadelphia. Appropriate containers will be provided for the mailing of these specimens and the data.

The specimens and data will be assembled and classified in the State Department of Health for periodic review and the information derived will be distributed through the Medical Society of the State of Pennsylvania and its Cancer Commission for recommendations as to better organization and correlation of c a n c e r treatment facilities in the State. A final check will be made with the death certificates as they are collected in the Bureau of Vital Statistics.

In all cases in which an autopsy is performed, microscopic sections of the growth and data are to be sent to the same place.

Pathologists occupy the key position in this accumulation of data because the best means of diagnosis of cancer is by pathological examination. To cover the cost of preparation of extra slides and of filling out blanks, the sum of 50 cents will be paid for each slide plus blank received.

This will not be a diagnostic service, nor will the diagnosis of individual pathologists be criticized or superseded. In cases of differences of opinion, these will be recorded on the cards in the files for final disposal on the basis of further data, or as a result of conferences. These conferences, to be attended by pathologists and others interested, will be held at stated times, tentatively set at once a year, preferably at the time of the meeting of the Pennsylvania State Medical Society.

All individual cases, rare or commonplace, remain under the jurisdiction of the physicians in attendance on the patient, and will not be used except as part of mass statistics.

Obviously, the names of patients are essential for proper disposal and classification of data. Assurance is given to all clinicians and patients that names will be held inviolate and will be used only for the necessary cataloging and by only such few persons as are necessary for this purpose, who will be honor-bound to hold inviolate the names of patients.

Such a fact-finding procedure will:

1. Make for keeping better records.
2. Answer numerous immediately important practical questions, such as radiation before and after breast cancer surgery, delay-times, surgery vx. radiation in lip cancer, etc., etc.
3. Stimulate the taking of biopsies.
4. Make for better pathological diagnoses.
5. Raise all standards of diagnoses and treatment.
6. Educate doctors and lay people.
7. Provide data to determine the part heredity p l a y s in the incidence of cancer.

This collection of slides and data will be available to any qualified person for study and correlation, at the discretion of the Secretary of Health. We urge your wholehearted cooperation in filling out the official cards because the success of this investigation depends entirely u p o n complete answers to e v e r y question in the questionnaire.

The magnitude and importance of this work have resulted in the establishment, by the Secretary of Health, of a Division of Cancer Control in the Department of Health of the Commonwealth of Pennsylvania.

* * * *

It would appear from the above that the H e a l t h Department of Pennsylvania is carrying out the suggestions of their House of Delegates of their State Association and with the cooperation of the physicians of the State much will be accomplished toward cancer control.

NEW HEADQUARTERS

Plaza Court Building

Oklahoma City

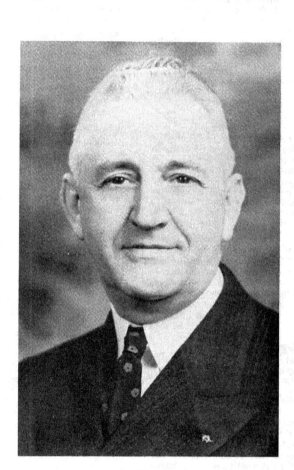

THE PRESIDENT

Doctor W. A. Howard
Chelsea, Oklahoma

Oklahoma State Medical Association, 1939-40

THE JOURNAL
OF THE
Oklahoma State Medical Association

Issued Monthly at McAlester, Oklahoma, under direction of the Council.

Copyright, 1939, by Oklahoma State Medical Association, McAlester, Oklahoma.

Vol. XXXII	MAY	Number 5

DR. L. S. WILLOUR...............................Editor-in-Chief
McAlester, Oklahoma

DR. T. H. McCARLEY...............................Associate Editor
McAlester, Oklahoma

Entered at the Post Office at McAlester, Oklahoma, as second-class matter under the act of March 3rd, 1879.

This is the official Journal of the Oklahoma State Medical Association. All communications should be addressed to The Journal of the Oklahoma State Medical Association, McAlester Clinic, McAlester, Oklahoma. $4.00 per year; 40c per copy.

The editorial department is not responsible for the opinions expressed in the original articles of contributors.

Reprints of original articles will be supplied at actual cost provided request for them is attached to manuscripts or made in sufficient time before publication.

Articles sent this Journal for publication and all those read at the annual meetings of the State Association are the sole property of this Journal. The Journal relies on each individual contributor's strict adherence to this well-known rule of medical journalism. In the event an article sent this Journal for publication is published before appearance in The Journal the manuscript will be returned to the writer.

Failure to receive The Journal should call for immediate notification of the Editor, McAlester Clinic, McAlester, Oklahoma.

Local news of possible interest to the medical profession, notes on removals, changes of addresses, births, deaths and weddings will be gratefully received.

Advertising of articles, drugs or compounds unapproved by the Council on Pharmacy of the A. M. A., will not be accepted.

Advertising rates will be supplied on application.

It is suggested that wherever possible members of the State Association should patronize our advertisers in preference to others as a matter of fair reciprocity.

Printed by News-Capital Company, McAlester.

EDITORIAL

HEADQUARTERS IN OKLAHOMA CITY

It was impossible for the Executive-Secretary to abstract the minutes of the meeting which we have just concluded, in time for this issue of the Journal. The meeting was apparently a success in every way. Our Guest Speakers were well received and presented excellent material and the Scientific Sections were well attended.

The Council and House of Delegates dispensed with much important business, the most important being the change of headquarters to Oklahoma City where they will be under the direction of the Executive-Secretary. The Secretary-Treasurer-Editor was retained but is relieved of all detail work. An Editorial Board of the Journal, composed of Drs. Ned Smith, L. J. Moorman and L. S. Willour, was elected by the Council and authorized the present Editor to continue in that capacity for the present, the Journal continuing to be published in McAlester.

It is important that all Secretaries of the County Medical Societies, having business with the Association, be familiar with the fact that the headquarters are now in the Plaza Court Building, Oklahoma City, and that all correspondence be so directed.

This looks like a very happy solution of the problem and with the full-time Executive-Secretary memberships should be increased and the activities of the Association greatly widened.

Let every member give the new Executive-Secretary their fullest cooperation and make every effort to make it a banner year of the Association.

---o---

THE EDITORIAL BOARD ORGANIZES

The Editorial Board, as provided for in the recently adopted By-Laws and elected by the Council, composed of Doctors Ned Smith, Tulsa, L. J. Moorman, Oklahoma City, and L. S. Willour, McAlester, met in McAlester, May 11th, and organized, electing Dr. Willour Chairman.

The Editorial policy of the Journal was discussed and some division of the work was adopted. Mr. R. H. Graham, Executive-Secretary, was present and as provided in the By-Laws will accept all of the business management of the Journal. It was apparent from the discussion of the Board that there will be no radical changes made in the editorial policy of the Journal but the high standard of both the scientific and advertising material will be maintained and Mr. Graham said, if a decrease in the cost can be obtained with maintenance of the quality of the product, that this will be accomplished.

Bids for the publication of the Journal will be received by Mr. Graham and the Association may feel sure that he will accomplish any economy possible and still maintain the Journal's high standard.

Editorial Notes—Personal and General

DR. E. RANKIN DENNY, Tulsa, was guest of the Pittsburg County Medical Society at their meeting April 21st. His subject was "Chemotherapy in Bronchial Asthma."

DR. J. T. LONEY, Tishomingo, was re-appointed County Health Superintendent of Johnston County.

DR. L. G. LIVINGSTON, Cordell, has returned from New Orleans where he took post graduate work at Tulane University.

DR. J. F. MARTIN, Stillwater, who has been seriously ill at his home, is reported improved.

News of the County Medical Societies

DR. GEORGE H. KIMBALL made a talk at the meeting of the Tulsa County Medical Society at Tulsa on Monday, April 24, 1939. Dr. Kimball's subject was "Common Problems of Plastic Surgery" and the talk was accompanied by various interesting slides.

The Southern Oklahoma Medical Association will hold their next meeting Tuesday afternoon and evening, June 6th, at the Veterans Hospital, Sulphur, Oklahoma. One of the highlights of the program is the address by Dr. Arthur E. Hertzler, of Halstead, Kansas, on "Goitre."

RECENT DEATHS

(Insufficient Data For Obituaries)

Dr. J. H. Logan, Madill, May, 1939.

Dr. W. W. Campbell, Tulsa, April, 1939.

Dr. J. B. Carmichael, Duncan, April, 1939.

Dr. J. E. Hollingsworth, Strang, April, 1939.

Dr. E. L. Bagby, Enid, died May, 1939.

Michigan Society Acts On Medical Care Plans

The House of Delegates of the Michigan State Medical Society, at a special session held in Detroit on January 9, approved the principles of group hospitalization and group medical service and empowered the Society's Council, in cooperation with hospitals and civic groups, to proceed with the establishment of plans for the formation of non-profit organizations to provide these two types of service.

The group protection would take the form of insurance with rates and benefits fixed according to actuarial studies. Rates for the hospitalization plan would probably range, for care in a ward, from 60 cents a month for a single subscriber to $1.25 for a family. Benefits would include 21 days' hospital care for the first year.

For the suggested medical service plan, an employed subscriber would be entitled to a maximum block of units of service, with an alternative plan based on a time consideration.

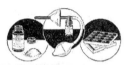
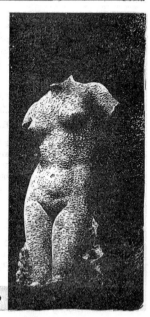

ABSTRACTS : REVIEWS : COMMENTS
and CORRESPONDENCE

SURGERY AND GYNECOLOGY
Abstracts, Reviews and Comments from
LeRoy Long Clinic
714 Medical Arts Building, Oklahoma City

"Studies on the Endometrium in Association With the Normal Menstrual Cycle, With Ovarian Dysfunctions and Cancer of the Uterus," by Wallace E. Herrell, M.D.; American Journal of Obstetrics and Gynecology; April, 1939, Vol. 37, No. 4, page 559.

This is a very practical review of the findings in the endometrium in relation to the ovarian activity and especially ovarian dysfunction. There is also included a study of 50 cases of carcinoma of the uterine fundus with the conclusion that this disease is associated with an unapposed action of estrin and, therefore, persistent proliferating type of endometrium with cystic changes.

The activity of the ovary is reflected in the activity of the endometrium. For the purposes of classification this author has divided the normal endometrial cycle into five phases, (1) the menstruating phase, (2) a phase of early proliferation (based upon the action of the follicular hormone. estrin), (3) a phase of late proliferation (based upon continued and more abundant action of estrin), (4) a phase of early differentiation (based upon early effect of the corpus luteum hormone, progestin), and (5) a phase of late differentiation (based upon continued and more abundant action of the corpus luteum hormone, progestin). These last four phases correspond roughly to the first four weeks of a normal menstrual cycle in the order named. When there is an abnormal ovarian activity, there results an abnormal endometrial cycle with an arrest of the cycle in any of the phases enumerated above. He has called the phase of arrest the persistent phase and has pointed out again that the stage of arrest in the endometrial cycle depends upon the degree and the kind of ovarian dysfunction—that is, an increase or a decrease in either estrin or progestin secretion or an increase or a decrease in both. This is thus a very simple classification for correlation of the study of the endometrium with the ovarian activity in a patient.

He has likewise extended his clinical classification of ovarian dysfunction into a primary and secondary group. The primary ovarian dysfunctions lie upon the basis of failure in the ovary itself. The secondary dysfunctions are due to changes in the ovary which follow or accompany failure of the thyroid or pituitary functions. He emphasizes that the endometrium reflects only the activity of the ovary whether the ovary is primarily at fault or whether its dysfunction is due to the action of the thyroid or pituitary dysfunctions or to general metabolic disturbances.

From his studies of the endometrium he has also drawn certain conclusions as to significance of cystic changes in the endometrium. "When cystic changes are present in the proliferative phase of the cycle, the tendency is greatest toward bleeding dysfunction and to a lesser degree toward sterility. On the other hand, when cystic changes are associated with the differentiative phases, the tendency is greatest toward sterility, while the tendency toward bleeding dysfunction is almost entirely absent."

In his study of 50 patients with carcinoma of the body of the uterus the adjacent endometrium was practically always in the proliferative stage and was usually cystic. He objects to the term "hyperplastic endometrium" and feels that this endometrium is due to the unapposed action of estrin and from the absence or failure of activity of the corpus luteum. In support of the thesis that carcinoma of the endometrium is due to an unapposed action of estrin, he has the following reasons: (1) the ovaries associated with the fundal carcinoma specimens contained cystic portions lined with typical granulosa cells which he feels are probably the source of estrin in at least 90 per cent of the cases of carcinoma; (2) in the cases of carcinoma of the body of the uterus estrin was found in the urine of these patients; (3) the endometrium in patient with carcinoma of the endometrium was of a persistent, proliferative phase and was not true atrophic endometrium; (4) "Carcinoma of the body of the uterus never has been seen as far as I have been able to determine, if an individual has been previously castrated."

Comment: This is an important contribution to medical literature because it crystalizes much of the present knowledge of ovarian effect upon the endometrium into a simple clinical classification which is necessary for proper diagnosis and application of the treatment of the patient including the proper choice of ovarian hormone therapy.

Too much emphasis cannot be placed upon the fact that changes in the endometrium and, therefore, menstrual irregularities are but a direct reflection of the ovarian activity and quite frequently this ovarian dysfunction is upon the basis of other glandular or general disease. It becomes at once obvious that in treating patients with ovarian dysfunction one must use every means to disprove thyroid or pituitary dysfunction or other metabolic disturbance as the cause for ovarian dysfunction prior to the institution of ovarian hormone therapy. Naturally, if the ovarian dysfunction is secondary in type, the therapy will not be curative of the cause and will only temporarily influence the endometrial changes and probably the ovulatory activity of the ovary.

Having once determined that ovarian hormone therapy should be employed because the ovarian dysfunction is primarily in the ovary, one should use every means possible to select the proper hormone for administration. Otherwise, it will be of little effect and probably considerable harm. It is in this direction that such study of endometrial tissue, a true mirror of ovarian activity, will be of benefit preceding ovarian hormone medication.

The observations made by Dr. Herrell in relation to the etiology of carcinoma of the cervix resting at least in part upon the continued activity of estrin is an extremely important one. Though he disagrees with the term "hyperplastic endometrium," his observations are but a refinement of the feeling of Meyer, Taylor, Novak, and others who have felt that endometrial activity past the

menopause was in a degree responsible for endometrial carcinoma. Most arresting is his observation that he has not heard of a case of carcinoma
of the endometrium in the uterus of a previously
castrated individual.

Wendell Long.

———

"Acute Intestinal Invagination in the Grown-up
Child, with Two Observations, in One of Which
There Was a Meckel's Diverticulum (L'Invagination Intestinale Aigue de la Seconde Enfance,
Deux Observations Dont Une Avec Diverticule
de Maeckel)," by Charles Lefrancois, Chirurgien
de l'hopital Saint-Luc, Montreal; L'Union Medicale du Canada, April, 1939, Vol. 68, No. 4, page
387.

The author makes a very interesting and instructive report about two grown-up children (seconde
enfance), remarking that intestinal invagination
at that age is more rare than in infants.

Intestinal invagination in the grown-up child
is not usually as grave as in the case of the infant.
Ordinarily, the invagination in the grown-up child
is chronic or at least subacute, and the surgeon is
able to spend some time in making a decision.

At the same time, there exists in the intestinal
invagination of older children acute and subacute
forms that may become rapidly fatal if diagnosis
is delayed so that an early operation cannot be
done.

In the intestinal invagination of the grown-up
child, if it is acute, the beginning is sudden.
Briefly, the symptoms are the classic symptoms of
intestinal invagination of the younger child—that
is, pain that appears in crisis of an atrocious
character, separated by intervals of relief; early
vomiting. Bloody stools are not as frequent as in
infancy, and for that reason it is important to
make a digital examination of the rectum in order
to determine, if possible, if there is evidence of
either a tumor or of blood. Very often there is no
evidence of blood at all at the beginning of the
difficulty. At the same time, there is complete
obstipation.

The author directs attention to the extreme importance of a palpable tumor in the abdomen. He
remarks that this abdominal tumor nearly always
exists in the case of intestinal invagination in
the grown-up child, and that it is one of the most
important evidences of invagination at its beginning. ("Cette tumeur abdominale qui existe
presque toujours est un des plus precieux symp-
tomes pour identifier l'invagination a son debut.")

There are two case reports as follows:

(1) A boy of 10 years entered hospital 4:00 p.m.
on a certain day because of violent abdominal pain.
The difficulty began at 10:00 a.m. the same day.
At first the pain was more violent on the right
side of the abdomen. He was put to bed at once
and a physician was summoned. There were
periods in which he appeared to have some relief,
but always the pain would reappear with equal
violence. These intermittent crises continued until
he was admitted to the hospital. In the meantime,
there had been vomiting on two or three occasions.

The patient was a well-developed boy of 10 years.
His health had always been good. He appeared to
be very sick, and responded with difficulty to questions. At intervals there would be attacks of pain,
at which time he would cry in a distressing manner.

The pulse was 134, temperature 97° F.

On palpation, there was extreme tenderness in
the right lower abdomen, the tenderness remaining
between the crises of pain. However, there was no
muscular rigidity. The abdomen was slightly distended.

In palpating the abdomen, a mass about the
size of an orange was felt rather deeply in the

right lower abdomen near the flank. It was slightly movable, and was extremely tender.

Suspecting an intestinal invagination of an acute
character, a rectal examination was made. There
was no particular tenderness in connection with
this examination, and there was no evidence of
blood. No mass could be felt by rectum.

The blood count showed hgb. 50 per cent, R.B.C.
3,500,000, W.B.C. 19,700, polymorphonuclears 97 per
cent.

Operation was done through a right pararectus
incision below the umbilicus eight hours after the
beginning of the attack. As soon as the peritoneum
was opened the mass was found. It was very clear
that there had been an ileo-colique invagination
.—that is, an intussusception.

It was decided to attempt a reduction of the
invagination. This was carried out with considerable difficulty, the assistant exerting very light
traction on the ileum, while the operator maneu-
vered the mass from the distal point. Fortunately,
after 15 minutes the invagination was reduced.
It showed that there had been an invagination of
about 30 centimetres of the ileum. There was
some infiltration here and there with a few ecchy-
motic areas, but, on the whole, the intestine was
in very good condition.

The appendix was removed simply as a prophylactic measure. The terminal ileum was fixed by
five or six sutures to the surrounding peritoneum
as a preventative measure. The abdomen was
closed without drainage.

The postoperative course was excellent. The
child was discharged from hospital on the ninth
day after operation, his condition being good at
the time.

(2) The second patient, the case of which is
reported by the author, was a boy 13 years of age.
While eating supper at about 7:00 p.m. December
24, 1937, there was sudden severe pain in the
abdomen. The pain was so severe that the parents
became alarmed at once, and took him across the
street to the family physician who happened to
live near them. The physician ordered him to bed,
put ice on the abdomen, and told the parents he
would see the child a little later. He went by to
see the child at 10:00 p.m., at which time the complaints were very much more pronounced than
when he had seen him at first. In fact, he was
so alarmed about him that he took the child in
his automobile and transported him some distance
to a hospital. In the meantime, there had been
extremely severe, intermittent pain, when the child
would cry out, notwithstanding he had had some
morphine hypodermatically. He had vomited two
or three times before he reached the hospital.

In this case it was learned that the boy had had
a somewhat similar, but much milder, attack —
possibly several such attacks before.

At the hospital, the boy showed evidence of acute
suffering. He was agitated, and cried out spas-
modically.

On palpation, the abdomen was soft, and there
was nothing about the right iliac area that would
cause suspicion. However, near the umbilicus one
could feel a mass that seemed to extend across
the abdomen at that point. The tumor was movable, but manipulation caused extreme pain. Rectal
examination was negative, both in connection with
the presence of blood or the existence of a tumor.
Pulse was 66, temperature 97.

There was a tentative diagnosis of intestinal invagination, but one considered, also, the possibility of an intestinal infarction.

Surgical operation was done seven hours after
the beginning of the attack. The approach was
through a low median incision. The mass was
found at once. The head of it was some 10 cm.
from the cecum. It was decided to try to reduce

the mass. This was carried out with extreme difficulty, and required much patience and gentle handling. Finally, after a manipulation over a period of about half an hour it was reduced. At that time it was seen that there existed in connection with it a Meckel's diverticulum which had become invaginated into the intestinal tract. The intestine was, fortunately, in very good condition. The Meckel's diverticulum was about 2½ inches long and its diameter a little greater than the intestine (ileum). At the point of insertion of the diverticulum the intestine was not narrowed, as is frequently the case. On the contrary, it was dilated which made it possible to carry out a simple resection of the diverticulum, with closure of the opening by three layers of sutures. After placing a cigarette drain, the abdomen was closed.

The postoperative course for two days was alarming. There was difficulty in connection with the lungs, it being pretty clear that there was a distinct pulmonary congestion. Fortunately, after two days there was improvement, and the patient was discharged from the hospital 15 days after admission, his condition being good at the time.

The author makes some very interesting comments in connection with the diagnosis and proper treatment of acute intestinal invagination in the grown-up child, indicating in a very clear way that an early operation is of even very much greater importance than an early operation in acute appendicitis, because after 12 or 15 hours it is quite probable that one would not be able to reduce the invagination, thus making resection necessary—an operation that carries with it a very high mortality.

Altogether, this is a very important and a very practical contribution. It is a contribution that shows us the tremendous importance of the problems in connection with the "acute abdomen." Moreover, reports like these show how futile and dangerous it is for one to play the role of an "abdominal surgeon, limited." The reports show, too, the salvation to be derived from prompt and intelligent cooperation of the attending physician and the surgeon.

LeRoy Long.

"Prothrombin Deficiency and the Effects of Vitamin K in Obstructive Jaundice and Biliary Fistula." John D. Stewart, M.D., Boston, Mass. Annals of Surgery, Vol. 109, No. 4, April, 1939, page 588.

When Dam, in 1935, showed that the lack of a fat-soluble substance which he called vitamin K in the diet of chicks led to fatal bleeding, he opened a new approach to the study of pathologic bleeding. Investigation of a hemorrhagic disease of cattle resulting from eating spoiled sweet clover had led to demonstration of low plasma prothrombin as the etiologic factor, presumably due to toxic effect on the liver. Improvements in methods of determining plasma prothrombin were followed by observation of low plasma prothrombin in animals with experimental liver poisoning and biliary obstruction, in chicks with hemorrhagic disease from vitamin K deficiency, and in patients with obstructive jaundice.

Another link in the chain was supplied by the experimental proof that fat-soluble vitamins are not absorbed from the intestine in the absence of bile salts. Practical application of these facts has led to successful treatment of prothrombin deficiency in patients with liver disease by means of extracts containing vitamin K. Considerable progress has been made in the purification of vitamin K, although a preparation suitable for parenteral use is not yet available. Much study has been given to developing better methods of assaying the vitamin K content of various animal and vegetable fats, but a method based on the protective or curative effect on chicks must still be used.

Data included in this article were obtained in the study and treatment of patients with obstructive jaundice or biliary fistula on the Surgical Services of the Massachusetts General Hospital during the past year. The author states that this is to be regarded as a preliminary report, given because his results are so striking.

He sets forth in detail the laboratory procedures carried out such as the method for determination of plasma prothrombin percentage, etc.

The average increase in plasma prothrombin under vitamin K therapy was 32.8 per cent.

The frequency with which plasma prothrombin is reduced in obstructive jaundice is striking. During the course of this study only one case was seen in which obstruction to bile flow for over a week had not been associated with plasma prothrombin levels of less than 84 per cent. In this case the author says that the patients' appetite had remained remarkably good and the biliary obstruction was not complete. In the preoperative group the response to vitamin K-cholic acid has been invariable. It seems to be true, however, that the more severe the liver damage the less marked is the prothrombin recovery. Little, if any, correlation is discernible between the degree of depression of plasma prothrombin and the plasma bilirubin level. This is not surprising since the excretory function of the liver is only one of the factors concerned in the maintenance of plasma prothrombin. Also, even when bilirubin is being excreted, bile deficient in cholic acid and hence less effective in promoting absorption of vitamin K may be formed by the damaged liver.

A drop of 20 to 40 per cent in plasma prothrombin concentration immediately after operation is to be expected, dependent perhaps on such factors as blood loss and dilution of plasma, clotting, and depression of liver function by anoxemia and anesthesia. The fall is transitory, however, if vitamin K-cholic acid feeding is resumed at once.

It is apparent that the plasma prothrombin level is quickly responsive to change in metabolic conditions, suggesting the absence of prothrombin reserves in these patients. A safe preoperative plasma prothrombin level, preferably above 75 per cent, is highly desirable. Since the prothrombin level may change quickly, the need for frequent determinations in the early postoperative course is obvious.

There were five cases of postoperative hemorrhage. Two of these created an interesting experiment by refusing to take the vitamin K-cholic acid capsules after operation on grounds that they caused epigastric distress. In both cases a steady drop in plasma prothrombin with subsequent massive hemorrhage resulted. Thereafter, the patients cooperated in taking the mixture and rapid restoration of plasma prothrombin and cessation of bleeding followed. In one patient the biliary obstruction continued only partially relieved after operation because of cholangeitis, and bleeding set in as late as the sixteenth postoperative day. The author feels that the vitamin K, taken for eight days after operation, postponed the bleeding, for, as a rule, bleeding from prothrombin-lack occurs within the first week after operation. He feels that a most interesting question, which deserves study, is the influence of infection on plasma prothrombin. There is evidence that the liver may react sensitively to extra-hepatic inflammation, for example, the rise in plasma fibrinogen occurring in the course of abscess formation and in pneumonia.

Blood transfusion appeared to be a rather inefficient method of combating the bleeding tendency due to hypoprothrombinemia, as the effect on the recipient's plasma prothrombin is slight and transitory. The author has found a measurable increase of only 6 per cent occurring in one adult patient whose plasma prothrombin level was determined before and after transfusion of 600 cc. of blood. He feels that blood transfusion is needed to replace lost blood, but vitamin K-cholic acid therapy is indicated in order to prevent further bleeding.

The conclusions drawn by Dr. Stewart are as follows:

"1. In obstructive jaundice and biliary fistula the plasma prothrombin level may be low.

"2. Following operation upon such patients, further reduction in the plasma prothrombin may occur.

"3. Dangerous bleeding may take place with plasma prothrombin concentration of less than 50 per cent normal.

"4. No correlation can be made out between plasma fibrinogen and prothrombin concentrations.

"5. Administration of a mixture of vitamin K and bile salts, through a jejunostomy if necessary, leads to a restoration of plasma prothrombin and control of the bleeding tendency.

"6. Plasma prothrombin level depends on the functional capacity of the liver as well as absorption of vitamin K from the intestine."

LeRoy D. Long

---o---

INTERNAL MEDICINE
Edited by Hugh Jeter, M.D., 1200 North Walker, Oklahoma City

A Preliminary Report of the Blood Picture in Brucellosis. Myrtle Munger, B.S., and I. Forest Huddleson, Ph.D., East Lansing, Michigan. (The Journal of Laboratory and Clinical Medicine, March, 1939, Vol. 24, No. 6.)

Herein is a preliminary report of the blood picture in Brucellosis. This report is based on the study of the blood on a number of acute undulant fever cases from which Brucella melitensis was recovered. All patients were showing symptoms of the disease at the time of examination and the blood examinations were made from two to four weeks after the onset of the disease. The authors found in this study of Brucella melitensis infected individuals that the blood picture reveals a leucopenia with a relative lymphocytosis and monocytosis. Red blood cells tend to be slightly smaller than normal. However, some patients show macrocytosis. One interesting point that has not been noted before is that many of the mature small lymphocytes are much larger than normal which is similar to the infectious mononucleosis type of lymphocyte. These have been termed "pathologic lymphocytes." "Liver damage cells" were found consistently in these patients. The "liver damage cell" of Isaacs is a cell averaging 15 x 13 microns with an oval nucleus, rather dense chromatin, foamy blue staining cytoplasm, but with absence of minute red staining granules of the monocyte and no perinuclear clear zone as in the lymphocyte.

It is found in disease associated with liver pathology.

Another interesting point that is noted is a marked basophilia of the granules of the neutrophiles. The authors believe that this phenomenon may be associated with the temperature elevation that the patients experienced and believed that it is characteristic of the Brucella melitensis infection since it was not encountered in the Brucella suis and Brucella abortus infections.

Visualization of the Chambers of the Heart, the Pulmonary Circulation, and the Great Blood Vessels in Man; A Practical Method. By George P. Robb, M.D., and Israel Steinberg, M.D., New York City. (The American Journal of Roentgenology and Radium Therapy, January, 1939, Vol. 41, No. 1.)

In this the authors present a method of visualizing the chambers of the heart, the pulmonary circulation and the great blood vessels.

The method consists of two essential parts: The injection of enough radiopaque substance into the blood entering the heart to make the chambers and important thoracic blood vessels opaque to the roentgen-ray during the first circulation and the making of roentgenograms of these structures at the time of opacification. A full description of the exact procedure is presented as well as pictures with descriptions of the apparatus used.

A total of 238 injections were made in 127 patients of whom 42 were normal, 47 had pulmonary disease and 38 cardiac disease. The important practical features of this method are the 70 per cent of diodrast, adequate dosage, rapid intravenous injection, accurate determination of the time for exposure and the proper position during roentgenography. The radiopaque substance, diodrast, was used because of the mildness of its pharmacological action. It is not radioactive.

The authors conclude from this work that visualization of the heart and the thoracic blood vessels is a practical procedure. The method provides information regarding the anatomy and the physiology of the normal and diseased cardiovascular system heretofore unobtainable. It is possible to determine the site of stenosis or occlusion of the superior vena cava and its tributaries and the course and extent of the collateral circulation. The vascular nature of the hilum may be demonstrated and these vessels differentiated from adjacent structures. Accurate studies of the arterial and venous patterns of the lung can be made. The internal structure of the living heart has been revealed for the first time and abnormalities due to disease have been observed.

Comment: One of the authors (Dr. Robb) read a paper before the American College of Physicians in New Orleans this month reviewing material of this article with some added cases. The procedure has its limitations because in only selected cases may it be expected to prove of value. The author emphasizes the fact that it is not a procedure intended for use in the routine examination of heart cases or cardiovascular disturbances, but is one which should be used as an aid in selected cases, especially those in which there is expected to be a thoracic obstruction of the venous system. More experience with a greater variety of cases may

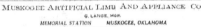
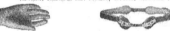
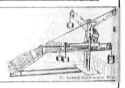

prove of value in the diagnostic study of various types of cases in which there is a necessity for tests of precision in connection with the cardiovascular system. This paper was received very favorably at the meeting in New Orleans.

———————o———————

PLASTIC SURGERY
Edited by
GEO. H. KIMBALL, M.D., F.A.C.S.
404 Medical Arts Building, Oklahoma City

"The Management of Arteriovenous Aneurysms in the Extremities." Louis G. Herrmann, M.D. and Mont R. Reid, M.D., Cincinnati, Ohio. From American Journal of Surgery, April, 1939.

The authors have outlined a practical means of dealing with this condition. They have so written the technique relating to the problem that the average practicing surgeon can follow the details. The discussion deals especially with those cases having a single communication between artery and vein. Such abnormal vascular communications are usually the result of penetrating wounds, such as gunshot or stab wounds, although occasionally a single arteriovenous communication of this type is either spontaneous or congenital in origin.

Diagnosis is often difficult in the presence of a large hematoma, especially the first few days after injury. After several days a thrill and bruit may appear. Auscultation elicits a to and fro murmur over the fistula if it is unimpeded. Palpation elicits a thrill. Superficial veins usually enlarge about the site of the communication. Cardiac embarrassment may become so severe that early operation is precipitated. This embarrassment is accompanied by rapid pulse, shortness of breath, peripheral swelling, and enlargement of the heart. Hematoma about the site of the injury may be so severe as to result in gangrene. Infection within the hematoma is a serious complication.

Surgical Treatment: During the evolution of an arteriovenous aneyrysm from the time of the original traumatization of an artery and a vein in an extremity to the late stages associated with serious cardiac damage, there may be many different indications for surgical intervention either as emergency or lifesaving procedures or as elective and curative surgical operations. Massive hemorrhages into tissue of an extremity or the formation of a large hematoma may occur as an early complication of such vascular injuries. The compression of collateral arterial pathways in such an extremity may be so complete that the nutrition of the tissues distal to the injured vessels is seriously impaired. Early surgical operations with the evacuation of all clots of blood should be carried out to relieve as much tension as possible on the vital structures of that extremity. The use of a tourniquet on the proximal side of the injury to the great vessels is usually necessary and a large incision in the skin and superficial tissues is recommended to provide an adequate exposure of the injured vessels. After all clots of blood have been washed out of the wound by careful irrigation with

warm saline solution, the glistening intima of the injured artery is usually detected without difficulty. After all the bleeding has been controlled, the skin and superficial tissues external to the fascia should be brought together loosely by widely spaced interrupted sutures. A sterile gauze sponge moistened with warm saline solution should be placed directly on the sutured wound and the entire area then covered with some waterproof material to retard the dessication of the wound and the dressing. The capillary action of the saline solution within the meshes of the gauze sponge helps to draw the old blood and serum out of the wound through the space between the sutures.

In those cases in which the artery has been completely severed it is usually unwise to attempt to restore its continuity by suturing together the injured ends of the vessel. When the injury to the artery is so extensive we believe that the proximal and distal ends should be isolated carefully and then ligated with heavy braided silk or narrow cotton tape. The choice of the suture material and its size should be governed by the caliber and activity of the artery which is to be ligated. If the surgeon is skilled in the use of the Tuffier tubes it may be possible to restore the blood-carrying function of an injured artery for a sufficient length of time to permit the spontaneous development of an adequate collateral arterial circulation in the affected extremity. After an artery has been repaired by sutures or after the continuity of the injured artery has been restored by the insertion of a Tuffier tube, it may be wise to prevent further intravascular clotting of the blood from taking place by the administration of purified heparin according to the method suggested by Murray, Best and their associates in Toronto.

Since we also have available an active means of stimulating the flow of blood through existing collateral arterial pathways by the rhythmic alternation of the environment pressure about the extremity in the form of passive vascular exercises, we have ceased to worry about severe degrees of ischemia which occasionally make their appearance after these extensive surgical operations upon the vascular system. If the need arises we can usually restore the arterial circulation to an adequate level by this physical means and thus prevent the occurrence of degenerative changes in the distal part of the affected extremity. When the small arterial and arteriolar network is structurally normal only a few days of intensive passive vascular exercise treatment are necessary to get the flow of blood started through the existing collateral arterial pathways. This method of overcoming acute ischemia of the tissues distal to the injured vessels of an extremity must be considered as a valuable adjuvant and should be kept ready for immediate use during the active phase of surgical treatment. It has given us the added courage necessary to perform very radical surgical procedures upon the peripheral vascular system when such operations are absolutely necessary for the cure of the arteriovenous aneurysms. In those acute cases where a tourniquet cannot be applied proximally to the injury of the vessels it is essential that some form of temporary occlusion of

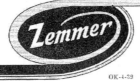

the major artery proximal to the aneurysm be performed before any attempt is made to cut into the aneurysm. Severe hemorrhage may result even when the incoming artery is temporarily occluded but the bleeding can usually be controlled by digital pressure after the clots of blood are rapidly removed from the wound. The ligation of the incoming artery should never be employed as a means of giving permanent relief. This proximal occlusion of the artery interferes greatly with the collateral arterial circulation and it is almost certain to lead to gangrene of some distal part of the extremity. The injured artery should be ligated immediately above and below the injured area in order to preserve as many of the collateral as possible.

The authors continue in detail about the emergency operation indicated if signs of infection make their appearance in the hematoma about the injured vessels. They give a comprehensive detailed report of the recommendations in such indications.

Remarks by authors:

The most essential fact concerning the elective operations for arteriovenous aneurysm is the absolute necessity of doing some surgical procedure which will completely prevent blood from passing through the fistula from the artery into the vein. In general, any operation which does not accomplish the occlusion of the abnormal communication will certainly not be a permanent cure of the aneurysm. We cannot condemn too strongly the procedure of simple ligation of the involved artery at any point proximal to the fistula. This operation is still commonly used in spite of the fact that it carries with it a high incidence of gangrene of the affected extremity. The procedure simply cuts off the main force of the arterial stream so that the small amount of arterial blood which finds its way around the collateral arterial pathways into the distal portion of the major artery immediately takes the path of least resistance by passing through the fistula and back to the heart, this depriving the rest of the extremity of its proper nourishment.

We prefer to allow a period of from four to six months to elapse before performing any elective operations for the cure of arteriovenous aneurysms in the extremities since experience has shown that the collateral arterial circulation which develops spontaneously will greatly reduce the risks of complication resulting from serious arterial insufficiency in the distal parts of the affected extremity. This delay also permits the extravasated blood to become completely absorbed and the tissues to return to more or less healthy condition and appearance thereby greatly reducing the probability of stirring up any old infection in the wound. When all of these dangers are removed the surgeon can freely choose from the numerous curative surgical operations that one which is best suited to his particular case and carry out the procedure without any fear that some serious complication will eradicate all his hopes for success. It is well to remember, however, that the surgical operations upon arteriovenous aneurysms are frequently very difficult and usually demand the greatest surgical skill, linked with sound surgical judgment. The execution of such operative procedures should not be attempted by any surgeon who has not had considerable experience with the suturing and ligation of large blood vessels.

Comment: For a great many years I have regarded Dr. Reid especially as a reliable authority on the subject of management of arteriovenous aneurysms. It has been my privilege to hear Dr. Reid discuss this subject and I have always learned considerable about the conditions from him. It must be remembered that this type of surgery involves several dangers: viz, loss of part by gangrene, infection and secondary hemorrhage.

Anyone undertaking such an operation should be thoroughly acquainted with the facts of the situation together with having proper instruments at hand to deal with the problem competently.

———————o———————

ORTHOPAEDIC SURGERY
Edited by Earl D. McBride, M.D., F.A.C.S.
717 North Robinson Street, Oklahoma City

"Recurrent Anterior Dislocation of the Shoulder," Burgh S. Burnet, Hot Springs National Park, Ark. Jr. Bone & Joint Surg., Vol. XX, No. 4, October, 1938.

The author describes 11 cases treated by the method of Roberts, of traumatic recurrent dislocation of the shoulder. He describes a number of techniques for correction of habitual dislocating shoulder; among them that of Thomas' operation of plication of the capsule; the tenosuspension method of Henderson; the biceps-tendon fixation operation of Nicola; and the deltoid-sling operation of Clairmond and Ehrlich. Roberts' technique is almost identical with that of Nicola's method with certain exceptions which to the author makes the procedure much more simple. The usual anterior approach to the shoulder is made with an incision beginning just below the anterior tip of the acromion and continuing down in the direction of the antecubital fossa for about four inches. By blunt dissection the anterior fibers of the deltoid are obtained and retracted laterally. The long tendon of the biceps is identified and removed from its groove. With a gouge, the bicipital groove is deepened, all cartilage removed, and the groove then extended upward into the humeral head for about three-fourths of an inch.

After roughening the long tendon of the biceps it is replaced into the groove. Two or three chromic catgut sutures are taken through the transverse humeral ligament, anchoring the long tendon of the biceps in place. Closure is in the usual manner. The arm is held in a triangular sling tied tight enough to support the elbow, over which a muslin bandage is applied to hold the arm and body. The sling and body bandage are discarded after the twenty-first day, and active exercise, baking, and massage are commenced.

With this technique the author has not had a recurrence in the 11 cases.

Comment by abstractor: It is to be noted that this procedure is almost identical with the Nicola procedure, with the exception that instead of drilling a hole through the upper end of the humerus in the line of the bicipital groove, that the groove is deepened and the tendon is laid in this instead of having to be divided as in the Nicola operation, and pulled through the hole that has been created. In the Nicola operation the tendon is then resutured. The abstractor has had no personal experience with Roberts' technique, but it seems to him that the only criticism to offer would be the same as has happened in certain cases of the Nicola operation; i.e. failure of the tendon to unite solidly to the bone so that recurrence is possible by the tendon of the biceps sliding through the groove or tunnel as it may be. We feel this procedure is much simpler than that of Nicola and is worthy of trial.

THE JOURNAL
OF THE
OKLAHOMA STATE MEDICAL ASSOCIATION

| VOLUME XXXII | McALESTER, OKLAHOMA, JUNE, 1939 | Number 6 |

SEPTICAEMIA*

GEORGE A. LaMOTTE, M.D.
OKLAHOMA CITY, OKLAHOMA

Introduction: "When we are born, we cry that we have come to this great stage of fools." Mankind develops, matures and declines more or less intimately associated with various proved septic microorganisms, since the latter for practical purposes are ubiquitous. Self preservation f r o m septicaemia primarily depends upon the resistance of the host, the dose and virulence of organisms accidentally or otherwise inoculated into the circulation.

HISTORY

Hippocrates r e c o g n i z e d complicated wound infection.

John Hunter, 1774, discussed the factor of suppurative phlebitis.

Virchow, 1856, credited metabolic abscess to infected emboli.

Pasteur taught puerperal sepsis was of bacterial origin, confirming the ideas of Oliver Wendell Holmes and Semmelweis.

Leube, 1878, described cryptogenic septicaemia.

BACTERIAL ETIOLOGY

In order of their frequency: Streptococcus, staphylococcus, pneumococcus, colon b a c i l l u s, gonococus, meningococcus, anthrax, gas b a c i l l u s, pyocyaneus, diphtheria and influenza.

PORTAL OF ENTRY

Skin lesions rank first, puerperal origin second and focal infections third; e.g. the

*Read before the Section on General Surgery, Annual Meeting, Oklahoma State Medical Association, Oklahoma City, May 2, 1939.

l a t t e r includes tonsils, sinuses, mastoid, respiratory and genito urinary tract, the intestines, l i v e r, gallbladder, bone and teeth.

PREDISPOSING CAUSES

Arise by virtue of lowered resistance, as exposure to cold, malnutrition, fatigue and chronic disease. However, the dose and virulence remain important factors, besides certain bacteria may become resistant to the individual's protective agencies, and become aggressive, while many less toxic members of their species would have succumbed. Flexner states a bacteriaemia is demonstrable in 20 per cent of the cases of chronic kidney and heart disease. Preagonal diminution of immune bodies permits 84 per cent of all deaths to result with some t y p e of terminal infection. It is therefore evident the preexisting condition of the host is a primary factor in allowing septicaemia to develop.

DEFINITION WITH QUALIFICATIONS

Septicaemia is best defined as a symptom complex, since the symptoms and complications result from the bacteriaemia; besides, it is not strictly speaking a definite disease entity, inasmuch as the etiology is variable. Transient bacteriaemia is very common, but in practice rarely produces constitutional phenomena, save in those disease entities in which the bacteriaemia appears early but eventually ceases in the natural history of these diseases by virtue of antibody formation, e.g. typhoid fever, pneumonia, a n t h r a x, malta fever and plague. Fortunately, such disease entities develop other definite characteristic clinical and laboratory phenomena different from pyogenic septicaemia that will help make a differential diagnosis. These and similar disease entities will not enter into my discussion, nor these other purely local infectious processes of haemotogenous origin, e.g. perinephric abscess and gonorrhoeal arthritis, since the normal circulating blood is capable of freeing itself of these bacteria. Generally speaking, the modern concensus of opinion holds bacteria are unable to multiply in the blood stream save in many terminal states, after most anti-bacterial mechanisms have broken down; except possibly in the stagnant capillaries of the liver, spleen and bone marrow. (Tileston.)

Bacteriaemia in a limited degree frequently occurs without symptoms or material damage and ends in complete recovery; but when resulting from some focal infections, that by virtue of a sensitization permits these pathogenic bacteria to reproduce in distant places and develop destructive lesions, e.g. pneumococcic meningitis and arthritis, we recognize a well known exception and that often proves itself obstinate.

PATHOGENESIS

We believe a small dose must be oft repeated, or a massive toxic dose must have entered the blood stream, e.g. following ill-advised surgery in streptococcic lymphangitis. The natural normal defenses appear competent to dispose of a non-repeated small dose, while polymorphoneuclear leukocytes and the reticuloendothelial system notably those cells in the liver and spleen, are prone to come to the rescue with efficient phagocytosis. In practice we have observed septicaemia commonly a r i s e s from a lymphangitis under c o n d i t i o n s where the lymphatic glands are inadequate to block fully the ingress of repeated doses of toxic bacteria. Likewise it often arises from a septic thrombophlebitis persistently discharging septic e m b o l i, that in turn c a u s e metastatic pulmonary abscesses, which eventually spill their contents into the blood stream, either too frequently or in too large quantities for the natural defense processes to effectively destroy or eliminate these doses.

MORBID PHYSIOLOGY

Early symptoms arise from the toxaemia, haemolysis and embolic processes with deranged systemic functions. We are taught if this picture is not early recognized and successfully treated, multiple visceral degenerative processes will eventually ensue and the case becomes too advanced for any known successful management.

MORBID ANATOMY

The spleen enlarges, c l o u d y swelling with fatty changes in the viscera eventuate with numerous foci of necrosis. The serous membranes and joints are especially vulnerable. Nephritis, metastatic abscesses and infarcts are common. Endocarditis occurs in 50 per cent of staphylococcus cases, 25 per cent from pneumococcus and only 8 per cent from streptococcus. Various skin eruptions are common and may be petechial, papular, pustular, bulbous or hemorrhagic. Progessive anaemia follows unless transfused. Haemolytic jaundice may eventuate. Leukocytosis, with excess of polymorphoneuclear cells, ranges from 10,000 to 50,000 per cubic millimeter and when persistently below 10,000, is considered of serious prognostic omen. Empirically multiple accessible external metastases augers a favorable immunological phenomenon.

MORTALITY

Mortality is somewhat higher when over 25 years of age; streptococcus 66 per cent, staphylococcus 71 per cent. The number of colonies from cultures are not especially prognostic, but the o u t c o m e depends largely on whether or not the etiological focus is amenable to competent and intelligent surgery; secondarily, on the availability of specific sera, and to no small degree on competent general management.

CLINICAL TYPES OF PYOGENIC SEPTICAEMIA

1. Fulminating: Results from an overwhelming dose of virulent bacteria in patients with low resistance. Usually fatal in a few days regardless of surgery and medical treatment.

2. Acute: Normally runs a course of a few weeks and may recover if the focus was amenable to surgery and the necessary specific serum was available.

3. Subacute cases: May be indefinite in their course. Death, when it results, is

from complications, because bacteria appear to acquire a super-resistance or results from ultimate degenerative pathology of important viscera. The acute and subacute types may assume a typhoid state, resemble meningitis with marked delirium or coma, or may closely simulate acute rheumatic f e v e r with endocarditis and polyarthritis.

DEFINITION FROM CONCENSUS OF OPINION

Pyogenic septicaemia is a morbid condition resulting from the p r e s e n c e of pathogenic bacteria and their associated poisons in the blood stream. The bacteriaemia persists because bacteria are continuously being fed into the circulating blood. In all cases, septicaemia is a disease of surprising vicissitudes and uncertainties.

DIAGNOSIS

The probable etiological history offers us our first dependable clue. Positive cultures are possible, along with the early toxaemic symptoms. The blood specimen is best taken during the rising stage of the fever or chill. Full cooperation with a well equipped medical technician is indispensable for a c c u r a t e information and proper typing of positive cultures. Accuracy of leukocyte counts and percentages of each type is likewise mandatory. The onset varies but may be acute, with chills, irregular fever, stupor, delirium or coma. The pulse is rapid and systolic cardiac murmurs are common. Some have anorexia, nausea, vomiting, febrile albuminuria and retinal hemorrhages. High leukocyte c o u n t with preponderance of polymorphoneuclears are expected. Later, e m b o l i c processes with metastatic abscesses, arthritis, osteoarthritis, etc., clears the picture sufficiently for tyros. Irregular fever and chills, a s s o c i a t e d with drenching sweats and a rapidly developing anaemia with emaciation, are almost pathognomonic.

DIFFERENTIAL DIAGNOSIS

1. Typhoid fever presents a relatively slow pulse, leukopaenia, dull facies, rose spots in crops and intestinal hemorrhage.

2. Rheumatic fever: shifting, non suppurating arthritis, pain y i e l d s to salicylates; no emboli or enlarged spleen.

3. Malaria: plasmodia demonstrable and yields to quinine.

4. Miliary tuberculosis: probably demonstrable f o c u s, dyspnoea, cyanosis, tubercles in the choroid and a lymphocytic leukopaenia.

5. Likewise pyelitis, Charcot's f e v e r, perinephric abscess, undulant fever and Hodgkin's disease have sufficient clinical characteristics, along with laboratory findings, to render their diagnosis reasonably certain; however, we fully realize septicaemia may complicate or co-exist with o t h e r disease entities, and not uncommonly arises from ill advised surgery producing favorable entrance and spread of pyogenic bacteria to the blood stream. The clinician has learned when he observes small vesicles presenting a red halo and rapidly becoming pustules, the staphylococcus is the probable etiologic f a c t o r. The pyocyaneus c a s e s present hemorrhagic spots becoming necrotic and suppurating at the center. Streptococcic invasion rarely obtunds the mind early, but victims are mentally alert and scrutinize the physician's attitude unusually closely.

TREATMENT

Physicians and surgeons should invariably endeavor to aid the patient intelligently, and not at any stage to hamper recovery through natural processes by ill advised exhibition of questionable and unproved remedies or procedures. They both fully realize progress in the management of pyogenic septicaemias has already, far too often, been retarded by tradition, superstition, half truths and untruths. They have also learned their lesson and fully realize symptoms ordinarily antedate serious structural changes and are therefore alert to establish the diagnosis and use intelligent management before irreparable damage occurs. The intelligent physician prefers to cooperate with a trustworthy surgeon and competent medical laboratory technician, before he outlines specific procedure or finally evaluates his prognosis. He furthermore fully realizes that immunity, natural or acquired, is never absolute but rather tends to vary with the individual at different times. After having consulted all his available authorities he also regretfully concludes our factual knowledge is still problematic, and the opinions of authorities still vary concerning the m o d u s operandi of immunological processes.

However, the p r a c t i c a l, conservative physician does know empirically that the successful management of pyogenic septicaemias depends primarily on his being able to modify such morbid physiology that exists in accord with what is normal in order that he might produce unfavorable environment for these bacteria; rather than implicitly follow his desire to kill or neutralize this type of bacteria with over advertised commercial specific d r u g s or serums.

GENERAL PRINCIPLES OF MANAGEWENT

1. Intelligent and competent surgery; when possible, remove, drain or isolate the distributing focus.

2. Ample r e s t and comfort, sedation, oxygen and vitamins when indicated.

3. Observe closely the intake and output of fluids, with minimum quantity per day of 3,000 c.c. as necessary, fluids parenterally as indicated.

4. High caloric diet relatively rich in proteins, symptomatic and expectant treatment to aid digestion and reasonable elimination.

5. Multiple s m a l l transfusions, with whole blood or serum, depending on existence and type of the anaemia; use immune donors when obtainable.

6. Administer suitable stimulants when indicated, best selected according to the presence of morbid physiology of the various systems, e.g. cardiovascular, respiratory and nervous system.

7. No antipyretics should be used, but hydrotherapy for fever moderation as well as cleanliness and c o m f o r t. We regard fever as a defense mechanism; realizing it will increase metabolism, change the albumin globulin ratio favorably to fibrinogen and globulin, lessens the suspension stability of the blood and decreases platelets, but increases leukocytosis, water retention and favors agglutination.

SPECIAL MEASURES FOR THE SPECIFIC INFECTION

1. Staphylococcic Septicaemia: We believe meticulous carrying out of the general principles already enumerated with judicious use of transfusions, offers about all that has proved advantageous. However, alert, competent and radical surgery should be emphasized. Thrombophlebitis

about the etiologic focus is preferably removed in toto, also ligation of veins likely to carry infection when feasible. Serums and bacteriophage are neither condemned or condoned by the authorities, but if used, the usual sensitization tests should be made before their use and we have learned by experience unfavorable reactions are less apt to occur if they are administered while the patient is under anesthesia.

2. Streptococcus Haemolyticus: S i n c e the v a r i o u s strains of streptococci are numerous and not fully worked out, the use of specific sera is problematic, but favorable agglutination tests of cultures from the patient will help determine if those serums available should be administered.

The reasoning is a n a l a g o u s to use of serums for pneumococcic infection, except we have less definite information concerning the types involved. Justification in the use of polyvalent serum exists, particularly if improvement e n s u e s with the first few doses, it may be advantageously continued, but if not, discontinue its use and change to some other company's product. It is very easy for one's wishes to overrule his judgment in the use of serums, since we are prone to forget nonspecific serums for the case in hand might readily prove harmful. Pyogenic bacteria require an antibacterial serum and materially differs from the use of antitoxic sera that have proved so effective, e.g. in diphtheria and tetanus which act by neutralizing toxins, comparable to the well understood acid base neutralization in chemistry. Sera, to overcome bacteria with endotoxins must also c o n t a i n ingredients comparable to those existing in immune serum, i.e. praecipitans, agglutinins, bacteriocidal and bacteriolytic substances which will in some way subject this particular strain of bacteria m o r e readily to phagocytosis with ultimate destruction or neutralization by proteolytic enzymes.

The anaerobic streptococcus putrificans so common in s e p t i c abortions, when p r o v e d present, may be rendered less harmful by gently dilating the cervix and thoroughly washing out the uterine cavity with oxydizing agents as taught by Dr. Otto Schwarz, nevertheless is disapproved by other equally prominent obstetricians.

SURGERY

When dealing with known streptococcic pathology, e.g. lymphangitis, the more conservative the surgeon the better, the existence of fewer avenues for dissemination with nature's protective exudates intact outweighs the advantage of free drainage from early incision even though done with the cautery..

SULPHANILAMIDE

At present has popular approval and does seem promising, but as yet we are not fully informed concerning its contra-indications. The dose recommended as 1 Gm per nine Kilos daily, best given in divided doses per oram, or parenterally. Direct application, or injection into cavities as empyema is permissible. Ninety per cent show cyanosis to some d e g r e e; nausea, dizziness, tinnitus and diarrhea may develop. Rarely nitroid reactions occur, e.g. dermatitis, eczema, hepatitis, or optic atrophy. "It produces in some patients a stimulation and in others depression of leukopoetic activity." (Krache.)

This drug should not be administered so promiscuously as is done at present, and it is safer to hospitalize such cases so the proper dosage may be maintained, i.e., approximately 10 M. Gm to 100 c.c. of blood, proved by laboratory methods. Besides, take frequent white counts to avoid serious leukopaenia and agranulocytosis, also make tests for N.P.N. and when found below 15 or 20 milligrams per cent, discontinue the drug. It is thought by some that the newer derivatives of sulphanilamide, e.g. neoprontosil produce less toxicity and are possibly m o r e efficacious in bacteriocidal action.

Many other antiseptic drugs and dyes have been in the past highly recommended, but to administer them in the hope of performing miracles, is not at present tenable; since without exception they have been weighed in the balance of experience and found wanting.

Autogenous vaccines and bacteriophages are permissible particularly in subacute and chronic infection and both have the indorsement of some reliable authorities.

Artificial fever by foreign proteins or other methods is not to be considered because the extreme continued hyperpyrexia necessary to kill the pyogenic b a c t e r i a would be lethal to the host.

THEORETICAL AND EXPERIMENTAL CONSIDERATION

If the physician institutes proper management, it is necessary for him to understand the patient and be able to visualize all co-existing and correlated pathological conditions, with their morbid physiology, as well as to diagnose and evaluate the status praesens from the superadded disease entity. He furthermore fully realizes and takes cognizance of the fact that constitutional and hereditary factors of any human being cannot escape the germ plasm of which they are made and furthermore, environment might mitigate but it can not change the general trend; also his ability to be of service will depend more on bringing about favorable changes in the patient's reactions, rather than theoretical modification of the bacteria. In some respects all patients appear alike in their morbid reactions, while in others, e.g. immunological reactions, they may be vastly different, as observed when allergic states present themselves, apparently out of a clear sky, with explosive exudates and outpouring of fluids. These allergic problems here presented have as yet not been clearly explained or very satisfactorily met by the symptomatic relief afforded from adrenalin, ephedrin, a t r o p i n e, calcium, auto transfusion, etc. This phase is mentioned merely to emphasize the hazards that may arise with serum therapy and places responsibility on their giver to the extent that he should be familiar with sensitization tests, use due caution concerning proper desensitization in susceptible individuals; be p r e p a r e d to meet anaphylactic reactions, thermal reactions and serum sickness intelligently.

Such research tests that are requested should, in my opinion, be evaluated somewhat on your confidence in the technician; non-medical technicians are at times too p o s i t i v e, probably because they fail to realize fully dead specimens may r e a c t differently from what they would were they yet bioplasm, besides they may not fully comprehend all the phases of the problem presented to the physician. A comprehensive consideration of problems concerning pyogenic septicaemia brings us face to face with the parting of the ways from s t r i c t l y scientific procedures and proved facts, to the reasoning by analogy followed by experimental dreamers. The facts are, with reference to pyogenic septicaemias, that if truth is ever to disrobe herself entirely, her underclothes will most likely be in the proud possession of an experimental dreamer.

Dr. Fred T. Cadman of Winnipeg, Canada, has to his credit the following:

He kept a large colony of rabbits injected twice weekly over a period of months with pyogenic bacteria. Whenever he had a case of pyogenic septicaemia, he made a vaccine with a heavy culture from this patient; this process took only 48 hours, including injection of this specific vaccine into a few of his prepared rabbits and after 24 hours, bleeding them from the heart and using this serum for the patient, claiming the titer is very high in antigen. For the ambocepter he makes use of commercial serums, besides furnishes more compliment from human serum, claiming it acts better than transfusion with whole blood by seeming to activate further the patients compliment, that has been found by him to drop materially after the first transfusion of whole blood, and is not much increased by subsequent transfusions. So far, Dr. Cadman has treated 100 cases in this manner and reports a mortality of only 15 per cent.

O. H. Robertson, M.D., observed that in experimental pneumonia the animal always dies unless there exists macrophage immune bodies in their lungs and their blood is also capable of destroying the pneumococci. While we do not fully understand the reticulo-endothelial system, we are taught its cells develop from special types of endothelium located in various organs, e.g. spleen, liver and bone marrow, also from the wandering cells of the reticulum. We think the monocytes are these cells that have entered the circulation and are so efficient in disposing of b r o k e n down red cells, which products finally eventuate into bilirubin, iron and globin. Besides exercising an all important phagocytic f u n c t i o n, the reticulo-endothelial system in some way influences metabolism as exemplified by Gauchers and Nieman-Picks disease as well as the Hand-Christian Syndrome and Xanthomatosis.

Most authorities grant active phagocytosis is a major part of our immunological reactions and the presence of opsonins is essential in preparing b a c t e r i a for the phagocytes. These phagocytes seem eager to ingest the crudest of food substances, notably particulate matter and the colloids. Moreover, they are able to digest or render most toxic substances harmless through the action of their proteolytic enzymes; at all events, no metabolic or functional disturbance follows their death.

Metchninkoff went so far as to teach that both immune bodies and compliment are derived from the leukocytes. Whenever the reticulo endothelial system becomes partially blocked with colloids, n a t u r e proceeds to unblock it by a further rapid hyperplasia, which produces more platelets and fibrinogen thereby shortening the coagulation time.

Diaz claims this system can be stimulated by the use of 10 c.c. of 1 per cent Congo-red in distilled water. The question naturally arises, are we sleeping on our rights in neglecting to bring this important reticulo endothelial system actively to our assistance? Or would we by so doing, wave a two-edged sword capable of producing u n k n o w n conditioned toxicities, analogous to harmful acquired allergies, or idiosyncrasies? At all events, reasoning by analogy, we do realize there are conditioned reflexes of the nervous system.

Human nature is most sorely tried when we physicians are forced to surrender to the inevitable; after due consultation and with conscientious prolonged effort to rescue our friends from pyogenic septicaemia. There arises in me a temptation somewhat analagous, I imagine, to the state of mind of a broke merchant endeavoring to recoup his losses by a last frantic effort in staking his possessions on the possibility of pyramiding in a freakish m a r k e t. Like his chances, the possibilities of cure are scant, but when in this frame of mind, I still at l e a s t talk about fixation abscesses, replacement transfusions and unblocking the reticulo-endothelial system.

CONCLUSIONS

We are at present possibly overtreating our septic patients; since the existing potential sources of septicaemia are so numerous, it is reasonably safe to conclude natures methods cure all this multitude of those cases that are undiagnosed. Intelligent and competent surgery is imperative, specific serums are advantageous, and general principles are a l w a y s helpful, but when doubt arises in your own mind, hesitate and don't u n w i s e l y interfere with natural processes.

BIBLIOGRAPHY

Tileston, Wilder: Septicemia. Oxford Medicine, Oxford University Press, Vol. IV, Part II, Page 895.

Rosenow, E. C., Jr., and Brown, A. E.: Review of Cases 1934-46 Inclusive, Proc. Staff Meet., Mayo Clinic, 13:89-93, February 9, 1938.

Allen, H.: Modern Advances in Therapy. J. Mo. M. A., 35:35-37, February, 1938.

Reed, E. B.: Question of Septicemia. Neb. M. J., 23:201-206, June, 1938.

Robinson, S. S.: Septicemia Eruptions, With Special Reference to Differentiation of Septic and Drug Eruptions. Urol. and Cutan, Rev., 41:490, 1937.

Sacks, M. S.: Fulminating Septicemia Associated With Purpura and Bilateral Adrenal Hemorrhage. Ann. Int. Med. 10:1105, 1937.

Gill, E. G.: Management of Blood Stream Infection With Special Reference to Immunized Blood Transfusions. So. M. J., 30:496, 1937.

Text Books, Last Editions, Makins, Musser, Christian, Cecil, Conybeare, Emerson.

* * * *

DISCUSSION

Dr. Horace Reed: From the moment we are born until death overtakes us, we live constantly in close proximity to danger. When we contemplate how n a r r o w the threshold really is, we may easily become morbid. With coolness and precision, so far as our knowledge permits us to go at this moment, the essayist has discussed the danger to which I refer, namely, septicemias. There are only two factors which serve to protect us from that danger. One is anatomic, or more strictly hystologic, because the barriers which every moment of our lives protects us from the invasion of the pathogenic organism is microscopic in dimension. The other factor may be called physiological, or p e r h a p s more strictly speaking, biological. A substance which also may be infinitesimal in quantity, namely, antibodies.

Dr. Lamotte has presented us with a thesis on the subject of septicemia. So far as I have been able to determine, he has presented us nothing but facts which are historical, or with theories which have been thoroughly proven, and when he has entered the field of speculation he has been judicious and conservative. In other words, it is difficult for one to add to or disagree with what he has presented, so thoroughly has he considered every phase of the subject. In doing this he has exhibited a profound insight into the art of the practice of medicine.

The bacteriologist more than a half century ago opened the door which let in the light by which we could see the causative agents of septicemia, namely, the "ubiquitous microorganisms," and since we have known the cause, we have been giving more and more attention to the laboratory in searching for the cure and, correspondingly, more and more have been neglecting the patient. Long before there was a science of bacteriology, physicians treated septicemia. There were no laboratories, hence, the physician himself treated the patient. Since laboratories have become so common, the tendency is to neglect more and more the patient and treat the disease.

Dr. Lamotte has demonstrated in his presentation how important it is not to neglect the patient, who, because of his affliction, is possessed with a morbid power of reasoning. The products of that which affects him make him mentally sick. Well may we pause to inquire as did Macbeth, "physician, canst thou not minister to a mind diseased?" Truly this art in the practice of medicine is being sadly neglected. There is no panacea or true specific in the treatment of septicemia, and the essayist has made this clear. Of course, in covering the subject of treatment, which has been done so thoroughly, he had to resort to brevity.

In discussing treatment, therefore, one can only hope to add to the value of this paper by emphasizing those points, the value of which are so well proven. The first of these that I would emphasize would be *rest*. The value of rest in treatment of septicemia, rest w h i c h is physiological, would be a subject well worthy of a thesis of itself. Nearly a century ago, Hilton delivered a series of lectures on rest and pain which, when collected, form a good sized volume. Every physician who assumes to treat anyone afflicted with an infection, it matters not what the causative agent may be, should have read Hilton on "Rest and Pain." In overwhelming infections produced by those organisms which are commonly found in what we call septicemia, the value of rest should be emphasized more than anything else, for without it all other m e t h o d s of treatment will surely be disappointing. With rest as the foundation upon which to build the management of a patient with septicemia, the outcome will be less likely to be disappointing. But even with rest thoroughly carried out, and all the other known and tried adjuncts in treatment, septicemia remains a dangerous disease.

Next to rest is nourishment. If the patient is to combat successfully the invasion of the hordes of organisms and their nefarious cohorts, the virulent toxins which they generate, he must be well sustained. Food of appropriate kind furnishes fuel by which he may develop reserves to carry on the fight. Well may it be said that the patient fights on his belly as does a successful army.

Next in the line of treatment may be mentioned repeated, even though small, blood transfusions. Sufficient t i m e has elapsed since transfusions have been used, and the results obtained have proved beyond a doubt that this in many cases is most beneficial. Theoretically, at least, if a donor could be used who has successfully overcome and fully recovered from this disease, the results should be more beneficial.

Dr. Lamotte has not overlooked the new panaceas, but we are pleased to note with what caution and conservatism he mentions them. Some of us "whose blood and judgment" are not so well commingled, would have blatantly described some of the newer remedies, particularly sulfanilamide and its allied chemicals. One of the discouraging things in later years is to note how increasingly gullible we as physicians are becoming. How many cure-alls of biologicals and serums have literally blazed across the sky in the last 20 years, only to disappear behind the horizon of gloomy disappointments. Who of us can still remember one of the e a r l i e r ones which was heralded as a most outstanding cure-all in infectious conditions, namely phylacogen. I, personally, missed by a hairsbreadth becoming one of its most ardent supporters. Having been asked to see a patient in consultation who was suffering from childbed fever, in whom the doctor had employed every known facility or remedy which up to that time had produced no apparent improvement, except phylacogen, I recommended it, even though I had never personally employed it. However, I had read the very exciting and alluring literature which was in all the medical publications at that time. Fortunately, or unfortunately, such was the demand for the product that it was not available. Three or four days later the patient's temperature dropped to normal from which point her recovery was rapid and uneventful. Had my pet remedy been available, what a wonderful cure it would have produced, assuming, of course, it did not of itself produce harm.

Sulfanilamide and its kindred products are just at this time blazing through the skies as the great cure-all of most of the known ills caused by infection. Let us hope that in the end the e f f e c t of the remedy itself will not prove to be as bad, if not worse, than the diseases for which it is being so injudiciously used. There is no doubt that it gives hope of the coming of a very valuable addition to our armentarium, but because it does give promise, let us jealously guard it against abuse until its possibilities have been made known.

————————o————————

Common Cold May Cause Infections In Sinuses

The common cold can cause infection in the sinuses, other parts of the respiratory tract and ears, Sidney N. Parkinson, M.D., Oakland, Calif., says in The Journal of the American Medical Association for January 21.

Nasal congestion during a cold interferes with circulation about the openings of the sinuses. This increases swelling and congestion within the sinuses and permits accumulation of mucopus which the hair-like projections in the respiratory tract are unable to remove. This complication is unfavorable to tissue defense.

"The purpose of local treatment during acute infection is ventilation in order to improve drainage," the author says. Shrinkage of the nasal mucous membranes with drugs opens the air passages. Free drainage then takes place if in the process of ventilation the hairlike drainage mechanism has not been damaged. This is why the selection of a physiologic drug is so important. Ephedrine in Locke's solution or its equivalent constitutes an efficient harmless agent for shrinkage.

The drug best reaches the membranes of the air passages with the patient lying on his side with his head bent downward exactly sidewise, using the shoulder as a fulcrum.

After from three to five minutes the head is rotated to face down to permit the nasal contents to escape from the nostrils. The head-low posture permits all important structures within the nose to come in contact with the medication and obviates any injury.

Remarks on Treatment of Dacryocystitis*

D. L. EDWARDS, M.D.

TULSA, OKLAHOMA

It is not my intention to present anything new in the treatment of inflammation of the tear sac, but the subject has not been reviewed before this section for some time and perhaps a few remarks concerning it are thereby appropriate to promote discussion and this explanation might serve as an apology for the rather didactic remarks to follow.

Dacryocystitis is somewhat unique in that the usual procedure of an acute process incompletely healed resulting in a chronic state of inflammation is exactly reversed. Acute dacryocystitis r e s u l t s from a chronically infected sac, and we should therefore discuss the chronic sac first.

"Chronic dacryocystitis is an inflammation of the mucous membrane of the lacrimal sac due to impeded outflow and consequent stagnation of the tears." This is the sum and substance of the pathology of this condition and is taken verbatim from Fuchs. The nasolacrimal d u c t becomes narrowed or completely occluded by cicatricial contraction, congenital conditions, obstruction by mucoid or mycotic plugs of material, or by extrinsic pressure by tumors in the region of the sac; very frequently polyps in the nose obstruct the terminal opening. This leads to stagnation and infection, the same as in a kidney pelvis with ureteral obstruction or a gallbladder with cystic or common duct obstruction. It is a truly chronic condition and lasts for years. Actual suppuration may be present in the early stages but soon gives way to a mucoid type of secretion or in the late stages merely watery tears.

The obstructions seen in young children due to congenital conditions are usually due to groups of epithelial cells within the duct or thin membranes, most often in the region of the nasal opening beneath the inferior turbinate. Pressure over the sac

*Read before the Section on Eye, Ear, Nose and Throat, Annual Meeting, Oklahoma State Medical Association, Oklahoma City, May 2, 1939.

by the physician together with instruction of the mother in the procedure to be repeated several times daily empties the sac through the puncta and so prevents stagnation; but it also is frequently successful in breaking down the obstruction by increasing the pressure through the nasolacrimal duct and so m a k i n g the duct patent. I seldom have found it necessary to pass a probe in an infant when this procedure is thoroughly carried out. General anesthesia is, of course, necessary for this procedure.

Chronically infected tear sacs are always dangerous. The bacterial content can be any of the pathogenic organisms found in the conjunctival sac; they are opportunists, awaiting a break in the surface epithelium to begin their work. I was struck by the large number of references in the foreign literature to mycotic infection of the tear sac and the scarcity of it in English articles. We perhaps do not study the bacteriology of the sac as well as we should. Tuberculosis, trachoma and syphilis may be harbored there. The pneumococcus is a frequent offender; hemolytic staphylococcus and streptococcus are frequently present. Routine conjunctival s m e a r s should include firm pressure over the lacrimal sac to express some of its contents, for many t i m e s an apparently negative conjunctiva contains pathogenic organisms in its sac.

I have spoken before of the procedure advocated by Green with reference to the lacrimal sac in c a s e s of corneal foreign bodies. In those cases in which the foreign body has penetrated through Bowman's membrane and involves the true corneal substance we know that healing will be delayed for 36 to 48 hours. Here is an excellent opportunity for organisms present in an infected sac to set up infection and result in a severe corneal ulcer. In these cases one makes firm pressure over the tear sac, and if it is at all suspicious of increased content, one fills the canaliculus and sac with White's ointment, using an ordinary Record s y r i n g e and lacrimal needle for this purpose. The antiseptic is dissipated slowly and two fillings usually will carry one beyond all danger of infection. It is my belief that this procedure is a good safeguard against the possibility of a severe corneal ulcer following corneal injury.

It is of course unnecessary to discuss the a b s o l u t e need of clearing up any chronic infection before all intra-ocular operations.

Non-surgical methods of treatment include probing and irrigating. A s o u n d should always be passed gently and cautiously because of the danger of creating a false passage. Too much should not be attempted at one sitting. I am sure that we younger men are not as adept in this procedure as the older eye doctors are for it apparently is not used as frequently at this time. Nevertheless an attempt should be made to re-establish patency by judicious use of the probe, and if successful, passage of the sound at intervals will often solve the problem.

Every known antiseptic solution has at some time, in some hands, been used as irrigation in this condition. In the duct with partial obstruction it is my opinion that normal s a l i n e is as good as any, though I have used many of the mercurial preparations and feel that Pregl's iodine solution has been of definite added benefit in some cases. Many patients will refuse surgery and irrigation must be continued.

In the case of complete or almost complete obstruction, not overcome by probing, surgery is indicated to r e l i e v e the constant epiphora and danger of infection of other ocular structures, particularly the cornea.

Removal of the sac has been practised for many years and every man was trained in the landmarks of anatomy and steps of the p r o c e d u r e. But this apparently simple extirpation more often than not turns out to be a formidable one. Bleeding can be severe, especially when one is working in the region of the superior portion of the sac and it is easy to leave a small portion of the sac lining in this area with a poor end-result. After its completion only one of the benefits has been accomplished however, that is, removal of

the danger of infection. Annoying epiphora is still present and in most cases many years are still ahead of the patient and the constant tearing often results in excoriation of the skin, a very annoying condition.

In choosing an operation upon the tear sac, one desires to restore the physiological function, i.e. to allow the free drainage of tears from the conjunctival sac, through the canaliculus and tear sac into the nose.

The method of treating chronic dacryocystitis by creating an artificial passageway into the nose is an ancient one, for Celsus and Galen before the third century treated this condition by plunging a red hot cautery through the lacrimal bone into the nose. Refinement has taken p l a c e through the work of Montaigne, Dupuy-Dutemps, Polyak, Toti, West, A r r u g a, Mosher, Poulard and many others. All have as their object to drain the contents of the lacrimal sac directly into the upper nasal cavity. In order for the operation to be successful, there must be some of the lacrimal sac remaining and there must be an opening from at least one of the lacrimal puncta into the tear sac. This operation can not be performed therefore after removal of the sac, whereas if unsuccessful, removal of the sac is possible as a last resort.

An intranasal approach as in the West operation can be used, but I have had no experience with this technique. The external operation, particularly that of Toti, modified by Mosher, is in my opinion more easily performed and has been successful in my cases. Marked nasal deformities such as deviated septum should be corrected before the operation and fracturing of the middle turbinate to give more room in the meatus above it often helps. It can be done under local anesthesia or in combination with avertin in cases where this is indicated. Failures by either technique are usually due to the formation of dense scar and granulation tissue in the nasal opening. Another complication that must be borne in mind is delayed and severe hemorrhage which may occur from the anterior ethmoidal arteries.

Acute dacryocystitis is a cellulitis of the connective tissue surrounding the sac, a result of infection from a chronic one entering by way of a break in the mucous membrane. It may therefore be a complication of probing that results in a false passage. Oftentimes it occurs with no preceding manipulation and in these is probably due to ulceration or necrosis of the lining. The phlegmon goes on to abscess formation necessitating incision. Measures to abort this abscess formation should be taken early, for incision almost invariably results in fistula formation which is difficult to close. Sulfanilamide in cases of appropriate bacteriology should help in some cases and if used early, X-ray irradiation can be used.

After the acute inflammation of the tissues have subsided, the underlying chronic sac must be dealt with for stenosis of the lacrimal duct was originally present. In many cases the fistula remaining will not close until the flow of tears into the nose is re-established. One of the procedures mentioned must be carried out and very frequently surgery, either extirpation or dacryocystorhinostomy must be done.

In conclusion, dacryocystitis is a condition presenting m a n y difficulties in its management. The improvements in the technique of dacryocystorhinostomy has made its management much easier for the ophthalmologist and patient alike.

---o---

Diverticulum of the Bladder*

J. HOLLAND HOWE, M.D.
PONCA CITY, OKLAHOMA

Diverticulum of the bladder is a condition which has not received clinical recognition until recent years. It was known to MORGAGNI, and several cases were reported as internal cystocele by CHOPART and CIVIALE. Already in the early 19th century the associated causal relationship of prostatic hypertrophy and increased intracystic tension was recognized.

The modern era began with the introduction of the cystoscope, and in 1901 DURRIEUX reported 200 cases collected mostly from postmortem autopsies. Later, radiology was applied to urology with complete visualization of the diverticula by means of cystograms. PEAN and CZERNY were the first to operate for this condition. YOUNG, in 1906, reported successful operation cases, and described new technique, which, with slight modifications, has stood to this day.

The diverticulum itself is a sac communicating with the vesical cavity and comparable with the condition seen elsewhere in the colon and pharynx. Diverticula may be large or small, single or multiple. Cases are reported of the sac containing more than a gallon of urine. As a rule, the orifice is quite small and out of proportion to the size of the pouch.

In the female the diverticula are not common. They may be associated with old standing pelvic inflammation with adhesions. These are traction diverticula, and may develop in any area of the bladder.

The pathological changes noted in diverticula of the bladder are atrophy and progressive chronic inflammation which may lead to cancer. The wall is tough and sometimes a l m o s t parchment-like. The inner surface is lined with a fine velvety membrane. Phosphatic calculi are very frequently found in the lumen of the diverticula. In the microscopic examination the mucous membrane is atrophied and may show extensive areas of superficial erosion. The bulk of the wall consists of fibro-granulation or fibrous tissue. Strands of muscle tissue are present. In the early stages the muscle may be well marked, but in old standing cases the muscle is broken up and may be f o u n d in many parts of the wall. A fine scar tissue is frequently noted, particularly under the mucous surface. There is very considerable infiltration of the wall with round ·cells.

*Read before the Section on Genito-Urinary Diseases and Syphilology, Annual Meeting, Oklahoma State Medical Association, Oklahoma City, May 2, 1939.

This is most prominent under the mucosa, and, in association with the large vessels in the outer layers, eosinophil cells are very noticeable. The fine capillaries near the surface are engorged and small extravasations of blood are frequent.

The origin of these diverticula is uncertain. By many it is held that, although they may not manifest themselves till late in life, they are always due to congenital predisposition. It is pointed out that they most frequently occur at certain places in the bladder which are developmentally weak, namely, just above the ureteric orifices, in this position being often symmetrical, or less commonly just behind the interureteric bar. In the course of routine cystoscopies it is not rare to find small recesses in the mucosa above and behind the openings. These may well be the precursors of true diverticula which develop later in life when some obstruction has occurred to the outflow of urine from the bladder. Another view is that they are formed from accessory ureteric buds.

When diverticula occur apart from any obstruction to the outflow of urine from the bladder they must certainly be congenital; but even when o b s t r u c t i o n is present it may well be argued that this has merely made obvious the presence of a pre-existing pouch by causing a great increase in its size or perhaps an infection of its c o n t e n t s. It has been, however, proved that true diverticula can also result from obstruction alone, such as a narrow urethral stricture lasting for several years.

Diverticula have been produced experimentally in dogs by a combination of increased intravesical tension and localized injury to the bladder wall. The production was facilitated by the onset ef infection. Infection easily develops since the urine stagnates in the diverticula.

The more moderate-sized diverticula do not, as a rule, give rise to symptoms unless they become infected. The larger diverticula, even before infection o c c u r s, usually give the patient sufficient discomfort to cause him to seek medical advice. A quite common sign of bladder diverticulum is hematuria, which may be due either to the inflammation to the sac, or to calculus in it, or the rare association of tumor with diverticulum. Hematuria, of course, may be due also to the coincidence of an enlarged prostate.

More frequent than hematuria are the t r o u b l e s of micturition. After voiding there is usually a second stream of foul urine which, however, occurs also in tabetic affections of the bladder and urethra, and is not pathognomic of v e s i c a l diverticulum. Frequency of micturition is often met with, and this common symptom is usually explained by the cystitis which so often r e s u l t s from the presence of the pouch; in other cases it may be due to an enlarged prostate. Difficulty of micturition often results from the association of an enlarged prostate, or stricture, but may be produced by the diverticulum itself. Retention of urine may result if the diverticulum interferes with the proper action of the trigonal musculature.

Pain is a symptom usually present when inflammation has developed. It is usually related to urination. Sometimes the diverticulum itself may cause pain which is felt particularly in the groin, and to a less degree in the perineum. Such pain may probably be due to the forcing of urine into the diverticulum and the stretching of the adhesions which, as is so often the case, surround the diverticulum.

The chief complications of bladder diverticulum are: 1. Involvement of a ureter. 2. Calculus formation. 3. Abscess formation within the diverticulum. 4. Neoplasm within the diverticulum. 5. Diverticulum in a hernial sac. 6. Compression of a ureter with resulting hydronephrosis and renal infection. 7. Constipation from pressure upon the rectum.

The most important aids in diagnosis are: 1. Cystoscopy. 2. Cystogram. Cystoscopy readily identifies the orifice of diverticula of any size. The location where it may be missed is at the summit of the bladder, at the urachal attachment. Some rough estimate of the capacity of a diverticulum may be had by passing a ureteric catheter into the sac. The most accurate information may be obtained by use of the cystogram. The bladder is filled by catheter and syringe or funnel with a sterile solution of 10 to 12½ per cent sodium iodide. It is very useful to watch the filling under a screen, but is not necessary. One hundred and fifty to 200 c.c. of fluid is u s u a l l y sufficient and then take cysto-

grams in whatever positions are best calculated to show the form and extent of
the pouch. Other radiograms should be
taken after the catheter has been allowed
to drain, or the patient allowed to mictur-
ate. Radiograms s h o u l d also be taken
apart from cystography, for, as mentioned,
they may reveal calculi whose existence
would otherwise not be suspected.

According to the cystogram, diverticula
may be separated into two groups:

1. Non-retentive.
2. Retentive.

In the first group, which empty fairly
w e l l with the act of micturition, and in
which there is little or no retention within
the sac, no treatment is required. After
relief of the raised intracystic tension the
pouch tends to egress. If the bladder is
for any other reason opened, it will be
good to stretch the orifice of the sac with
the fingers to enhance drainage into the
bladder.

In the second group there is often considerable retention, usually several ounces.
This is typically the large, flaccid, fibrous
sac with a narrow, rigid orifice. It contains foul, decomposing urine. It is often
prevented from emptying by adhesions to
other structures. Surgery is indicated.

Such surgical cases may be further sub-
divided into two groups:

1. Retention diverticulum without vesical neck obstruction.
2. Such with vesical neck obstruction.

In the first group the sepsis can be cleared up well enough by an indwelling urethral catheter to permit removal of the
sac. The performance of any suprapubic
drainage operation in these cases is to be
avoided.

In the second group the sepsis can be
overcome but r a r e l y by the use of the
urethral catheter to permit a safe operation on the bladder neck, either resection
or prostatectomy. Suprapubic drainage is
then necessary. The sac can be removed
at the first operation, if the patient is fit
for such procedure, so that the second operation will be the removal of the obstruction at the bladder neck alone.

There are two chief methods of dealing
with the sac itself: 1. Radical excision of
the entire sac after inversion. 2. Inversion

of the sac within the bladder with removal
of the lining mucosa, closure of the orifice,
and extra-vesical drainage of the residual
shut-off pouch.

The excision of a bladder diverticulum is
always an interesting and sometimes a difficult operation. Of course, excision of
the diverticulum alone will not be sufficient in the majority of cases. An obstruction should always be suspected until its
existence can or cannot be proved.

For the non-surgical cases the best form
that palliative treatment can take is to encourage the patient to find some position
in which he can perform miction in two
parts. Inoperable cases need irrigations
of the b l a d d e r. The complications are
treated according to their nature.

* * * *

CASE HISTORY

Patient: Mr. L. C. Was seen first on
May 28, 1936. Age 31. Barber.

General health fair. Very nervous and
irritable. Chronic constipation. Has had
usual diseases of childhood with uneventful recovery.

For 12 years patient states he has suffered from bladder trouble, itching and
burning sensations during urination, nocturia two to three times, and low back
pains, occasionally passing blood and pus.
Had a great deal of treatment. At one
time was treated for gonorrhea that he did
not have with no improvement in his condition.

On cystoscopic examination: A No. 24
Brown Buerger cystoscope was passed with
difficulty into the bladder, tightness being
noted in the posterior u r e t h r a. The
bladder contained a great deal of inflammatory exudate. The left ureteral orifice
appeared distended and partially obliterated; however, it was easily catheterized
with a No. 6 catheter. With Indigo Car-
mine in the vein each kidney functioned
normally. Examination of the specimens
from either kidney showed 1-5 w.b.c. from
the left kidney, about the same from the
right kidney, and a few r.b.c., which were
probably due to catheter trauma.

Roentgenologic examination: Flat plate
showed the kidneys to be in normal position and no suspicious shadows. A small
opening was noted to the left of the left
ureteral orifice. A cystogram was made

with 150 c.c. of 12½ per cent sodium iodide solution; showed a moderate sized diverticulum at that point, with no retention.

On September 14, a suprapubic cystotomy was done. The entire sac was pulled into the bladder by suction and removed. The muscular opening of the bladder wall was closed with chromic No. 1 pursestring s u t u r e and reinforced with interrupted chromic; the bladder was closed with a hard rubber drainage tube, and the perivesical space drained with cigarette drains. The cigarette d r a i n s were removed the fourth post-operative day, and the suprapubic vesical drains removed the seventh post-operative day. He was dismissed from the hospital on the tenth post-operative day; made a most satisfactory recovery. However, he was in about 10 days ago (after three years) complaining of burning on urination, and a cystogram was made in which the antero-posterior position was normal, but lateral visualization showed a small diverticulum posteriorly. He will now come in regularly for dilatations of the urethra to try to bring about an egression of the sac.

* * * *

Dr. Howe—In Closing

Obstruction is generally conceded as the exciting cause. Ninety per cent of all diverticula (in children) are found near the posterior angles of the trigone or in the dome, or vertex, the latter probably coming from an incomplete urachus cyst. With increased intracystic pressure t h e r e is trabeculation and the formation of cellules and saccules. Frequently by enlargement of a saccule a diverticulum may develop. The muscular component is usually scant or feeble; because of this a diverticulum is rarely able to empty itself, and, by the maintenance of a pool of stagnant urine, perpetuates infection and predisposes to the formation of stones. CAMPBELL says vesical diverticula are almost always congenital or are immediately secondary to congenital obstruction. In children the sex ratio is 5 to 1, in adults 10 to 1. ENGLISH reported diverticulum complicated by calculus in a boy eight days old. In the babies' hospital a diverticulum was found in a boy seven days old, and HYMAN performed a diverticulectomy on a child nine months of age. OCKERBLAD reports a tumor in a diverticulum, a couple of cases of stone, and one with a ureter opening into a diverticulum. In the latter case the patient complained of pain in the l o w e r quadrant, which was relieved by dilatation of the opening.

---O---

A Bug Full of Tricks*

LEWIS J. MOORMAN, M.D.
OKLAHOMA CITY, OKLAHOMA

The above title refers to a despicable little parasite now known as the tubercle bacillus. This microscopic wax covered bit of protein and sugar was plaguing humanity long before the days of recorded history. In subtle, evasive, insinuating fashion, this stealthy enemy of mankind plied its nefarious trade and paradoxical as it may seem, it boldly recorded its own ravages as revealed in exhumed prehistoric skeletons and E g y p t i a n mummies. These angular spines and distorted joints served as stimulating question marks, accentuating the intricate mysteries of a

*Read Before the Oklahoma City Academy of Medicine, April 3, 1939.

deadly disease, which has followed its host with the ardor of a well-known Biblical character, s i l e n t l y decreeing, "Whither thou goest I will go, and where thou lodgest I will lodge, Thy people shall be my people." So it is unto this day. In spite of all our accumulated knowledge, our destiny is still intimately identified with the tubercle bacillus.

Passing on to the serious study of recorded history, we find that the code of Hammurabi, written more than 2,000 years B.C., indicates a knowledge of tuberculosis. In Deuteronomy, the 15th century B.C., it is said, "The Lord shall smite thee with a consumption and with a fever and with an inflammation." In the fifth century B.C., Hippocrates and other Greek writers recognized the essential clinical features of the disease and described them well. They observed its wasting proclivities and appropriately called it "phthisis." Aretaeus, in the second century A.D., gave accurate c l i n i c a l description of tuberculosis and suggested routine treatment similar to that e m p l o y e d today. Galen accepted the teachings of Hippocrates and recorded his own observations.

In spite of their keen powers of observation and their illuminating clinical descriptions, it is obvious that Hippocrates, Aretaeus and Galen were groping for light while hopelessly submerged in the occult phenomena caused by this baffling bacillus. Apparently Galen never suspected that his own "side stitches" represented a pleuritic manifestation of phthisis. For more than 2,000 years, successive generations suffered and died in the dim light supplied by these renowned Greek physicians. During this long period there was much confusion about the pathological and clinical manifestations of the d i s e a s e. Scrofula and pleurisy were not recognized as of tuberculous origin and many other extra-pulmonary manifestations p a s s e d without identification. Bizarre beliefs and practices befogged the issue, and finally, the many a b s u r d therapeutic measures were climaxed by the royal touch for scrofula, and o n l y occasionally a flickering light appeared on the dim horizon to encourage further investigation.

In 1543, Vesalius published his monumental work on anatomy. In 1546 Fracstorius suggested the modern conception of contagion through microorganisms and expressed the belief that phthisis is due to invisible germs. In 1553 Servetus discovered the lesser circulation; in 1567 Paracelsus wrote about miner's phthisis and boldly broke away from Galenic teachings, becoming one of the f i r s t advocates of chemistry in medicine. In 1590, the compound microscope was introduced by Hans and Zacharis Janssen; in 1616 William Harvey announced his discovery of circulation of the blood; in 1650 Franciscus Sylvius declared that tubercles are the cause of phthisis and sensed the connection between scrofula and phthisis. In 1683 Leeuwenhoek described microorganisms and initiated the s t u d y of bacteria; in 1689

Richard Morton published a voluminous treatise on consumption, entitled "Phthisiologia." He stressed the teaching of Sylvius that tubercles are connected with and precede phthisis. In 1700, Manget gave the first postmortem report of miliary tuberculosis. A b o u t this time Morgagni (1682-1772). was laying the foundation for the study of gross pathology, but refused to perform autopsies on the victims of phthisis because of his fear of contagion.

About the middle of the 18th century, the tuberculosis d e a t h rate reached its highest point in statistical columns. This peak of mortality in the midst of universal confusion with reference to clinicopathological manifestations, was coincident with rapidly increasing facilities for the acquisition of knowledge and may have inspired the dawning urge for more specific investigations.

In 1761 Auenbrugger, though unheeded at the time, made an epochal contribution through his *Inventum Novum*, which described immediate percussion. In 1765, William Stark, fresh from the University of Edinburgh, came to London to study pathology under the renowned Dr. John Hunter. He devoted his energy almost entirely to the study of the pathology of phthisis. Contemporaneous with S t a r k, Robert Whytt described tuberculous meningitis, and Percival Pott first described tuberculous caries of the spine, w h i c h justly took his name but remained to be proven of tuberculous origin by Delpech in 1816. S o o n thereafter, Marc-Antone Petit described tuberculosis of the larynx and Portal suggested a definite connection between engorgement of lymphatics and pulmonary consumption. William Stark, at the early age of 29, died of miliary tuberculosis as the result of an a u t o p s y wound. Matthew Baillie, having recently graduated in medicine, received an appointment to St. Georges Hospital to work in the autopsy room where Stark had received his fatal infection. No doubt Baillie was inspired by the work of young Stark and sought the opportunity of pursuing the latter's pathological researches under his famous uncle, John Hunter. For 18 years Baillie diligently followed his postmortem studies of diseases of the chest, and made valuable contributions to our knowledge of tuberculosis. He also received an infection of the hand while performing an autopsy but died of advanced pulmonary tuberculosis at the age of 62. His work on "Morbid Anatomy" was published in 1795. His investigations clarified our knowledge of tubercle and differentiated nodular and infiltrating pathological types.

At the turn of the century Robert Willan discussed the relationship of erythema nodosum to tuberculosis, Thomas Beddoes, in his Pneumatic Institute at Clifton, England, was doing interesting work with provocative reports of his investigation, and Benjamin Rush was making valuable contributions in America. Bichat progressed from the organ pathology of Morgagni to tissue pathology within the organ, which was soon to be supplemented by the cellular pathology of Virchow.

After painstaking researches in pathology, Bayle described tuberculosis as a constitutional disease caused by tubercles. He also recognized extra-pulmonary tubercles and gave them proper consideration in connection with phthisis. F l i c k e says, "Bayle's life and work might be termed a melancholy romance of science. Born in 1774 he died of tuberculosis, probably contracted at the autopsy table, in 1816 at the age of 42." What he accomplished in a short time brought the knowledge of tuberculosis further forward than all that had been done before him.

In a volume on *Pulmonary Phthisis*, he carefully presents the results of his clinical observations, checked by autopsies on more than 900 individuals dying of consumption. His exhaustive studies at the bedside and in the dead room enabled him to have a better understanding of tuberculosis in all its stages and varied pathological phases, than any of his predecessors. He divided the disease into four stages: (1) occult; (2) incipient; (3) confirmed, and (4) advanced. He exhibited advanced knowledge of pleurisy and pleural adhesions but did not understand the relationship as we know it today.

Early in the 19th c e n t u r y, Covisart translated Auenbrugger's *Inventum Novum* and popularized percussion, which in spite of a previous French translation, had never achieved general r e c o g n i t i o n. Strange to say, Covisart first learned of percussion, not through the French translation of 1770, but through the influence of

Maximilian Stoll, who had succeeded de Haen as director of the Clinic in the Allgemeines Krankenhans, University of Vienna. In addition to his wide influence in the field of clinical investigation, Stoll manifested a special interest in tuberculosis, perhaps because of its ravages in his own body to which he succumbed at the early age of 46. Covisart's greatness is attested by the following quotation from his brief preface to the translation of Auenbrugger's pamphlet.

"I know well how little reputation nearly all translators and most commentators earn and hence I might have secured for myself an authorship if I had published a work on percussion based upon a recasting of the writings of Auenbrugger. I then would have sacrificed the name of Auenbrugger to my own vanity; that I did not wish to do; I wanted to snatch him and his beautiful, regularly m a d e discovery which he with entire propriety called a new invention, from forgetfulness."

Later Piorry introduced the ivory pleximeter which was soon to be replaced by the more satisfactory use of the fingers. Piorry's mediate percussion, combined with Laennec's new methods of auscultation, e x e r t e d a profound influence upon the progress of physical diagnosis.

We now come to the significant awakening with reference to clinical and pathological investigations with Portal, Stark, Baillie, Bichat, Bayle and Covisart supplying a stimulating background for the unprecedented work of Laennec and Louis in the first quarter of the 19th century. Laennec promptly grasped the significance of the clinicopathological implications and with an avid genius, he appropriated all previous scientific advances as he entered upon his monumental career. In spite of the handicap of progressive tuberculosis in his own person, he worked with remarkable industry and conspicuous discrimination. Before he was 22 years of age he had drawn up a minute history of nearly 400 cases of disease, which served as a foundation for his future researches and discoveries. When Laennec c a m e upon the scene, the diagnosis of diseases of the lungs and heart was still more difficult than that of other internal organs. In a short time he had made the most exacting diagnostic tasks relatively easy. In half the time now allotted for a medical education, virtually without chart or compass, he "Observed, recorded, tabulated and communicated" practically all that is now taught with reference to the physical diagnosis of diseases of the thorax. His voluminous work of nearly 800 pages on auscultation and diseases of the chest was published in 1819 and translated into English by Forbes in 1821.

After giving full credit for Covisart's revival of Auenbrugger's neglected invention, it is doubtful whether the remarkable advances of the 19th century would have followed each other so rapidly without the stimulus of another famous invention, the stethoscope. Immediate auscultation in haphazard fashion had been practiced since the days of Hippocrates, but it remained for Laennec, through his ingenious invention, to perfect this method of examination and to extend and record its diagnostic possibilities. Quoting from a recent article by Korns, "The great merit of Laennec's invention lay not so much in the instrument itself, as in the fact that it served to focus the attention of the entire medical world on the auscultatory method. Rolleston, in his Harveian oration (1928), expresses this idea as follows: "though the stethoscope has some obvious advantages over the naked ear, the enormous advances that followed its introduction were not so much due to the stethoscope as a mechanical instrument, as to the psychological effect that this new method exerted on Laennec, who otherwise would not have so ardently pursued auscultation as a means of diagnosis."

At the age of 45, on August 13, 1826, Laennec died of advanced pulmonary tuberculosis with associated tuberculous enteritis. In keeping with his genius for independent accomplishment, two hours before his death he removed the rings from his fingers in order to save others the trouble.

The great clinician, Louis, who was contemporary with Laennec and survived him by many years, also suffered from tuberculosis, but lived to be 85 years of age. Louis made use of the facts Bayle and Laennec had brought to light and gave them added significance through his own observations, his writings and his wonderful influence as a teacher. He carefully correlated the symptoms and the pathology of tubercu-

losis; he continued and amplified the study of clinical manifestations in the light of autopsy findings. Finally, when 34 years of age, he gave up general practice in order to more satisfactorily pursue his scientific investigations. Louis established the numerical or statistical method of investigation in medicine. Through his teachings and his pupils, he was largely responsible for the establishment of clinical medicine, with a special interest in physical examination, throughout the world. The results of his studies were published in a volume of 600 pages under the title, *Louis' Researches on Phthisis.* His influence is evident wherever the principles of clinical medicine are taught. In the United States, his teachings were perpetuated through such pupils as James Jackson, Jr., Oliver Wendell Holmes, George C. Shattuck, William Pepper, Gerhard, Stille, Power, Swett and Clark.

Contemporary with Louis, Virchow, advancing from Bichat's tissue pathology to cellular pathology, made valuable contributions to our knowledge of tuberculosis. However, he joined the dualist Schonlein, who coined the word "tuberculosis," in order, as he thought, to differentiate the nodular tubercles from the cheesy patch characterizing phthisis. Thus is seen the perspicacity of Laennec with reference to the "unity of phthisis" blocked by the unfortunate and misguided application of a scientific advance. Not until the discovery of the tubercle bacillus were the dualists routed and the unity of tuberculosis finally established.

In the University of Vienna the eccentric, impetuous Skoda (1805-1881), taking his cue from the French school, enthusiastically pursued the study of percussion and auscultation, with emphasis upon the investigation of tonal or sonorous phenomena. Skoda's skill in diagnosis so inspired Turkheim, minister of medical education, he established a special department on chest diseases with this great clinician in charge. Skoda's appointment as professor of medicine in 1846 and his skill in physical diagnosis attracted students from all parts of the world. However, the magnetic attraction of the University of Vienna for students of clinical medicine was shared by an illustrious contemporary of Skoda. The rapid rise of this school to the highest rank was largely due to Rokitansky (1804-1878), the world's greatest clinical pathologist. Skoda's w o r k was brilliantly complimented by the latter's illuminating demonstrations in the dead room. Rokitansky handled 1,500 to 1,800 autopsies annually. It is said that he performed over 30,000 postmortem examinations annually.

By the middle of the 19th century the stage was set for a great scientific awakening. In 1865 Villemin demonstrated the specific nature of tuberculosis through inoculation. Five years later, Gerlach proved that milk from tuberculous cows conveyed the d i s e a s e, and in 1873, Edwin Klebs, through feeding experiments, produced bovine tuberculosis. Medicine was moving into a new era. The consolidated methods of clinical, anatomical a n d pathological studies were soon to be supplemented by modern laboratory methods.

It seems worthy of note that much of the p r o g r e s s in physical diagnosis and pathology has been evolved through a sustained desire to solve the mysteries of tuberculosis. It is equally interesting to note that a large percentage of the most zealous investigators have suffered from tuberculosis; some apparently experiencing an excitation of genius which spurred them on to greater accomplishments, thus partially compensating for an early surrender to the enemy they so ardently pursued. It seems that the tubercle bacillus, in spite of its magical powers of evasion and deception, was preparing the way for its ultimate discovery and the gradual surrender of many of its secrets.

In 1856 Virchow, in the city of Berlin, established the first pathological laboratory. It served as a model for nearly all laboratories in Germany and in o t h e r countries. The first hygienic laboratory was opened by Pettenkofer in 1878. Robert Koch, stimulated by the discoveries of Pasteur, had already begun his epochal researches. Allen K. Krause, discussing Robert Koch's r a p i d and uninterrupted march from obscurity to universal fame, says: "Just before Koch emerged from Posen, Cohn, in writing his great work on botany, had scrapped what was then known about bacteria into the nondescript genus of *chaos*: when, in almost a trice and out of a most unexpected source, was born a new science, *bacteriology*. Stone by stone the builder raised his structure, year by year the new science took on form and fullness: from the cause and nature of anthrax in 1876; to the smear-preparation and staining methods of '77; the parasitic excitants of wound infection in '78; and then the crowning and astonishing plate-isolation method to signalize his assumption of the reins on *Luisenstrasse* in 1881. Already had been forged the tools to lay bare the gonococcus (Neisser, 1879), the pneumococcus (Sternberg, 1880), the typhoid bacillus (Eberth, 1880), the glanders bacillus (Loeffler, 1882)—bacteria of disease, as Koch put it, falling into his and his pupils' laps "like ripe apples from a tree." On his first trip to Breslau he had met Weigert, Cohnheim's associate, and the former's young cousin, Paul Ehrlich; and Ehrlich was doing a little more than *play* with aniline dyes, whose possibilities had long intrigued his pathologist-cousin Weigert—he was making thin smears of blood on cover-slips and staining these to study the cells.

So the stage was set for progression from Weigert to Ehrlich to Koch; and we follow the chain from Weigert's methylene-blue and Ehrlich's thin heat-fixed smears to Koch's stained smear-preparation, to demonstrate those early pathogenic bacteria. Gelatine, solid and transparent, was the culture medium, streaked with the material to be studied. And until 1882 these simple methods, fortified now by the plate-isolation process, promised to disclose the causes of all infectious diseases.

Then Koch struck a snag.

He began the search for the cause of tuberculosis in the year 1881. He got busy on known tuberculous t i s s u e s with his trusty ordinary methylene-blue, and saw— nothing; that is, nothing that might be imagined to be an adventitious product— a germ; no round dots as in wound infections and gonorrhoea, nor rod-like particles as in typhoid fever and anthrax. But, supreme adepter and borrower that he always was, he soon had recourse again to a Weigert tissue-stain method: he "fortifies" his methylene-blue stain with potash, dips in the mixture a fresh section of tissue, and now, first of mankind, beholds within the blue background of tissue elements the fine blue streaks that by this time had come to mean "germs." Thus ended step number one, the demonstration of something extrinsic to tissue and its degradation products, the presumption that Koch was gazing at the physical cause of consumption. The perfection of this f i r s t step, the refinement of the method by adding a counterstain, Bismarch-brown, was a mere detail to be worked out presently."

There were other snags but the story of Koch's "step-by-step proof of the specificity of the tubercle bacillus" is so well known it is not necessary to repeat it here. It is important to note that the snags encountered were due to the fact that the tubercle bacillus is a non-conformist and only a Robert Koch could have successfully accomplished the task. Again quoting Krause: "Given the s a m e circumstances, the same pioneer quest, the same l i m i t e d knowledge of possibilities, the same imperfection of initial media—and the view is almost compelling that only the r a r e s t of investigators would have maintained the prolonged and heartbreaking vigil for the earliest "showing through" of minutest particles that belonged, as yet, only to the shadowy realm of "working hypothesis."

This perfect performance which marked the zenith of Koch's career and its presentation in irrefutable terms, silenced the dualists and forever established Laennec's claims for the unity of tuberculosis. Even Virchow, still supporting the dualists and ever ready for controversy, quick of mind and body, remained speechless and immobile, thus accentuating the profound silence that followed Koch's dramatic presentation of the world's most perfect bit of research. Something new to mortal ken had sounded the death knell of dualism, and to the war horse of pathology, it was like the p a s s i n g of a cherished child. Though, on this occasion, he left the Berlin Physiological Society without a word of response, it is worthy of note that in the language of Krause, "When, full of years and every honor that a man of medicine can accumulate, he passed on to eternal peace, he could not reconcile himself to the idea of the all-embracing and unified cause of that appalling diversity of effect that tuberculosis comprehends."

The discovery of the tubercle bacillus in 1882 did not satisfy Robert Koch. His dauntless spirit was soon busily engaged in search of a cure for tuberculosis. In 1890, his announcement of t u b e r c u l i n

caused a furor throughout the m e d i c a l world.

Koch, having discovered the s p e c i f i c c a u s e of tuberculosis, and, as he first thought, having found a cure in tuberculin, it then seemed reasonable to anticipate the end of humanity's greatest scourge. Unfortunately, we were doomed to descend from this hopeful height, but the settling point left us far above the level attained by Laennec and Louis. Koch's discoveries led to many valuable epidemiological, d i a g n o s t i c, therapeutic and preventive principles, and initiated a sustained search for additional knowledge which has reached an astounding magnitude.

Though disappointing as a cure, tuberculin p r o v e d to be a valuable diagnostic agent and helped to stress the ubiquitous presence of the tubercle bacillus. Through Roentgen's discovery of the X-ray, the value of inspection was immeasurably increased. Later the bronchoscope extended our scope of vision and revealed pathological manifestations of tuberculosis not previously suspected.

Time will not permit a detailed discussion of therapy, but a brief reference to its development with its present sad limitations, is sufficient to further emphasize the baffling problems of the tubercle bacillus and its protean manifestations.

Immediately prior to Koch's epochal discoveries, Boddington, Brehmer, Dettweiler and Trudeau pioneered in sanatorium management, which has been so successfully pursued with untold benefit to patients, a wealth of accumulated clinical, pathological a n d therapeutic knowledge, and statistical data difficult to estimate. Collapse therapy, with its multiple surgical possibilities, is now a matter of common knowledge.

In spite of all that has been accomplished, the unsolved problems in the field of tuberculosis are infinite and in the words of David Riesman, "No matter what we take away from infinity, infinity remains."

To briefly refer to the problems now in the s c o p e of our consciousness, to say nothing of those not yet conceived, would require a large volume. To merely enumerate the research projects, now devoted to these problems, would fill another great volume. The bibliography on the tubercle bacillus and tuberculosis, as reflected in the quarterly Index Medicus, now occupies 25 times the space devoted to these subjects 30 years ago. The space devoted to tuberculosis is 12 times that allotted to the, now popular, subject of pneumonia, and four times that given to syphilis.

This voluminous literature on tuberculosis i n d i c a t e s that constantly we are making new observations of age-old conditions in this infinite field which still intrigues all investigative minds.

Even t h o u g h our command over the course of natural phenomena has speeded up immeasurably since Harvey urged us to travel in the path which "nature walks," we are unable to find our way to a full understanding of the t u b e r c l e bacillus. With all our studies of immunity and infection; the chemical fractional analysis of the tubercle bacillus; the cultural mutations with their v a r i e d morphological forms; our modern advances in diagnosis and therapy; tuberculosis still goes where we go, lodges where we lodge, and remains the greatest killer during the most useful period in the cycle of life.

----------o----------

Perforation of Hollow Viscus*
Roentgen Aspects

EDWARD D. GREENBERGER, M.D.
McALESTER, OKLAHOMA

The first single case report of the value of X-ray in the diagnosis of perforation of stomach and intestine was presented in 1915. The first statistical series of cases on the frequency of spontaneous pneumo-peritoneum occasioned by peptic ulcer were published by Singer and Vaughan in 1925 and another more complete series in 1929[1]. These authors stated then, "we know of no single symptom or sign in perforated peptic ulcer which is so constant or so free from possible misinterpretation as spontaneous pneumo-peritoneum."

The frequency of air u n d e r the diaphragm in perforated peptic ulcers, as reported by various authors, varies from 60 to 90 per cent. In Singer's and Vaughan's series of over 80 cases, 85 per cent of all their cases showed roentgen evidence of perforation, verified by operation or postmortem. A more recent series, reported by Dr. S. E. Johnson[4] of Louisville City Hospital of Kentucky, showed 83 per cent of his cases of proven perforated peptic ulcer to have been diagnosed by X-ray. Dr. G. Petren[7] of the Surgical Clinic of Lund, Germany, found but two-thirds of his proven perforated cases to show free air in the peritoneal cavity.

We know that no other abdominal catastrophe requires a more prompt diagnosis and treatment than does intestinal perforation. The surgeon today recognizes the value and is often guided by the roentgen findings in intestinal perforation. S i n c e the recognition of a spontaneous pneumo-peritoneum is so pathognomonic of perforation, why are we not able to demonstrate this pneumo-peritoneum in over 90 per cent of the perforated intestinal cases submitted to X-ray examination? Is it due to improper technique or insufficient study? Is it due to the fact that the lesion is walled off by adhesions at the time of rupture? Is spasm a factor? Is it due to the size or location of the perforation? To the interval of time between the perforation and time of X-ray?

An attempt to answer these questions prompted me to write this paper.

A few months ago, a middle aged salesman entered the hospital in the typical jack-knife posture, four hours after his perforation. At *no time* since the perforation did he or could he lie down. The X-ray studies were made as soon as the patient entered the hospital, in the sitting-up position. No air under the diaphragm was visualized. A large amount of air was present in the magenblasse of the stomach.

*Read before the Section on Dermatology and Radiology, Annual Meeting, Oklahoma State Medical Association, Oklahoma City, May 2, 1939.

At operation, a perforation eight mm. in diameter was found on the lesser curvature side of the pars pylorica. No adhesions of the omentum or liver, no exudate or fibrin was seen over the site of perforation. I therefore assumed that the failure to prove the presence of the perforation by X-ray in this case was due to my failure to place this patient on his left side in supine position, before I did the X-ray examination. The large amount of air in the stomach was trapped in the cardia, and never had the chance to get to the site of the perforation, which would have been the case if he had assumed the above mentioned position.

I thought I had stumbled on an additional aid in roentgen diagnosis of peptic ulcer perforations. On review of the literature, I found that Singer and Vaughan made this same observation 10 years b e f o r e. When their original examination on admission failed to prove the perforation, these authors were able to demonstrate free air in the peritoneum in several of their cases, after the patient was placed in the left supine position for a half hour to several hours.

Proper X-ray techique will therefore undoubtedly increase the percentage of cases of peptic ulcer perforations that are roentgen positive. But there are several other factors in 10 to 15 per cent of cases that prevent the leakage of air through the perforation, as:

1. *Spontaneous spasm* at the site of perforation. The importance of this factor was demonstrated by Dr. Poas[9]. He produced in dogs an artificial tear in the anterior duodenal wall close to the pylorus. The pyloric spasm that was produced persisted for s e v e r a l hours and prevented the passage of gastric contents i n t o the duodenum and thus into the peritoneal cavity.

2. Deposition of fibrin over the perforation, adhesions of omentum or neighboring organs to site of ulcer, and impacted m u c o u s plugs are o t h e r causes for spontaneous closure of the perforation soon after the rupture.

A common explanation that I have heard radiologists offer to referring physicians when the radiologist could not demonstrate the perforation by X-ray was that the lesion was probably a walled-off penetrating ulcer that had perforated. At the operating table, this type of walled-off perforation is rare, less than two per cent of all cases.

3. The size of the p e r f o r a t i o n—The smaller the hole, the more likely the possibility of a spontaneous closure before the air has had a chance to get through into the peritoneum.

4. The site of the perforation—In about 121 cases reported by the Russian Sosnyakov[3] of Leningrad, the perforations were localized in all their cases on the anterior wall of the stomach and duodenum; only in one case was the perforation found on greater curvature side and in only five cases near the cardia of the stomach. Since 90 to 95 per cent of all ulcer perforations occur at the pylorus and duodenum, the procedure of placing the patient in left supine position for a short period of time prior to X-ray study, will undoubtedly increase the number of roentgen-positive cases.

The clinician does not usually need the X-ray to diagnose a perforation of a posterior wall duodenal ulcer. The marked gastric hemorrhage and melena are characteristic. The site and nature of other peptic ulcer perforations are determined by m e a n s of barium meal X-ray study.

5. The interval of time between the perforation and X-ray study — In most cases, this is not a definite factor in the roentgen diagnosis. Most c a s e s will show free air in the peritoneum soon after the perforation. Placing the patient in the left supine position for a half to several hours after the first roentgen examination is negative, will reveal in many cases a *delayed pneumo-peritoneum*, i.e., in small perforations where the spasm is relieved or the plug dislodged.

TECHNIQUE

1. Sitting up position, posterior-anterior view. The patient should sit up for a few minutes before the film is taken in order to permit the free air in the peritoneum to a s c e n d to the diaphragm. The voltage and time of X-ray exposure should be slightly more than is required for a chest film.

2. Lateral position—The patient lies on his left side, right side up, film placed along lower right ribs, X-rays directed perpendicular to the body.

3. The majority of perforations will be demonstrated by the above positions. If the X-ray findings are negative by above, then the left supine position for one to several hours, and X-raying at intervals, as advocated by Singer is recommended. The X-ray studies that I have made reveal that the left s u p i n e *Trendelenberg* position will permit a much larger amount of air to collect in the pars pylorica. In the straight left supine position, X-ray studies by means of barium meal reveal most of the air to be collected in the esophageal end of the stomach and only a small amount on the lesser curvature side of the pars pylorica.

If there is no air in the stomach at the time of perforation, no air of course could go into the peritoneum. When X-ray studies show such an absence of air in the magenblasse, I have my patients swallow some air, and then use the above technique.

4. Fluoroscopy of the patient while on the stretcher in sitting-up p o s i t i o n should supplement the film studies. In several of my cases, the fluoroscopic study revealed a small sub-diaphragmatic collection of air that was not observed in the films. In many cases, the thin air collection was seen in expiration and not in inspiration. Often the oblique view shows the air collection best. Again, the free air is often hidden behind the air in the cardia.

The fluoroscopic study is of value in differentiating the free collection of air in the peritoneum from air within the colon or stomach, from emphysematous air pockets at base of the lungs, etc.

CLINICAL TYPES OF PEPTIC ULCER PERFORATION

Some of you have encountered surgeons who claim they never require roentgen aid for a diagnosis of intestinal perforation. These surgeons apparently have seen but few cases, and are familiar only with the classical text-book picture of perforation. It is therefore essential that the surgeon and radiologist consider and recognize the clinical types of peptic ulcer perforation:

1. Classical type — The patient experiences sudden excruciating pain in the abdomen, causing him to assume the jack-knife *sitting-up* p o s t u r e. The rigidity and abdominal tenderness is not equaled by any other abdominal catastrophe. The patient's attitude and symptoms remain unabated until operation.

2. Singer and Vaughan in 1933, designated this second type as the "formes fruste" case. The patient experiences the same sudden knife-like abdominal pain at the time of perforation. But within one to several hours, the patient's symptoms have abated and he is often ready to discharge the surgeon. Mild to moderate rigidity and tenderness are the only clinical findings at this time. In this type of case, the roentgen demonstration of a spontaneous pneumo-peritoneum achieves its greatest diagnostic value.

3. The explanation for the c h a n g e of symptoms in "forme fruste" cases is that the perforation has spontaneously closed. Under judicious care as by continuous gastric siphonage and parenteral feeding the perforation stays closed without operation. But if the above condition is not recognized and the patient overloads his stomach, the perforation again becomes patent with a repetition of acute symptoms. A third and even a fourth similar episode may occur, before the classical picture of p e r f o r a t i o n occurs. Singer and Vaughan first described this type of case in A.M.A. in 1934, under the title of *"Intermittent Leakage From Perforation of Peptic Ulcer."*[3] I refer you to their paper for further details.

4. The fourth type — The perforating peptic ulcer simulating the g a s t r i c crises of Tabes, is described in a recent n u m b e r of Staff Meetings of Mayo Clinic[5]. This type of ulcer syndrome is caused by deep penetration of the ulcer with invasion of tissues contiguous to stomach and intestines. This type is, of course, rare. Diagnosis is proven by X-ray studies by means of barium meal.

Other types of clinical pictures occur, being often confused and therefore must be differentiated from (1) perforated gall bladder, (2) pancreatitis, (3) acute coronary occlusion, (4) mesenteric obstruction, and (5) intestinal obstruction.

Spontaneous Pneumoperitoneum due to perforations other than peptic ulcers:

1. Perforations of colon and s t o m a c h after gunshot wounds or other missiles. A perforation of the small bowel by a foreign object does not p r o d u c e pneumoperitoneum, s i n c e the small bowel normally does not contain air.

2. Perforated carcimona of stomach or colon.

3. Leakage from enterostomy, colostomy, and anastomosis, etc.

4. Typhoid or tuberculous perforation of small bowel, perforation of appendix (occasionally).

5. Perforation from diverticulae or polypae of the large bowel or duodenum.

6. Perforation of the uterus in abortions.

Spontaneous Pneumoperitoneum occurs in other conditions other than perforations, as:

1. Following recent operations or trauma to abdominal wall by knife, gun, etc.

2. Abdominal paracentesis.

3. Tubal insufflation in Rubin test.

4. Previously i n d u c e d pneumoperitoneum.

Pneumoperitoneum must be differentiated from gas-containing organs around the diaphragm, as:

1. Hepato-diaphragmatic interposition of the large intestines. A good series of such cases was recently reported by Dr. Kolju[6].

2. Mobile pylorus of the stomach and mobile colon that intermittently assume a sub-diaphragmatic p o s i t i o n. This type of case was recently reported by Dr. Singleton of Toronto.

3. Sub-phrenic abscess, characterized by small transparent area within an area of increased density. This collection of air between the liver and diaphragm is fixed, whereas the air in perforation changes its position with change of patient.

(Lantern Slide Demonstration)

CONCLUSIONS

1. Four major clinical types of peptic ulcer perforation should be recognized —the classical type, forme fruste, intermittent leakage type, and gastric crisis type. X-ray is of greatest diagnostic value in second and third type.

2. The factors responsible for closure of the perforation or failure to show a spontaneous pneumoperitoneum were discussed. But with p r o p e r X-ray technique, at least 85 per cent of all cases of peptic ulcer perforation can be diagnosed by X-ray. The X-ray technique is described.

3. Air containing viscus under the diaphragm and various types of recently induced pneumoperitoneum are the roentgen findings to be differentiated b e f o r e making a positive roentgen diagnosis of intestinal perforation.

BIBLIOGRAPHY

1. Roger T. Vaughan and Harry A. Singer: "Value of Radiology in the Diagnosis of Perforated Peptic Ulcer." Surgery, Gyn. and Obst., November, 1929.

2. Same authors: "Further Observation of Value of Radiology in Diagnosis of Perforated Peptic Ulcer." Am. J. of Surgery, September, 1933.

3. Harry A. Singer: "Perforated Peptic Ulcer With Intermittent Leakage." J. of A.M.A., January, 1934.

4. Sydney E. Johnson: "Frequency of Air Under the Diaphragm in Perforated Peptic Ulcer." J. of A.M.A., January, 1937.

5. W. S. Sosnyakov: "Gastro Duodenal Perforation." (Abst) J. of A.M.A., page 1,678, 1937.

6. K. J. Kolju, Siberia: "Hepato Diaphragmatic Interposition of the Large Intestine." A. J. of Roentgenology, June, 1938.

7. G. Petrin, Germany: "Free Gas in Peritoneal Cavity." (Abst) A.M.A., page 2,083, 1937.

8. "Perforating Peptic Ulcer Simulating the Gastric Crisis of Tabes." Proceedings of the Staff Meetings of Mayo Clinic, March 29, 1939.

9. Dr. Poas: "Gastro-duodenal Perforation." (Abst) A.M.A., page 2,096, December, 1936.

———o———

O.U. Medical Alumni Directory

The University of Oklahoma Association has started preparation of a Medical Alumni Directory to be published as the August issue of Sooner Magazine, the monthly publication of the alumni association.

The directory will contain alphabetical and geographical lists of all graduates of the University of Oklahoma Medical School, and also will contain names of former O.U. students who obtained medical degrees elsewhere and are now in the medical profession.

All alumni of the medical school and former students now in the profession, are urged to report their correct addresses to the Alumni Office, University of Oklahoma, so that they will be properly listed in the directory.

Copies will be sent to all members of the University of Oklahoma Association, and a few extra copies will be printed for sale to others desiring the directory. Orders for individual copies must be placed in advance, however, and accompanied by payment of $1.00 per copy.

Perinephritic Abscess*

CHARLES M. O'LEARY, M.D.
Department of Surgery, University Hospital
REX BOLEND, M.D.
Head of Department of Urology, University Hospital
OKLAHOMA CITY, OKLAHOMA

The records of 33 patients with perinephritic abscess were studied. In 30 cases the diagnosis was corroborated by surgical findings, while in three, the pathology was disclosed at autopsy. The group presented themselves at the University Hospital during a period of 17 years. In this interval 95,000 hospital admissions were recorded.

The anatomical peculiarities of the perirenal structures predispose the presence of pathological variations. The kidney is surrounded by a pale layer of fatty tissue, more abundant posteriorly and inferiorly. Continuous with a similar layer about the ureter, this fatty tissue extends into the pelvis and is circumscribed by the renal and ureteral fascia. The possibility of extension of infection within the periureteral f a s c i a must be emphasized. Rolnick[1] demonstrated such ease of dessimination by injections of radiopaque medium within the periureteral fascia of postmortem specimens. Downward extension followed injections near the renal pelvis. An upward dessimination occurred along the ureter when injections were made at the base of the bladder. A somewhat similar process may have occurred in the patients herewith described:

Case No. 88954, Mrs. E. M., white, age 32. On the seventh postoperative day following a left salpingo-oophorectomy and appendectomy, the patient suffered a rather rapid onset of severe pain in the right posterior lung base. The temperature and pulse, which had been normal, rose to 101.6° and 120 respectively. Thereafter daily temperature elevation was 101°, and pulse rise 120. The respirations remained normal. Five days after onset a mass was palpated in the right costo-iliac

region. Four urinalyses s h o w e d a moderate number of white blood cells. The leucocytes were 13,000 with neutrophiles 86 per cent. Eight days after the onset an incision and drainage of the right perirenal s p a c e was performed. There was an extensive abscess at the inferior pole of the right kidney with indications of pelvic connection. Postoperative recovery was uneventful.

Case No. 79,107, Master J. M. W., white, 19 months of age. There had been pain in the left hip of one month duration, fever, and inability to bear weight on the left lower extremity. A gradual flexion deformity of the left thigh on the abdomen had developed. An outpatient diagnosis of infectious arthritis of the left hip was made and admission requested. After admission, four days later, careful examination disclosed a mass in the left subcostal and costo-iliac r e g i o n s. There was tenderness and muscle spasm in the left costovertebral angle and evidence of psoas spasm. There were daily elevations of temperature to 103.6°, of p u l s e to 128 and of respiration 28. Urinalysis showed one plus albumin. The leucocytes were 17,000 with neutrophiles 86 per cent. X-rays of the dorsal and lumbar spine were negative. Incision and drainage of the left perirenal space disclosed an abscess containing 100 c.c. of thin purulent material and located inferior to the kidney. Recovery was uneventful.

The first case presents the possibility of an upward dessimination while the latter, because of downward extension caused the clinician to attribute the pathology to the hip joint. The renal fascia is closely attached to the kidney pedicle, thus preventing any transverse spread of an infection.

*Read before the Section on Genito-Urinary Diseases and Syphilology, Annual Meeting, Oklahoma State Medical Association, Oklahoma City, May 3, 1939.

The retrorenal portion is more commonly known as the fascia of Gerota. Posterior to the fascia of Gerota is a second fatty layer situated in close proximity to the muscles and fascia of the posterior abdominal wall.

The blood supply of the perinephrium is derived from branches of the main renals, the adrenals, spermatics, and the first lumbar, combining to form a vascular network about the kidney. The intercolumnar arteries of the renal cortex after penetrating the capsule contribute to this vascular network. Hence the perirenal fatty layer may be involved by a blood b o r n e infection from suppuration existing at any place in the body and without p r i m a r y kidney pathtology.

The l y m p h a t i c s of the perinephrium communicate freely with the subcapsular kidney group and drain into the upper lateral lumbar nodes.

Perirenal suppuration may ensue from three sources: an extrarenal direct blood borne infection, rupture of single or multiple cortical abscesses, and secondary to severe kidney infections. The latter may transpire by blood or lymphatic anastomoses or direct extension. An abscess of extrarenal direct blood borne origin as from foci of infection is most likely to be diffuse, unilateral and fairly extensive. It is usually situated posterior to the kidney, at the mid and inferior portions. The fatty t i s s u e at the superior pole is of small amount and not often involved by a blood borne infection.

Secondary extension from a cortical abscess may occur at any point in the perinephrium. The involvement is frequently small and resolution often results from conservative management. Perinephric abscess arising from a pyelonephritis is fortunately less frequent. Predominant kidney pathology masks the diagnosis of the complication. Three perinephric abscesses found at autopsy were secondary to a severe pyelonephritis. Obstruction at some point in the urinary tract contributed to the kidney infection. One patient had a large hypertrophied prostate, the second an impassable urethral stricture and the third, incarceration of the u r e t e r by a parametrical extension of a carcinomatous cervix.

The more extensive perirenal abscesses usually rupture the fascia of Gerota and underlie the fascia and muscles of the posterior abdominal wall. Occasionally pathological processes of nearby organs secondarily involve the peri and pararenal tissues. Important sources of such involvement are perforated ulcers of the posterior d u o d e n a l wall, a neglected retrocecal, retroperitoneal appendicitis, a n d a ruptured liver abscess of the dome with subphrenic spread and secondary extension.

In the direct blood borne extrarenal infection of the perinephrium, the most common p r i m a r y foci of suppuration are furuncles, carbuncles, paronychia and less often osteomyelitis and gonorrhea. Upper respiratory infections, scarlet fever, influenza and other g e n e r a l infections contribute to the etiology. Fifteen of 30 patients had a history or physical findings of a previous or existing infection as a possible primary foci. The history was questionable in five and not listed in eight records. In six patients trauma seemed to play an important role. Two were injured in the respective costo-iliac areas during wrestling matches. One was thrown from a horse striking the side. Another delivered ice for his livelihood, with symptoms on the side that the ice was carried. The fifth was kicked in the kidney region during a fight and the sixth strained the respective costovertebral area during lifting.

Hemorrhage into the renal retroperitoneal area from trauma predisposes to bacterial invasion and in this event may result in a traumatic abscess.

TABLE I

Etiological factors contributing either singly or in combination to the development of a perinephritic abscess.

Types of Infection	Number of Patients
Furuncles	5
Influenza	5
Questionable	5
Gonorrhea	2
Measles	1
Typhoid	1
Known direct extension	3
Trauma	
Strains	4
Direct injuries	2
Postoperative	1

Twenty-one of the 33 patients were between the ages of 20 and 40. The youngest was 19 months and the oldest 63 years of age.

TABLE II
Distribution of patients in age groups.

Decades	Number of Patients
0-10	2
10-20	5
20-30	13
30-40	8
40-50	3
50-60	1
60-70	1

Twenty-six patients were of male and seven of the female sex. One was of the colored race. One patient had bilateral involvement, secondary to bilateral pyelonephritis. Thirty-two presented a unilateral abscess, 21 on the right and 11 on the left.

The symptomatology of the perinephric abscess in its early stages is confusing. Eleven of the 26 had had symptoms for four weeks or longer prior to hospitalization, and one for five months.

TABLE III
Duration of symptoms before hospitalization.

Duration	Number of Patients
1-7 days	4
7-14 days	2
14-21 days	9
21-28 days	3
28-35 days	2
35-42 days	2
42-49 days	2
8 weeks	1
5 months	1

It was necessary to keep some patients under observation in the hospital for a considerable period. In 18 of 28 the observation extended beyond three weeks, and in two as long as two months.

TABLE IV
Hospital days before surgery.

Days	Number of Patients
1-7	1
7-14	2
14-21	7
21-28	5
28-35	7
35-42	
42-49	4
49-56	2

At onset, the majority of patients will complain of pain in the corresponding costovertebral angle, more in the nature of a dull ache. Twenty-three of 33 recalled low grade pain as the first symptom. Seven had abdominal and one hip joint pain. Chills and fever were the first symptoms in one and in another, urinary retention. Usually the onset in those cases not attributed to trauma is gradual with a continuous persistent fever. In the six patients with a history of trauma, the symptoms gradually subsided for five to ten days. Pain and tenderness then reoccurred associated with evidence of infection. The presence of abdominal pain may be misleading. The pathology is often attributed to the gall bladder, appendix or other organs. In an abscess about the lower pole of the kidney, the symptoms may resemble those of a retrocecal appendicitis. As an example of such a diagnostic problem:

Case No. 70166, Mr. J. C., white, age 22. Three weeks prior to admission an aching pain was noted in the right hip aggravated by movement and riding in an automobile. Gonorrhea developed one week before admission and treatment was received. The patient had remained constantly in bed. There had been a persistent diarrhea for three days. More relief was noted with both thighs flexed on the abdomen. Admission temperature was 102.4°, pulse 138, and respiration 24. The patient was toxic and dehydrated. Tenderness was present in the right lower quadrant, less pronounced in the right upper quadrant and marked in the right costovertebral angle. Rigidity presented in the right lower quadrant extending into the right costoiliac region. Repeated urinalyses were negative. The blood leucocytes were 18,100 with polymorphonuclears 93 per cent. A retrocecal appendicitis was feared; appendectomy was performed with a McBurney incision. The appendix was retrocecal and only mildly injected. The blood leucocytes dropped to 9,000; however, there was a daily postoperative fever to 101° or 102°. On the eleventh postoperative day pain increased in the right costovertebral angle and radiated to the epigastrium. Diarrhea continued and tenderness increased in the right costovertebral angle. Rigidity became quite marked at this point. Blood leucocytes were 26,200 with 90 per cent neutrophiles. Five postoperative urinalyses were negative except for a few red blood cells in one specimen. Sixteen days after hospitalization an incision and drainage of the right costovertebral angle disclosed a perinephric abscess.

A past history of urinary symptoms was given by six patients. At admission 13 complained of dysuria, frequency or nocturia. Dysuria was the sole urinary symptom in nine. Eleven complained of nausea and vomiting and seven had had chills. One had pronounced night sweats and another a persistent diarrhea.

In the typical case of perinephritic abscess, the physical findings will vary with the duration of the disease and the location of the process. Authors agree that occasionally two months or longer may transpire before the correct diagnosis is apparent. In other instances the physical findings will be characteristic within a few days. This occurred in the following case:

Case No. 94162, Mr. R. B., white, age 17. Symptoms had been present for six weeks but more pronounced during the last three weeks. Paroxysms of severe sharp pain would occur in the right lumbar region, more severe at night and of variable duration. The pain often radiated to the right inguinal region and upper inner thigh. The attacks were followed by slight dysuria and frequency. The admission temperature was 100.6, pulse 88 and respiration 20. Complete p h y s i c a l examination was negative except for slight tenderness to percussion in the right costovertebral angle. Ureteral calculus, right, was t h o u g h t to be present. Seven urinalyses were negative e x c e p t for red blood cells and white blood cells in two specimens. Blood chemistry, hemaglobin and red blood count were normal.

The Wasserman and malarial smear were negative. The white blood count was 12,900 with polymorphonuclears 90 per cent. Cystoscopic, u r e t e r a l catheterization with u r i n e cultures and retrograde pyelograms were negative. Eight days after admission the pain and tenderness increased in the right costovertebral angle. D i r e c t questioning elicited a history of furunculosis during the last three months. Examination showed evidence of a right psoas spasm with pain to hyperextension of the right hip. The patient was more comfortable with the right hip flexed. There was fullness of the right costovertebral angle and

scoliosis of the spine with convexity to the left. Increased abdominal reflexes on the right and some hypersensitiveness of the right first lumbar nerve distribution were found. Perinephritic abscess, right, was suspected and incision and drainage in the right lumbar region corroborated the diagnosis.

A definite conclusion after one examination is not often possible. Repeated examinations are usually necessary in both horizontal and upright positions. Only 12 of the 30 operative cases were diagnosed correctly at admission.

TABLE V
Impression received by the clinician after one examination.

Impression	Number of Patients
Perinephritis Abscess	12
Pyelitis	6
Psoas Abscess	3
Pyelonephritis	2
Ureteral Calculus	2
Acute Appendicitis	2
Postoperative Pleurisy	1
Infectious Arthritis of Hip	1
Renal Calculus	1

Physical findings will include scoliosis of the spine with convexity toward the opposite side, spasm of the corresponding erector spinae muscle group, marked tenderness to percussion in the related costovertebral angle and palpable or percussion tenderness extending into the costo-iliac region with variable spasm of the underlying muscles. The patient seeks to keep the hip joint flexed and pain is experienced to extension and hyperextension. There will be a variable d e g r e e of voluntary rigidity of the paraumbilical and mesial anterior costo-iliac region. A mass may be palpated fading into the costo-iliac area. If investigated, skin parasthesias usually are elicited in the right lower quadrant and upper inner thigh, due to irritation of the ilioinguinal and iliohypogastric nerves. Often wth a low lying extensive abscess hypersensitiveness is present on the superior lateral aspect of the thigh, caused by irritation of the lateral cutaneous nerve. Actual swelling or edema of the lumbar region is a late sign.

In abscess about the upper pole of the kidney the diagnosis may be more difficult. Rigidity and tenderness are frequently absent, or present to a slight degree. If the abscess perforates the renal fascia and comes to underlie the diaphragm the signs and symptoms of a subphrenic abscess are superimposed.

On admission all patients had fever, in 28 the d a i l y r i s e was 101° or above. Twenty-five had a daily pulse rise to 100 or more.

TABLE VI

Daily elevations of temperature and pulse.

Degree of Temperature	Number of Patients	Pulse	Number of Patients
99-100	1	80-90	5
100-101	4	90-100	3
101-102	17	100-110	10
102-103	7	110-120	9
103-104	4	120-130	5
		130-140	1

Twenty-two of the 30 patients had a history of some degree of weight loss, nine losing over 20 pounds and 13 less than 20. The appetite was good in one, fair in 14 and poor in 18 cases.

TABLE VII

Degree of weight loss in 22 patients.

Pounds	Number of Patients
10-20	3
20-30	1
30-40	3
Marked weight loss	5
Some weight loss	9

The urinalysis is of little assistance in arriving at the diagnosis. Albumin was present in seven, pus cells in appreciable amounts in nine, and red cells in four.

A definite leucocytosis was present in the majority of the patients. Thirty had a white blood count ranging above 10,000 white cells. The lowest white blood count was 4,000 and the highest was 34,000. In 24 the differential polymorphonu c l e a r count was above 80 per cent.

TABLE VIII

A study of the degree of leucocytosis.

White Blood Count	Number of Patients
4- 6,000	1
6- 8,000	1
8-10,000	1
10-12,000	2
12-14,000	6
14-16,000	6
16-18,000	3
18-20,000	5
20-22,000	5
28-30,000	2
32-34,000	1

Some degree of secondary anemia was present in 11 of the 30 patients.

TABLE IX

A study of the degree of anemia present.

Red Blood Count	Number of Patients
2-2,500,000	1
2,5-3,000,000	1
3-3,500,000	4
3,5-4,000,000	5
4-4,500,000	7
4,5-5,000,000	10
5-6,000,000	2

The blood chemistry was elevated in two cases, both having definite kidney pathology.

Urography, cystoscopy and u r e t e r a l catheterization are of more value in the differentiation of a kidney lesion. Retrograde pyelograms in 10 cases demonstrated on the side of the lesion: ureteral stricture in three, some distortion of calyces in two, upward displacement of kidney in one and negative findings in f o u r. Intravenous pyelograms in eight cases showed on the involved side: poor function in four, upward displacement of the kidney in one, and negative findings in t h r e e. In the lateral view a forward displacement of the contrast filled kidney is helpful. Hilgenfeldt[2] emphasizes the v a l u e of the two films exposed at opposite extremes of the respiratory cycle for comparison of kidney mobility. Normal renal respiratory mobility v a r i e s from 1.5 to 6 cm. Mathe[3] stresses the importance of the lack of renal mobility as may be seen in the comparison of pyelograms taken in the supine and upright positions. Three centimeters is taken as a normal figure. An X-ray of the abdomen may show the kidney and psoas shadows to be indistinct or completely obliterated. Nine of 15 cases demonstrated this finding. Scoliosis of the lumbar spine with concavity toward the side of the lesion was less often present, being evident in seven of 15 X-rays. Occasionally the colon is displaced as is evident by the contained gas. Two such instances were recorded.

Dissimilar conditions may give rise to the erroneous impression of perinephric suppuration. Such pathology as colecystic disease, osteomyelitis of the twelfth rib, tuberculosis of the spine and hip, saccular aneurysm of the abdominal aorta, severe kidney infection, stone or malignancy, lumbar hernia, lumbar arthritis and retrocecal appendicitis may resemble a perinephric abscess in many respects.

No complications were encountered in

this series arising before incision and drainage. The danger of untoward extension of the neglected perinephritic abscess is ever present and is an added incentive for early diagnosis.

The prognosis of the operated perinephric abscess is good. The presence of kidney pathology will increase the operative hazard. One of the 30 operative patients expired. Simple incision and drainage was the procedure in all instances. In 19 the temperature was n o r m a l by the fifth postoperative day. No postoperative complications were encountered.

BIBLIOGRAPHY

1. Rolnik, H. D.: Archives of Surgery. 26:41-49, January, 1933.
2. Quoted from—Bacon, Ralph D.: Pennsylvania Medical Journal, 41:992, August, 1938.
3. Mathe, Charles Pierre: The Urologic and Cutaneous Review, September, 1934.

---o---

New Books

PRINCIPLES OF HUMAN ANATOMY, With Synopsis and Bibliography. By Chas. F. DeGaris, M.D., Ph.D. (Hopkins), Professor of Anatomy in the University of Oklahoma School of Medicine, Oklahoma City, Oklahoma; Formerly Associate in Anatomy at Johns Hopkins Medical School, Baltimore, Md. Ernst Lachmann, M.D., (University of Breslau), Assistant Professor of Anatomy in the University of Oklahoma School of Medicine, Oklahoma City, Oklahoma. And Ralph E. Chase, A.M., (University of Oklahoma), Instructor in Anatomy in the University of Oklahoma School of Medicine, Oklahoma City, Oklahoma. 239 pages, Cloth, $2.50 net. Lea & Febiger, Philadelphia, 1939.

This compend on Human Anatomy, the authors of which belong to the anatomical department of the School of Medicine of the University of Oklahoma is prepared essentially for teaching purposes and of course will be of great value to the medical student, especially when preparing for examinations. It also makes an excellent reference book for the busy surgeon who wishes to look up some particular point. This of course sets forth the principles of anatomy as revealed by dissection of the human body and follows the course of anatomy as given by our Medical School.

CANCER OF THE BREAST and CANCER OF THE UTERUS by Marion Ellsworth Anderson, A.B., M.D., Clinton, Iowa. Second Edition.

This brochure of 100 pages on Cancer of the Breast and Cancer of the Uterus has been compiled from observations of the author during the past 30 years. It is not particularly adapted for the surgeon, gynecologist or pathologist; but to the general practitioner, a discussion of this subject in this form will benefit him greatly by its perusal. The bibliography is complete and many authorities are quoted.

---o---

The depth of the burn in the tissues is relatively not as important as the extent of skin surface involved.—Hygeia.

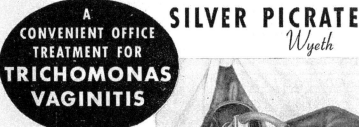
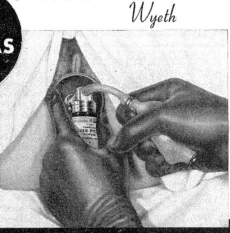
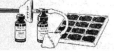

THE JOURNAL
OF THE
Oklahoma State Medical Association

Issued Monthly at McAlester, Oklahoma, under direction of the Council.

Copyright, 1939, by Oklahoma State Medical Association, McAlester, Oklahoma.

Vol. XXXII	JUNE	Number 6

DR. L. S. WILLOUR..Editor-in-Chief
McAlester, Oklahoma

DR. T. H. McCARLEY..............................Associate Editor
McAlester, Oklahoma

Entered at the Post Office at McAlester, Oklahoma, as second-class matter under the act of March 3rd, 1879.

This is the official Journal of the Oklahoma State Medical Association. All communications should be addressed to The Journal of the Oklahoma State Medical Association, McAlester Clinic, McAlester, Oklahoma. $4.00 per year; 40c per copy.

The editorial department is not responsible for the opinions expressed in the original articles of contributors.

Reprints of original articles will be supplied at actual cost provided request for them is attached to manuscripts or made in sufficient time before publication.

Articles sent this Journal for publication and all those read at the annual meetings of the State Association are the sole property of this Journal. The Journal relies on each individual contributor's strict adherence to this well-known rule of medical journalism. In the event an article sent this Journal for publication is published before appearance in The Journal the manuscript will be returned to the writer.

Failure to receive The Journal should call for immediate notification of the Editor, McAlester Clinic, McAlester, Oklahoma.

Local news of possible interest to the medical profession, notes on removals, changes of addresses, births, deaths and weddings will be gratefully received.

Advertising of articles, drugs or compounds unapproved by the Council on Pharmacy of the A. M. A., will not be accepted.

Advertising rates will be supplied on application.

It is suggested that wherever possible members of the State Association should patronize our advertisers in preference to others as a matter of fair reciprocity.

Printed by News-Capital Company, McAlester.

EDITORIAL

REPORT OF REFERENCE COMMITTEE ON THE WAGNER HEALTH BILL
By R. G. LELAND

There was considerable constructive legislation by the House of Delegates of the American Medical Association; however, the one outstanding action was taken relative to the Wagner Health Bill. This, of course, is published in the Journal of the A.M.A., but we feel that every member of the Oklahoma State Medical Association should read this document and we are consequently publishing it.

It is important that you read this and then it is important to do your part to see that the findings of the House of Delegates are carried out and each member can assist by bringing these findings to the attention of his Representatives and Senators. This is really constructive criticism.

* * * *

Your Reference Committee has carefully considered the Bill designated as S.-1620, "A Bill to provide for the general welfare by enabling the several states to make more adequate provision for public health, prevention and control of disease, maternal and child health services, construction and maintenance of needed hospitals and health centers, care of the sick, disability insurance, and training of personnel; to amend the Social Security Act; and for other purposes."

This bill was introduced by Senator Robert A. Wagner of New York, February 28, 1939, and is commonly referred to as the Wagner Health Bill. The bill itself provides that, if it be enacted, it may be cited as the "National Health Act of 1939." The purposes of the bill are sufficiently stated in the title, but the bill itself must be recognized as a proposed amendment to the Social Security Act of 1935. The bill is intended to make effective a national health program recommended by the Interdepartmental Committee to coordinate health and welfare activities.

The House of Delegates of the American Medical Association at its special session in Chicago, September 16, 1938, considered the National Health Program and adopted resolutions based on five recommendations contained in the program. It is important that this fact be borne in mind, for the bill, which was drafted long after these resolutions were adopted and at a time when the resolutions were presumably known to the proponents of this measure, does not recognize either the spirit or the text of these resolutions. Any criticism of this bill by the Association is not to be construed, therefore, as a repudiation of any of the principles adopted by the 1938 Special Session of the House of Delegates.

ANALYSIS OF THE BILL

S. 1620 proposes to amend Title V. of the Social Security Act—Grants to States for Maternal and Child Welfare—and Title VI —Public Health Work and Investigations —and proposes to add to the Social Security Act certain new titles; namely, Title

XII—Grants to S t a t e s for Hospital and Health Centers; Title XIII — Grants to States for Medical Care, and Title XIV— Grants to States for Temporary Disability Compensation.

Already some individuals and organized groups in the United States have appeared before the S e n a t e Subcommittee which has this bill under consideration and have urged its immediate enactment. Although the stated objectives of the Wagner Health Bill are generally recognized as desirable, your committee cannot approve the methods by which these objectives are to be attained.

Repeatedly, physicians and all o t h e r qualified professional groups have recommended the coordination and consolidation of the health activities of the Federal Government. The Wagner Health Bill leaves existing and proposed preventive and curative medical services widely s c a t t e r e d through several federal agencies.

This bill does not in any way safeguard the continued existence of the p r i v a t e practitioners who have always brought to the p e o p l e the benefits of scientific research and treatment.

It does not provide for the use of the thousands of vacant beds now available in hundreds of church and community hospitals.

The Wagner Health Bill proposes an extensive program in the field of "health, diagnostic, and treatment centers, institutions and related facilities," without defining their functions.

This bill proposes to make federal aid for medical care the rule rather than the exception, since it does not specifically limit its benefits to persons unable to pay for adequate medical care.

The Wagner Health Bill does not recognize the need for suitable food, sanitary housing and the improvement of other environmental conditions necessary to the continuous prevention of disease and promotion of health.

This bill insidiously promotes the development of a complete system of tax supported governmental medical care, thus undermining and debasing present standards of medical services.

The House of Delegates in September, 1938, urged compensation for the loss of wages during sickness. The W a g n e r Health Bill deviates from this suggestion by proposing to provide medical services in addition to compensation.

The Wagner Health Bill would authorize an enormous expansion of governmental medical services and therewith ultimately unlimited appropriations for its h e a l t h program. The funds necessary would be so great as to increase still further the present burdensome general taxation.

The Wagner Health Bill provides for supreme federal control. Rules and regulations must be promulgated by the Chief of the Children's Bureau in the Department of Labor, the Surgeon General of the Public Health Service, the F e d e r a l Emergency Administrator of Public Works, and the Social Security Board. These federal agents are given authority to disapprove plans proposed by the individual states.

The House of Delegates at its September, 1938, Session approved the expansion of preventive and other medical services when the need could be shown. The Wagner Health Bill prescribes no method for determining the nature and extent of the needs for which it proposes allotments of funds.

The provisions in the Wagner Health Bill that have never been considered by the House of Delegates are: the authorization of appropriations for studies, investigations and demonstrations, and the creation of federal and state advisory councils.

The Wagner Health Bill, as judged by the considerations that have been h e r e presented, is inconsistent with the fundamental principles of medical care established by years of scientific professional medical experience, and in the opinion of your committee it is, therefore, contrary to the best interests of the American people.

For years the health of the people of the United States, as measured by sickness and death rates, has been better than that of most foreign countries, and this improvement has been continuous. The fortunate h e a l t h conditions in the United States cannot be disassociated from the standards and methods of medical practice that have prevailed under the present s y s t e m of medical practice.

No other profession and no other organization has done more for the prevention of disease, the promotion of health and the care of the sick than have the medical profession and the American Medical Association. No other groups have shown more genuine sympathetic interest in human welfare.

The contribution of the individual members of the American Medical Association to medical care is universally regarded as monumental in total volume. The contribution of the American Medical Association, through a program of medical education and the activities of its numerous councils which safeguard medical service, give abundant proof of interest in the problems of the national health. It has given continued consideration to these problems, whereas others show concern with these proposals because of a present but, it is to be hoped, a temporary need for relief. These are the groups which request revolutionary legislative action as indispensable for the extension and further diffusion of health facilities.

In view of its record and in consideration of the responsibility which American social history and the nature of medical care have imposed on the medical profession, the American Medical Association would fail in its public trust if it neglected to express itself unmistakably and emphatically regarding any threat to the nation's health and well-being.

The American Medical Association must therefore, speaking with professional competence, oppose the Wagner Health Bill.

Nevertheless, recognizing the soundness of the principles stated in the resolutions adopted by the House of Delegates at its special Session in 1938, namely, the expansion of preventive medicine and public health where need can be shown, the extension of medical care for the indigent and the medically indigent where the need can be demonstrated, with local determination of needs and local control of measures to supply these needs, your committee would urge the development of a mechanism for meeting these needs within the philosophy of the American form of government and without damage to the quality of medical services.

This question, as it relates to the aid to be given by an individual state to its own counties, municipalities or other local political units, is not immediately before this Association. The answer is to be found in the individual state constitutions and state statutes. Counties, townships and municipalities are creatures of the individual states and can be molded and guided by the state for its own purposes. The individual state, itself, is not a creature of the Federal Government. The Federal Government is, as a matter of fact, a creature of the individual states.

The fundamental question is how and when a state should be given financial aid by the Federal Government out of the resources of the states as a whole, pooled in the Federal Treasury. Disasters, such as floods, dust storms, fire and epidemics, have long been recognized as justifying such Federal aid. No state or person has ever been heard to object to the use of funds out of the Federal Treasury for such purposes. No one has ever proposed, however, that because Federal aid is extended under such conditions to a state in distress, a corresponding aid must be extended to every other state, regardless of its need. Nor has anyone ever been heard to say that Federal aid to a state in distress, because of flood, dust storm, fire or epidemic, shall not be extended, unless and until the suffering state has produced from its own treasury a stated amount of money to aid in affording the relief. The development of such bizarre thinking may be traced to those who have originated within comparatively recent years the granting of Federal subsidies—sometimes referred to as "grants in aid"—to induce states to carry on intrastate activities suggested frequently in the first instance by officers and employes of the Federal Government. The use of Federal subsidies to accomplish such federally determined activities has invariably involved Federal control. Any state in actual need of financial aid from the Federal Government for the prevention of disease, the promotion of health and the care of the sick should be able to obtain aid in a medical emergency without stimulating every other state to seek and to accept similar aid and thus to have imposed on it the burden of Federal control.

The mechanism by which this end is to be accomplished, whether through a Federal Agency to which any state in need of Federal financial assistance can apply, or through a new a g e n c y created for this purpose or through responsible officers of existing Federal Agencies, m u s t be developed by the Executive and the Congress who are charged with these duties. Such method would afford to every state an agency to which it might a p p l y for Federal assistance to enable it to care for its own people without involving every other state in the Union or the entire government in the transaction, and without disturbing permanently the American concept of democratic government.

SUMMARY

1. The Wagner H e a l t h Bill does not recognize either the spirit or the text of the resolutions a d o p t e d by the House of Delegates of the American M e d i c a l Association in September, 1938.

2. The House of Delegates cannot approve the methods by which the objectives of the National Health Program are to be obtained.

3. The Wagner Health Bill does not safeguard in any way the continued existence of the private practitioners who have always brought to the people the benefits of scientific r e s e a r c h and treatment.

4. The Wagner Health Bill does not provide for the use of the thousands of v a c a n t beds now available in hundreds of church and community general hospitals.

5. This Bill proposes to make federal aid for medical care the rule rather than the exception.

6. The W a g n e r Health Bill does not recognize the need for suitable food, sanitary h o u s i n g and the improvement of other environmental conditions necessary to the continuous prevention of disease.

7. The Wagner Health B i l l insidiously promotes the development of a complete system of tax supported governmental medical care.

8. While the Wagner Health Bill provides compensation for loss of wages during illness, it also proposes to provide complete medical service in addition to such compensation.

9. The Wagner Health Bill provides for s u p r e m e federal control: federal agents are given authority to disapprove plans proposed by the individual states.

10. The Wagner Health Bill prescribes no method for determining the n a t u r e and extent of the needs for preventive and other medical services for which it proposes allotments of funds.

11. The Wagner Health Bill is inconsistent with the fundamental principles of medical care established by scientific medical experience and is therefore contrary to the best interests of the American people.

12. The fortunate health conditions which prevail in the United States cannot be disassociated from the prevailing standards and methods of medical practice.

13. No other profession and no o t h e r group have done more for the improvement of public health, the prevention of disease and the care of the sick than have the medical profession and the American Medical Association.

14. The American M e d i c a l Association would fail in its public trust if it neglected to express itself unmistakably and emphatically regarding any threat to the national health and well being. It must, therefore, speaking with professional competence, oppose the Wagner Health Bill.

15. The house of Delegates would urge the development of a m e c h a n i s m for meeting the needs for expansion of preventive medical services, extension of medical care for the indigent and the medically indigent, with local determination of needs and local control of administration, within the philosophy of the American form of government and without damage to the quality of medical service.

16. The fundamental question is how and when a state should be given financial aid by the Federal government out of the resources of the states as a whole, pooled in the Federal Treasury.

17. The bizarre thinking which evolved the system of F e d e r a l subsidies—sometimes called "grants - in - aid"—is used to induce states to carry on activities suggested frequently in the first instance by officers and employes of the Federal government.

18. The use of Federal subsidies to accomplish such Federally determined activities has invariably involved Federal control.

19. Any state in actual need for the prevention of disease, the promotion of health and the care of the sick should be able to obtain such aid in a medical emergency without stimulating every other state to seek and to accept similar aid, and thus to have imposed on it the burden of Federal control.

20. The mechanism by which this end is to be accomplished, whether through a Federal agency to which any state in need of Federal financial assistance can apply, or through a new agency created for this purpose or through responsible officers of existing Federal agencies, must be developed by the Executive and the Congress, who are charged with these duties.

21. Such a method would afford to every state an agency to which it might apply for Federal assistance without involving every other state in the Union or the entire government in the transaction.

22. Such a method would not d i s t u r b permanently the American concept of democratic government.

———————o———————

Transcript of Some Remarks Made by Dr. A. S. Risser before the House of Delegates at the State Meeting at Oklahoma City, May 3, 1939.

Mr. Speaker: It is my understanding that some 300 former members of the State M e d i c a l Association have not renewed their membership for the c u r r e n t year. This means that in a time of crisis, when we have had to make special efforts to prevent vicious legislation, when our expenses have been especially heavy, our income has been cut at the very outset some $3,000. (Besides these 300 there are almost 500 other physicians qualified to become members of our State Association but have never affiliated.) The members of our Legislative Committee, our Post Graduate Committee, the Councilors, and many other members in our organization besides paying their dues have given unstintedly of their t i m e, have sacrificed their own professional business to further the work of the organization while these 300 and the 500 others have refused both personal service and the service which the payment of their dues would furnish. This condition, men of the House of Delegates, seems manifestly unfair. You here are giving of your own time and are sacrificing "business" at home to take care of the business of the whole organization while these 300 probably remain at home to profit by your absence and by what you do here for organized medicine. Again I say, it is unfair. Personally I have never admired hitch-hikers nor their prototype, the men who rode the rods and the blind baggage on the railroad without paying for their transportation. If there ever was a time when organized medicine needs *all* qualified men *in the ranks* it is *now,* when in our own State a mass of vicious legislation is threatening and when the federal government is straining every nerve to foist State Medicine upon us. More than the dues of these laggards, their money, we need their *man power,* educated, coordinated, united. Each man in his own office and among his own clientele to explain to his patients the evils of letting down the bars to cults and commercialism, of lowering medical standards, the loss they will suffer if they accept the subterfuge of state medicine. At home, "at the grass roots," if you please, is where we must do our educating and win our votes for the good both of the people and of the profession. If we leave it to our legislators, human as they are and susceptible to influences which we can not offer, we have already lost the fight for high standards of medical service. Each of you must be a missionary henceforth to win these men and others into the organization, to help educate them, that they may help to educate the laity, that our work and high calling may not have been in vain.

Editorial Notes—Personal and General

DR. FOWLER BORDER, Mangum, attended clinics in New York and Rochester during May.

DR. GEORGE H. KIMBALL, Oklahoma City, attended the A.M.A. in St. Louis. He visited the Plastic Clinics at Barnes Hospital.

DR. E. H. SHULLER, McAlester, has recently been confined in Albert Pike Hospital and is now convalescing from an appendectomy.

DR. G. A. KILPATRICK, McAlester, has returned from New York where he attended the International College of Surgeons' Meeting.

DR. HOUSTON SPANGLER, who has been Superintendent of Valley View Hospital at Ada has accepted a position with the American College of Surgeons.

DR. W. K. HAYNIE, Durant, has returned from New Orleans, where he took post graduate work. DR. J. T. WHARTON, Durant, is taking post graduate work on diseases of the heart in New York. DR. JOHN A. HAYNIE, Durant, will spend the months of June and July taking post graduate work in diseases of children in the New York Post Graduate Medical School of Columbia University.

The Meeting of the American Medical Association was largely attended by the doctors from Oklahoma. We were officially well represented as the President, President-Elect, Secretary-Treasurer-Editor, Executive-Secretary, two Delegates, and two Alternates were present and all were quite attentive to the Sessions of the House of Delegates. We received much valuable information as to the workings of this body, the things which have been accomplished by the A. M. A., both in a constructive way and obstructive to some of the legislative proceedings which did not appear to be to the best interests and health of the people of this country or to the interests of the medical profession.

Southern Oklahoma Medical Association held their Forty-third Quarterly Session Tuesday, June 6, 1939, at Sulphur, Oklahoma, State Veterans Hospital, under the auspices of Murray County Medical Society.

The following secientific program was heard: 1:30 p.m., registration—State Veterans Hospital. 1:45 p.m., "Cancer of the Uterus; Illustrated by Lantern Slides"—Dr. C. P. Bondurant, Oklahoma City; discussion by Dr. E. C. Lindley, Duncan. 2:30 p.m., "Goiter: Its Types and Treatment"—Dr. Arthur E. Hertzler, Halstead, Kansas; discussion by Dr. F. L. Carson, Shawnee. 3:30 p.m., "Colitis" —Dr. Tate Miller, Dallas, Texas; discussion by Dr. J. M. Gordon, Ardmore. 4:15 p.m., "Management of Arteriosclerotic Heart Disease"—Dr. Russel C. Pigford, Tulsa, Oklahoma; discussion by Dr. Wm. F. Dean, Ada.

Entertainment: 5:30 p.m., Artesian Hotel, Kiwanis Rooms. 6:30 p.m., Chicken Barbecue Dinner at the Vendome in Platt National Park, music by Don Percell's Colored Band. Entertainment Committee for visiting ladies: Mrs. W. D. DeLay, Mrs. Ernest Rose, Mrs. Arthur Fowler.

Oklahoma Physician Honored

Dr. Henry H. Turner, Oklahoma City, was elected president of the American Therapeutic Association which met in St. Louis, May 12th and 13th.

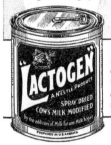

OBITUARIES

DR. E. L. BAGBY
From "The Bulletin," Enid, Oklahoma

Dr. E. L. Bagby was born in Plattsburg, Missouri, March 13, 1875, and died in Enid, Oklahoma, May 10, 1939, after an extended illness from Mitral Stenosis and Myocarditis. Dr. Bagby was a graduate of the Ensworth Medical College, St. Joseph, Missouri, with the class of 1898. After graduation he located in Oklahoma, practicing his profession at Ralston and Fairfax, later accepting a position on the staff of the Eastern Oklahoma Hospital. On the entry of the United States in the World War he volunteered his services and was commissioned as Captain, Medical Corps. In recognition of his previous training and experience he was assigned to the Neuro-Psychiatric unit at Camp Gordon, which assignment he held until the close of the war. After his release from military service he returned to Oklahoma and was appointed superintendent of the Western Oklahoma Hospital and continued in that capacity until 1931. In that year, due to a change in the personnel of the state administration, he was again assigned to the staff of the Eastern Oklahoma Hospital and remained there until his appointment to the superintendency of the Northern Oklahoma Hospital at Enid in 1935.

The report of his stewardship of the Northern Oklahoma Hospital received special commendation from those in authority and attracted state-wide attention. It was shown to be the most efficient and economically managed of any state institution, and without the sacrifice on any part of the care,

comforts or conveniences of the patients; on the contrary, all these were improved.

Early in 1939, realizing his health was failing, he entered a hospital in Kansas City, Missouri, for treatment. His condition gradually grew worse and realizing his days of usefulness were over he submitted his resignation to the Governor, put his worldly affairs in order and calmly awaited the event he knew was soon to come.

Dr. Bagby was a member of the Presbyterian Church, the Oklahoma State Medical Association, the Garfield County Medical Society, the Masonic Lodge at Fairfax, the Consistory at McAlester and the American Legion at Enid.

He is survived by his wife of the home, one daughter, Mrs. Milton Garber of Enid, and a brother, Dr. A. H. Bagby of Norman.

Funeral services were conducted at the First Presbyterian Church by the Rev. T. H. McDowell. Burial was in the Memorial Park cemetery, Enid.

> Sleep—sleep on, Doctor!
> Through the dark night, sleep on,
> Until the Master bids you waken
> To behold the glorious dawn.

———————o———————

ARE YOU LOOKING FOR A LOCATION? A county seat town of 3,000, county of 20,000, educational center, good agricultural territory, fruit growing, dairying and stockraising. Seven doctors in county, three over 70 years old. Good roads leading in every direction. Man with few years' experience could soon have an excellent practice. If you think you would fit into a small town and a general rural practice, write the Editor of this Journal for further information.

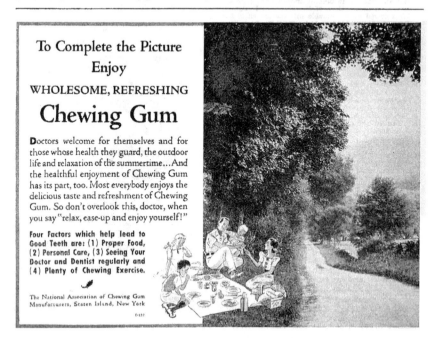

ABSTRACTS : REVIEWS : COMMENTS
and CORRESPONDENCE

SURGERY AND GYNECOLOGY
Abstracts, Reviews and Comments from
LeRoy Long Clinic
714 Medical Arts Building, Oklahoma City

Experiences With Employment of Suction in the Treatment of Acute Intestinal Obstruction, A Reiteration of the Indications, Contra-Indications, and Limitations of the Method: O. H. Wangensteen, M.D., F.A.C.S., C. E. Rea, M.D., B. A. Smith, Jr., M.D., and H. C. Schwyzer, M.D.; Surgery, Gynecology and Obstetrics, May, 1939, Vol. 68, No. 5, page 851.

I was at the Meeting of the Western Surgical Association in Omaha in December, 1938, when this paper was read to the Association by Dr. Wangensteen.

Seven years ago Wangensteen reported the successful decompression of three instances of acute mechanical intestinal obstruction by continuous suction applied to an indwelling tube. He then indicated that the chief role of conservative decompression in the management of mechanical obstruction of the bowel would probably be found to be in instances of adhesive obstruction in which drainage of the bowel would permit automatic reestablishment of luminal continuity. He asserted at that time that colonic obstruction accompanied by great distention and strangulating obstructions were absolute contra-indications to attempts at achieving release of the obstruction by suction.

He explained in the initial communication seven years ago that the idea that the small bowel when obstructed could be decompressed by an indwelling duodenal tube was no accidental observation but was the outgrowth of quantitative determinations of the gas and fluid escape through enterostomy tubes following operative relief of obstruction. It was observed that as soon as drainage of the bowel proximal to the obstruction permits reestablishment of intestinal continuity, the escape of gas and fluid through the enterostomy usually ceases.

He now feels that the indications and the contra-indications for the employment of suction applied to an indwelling duodenal tube in the management of acute obstruction have remained essentially the same during these past seven years. At this time he feels it necessary to reiterate a warning in relation to the indications for the employment of suction. "The practice of employing suction as a test procedure to indicate whether operation will be necessary leads only to deferment of appropriate treatment." He feels that neglect of this admonition is the most mischievous error into which one may fall in the application of suction to patients with intestinal obstruction.

He freely admits that suction in such instances is a "blind method" far more dim sighted than "blind enterostomy." It is highly important, therefore, that he who uses the method be acquainted not only with its shortcomings, but also with the intricacies and limitations of diagnosis of acute abdominal disorders.

In this paper he sets forth the experience of his

clinic with all types of mechanical obstruction of the small bowel over the seven-year interval between June 1, 1931, and June 1, 1938. The indications and contra-indications for the suction management of mechanical obstruction described in 1931 are reiterated and the lessons learned by him and his co-workers in the intervening years are reviewed. In this series among 156 patients treated for acute mechanical obstruction of the small intestine ,there were because of repetition of obstruction in some patients, 190 cases. There were 28 deaths in the entire group, a patient mortality of 17.9 per cent and a case mortality of 14.7 per cent.

In the group of cases in which suction was the primary treatment (though in a portion of these operation became necessary to effect a satisfactory decompression), there were 96 patients and 126 cases of obstruction. There were 15 deaths, a patient mortality of 15.6 per cent and a case mortality of 11.9 per cent. In those instances in which suction alone accomplished a satisfactory decompression and relief of the acute obstruction, there were 64 patients and 83 cases. Five deaths occurred, giving a patient mortality of 7.8 per cent and a case mortality of 6 per cent.

The suction group constituted 61.5 per cent by patient and 66.3 per cent by case of all patients treated for acute mechanical obstruction of the small intestine during the period under study. The number in which suction alone was the only direct attack employed for the relief of acute obstruction was 41 per cent by patient and 43.6 per cent by case of the entire group.

The conclusions reached by Wangensteen and his co-workers are as follows:

"Suction applied to an inlying duodenal tube has a definite role in the treatment of acute mechanical obstruction of the intestine. In suitable cases, complete relief of obstruction may be obtained through this agent alone. In a far larger group, suction is to be employed solely as an ancillary procedure, subordinate in importance to operative decompression or direct attack on the obstructive mechanism.

"The intelligent use of suction in the relief of acute intestinal obstruction rests upon the following:

"1. Ability to differentiate simple and strangulating types of obstruction.

"2. Ability to distinguish between acute obstruction of the large and small bowel.

"3. Appreciation of the importance of scout X-ray films for indicating the location of the obstruction and whether it is complete or incomplete, and for determining whether a satisfactory decompression is being obtained.

"4. Appreciation of the shortcomings of suction applied to an inlying duodenal tube in the management of acute intestinal obstruction.

"The experience of this clinic with the use of suction in the management of obstruction suggests that when employed on suitable indications and with full realization of its weaknesses and defects, it is a worth while addition to the available therapeutic agents, and that its rational use should lead to a definite, general lowering of the mortality of acute intestinal obstruction.

"The conservative decompression mode of management is a painstaking procedure which demands meticulous attention to detail. The limitations of the method demand also that patients accepted for treatment be passed upon by trained observers. Frequent periodic resurvey of the status of a patient being treated conservatively is mandatory. The consistently best results in the treatment of acute intestinal obstruction will be obtained in hospital practice when the management of all such cases is concentrated in the hands of a few individuals who are interested in and willing to devote time and energy which such cases should rightfully command."

LeRoy D. Long.

Primary Streptococcus and Pneumococcus Peritonitis in Children. A Study of 61 Cases with the Report of Two Interesting Recoveries: Edward T. Newell, Jr., M.D., Chattanooga, Tennessee. Surgery, Gynecology and Obstetrics, April, 1939, Vol. 68, No. 4, page 760.

The article begins with the following statement: "The idiopathic or so called 'primary' cases of peritonitis, caused by the Beta streptococcus and the various types of the pneumococcus, while not common in children, occur with greater frequency than is generally recognized." The lack of uniformity of management is indicated, some believing in surgical operation, while others depend upon non-surgical procedures. A significant statement is that "the question of the portal of entry remains obscure although the point has been much discussed."

The study is based upon an analysis of the cases of patients in Johns Hopkins Hospital (Harriet Lane Home for Children), and from the department of surgery over a period of 25 years. During that time there were 25 patients who had primary streptococcus peritonitis and 36 primary pneumococcus peritonitis, these being proved by both bacteriological and pathological study. The mortality in the streptococcus group reached the astounding figure of 92 per cent, and in the case of the pneumococcus group the mortality was 61.1 per cent. There were autopsy studies in the case of 36 of the unfortunate patients who succumbed.

The author indicates that he prefers to abandon the classification of pneumococcus peritonitis into two groups, as has usually been done—that is, fulminating and subacute. He suggests that pneumococcus peritonitis be divided into three groups. The first one he would call "idiopathic," apparently because there is no demonstrable cause. In the group studied there were just 12 children. The mortality was 50 per cent. In the second group he includes patients where the peritonitis is associated with an upper respiratory infection. In the entire group upon which this analysis is based, there were eight patients in this class. In this connection, he says: "The upper respiratory infection usually preceded the peritonitis, but when pneumonia developed, the pneumonia was usually secondary to a fulminating pneumococcal peritonitis." In this group—that is, the second group in the classification employed by the author—the mortality was 62.5 per cent. The third group consisted of 16 patients who had nephrosis as a predisposing cause. The mortality in this group was 68.7 per cent.

The grouping suggested by the author seems to be a rational one.

In children, pneumococcus peritonitis occurs most often from the first to the tenth year, while streptococcus peritonitis occurs frequently from six months to two years.

The author has not observed that there is any particular predilection for the development of pneumococcus peritonitis in females.

Abdominal pain is the most frequent early symptom. It may or may not be diffuse. Quite often it may be noticed first in the right lower abdomen. "Other important symptoms are loss of appetite with nausea, and persistent vomiting; fever and diarrhea are also common."

As a rule patients are admitted to hospital from one to four days from the beginning of the attack. In this connection the author makes the following statement: "There is a small group of patients who have been seen two to six weeks following an attack of abdominal pain with vomiting and fever, and who, on examination, appear emaciated and have a large peritoneal abscess. These abscesses usually occur in the pelvic region, but sometimes occur in the epigastric region simulating a pancreatic cyst."

The most common finding is abdominal distention with tenderness on deep palpation. Muscular rigidity is not pronounced in the average patient. The temperature usually ranges from 101° to 104°, and the white blood count may be from 20,000 to 40,000.

In the doubtful case, it is advised that some material from the abdominal cavity be secured through the employment of a spinal puncture needle. The author says that the procedure has been described by Neuhof and Cohen, Danzer, Pollock, and others. He says that abdominal puncture as described by Neuhof and Cohen in 1926 is "simple and safe procedure." He emphasizes that it is necessary to secure only a drop or two of pus in order to make a differential diagnosis.

In connection with the management of pneumococcus peritonitis, it is advised that, in addition to surgical exploration, pneumococcus rabbit serum be administered. The cases of two children are reported, in one of which there was a total dose of 295,000 units of anti-pneumococcus rabbit serum, intravenously, at two-hour intervals over a period of 12 hours. This was the total dose, it being divided into fractions given intravenously every two hours. In the case of the other patient, 300,000 units of anti-pneumococcus rabbit serum was administered in fractional doses over a period of some hours. The last patient mentioned in this analysis was discharged from the hospital 24 days after admission, but the other patient had several severe complications that protracted the stay in hospital.

In connection with surgical treatment, it is indicated that it is not wise to undertake it until there has been localization.

To sum up, it appears to be the opinion of the author that when there has been a diagnosis of pneumococcus peritonitis operative procedure be deferred until there are distinct evidences of localization. The second interesting, and probably important, observation made by the author is the remarkably satisfactory results following the intravenous employment of pneumococcus rabbit serum, as indicated in the case reports referred to above.

Streptococcus peritonitis is even more dangerous than pneumococcus peritonitis. Streptococcus peritonitis has been divided into the so-called "idiopathic" group and the group associated with erysipelas. In the group of so-called idiopathic streptococcus peritonitis studied by the author, there was a mortality of 88.2 per cent. In the erysipelas group there was a mortality of 100 per cent.

The author says: "The most important symptoms in the cases of streptococcus peritonitis in the order of their frequency are: vomiting, diarrhea, and abdominal pain. Many of these children are too young to reveal pain except by fretfulness and crying, particularly when the abdomen is touched.

"The more important signs are an acutely ill,

often moribund, child with considerable abdominal distention. The abdomen is tender to palpation but not board-like. In several of the cases the umbilicus and surrounding area for about two centimeters were red and swollen. Unfortunately, this is a late sign, which usually is seen in moribund infants. The children may have evidence of a streptococcus infection elsewhere, such as a pharyngitis, a cellulitis of the skin, or an otitis media. Leopold and Kaufman quote Mordlund's series of primary streptococcus peritonitis in which 63 per cent of the cases have a preceding upper respiratory infection."

The temperature varies from 103° to 106°, and the white blood count ranges from 2,700 to 45,000, the low count being seen most often in the moribund child.

It appears that conservative treatment of streptococcus peritonitis is the better procedure. It is suggested that sulfanilamide might be of considerable service.

LeRoy Long.

Statistical Analysis of One Thousand Abortions: Jalmar H. Simons, M.D., F.A.C.S.; American Journal of Obstetrics and Gynecology; May, 1939, Vol. 37, No. 5, page 840.

Though the accuracy of the data obtained from patients having abortion is recognized as unreliable, the author was able to draw the following conclusions:

"1. There is evidence of increasing number of abortions, principally in the self-induced group.

"2. Religion does not seem to be a deterrent to induction of abortion.

"3. As Taussig states, 'Abortion is a problem concerned with the married woman,' both induced and criminal, and it is in this group that the high death rate is obtained.

"4. Most spontaneous and induced abortions occur under three months and most often under 30 years of age, increasing again in incidence after 35.

"5. The total abortion incidence is one abortion to 2.7 pregnancies and one abortion to 1.6 confinements."

The mortality rate in this series was 1.9 per cent.

The conservative treatment was followed in the septic cases unless complicated by hemorrhage. In their septic patients evacuation of the uterus was done later if necessary when there was an approximately normal leucocyte count and temperature for a period of at least five days. They found the sedimentation time of little value in this respect.

Their nonseptic cases were evacuated, "almost routinely," in order to conserve blood and shorten hospitalization.

Repeated transfusions were of particular value in the infected patients and in those with hemorrhage. Practically all patients with a hemoglobin of 60 per cent or less received one or more transfusions. There is no statistical data given about sulfanilamide except that the author feels that it gives promise of great assistance in the septic patients. .

The operative incidence in this series of 1,000 abortions was 51 per cent. This means that 51 per cent of the patients had an evacuation of the uterus.

In the discussion Dr. Ralph R. Wilson of Kansas City gave the statistical information of 1,200 abortion patients handled in the Kansas City General Hospital between the years 1923 and 1933 inclusive.

"1. The Kansas City series had an incidence of 25.3 per cent of septic cases as compared to 18.9 per cent in the Minenapolis cases.

"2. Death rate in the Kansas City series was 3.6 per cent as compared to 1.9 per cent for Minneapolis.

"3. Each city had one case due to Bacillus welchii and lesions in the uterus were obtained from an autopsy of the Kansas City case.

"4. Hemorrhage caused no deaths in the Minneapolis series while in the Kansas City series, four died from hemorrhage.

"5. Conservative, supportive, and symptomatic measures were the characteristic modes of treatment in both institutions."

There are two other interesting points in the discussion of this paper. The patients reported in the original article were examined by student clerks and interns and later by residents and the staff surgeon. Dr. J. L. Bubis questioned the advisability of so much manipulation.

The advisability of the use of pituitrin and other oxytocics was raised and it was Dr. Simons' opinion that pituitrin and ergot, especially pituitrin, might be harmful in inducting too much activity of the uterine muscle and thereby breaking down leucocytic barriers to infected areas.

Comments: As in all statistical reviews, there are certain sources of error, but, on the other hand, with a group as large as this one, it is possible to gain a splendid idea of the frequency of a condition and the merits of the various means and methods of treatment.

Taussig, who collected the available statistics on abortion in this country and abroad came to certain definite conclusions about proper treatment. It was evident from his statistics that the nonseptic cases did well with immediate evacuation. It was equally pronounced that the septic patients did not do well with immediate evacuation and that the complication and death rate was higher. The most important observation in this direction was to the effect that the septic and the nonsepic patients could not be differentiated when the patient first presented herself and treatment was instituted. He, therefore, came to the conclusion that expectant treatment was to be preferred until it was definitely demonstrated whether an individual patient could be classified in the category of septic or nonseptic. It is agreed by all that the septic patient should be treated conservatively and it is, I feel justly, concluded by Taussig that the nonseptic patients should be treated expectantly until they definitely demonstrate themselves to be nonseptic.

The use of ergot as an oxytocic has been frequently discussed and there have been theoretical objections, but from a practical standpoint it is my feeling that ergot is a very valuable drug in the treatment of abortion and should be employed. While there is the objection that it interferes with the leucocytic barrier and that it possibly pushes the infection in both directions, there is the equally potent theoretical argument that it contracts the uterus and forms a more solid barrier against invasion.

There would certainly be little argument about the advisability of infrequent manipulation of the pelvis. Pelvic examination should not be done for two or three days unless there is excessive hemorrhage after the patient has been placed in bed.

In this direction, many immediate evacuations are done upon the basis of hemorrhage on admission to the hospital whereas most of these patients will greatly reduce the amount of bleeding when placed in bed and kept quiet for a reasonable time.

Wendell Long.

Three Hundred Cases of Extensive Conization of the Cervix: Robert J. Crossen, M.D., and George J. L. Wulff, M.D.; American Journal of Obstetrics and Gynecology; May, 1939, Vol. 37, No. 5, page 849.

A modification of Hyams electrode was employed with the cutting wire on the electrode placed farther away from the central tube in order to permit the removal of all the infected tissue.

This series of 300 patients was operated upon by 12 members of the visiting staff of the Barnes Hospital and nine members of the house staff. In several instances the procedure was combined with radium therapy, supravaginal hysterectomy, and vaginal plastic operations.

In the 300 patients there were 17 who had postoperative bleeding and were all controlled satisfactorily by packing.

Both to control postoperative bleeding, and to encourage better healing, the authors feel that conization of the extensive type should preferably be done in the postmenstrual period so as to allow two or three weeks for healing before the onset of the following menstruation.

They also feel that the use of Sturmdorf suture anteriorly and posteriorly and if necessary laterally allows conization in the more extensive cases of chronic cervicitis where Sturmdorf operation would otherwise be the one of choice. They likewise feel that the suturing diminishes the possibility of postoperative bleeding and they condemn coagulation of bleeding points at operation as encouraging postoperative hemorrhage.

In their series of patients there was one stricture and there were three others with a tendency to stricture. The authors believe that a small rubber tube inserted into the cervical canal for seven days in the more extensive cases will prevent stricture.

In this group there have been 15 pregnancies following treatment with five full-term easy deliveries, seven miscarriages and three patients now pregnant.

Comments: This is an interesting contribution to cervical surgery and in conjunction with other reports such as that of Norman Miller emphasizes more strongly the fact that conization has a desirable place in the treatment of chronic cervicitis. Though it is not emphasized in this article, conization of the cervix in this extensive manner is entirely a hospital procedure. Conization cannot replace the other means of treating the cervix, but it has a peculiar adaptability in the treatment of certain selected patients.

Wendell Long.

———————o———————

EYE, EAR, NOSE AND THROAT
Edited by Marvin D. Henley, M.D.
911 Medical Arts Building, Tulsa

A Glareless Illuminated Holder for Visual-Acuity Test Charts with Variable Intensity of Light. C. E. Ferree, Ph.D., and G. Rand, Ph.D., Baltimore. American Journal of Ophthalmology, April, 1939.

This interesting article with its accompanying illustrations has the following summary by the authors.

Some of the faults in the present illuminated chart holders are: excessive glare from the lighting device; glare on the surface of the chart; a very uneven and poorly diffused illumination of the test surface; high light and brightness on the lateral edges of the chart and near to the illuminating units; an unstandardized and a too high intensity of light; and lack of portability.

The chart holder described in this paper was devised to remedy these defects. A simple mechanical provision is also made for varying the intensity of illumination in continuous change from approximately zero to full without change in the color, composition, or placement of the light.

The following are some of the situations in which there is an important need for such a chart holder. (a) In all cases where there is a problem of the accurate and reproducible testing of visual acuity; such, for example, as in motor-vehicle departments, in the testing of railroad employes, in the air service of the army and navy, and in the commercial air service. A particular and very important case of this need is in the testing of vision in the public schools, where customarily no attempt is made at a complete refraction correction and all knowledge of the pupil's eyes and all advances or recessions of any condition, refractive or otherwise, is dependent upon the testing of vision. Apparently this testing from the kindergarten through college is in a very unfavorable condition. A great variety of test equipment is being used and very little attention is paid to the standardization of the illumination of the test charts. Results obtained under these conditions are of little value from the standpoint of comparative ratings or the determination of anything approximating a set of norms. (b) In the correction of errors of refraction. By preference many refractionists still use and always will use a printed chart. The best test conditions, particularly for visual acuity, are given by a properly illuminated printed chart. With it, a better state of adaption may be had, a clearer definition of the test object, a better diffusion of light, and a better background for seeing the test object than can be had by any other type of test equipment. Provided with the feature of variable illumination, ideal conditions for testing vision and for detecting and correcting errors of refraction are obtained with the printed chart.

Role of the Tonsil in Experimental Endocarditis. Ira Frank, M.D., and Margery Blahd, M.D., Chicago. Archives of Otolaryngology, March, 1939.

"The advisability of removing the palatine tonsils as a prophylactic measure for the various forms of endocarditis has long been a subject of controversy among clinicians. The advocates of tonsillectomy point out the decreased incidence of chronic cardiac disease in tonsillectomized persons, as borne out by certain studies. Their opponents, basing their opinions on studies of other groups, maintain that routine removal of tonsils for the prevention of cardiac disease is not based on conclusive data. Furthermore, some clinicians contend that actual harm can be done by removal of the tonsils, not only in the operative mortality but also in respect to the development of infections of the respiratory tract."

Previously the results were reported by the author on 25 dogs which had intravenous injections of a virulent hemolytic streptococcus from a pneumonic lesion. Endocarditis developed in 40 per cent or 10 dogs. The method of transferring the infection is different in this group of 30 dogs.

In two of 30 dogs, after intratonsillar injection of virulent beta hemolytic streptococci acute endocarditis developed. The hemolytic streptococci used had previously produced endocarditis in 40 per cent of a series of 25 dogs. Endocarditis did not develop in any of 15 tonsillectomized dogs after repeated introduction of the same organism into the tonsillar bed and parapharyngeal regions. Furthermore, repeated blood cultures of the control dogs remained sterile. It is likely that the tonsils played a role in the development of bacteremia and endocarditis in these experiments. The results of the investigations cannot be applied too readily to the patient. However, these studies present experimental confirmation of the favorable clinical results reported in the literature in respect to prophylactic tonsillectomy for endocarditis.

Electrocoagulation of Tonsils. Meyer L. Niedelman, M.D., Philadelphia. Annals of Otology, Rhinology and Laryngology, March, 1939.

This is a subject over which there has been and still is much controversy. The strongest advocates are those who have used this method and the bitterest critics are those who have not used the method at all or used it in an ill advised manner. The indications as listed by the author are:

1. General medical conditions such as hypertension, endocarditis, nephritis, tuberculosis, or any other chronic pulmonary conditions and syphilis. In this class can be included any condition which would contraindicate active surgery.

2. Neurotics who are in need of tonsillectomy but will not submit to surgery. This embraces a large class who, because of fear of hospitalization, hemorrhage or other complications, absolutely refuse to submit to surgery.

3. Blood dyscrasias, such as hemophilia, moderate secondary anemia, and long bleeding and coagulation time.

4. Economy to the patient. There are many patients, especially during the recent period of economic stress and strain, who cannot undergo hospitalization and the outlay of an immediate sum.

5. Postoperative tonsillar tabs or remnants and small lymphoid growths.

6. Those above the age of surgical risk.

7. Lingual tonsil and varix.

8. Carcinoma of the tonsil.

9. Public speakers and singers. There are no voice changes, as the vocal structures are left intact.

Contraindications

1. Children. The ideal here is obtained by general anesthesia, plus any of the recognized methods of enucleation.

2. For those who would rather have the work done at one sitting by surgical methods.

3. Acute or recent infections of throat or tonsils. Outside of these I know of no contraindications for electrocoagulation of the tonsils.

The author's conclusions are:

This is a safe and efficient method.

It does not and should not replace surgical removal, but is an alternative method in the removal of tonsils.

It is used when surgical removal is contraindicated.

A thorough knowledge of anatomy and surgical principles is prerequisite to the correct use of electrosurgical technique.

A method of anesthesia is outlined.

Two Cases of Brain Abscess Secondary to Acute Otitis Media, with Unusual Symptoms, Operation; Recovery. N. Asherson, London. The Journal of Laryngology and Otology, March, 1939.

Case one is a girl, age 5½ years. Left-sided otogenic temporo-sphenoidal lobe abscess. The following unusual features were noted.

1. The development of symptoms of intra-cranial pressure, following an attack of acute otitis media which had not given rise to any ear discharge—though the tympanic membrane was still inflamed, at the end of three weeks. At this time the symptoms were headache and vomiting, with papilloedema.

2. The slight changes in the cerebrospinal fluid, coupled with the papilloedema, suggested the diagnosis of a temporal lobe abscess. This was supported by the high polymorph white cell count.

3. The problem of the precise localization of the abscess was solved spontaneously by the brain and dura rapidly herniating though the first breach in the squama-exploration of this protrusion disclosed a large abscess.

4. The vagueness of any focal signs, in view of the large abscess disclosed, is a matter of comment. This suggests that the anterior part of the temporal lobe is a "silent" area in which a large abscess may collect insidiously. Hence this region must be exposed and explored when seeking for a suspected temporal lobe abscess in the absence of any definite localizing signs.

5. The abscess was exposed and drained through the squama, and not through the mastoid process.

Two and a half years later the child is still well.

Case two was in a child age three years. Acute temporal lobe abscess (right) secondary to an acute otitis media; with Jacksonian convulsions as the first and only symptom. Four days following a myringotomy a huge swelling developed suddenly and rapidly in front of the right ear. Comment on this case is as follows.

1. Until the onset of the convulsions and coma, no complication — inter-cranial or otherwise — was suspected. The brain abscess developed insidiously, and reached a large size without producing any symptoms to suggest its presence.

2. The location of the abscess. This was situated exactly beneath the superficial abscess which had developed on the fourth day after the myringotomy, in the temporal fossa. The dura was congested at this site and enabled the abscess to be easily located at the first incision.

3. The child was examined (after the temporal lobe abscess was drained) by Dr. C. P. Symonds, neurologist to the hospital. He looks upon the Jackson convulsions as due to an extension of the abscess to the cortex. He also notes that in such cases as this in which a Jacksonian convulsion is a leading symptom of the brain abscess, the convulsion is apt to recur at later dates, without the abscess necessarily pocketing or recurring.

4. When the second convulsion developed, it was unnecessary to reopen the wound as the temporal lobe could easily be explored by needle and syringe through the healed intact skin over it.

5. The brain abscess was drained through the squama.

Bilateral Endophthalmitis Complicating Pneumococcic Septicemia; Case Report. Jacob Reber, M.D., and Harold G. Scheie, M.D., Philadelphia. Archives of Ophthalmology, May, 1938.

The first manifestation of a generalized septicemia was the appearance of the eye infection. This is the report of a case of a man age 48, who on December 1, 1937, ran a tack in his foot (he was an upholsterer). The usual swelling and lymphangitis was treated, apparently successfully. Two weeks from the time of the accident he had a severe frontal headache and complained of a dimness of vision in each eye. Swelling followed the next day with more pain and a chill with an elevation of temperature. A consulting ophthalmologist found a typical endophthalmitis-corneas hazy-pupils small, irregular and fixed-posterior synechiae-iris hemorrhagic-fundus could not be seen—vision reduced to light perception. He was admitted to the hospital with a temperature of 103. The family and past history were of no importance. W.B.C. 20,500 with 82 polys. X-ray showed some cloudiness in the ethmoids, which was ruled of no importance by the otolaryngologist. Other laboratory work was negative except the blood culture which showed type 16 pneumococcus. The patient ran a septic temperature (101°-105°). Culture from the nose showed staphylococcus aureus. The endophthalmitis gradually subsided —vision being only light perception. Medication consisted of sulfanilimide, daily transfusions and oral administration of ethylhydrocupreine hydrochloride, all of which were apparently of no avail. The patient died January 7, 1938. The blood culture remained positive. The autopsy showed among other things a phlebitis of the left femoral vein (the septic focus), the aspirated fluid obtained from the left cultured type 16 pneumococcus.

The unusual features of the case are that the ocular lesion was the first manifestation of a generalized septicemia and that there was an involvement of both eyes. According to Sherer systemic infections may show in the eye as iridocyclitis, metastatic ophthalmitis, septic retinitis of Roth and ring abscess of the cornea. In Groenouw's 166 cases reported in metastatic lesions of the eye from general sepsis, 85 per cent of the bilateral eye involvements were fatal.

"The physical factor for the production of the septic choroiditis or retinitis, as the case may be, is the lodging of the circulating organisms in either a ciliary or a retinal artery. These infected emboli set up a localized purulent inflammation, which, if it involves the coats of the eyeball and the surrounding orbital tissues, often results in spontaneous rupture of the sclera."

Some New Data Concerning the Pathology and Treatment of Ozaena. Dr. Geza Halasz, Budapest. The Journal of Laryngology and Otology, May, 1939.

This condition produces an inflammation and atrophy of the mucosa. Due to inadequate nutrition and degeneration the many glands in the nose become atrophic. There naturally follows that there is an insufficient supply of cleansing mucus in the nose. Then in the subsequent culture-media bacteria thrive and grow and there is present more pseudo-membranes and malodorous disintegration.

According to the author the ozaenous mucosa shows under the microscope a marked fibrosis, deficiency of cells, an additional amount of connective tissue and a shriveling of the turbinate bones. Mucous glands are diminished, the number of blood vessels are reduced, large collections of lymphocytes are to be found as well as hyaline and pigment-degeneration.

Atrophy is produced by general cachexia, inactivity, pressure and chemical injury but in this instance another factor enters, i.e. trophoneurotic troubles. The author demonstrated several years ago that in a pharyngitis after a tonsillectomy the infection was due mostly to an absence of a tonsillar endocrine function and could be cured by a subcutaneous administration of tonsillar extracts.

After a discussion of the relation of adenoids and tonsils in the increased amount of activity in a patient with ozaena, the author states that he believes that destruction or misdevelopment of the lymphatic ring is the primary cause of ozaena. He found that in his patients so afflicted the greater number had suffered from tonsillitis and subsequent pharyngitis in childhood and that their tonsils were scarcely visible, atrophic, pale and containing little lymphoid tissue. Adenoid vegetation was entirely absent. He states: "Hypoplasia of the tonsils and the adenoid tissue diminishes hormonal output, and the lack of hormone becomes manifest as ozaena."

After many experiments he prepared the following solution: Physostigmini gta. 0.005, Potassi Sulf. 0.075, Acidi phosphorici 0.01, Aqu. dest. bister, ad 10.0, an isotonic solution. Injection of 0.5 c. cm. every day or every other day was made in each tonsil of the ozaena patient. The technique is described and is very simple as the injection is made directly into the tonsil. The result was: the nasal mucosa recovered its normal color and the vessels filled with blood; false membranes and foetor disappeared. The injections were made at longer intervals, a week or in some cases a month apart, after the patient was well under control. He likens the treatment to that of insulin in diabetics.

Many of the conflicting theories of ozaena are enumerated with their authors. The author's short summary is as follows:

1. Ozaena is caused by lack of tonsillar hormone.

2. Tonsils are specific endocrine glands, which regulate the vessels of the upper respiratory tract. The hormone is a substance similar to acetylcholine.

3. Successful treatment of ozaena has been achieved by means of intra-tonsillar injections of potassium and phyostigmine which inhibit the action of cholin-esterase.

A bibliography is appended.

———o———

PLASTIC SURGERY
Edited by
GEO. H. KIMBALL, M.D., F.A.C.S.
404 Medical Arts Building, Oklahoma City

Painless Rendering Closure of Superficial Wounds. Michael Gosis, South Ozone Park, N. Y., American Journal of Surgery, May, 1939.

The author presents a method of closing superficial wounds and lacerations which he has found practical and fundamentally sound. He makes no claim to priority of discovery but relates in simple detail the method which he states is an outgrowth of the time honored procedure of closing small superficial wounds with butterfly strips of adhesive. He states that the latter is not very applicable when one desires perfect approximation, for the broad base needed for the adhesive to adhere to the skin prevents the use of many strips placed close together as would be required. Further closing a wound with a broad piece of tape causes irritation of the skin edges which does not

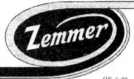

lend itself to the formation of hairline or almost invisible scars.

He states that out of 30 cases which he has done in the past two years, 29 of them had practically invisible resultant scars. After a few months during which time the initial erythema subsided, the scars were as satisfactory as those produced in plastic surgery.

The technique is described as used when there is no co-existent laceration of muscle or deep fascia. The wound is wiped dry and edges approximated. The adhesive is to be flamed before applying and then, skin over which it is to be applied should be painted with compound tincture of benzoin. The adhesive will adhere to the skin for at least 10 days with no appreciable loosening or irritation. The one-half inch strips of adhesive are placed one-fourth inch from the edge of the wound and extend to about three-fourths inch beyond the end of the wound. Wider strips may be used in case of longer wounds and narrower strips in case of small areas as nose and fingers.

The adhesive is then sutured with one continuous suture beginning outside the end of the laceration and running across from one strip of tape to the other the full length of the tape. It is best to have no elevation of the adhesive near the wound for insertion of needle and thread. Simply slip the needle between the skin and the superimposed tape without disturbing the bond between the two.

In irregular lacerations where sharp angles or corners of tissue must be approximated one might apply preliminary strips at the angles and then the tape as above outlined is sutured into place. Where the angle is not too acute strips may be placed parallel to the general direction of the wound edges without applying preliminary tension strips. Such lacerations may be about the fingers or palm of hand. In these cases the adhesive strips were placed parallel to the wound edges but they were made to hug the skin and invaginate at the creases. The first sutures taken in such situations are interrupted in order to approximate the crease marks, then the continuous suture is run along the length of the wound. After the sutures are in place it is sometimes advisable to place additional adhesive at right angles to the suture strips.

The author states that cleansing the wound with soap and water after picking out all gross contaminants and blood clots with thumb forceps, is sufficient. Where debris is found he states that a rubber drain may be placed into the depths of the wound and brought out at one end. This is left in for 24 hours. If debridement is necessary this method of wound closure is applicable, provided too much tissue is not removed. When deep tension sutures are not required for coaptation of skin edges suture of parallel adhesive strips with a broad base will serve as well.

The author states that when deep fascia and muscle lacerations are present requiring separate sutures, the wound cavity is filled with five per cent novocaine solution and the fluid allowed to remain there for about three minutes. This will anesthetize the deeper tissues and then the closure may be made in the manner described. Removal of sutures from five to seven days is the simplest

procedure. The adhesive is loosened at one end and is removed sutures and all at one sweep. There is none of the pain due to tugging at the usual type of skin sutures.

Conclusion: This method is advocated for use in suitable wounds. Relieving the patient from unnecessary pain is adequate compensation for the extra precautions taken. Wound healing in cases not grossly infected at the time of injury is promoted by lessening the a m o u n t of additional trauma inflicted on a wound by penetrating sutures. Should infection ensue there is no obstacle to self-drainage. Suture removal in the event of a clean or infected wound is rendered absolutely painless.

Comment: The author apparently has very good results with this method of wound closure. The illustrations are adequate for anyone interested in the procedure. Personally I close wounds with sutures. The pain that is associated with closure can be avoided by local anesthetic and the pain of removing sutures is not worth mentioning in my opinion if horse hair or waxed silk is employed. Most people seem to have more fear of the procedure of suture removal because of what they have heard other epople say. It is certainly exaggerated.

Immediate Full Thickness Grafts to Finger Tips. Jewett V. Reed, M.D., F.A.C.S., and A. K. Harcourt, M.D., Indianapolis, Indiana. S. G. and O. May, 1939.

The authors describe a minor operation to be used in certain types of injury to the finger end which averts necessity for amputation or its alternative, thin skinned, painful scar. This operation is applicable and is used considerably in workingmens' hand injuries where there is loss of soft tissues of the finger usually without loss of bone. The tissue loss may involve the distal tip, skin, and soft tissues sometimes exposing the bone. It may include one side of the whole distal phalanx sometimes involving the nail. It may remove the whole palmar pad.

The types of injury requiring the suggested graft to the finger tip are as follows: 1. Slice wound tip, not exposing bone. 2. Loss of one side of distal segment and nail. 3. Slice wound of pad without exposing bone. 4. Loss of soft tissues side of digit without injuring the nail. 5. Avulsion of pad of finger exposing palmar aspect of distal phalanx. 6. Loss of soft tissue exposing tip of phalanx.

The author has shown diagrammatic photos of each type above named and follows it with a chronological chart analysis of results in 53 cases, all patients being white males with two exceptions. Some of the injuries named are as follows: Mashed in steel girders, cut with steel chip pad amputated, cut with power saw, caught in joiner, caught in meat slicer, caught in gears, caught in punch press, caught in cogs, caught in bottle crowner, pinched between cable and drum, caught in food grinder, pinched in roller, etc.

A very comprehensive outline of the procedure used to transfer full thickness grafts to injured finger tips, is related by the authors. The suggested donor site in most cases is usually the volar aspect of the proximal fourth of the same forearm. In females the lateral aspect of the thigh

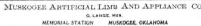
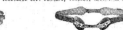
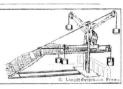

near the ilium is chosen in an effort to place the scar where it will be at all times covered. The pattern is outlined with a sharp scalpel. Near the margin of the graft care must be taken to separate the skin from subcutaneous tissue accurately. Graft is immediately transferred to the injured finger and set into place by means of very small cutting edge needles and "A" silk. Sutures should be interrupted as continuous sutures choke off blood supply.

The patient is advised to keep the hand dependent a part of the time after a dry gauze quare is placed over the graft and held in place with a moderately tight bandage. The dressings are not changed for five days. Sutures not removed from the perimeter of the graft for two weeks. Usually at the end of five days the graft is pink and dry and appears similar to the surrounding skin except that fine hairs transferred in the graft, may be seen.

The authors state instances and results in the practice of the Indianapolis Industrial Clinic and give an analysis table from an economic viewpoint. Under the Indiana Compensation Law specific permanent impairment allowances are made for the loss of each digit.

Conclusions: An immediate full thickness graft applied to a finger end suffering soft tissue loss, conserves length and averts painful scar. The technique is simple. The end results are satisfactory to the individual, to the surgeon and to the person or to the company liable for the injury.

———————o———————

ORTHOPAEDIC SURGERY
Edited by Earl D. McBride, M.D., F.A.C.S.
717 North Robinson Street, Oklahoma City

The April, 1939, issue of the American Journal of Surgery is devoted to a symposium on surgery of the extremities. It is the opinion of those abstracting that the information contained in this particular volume is invaluable to those interested in surgery of the extremities. It is impossible to abstract for the State Journal enough of the articles to be of more than brief interest. However, two articles will be abstracted to show primarily the value of the entire volume. These particular articles were chosen because this type of fracture is so frequently mistreated.

———————

"Fractures of the Carpal (Navicular) Scaphoid," Edward K. Cravener, and Donald G. McElroy, Schenectady, N. Y. Amer. Jr. of Surg. Inc. New Series, Vol. XLIV, No. 1, April, 1939.

The authors try to estimate the frequency of c a r p a l scaphoid or navicular fractures. They probably constitute around eight to nine per cent of all hand fractures. However, other writers give higher and some give lower incidences. The scaphoid bone is particularly valuable in that it is the wedge or keystone of the wrist arch. In the absence of this the wrist is very insecure. The bone is described as consisting of a body, constricting waist and a tuberosity, named in order from the proximal to the distal ends. The waist gives insertion to the radiocarpal ligaments and also to the blood vessels. This is particularly important in discussing healing.

Fractures through the tuberosities will heal even if somewhat neglected. Waist or body fractures are different and are the basis for the many treatments for fractures of the navicular. Many theories exist as to the cause of this; primarily that of embarrassed blood supply, or interposition of the radial-carpal ligament. However, the primary factor in union is complete prolonged immobilization.

In making a diagnosis of fracture of the navicular, first the X-ray is important. This is best when taken with the wrist slightly dorsiflexed. In this position the navicular is exposed its whole length and its overlying shadows are eliminated. This is done most easily with the fist clenched so that the wrist is kept slightly dorsiflexed and is firm. Any specific symptoms of navicular fracture are of no great importance since the advent of X-ray since any painful wrist after trauma should be submitted to X-ray examination.

Eight different types of fractures of this bone are described.

The authors recommended treatment as follows: In the case of tuberosity fractures, hold the wrist for three weeks in dorsiflexion and radial deviation. Fractures through the low waist should be kept in fixation at least eight weeks and then check for X-ray evidence for union before permitting free use of the wrist. In complicated old fractures through the upper waist or body, these must be exposed surgically and autogenous bone graft passed through from the distal to the proximal fragment. This has been modified some by making several drill holes through the fragments across the fracture line and pass the graft through one of these. This is not simple surgery and should not be undertaken by one not familiar with the anatomy of the wrist.

The authors feel that surgery is conservative treatment in this type of fracture in that the usual result will be a definitely painful wrist which may later require removal of a portion of the bone. They cite the fact that X-ray should be taken accurately and carefully. Plaster fixation is used, or possibly splint fixation only in tuberosity fractures. In low waist fractures, possibly plaster or splint fixation. In all high waist and body fractures drilling and bone pegging are used. In the case of a degenerated fragment resection is used. When speed and the assurance of a good result are desired, drilling and bone graft are advised except in fractures of the tuberosity, or in cases of degenerative arthritis.

———————

"The Diagnosis and Treatment of Fractures of the Pelvis and Their Complications," Grover C. Weil, Edwin M. Price and Harold W. Rusbridge. Pittsburgh, Pa. Amer. Jr. of Surg. Inc. New Series Vol. XLIV, No. 1, April, 1939.

This fracture is not a rare fracture in modern transportation methods and is estimated to include three per cent of all skeletal fractures. Any disturbed continuity of the pelvis and its normal anatomical relationship causes severe changes in body function and every effort should be made to secure perfect reduction. The high mortality from 10 to 30 per cent causes these fractures to be placed in the realms of major injury.

The anatomy of the pelvis is reviewed briefly and the functions, both of the viscera and the body as a whole; standing and sitting.

The three particular points of weakness of the pelvis are: (1) midway between the symphysis pubis and the acetabulum; (2) the symphysis pubis; and (3) a trifle external to both sacroiliac joints.

In the simpler forms of fracture involving one of the rami on either side, or a moderate separation of the symphysis, without loss of continuity of the pelvic ring, only mild physical complaints may be recorded. With the history of some form of trauma, one can find tenderness over some portion of the pelvic ring particularly in the perineal region, over the adductor muscles and the most typical sign is that of pain on compression of the iliac crests. X-ray is positive evidence. Occasionally intestinal ileus occurs in mild injury. In severer forms of injury the physical signs include those in the pelvis plus those from injury to the viscera.

The symptoms and physical findings in such cases include shock in varying stages, inability to demonstrate proper function of one or both lower limbs by voluntary elevation while reclining. This attempt is always painful about the groin, inguinal and pubic regions. The bladder may be found distened and the abdomen may show distension with muscular resistance. Lateral compression of the iliac crests or hip joints imparts a giving sensation, showing a lack of firmness and crepitus may be present. Pain may be produced by palpation along the pelvic ring, depending on the location of the fracture. There may be beginning paralytic ileus, especially in severe types.

Rectal examination may show a fragment to press upon the rectal wall or a sharp spicule of bone may rupture into the rectum. There is either anuria or definite rupture of the urethra. In case of rupture there always appears some evidence of blood at the urethral orifice. There may be extravasation of hemorrhage or urine into the soft tissues. Gas bacillus infection, developing after rupture of the rectal walls, appears early and the presence of bluish-brown, discolored form of cellulitis of the skin and subcutaneous tissues, spreading over the perineum, scrotum and abdominal wall, with emphysema, point definitely to its presence.

The authors have found that good first aid care followed by immediate treatment of the fractures offers the best solution for prevention of shock and after effects. The patients are transported carefully in splints; they are brought to the hospital. After careful preliminary examination, X-ray is made and if injury is not too severe the patient is put to bed, traction is applied to the limb and hammock adjusted as is necessary for the type of fracture. Intestinal ileus is anticipated and the patient is usually given cascara pills followed by enema, consisting of soap suds, glycerin and sodium bicarbonate, in cases where not contraindicated. Sedatives are given for rest at night. For severe types of ileus the usual surgical procedures are adopted such as turpentine stupes, surgical pitrutrin, physostigmine, pitressin and prostigmine. Often more heroic methods are necessary, with the use of paravertebral or intraspinal injections of novocaine. Continuous oxygen inhalation is helpful.

In reduction of the severe fractures, X-ray is necessary to determine the exact procedure and treatment is carried out according to this.

The most frequent and important complications are: shock, ileus, hemorrhage, rupture of the rectum, urogenital injuries and infections. It is important that these complications be kept in mind and treatment instituted immediately on the diagnosis of any of them.

All patients, except those with very minor fractures, are confined to bed for a period of eight to ten weeks, after which the patient is confined to wheel chair for two weeks, before allowing gradual body weight. Physical therapy, such as infra-red, massage or diathermy is instituted, after the second week.

* * *

It is the opinion of the abstractors that the volume of the American Journal of Surgery mentioned above, should be in the library of every doctor who does traumatic surgery or surgery of the extremities.

"Gas-Bacillus Infection as a Complication of Fractures," David M. Bosworth, New York City. Jr. Bone & Joint Surg., Vol XX, No. 4, October, 1938.

The author reviews the history of gas-bacillus infection, particularly that of the men who have discovered the various organisms and its effect during the wars. The bacteriology is then discussed, followed by the pathology. Diagnosis of this condition is made on the odor, which may or may not be present. "The most outstanding impression is that of a very sick patient, slightly disoriented, complaining of great pain if asked, but otherwise lying quietly with a flushed face, very rapid pulse and no great temperature." The patient is sick and toxic way beyond the bounds indicated by temperature alone. Percussion of the skin near the wound area usually gives a tympanites and crepitus. Discoloration appears gradually and later X-ray examination shows gas in the soft tissues. This is not positive, however, unless an increase of gas is seen on successive films. A smear from the wound will show anaerobic bacteria, which is absolutely diagnostic.

Treatment: The author feels first that prophylactic doses of tetanus and gas antiserum should be given in every case of compound fracture. In case of a positive infection, curative serum therapy is commenced immediately before even the bacteriological diagnosis is positive. The author uses 20 c.c. doses of refined polyvalent serum intravenously every two hours until the infection is under control. No intramuscular serum has been used. If the case is operative, drainage is usually sufficient through the wound. If only a compound wound is present it should be enlarged through the skin and fascial planes with due regard for vessels and nerves. Extensive debridement or removal of muscles should be avoided. Repeated massive infusions of glucose and saline are routinely used. Support of the part in metal splints with continuous moist dressings to encourage drainage is strongly advised. The author states that amputation is senseless and harmful and all reports to date will bear this out. X-ray therapy has been reported favorably and the author thinks that cannot do harm and may do good. However, this should not take the place of the antiserum.

The author cites three cases. One case received a total of 400,000 units of the antiserum before he was successfully healed.

Comment: It still seems reasonable to us in this part of the country to amputate in gas gangrene infections. However, I believe that as we study our cases we will likely depend more on our serum and less upon surgery. The final word in this has not yet been stated.

---o---

UROLOGY
Edited by D. W. Branham, M.D.
514 Medical Arts Building, Oklahoma City

Preoperative Prostatic Mortality. W. J. Engel, Cleveland Clinic, Cleveland, Ohio. Journal of Urology, April, 1939.

Dr. Engle has critically analyzed 54 cases of prostatic obstruction who died before surgery was performed in an attempt to determine the predisposing factors in his preoperative management that may possibly have favored such a result.

In his opinion 40 or 74 per cent were what might have been classified as unavoidable but 14 or 26 per cent could have been prevented by a different technique of preoperative care. He believes that the dangers attendant with the first catheterization and instrumentation of the patient and also the inlying urethral catheter condemned as a routine procedure for preoperative drainage is underestimated.

He summarizes his plan of preoperative management under four headings:

1. Patients who are in excellent condition as far as blood nitrogen without complete retention and a small amount of residual urine have surgery performed without preliminary catheterization.

2. Patients who have complete retention but are

in good condition otherwise are intermittently catheterized for a short while before surgery is performed.

3. Those patients whose condition requires preliminary catheter drainage have a suprapubic vesical puncture made which is followed by the insertion of a catheter.

4. Inlying catheters for those in whom a suprapubic puncture is contraindicated, such as, a badly infected bladder.

Since this plan of management has been introduced the author states that not only the mortality rate has been reduced but patients have a smoother convalescence following surgery.

A Task Of All the People. Ray Lyman Wilbur, M.D. Journal of Social Hygiene, March, 1939.

Excerpts from an address by Dr. Wilbur before the Committee of Fifteen in Chicago, February 13, 1939.

"We have now reached the stage where we know something of the costs of syphilis and gonorrhea. We have adequate remedies for their treatment. We know procedures that can protect many of the innocent. The problem is simply one of how to get started with the proper campaign and how to carry it on over the years in order that these diseases may be made at least rare, rather than common."

"When we realize that 50 per cent of venereal patients acquire these diseases innocently, accounting for the congenital cases and other accidental infections, and that the other 50 per cent is acquired through either public or clandestine prostitution, and sexual promiscuity, we see that we face a problem where we ought to make every effort for the protection of youth, at least."

"The greatest single disseminator of these diseases is the prostitute. The tavern with its present freedom gives her easy refuge and makes it easy for her to entice boys and young men. There have been all sorts of schemes to control the so-called "women of the street." None of them have been completely satisfactory. Experience has shown that the one thing that is most important of all is to make her difficult of access. In that way there is the most likelihood of giving protection to youth. We cannot stop the sophisticate but we can protect minors. No scheme of segregation or of medical examination of the prostitute has stood up as of value in the control of the spread of the gonococcus and the spirochete. A certificate of health given to a prostitute may be a death certificate with a delayed reaction for the young man involved."

"We have been slipping back steadily for over a decade, have become more careless in the control of prostitution, have done less to protect our children, have a wider spread of unsavory literature, and have more alcohol being consumed by our boys and girls."

"We cannot turn this job over to the government alone. But every good citizen, parent, teacher, church member, has a responsibility at least to youth in seeing that they obtain satisfactory education and sufficient information on these important and prevalent diseases."

Effect of Alcohol on Normal Kidney and Kidney of Bright's Disease. Maurice Bruger, M.D., S. Arthur Localio, M.D., and Nobel W. Guthrie, M.D., New York. The Journal of the American Medical Association, May 6, 1939.

Twenty-one patients were studied of whom five were free from renal diease, five had acute diffuse glomerular nephritis and five had arteriosclerotic nephritis. Alcohol was administered to these individuals in appropriate amounts under a standardized routine as far as rest and dietary intake was concerned. Various laboratory examinations of the urine were made as well as several different renal functional tests were performed to evaluate the effect of alcohol on the kidney.

Their conclusions were:

"Alcohol or whiskey in moderate doses rarely augments the proteinuria of patients with Bright's disease. Moderate diuresis may be induced even in the presence of marked impairment of renal function. Alcohol or whiskey has no deleterious effect on the kidneys of normal subjects, nor does it aggravate the renal lesion in patients with acute or chronic diffuse glomerular nephritis. In patients with arteriosclerotic nephritis (nephrosclerosis) the ingestion of alcohol or of whiskey is followed frequently by a transient increase in the number of red and white blood cells and casts excreted in the urine and by a temporary diminution in renal function."

Physiological Bladder Changes During Pregnancy and the Puerperium. S. Richard Muellner. Journal of Urology, May, 1939.

The effects of pregnancy on the upper urinary tract have been repeatedly demonstrated. The possibility that pregnancy might produce similar changes in tone and capacity of the bladder suggested this study. Fifty normal women in varying stages of pregnancy were subjected to cystometric studies.

Their conclusions were:

"The bladder undergoes progressive changes in tone and capacity during pregnancy and the puerperium.

Beginning with the third month of gestation there is a gradual increase of capacity and decrease in tone, reaching extreme levels in the last trimester. The tone improves before termination of pregnancy.

The bladder empties without residual during pregnancy.

Post partum, the bladder capacity is apt to be largest, and there is considerable decrease in tone as compared with the ninth month. Residuals are common and may be quite large during this period, and should be drained by catheter if infected.

The bladder returns to normal over a period of six to eight weeks.

The parallelism between the bladder changes and those of the upper urinary tract is pointed out and its significance is discussed."

Comment: A study such as this develops knowledge of a practical nature that one may apply in general practice. Many intractable infections of the female bladder date from infection contracted during and immediately following pregnancy. These infections develop because the obstetrician pays insufficient attention to the bladder as far as its complete emptying is concerned.

──────○──────

Only Fifteen Minutes Required In New Syphilis Test Method

A new test, requiring only 15 minutes, for the demonstration of the syphilitic organism is reported by Leon Friedman, M.D., Philadelphia, in "The Journal of the American Medical Association" for January 14.

The test is especially applicable in cases of gonorrhea in which syphilis is suspected and, in comparison with other tests, saves considerable time.

The principle of the test is centrifugation of the gonorrheal discharge, or any other body fluid capable of being collected in a capillary tube, at low speed. This gives a clear specimen of serum suitable for dark field examination.

The author isolated the syphilitic organism from the gonorrheal discharge in one patient 50 days before the blood test showed the organism and in two patients whose history was not suggestive of syphilis.　. . .

ROSTER

Oklahoma State Medical Association
1939

ADAIR

GREENE, E. P. ....Westville
SELLARS, R. L. ....Westville

ALFALFA

BEATY, C. SAM ....Cherokee
BUTTS, A. J. ....Cherokee
CLARK, Z. J. ....Cherokee
DUNNINGTON, W. G. ....Cherokee
HARRIS, G. G. ....Helena
HUSTON, H. E. ....Cherokee
LANCASTER, L. T. ....Cherokee
WEBER, A. G. ....Goltry

ATOKA

BATES, FRANK ....Coalgate
BRIGGS, THOS. HIRAM ....Atoka
CLARK, J. B. ....Coalgate
FULTON, J. S. ....Atoka
HIPES, J. J. ....Coalgate

BECKHAM

BAKER, L. V. ....Elk City
DENBY, J. M. ....Carter
DEVANNEY, P. J. ....Sayre
JONES, C. F. ....Erick
KILPATRICK, E. S. ....Leedy
McCREERY, R. C. ....Erick
McGRATH, T. J. ....Sayre
SPEED, Sr., H. K. ....Sayre
SPENCE, W. P. ....Sayre
STAGNER, G. H. ....Erick
STANDIGER, O. C. ....Elk City
TISDAL, V. C. ....Elk City
WINDLE, O. N. ....Sayre

BLAINE

BOHLEMAN, WM. ....Watonga
BROWNING, J. W. ....Geary
BUCHANAN, R. F. ....Canton
CLARK, BEN P. ....Okeene
OOX, A. K. ....Watonga
GRIFFIN, W. F. ....Watonga
KIRBY, L. R. ....Okeene
MILLIGAN, E. F. ....Geary
OLSON, VIRGINIA ....Watonga
RYAN, ROBT. O. ....Canton

BRYAN

BAKER, ALFRED ....Durant
CAIN, P. L. ....Albany
COKER, B. B. ....Durant
COLWICK, O. J. ....Durant
COLWICK, J. T. ....Durant
FUSTON, H. B. ....Bokchito
HAYNIE, JOHN A. ....Durant
MOORE, B. H. ....Perrine Bldg., Oklahoma City
MOORE, CHAS. F. ....Durant
PRICE, CHAS. G. ....Durant
RUSHING, G. M. ....Durant
SAWYER, R. E. ....Durant
SCOTT, GEO. W. ....Tishomingo

SHULER, JAS. L. ....Durant
TONY, S. M. ....Bennington
WANN, C. E. ....Albany
WELLS, A. J. ....Calera
WHARTON, J. T. ....Durant

CADDO

ANDERSON, P. H. ....Anadarko
CAMPBELL, GEO. C. ....Anadarko
CANTRILL, J. H. ....Lindsay
COOK, ODIS A. ....Anadarko
DIXON, W. L. ....Cement
HASLAM, G. E. ....Anadarko
HAWKINS, E. W. ....Carnegie
HAWN, W. T. ....Binger
HENRY, J. WORRELL ....Anadarko
HUME, CHAS. R. ....Anadarko
JOHNSTON, R. E. ....Bridgeport
KERLEY, W. W. ....Anadarko
McCLURE, P. L. ....Ft. Cobb
McMILLAN, C. B. ....Gracemont
MILES, J. B. ....Anadarko
PATTERSON, F. L. ....Carnegie
PUTNAM, W. B. ....Carnegie
ROGERS, F. W. ....Carnegie
SULLIVAN, C. B. ....Carnegie
WILLIAMS, R. W. ....Anadarko
WILLIAMS, S. E. ....Springdale, Ark.

CANADIAN

ADERHOLD, THOS. M. ....El Reno
BROWN, HADLEY C. ....El Reno
CATTO, WM. B. ....El Reno
CRADEN, PAUL J. ....El Reno
FUNK, G. D. ....El Reno
GOODMAN, GEO. LEROY ....Yukon
HEROD, PHILLIP F. ....El Reno
JOHNSON, ALPHA L. ....El Reno
LAWTON, W. P. ....El Reno
MILLER, W. R. ....Calumet
MYERS, PIRL B. ....El Reno
PHELPS, JOS. T. ....El Reno
PHELPS, MALCOM E. ....El Reno
RILEY, JAS. T. ....El Reno
RICHARDSON, D. P. ....Union City
STOUGH, Sr., D. F. ....Geary

CARTER

BARKER, E. R. ....Healdton
BOADWAY, F. W. ....Ardmore
CANTRELL, Jr., D. E. ....Healdton
CANTRELL, D. E. ....Healdton
CANTRELL, EMMA J. ....Healdton
CARLOCK, J. HOYLE ....Ardmore
COX, J. L. ....Ardmore
DARGATZ, F. E. ....Newkirk
HARDY, WALTER ....Ardmore
HATHAWAY, W. G. ....Lone Grove
HIGGINS, H. A. ....Ardmore
JACKSON, T. J. ....Ardmore
JOHNSON, G. E. ....Ardmore
JOHNSON, WALTER ....Ardmore
LOONEY, MacDONALD ....Marietta
MOXLEY, J. N. ....Ardmore

PARRISH, R. M. ....Ardmore
POLLOCK, J. R. ....Ardmore
SULLIVAN, R. C. ....Ardmore
VEAZEY, L. C. ....Arnore
VEAZEY, J. H. ....Ardmore
VON KELLER, F. P. ....Ardmore
WOODS, L. B. ....Ardmore

CHEROKEE

ALLISON, J. S. ....Tahlequah
BAINES, SWARTZ ....Tahlequah
BARNES, HARRY E. ....Tahlequah
BROWN, W. L. ....Hulbert
DYER, ISADORE ....Tahlequah
McINTOSH, R. K. ....Tahlequah
MASTERS, HERBERT A. ....Tahlequah
MATTHEWS, G. F. ....State Health Dept.,
Oklahoma City
MEDEARIS, P. H. ....Tahlequah

CHOCTAW

BOYER, H. L. ....Ft. Towson
GEE, ROBT. L. ....Hugo
HALE, C. H. ....Boswell
JOHNSON, E. A. ....Hugo
SWITZER, FRED D. ....Hugo
WATERS, FLOYD L. ....Hugo
WOLFE, REED .................................C.C.C. Camp, Oklahoma City

CLEVELAND

ATKINS, W. H. ....Norman
BERRY, CURTIS ....Norman
BOBO, C. S. ....Norman
BUFFINGTON, F. C. ....Norman
COOLEY, B. H. ....Norman
DORSEY, ELIZABETH ....Norman
FOWLER, W. A. ....Norman
GABLE, J. J. ....Norman
GRIFFIN, D. W. ....Norman
HADDOCK, Jr., J. L. ....Norman
HOOD, J. O. ....Norman
HOWELL, O. E. ....Norman
MAYFIELD, W. T. ....Norman
MERRITT, I. S. ....Norman
NIELSON, GERTRUDE ....Norman
PROSSER, M. P. ....Norman
RAYBURN, C. R. ....Norman
REICHERT, R. J. ....Moore
SCHMIDT, ELEANORA ....Norman
STEEN, CARL ....Norman
STEPHENS, E. F. ....Norman
THACKER, R. E. ....Lexington
TURLEY, L. A. ....Norman
WICKHAM, M. M. ....Norman
WILEY, G. A. ....Norman
WILLARD, D. G. ....Norman

COMANCHE

ANGUS, DONALD ....Lawton
ANTONY, JOS. T. ....Lawton
BARBER, GEO. S. ....Lawton
BROSHEARS, JACKSON ....Lawton
DOWNING, G. G. ....Lawton
DUNLAP, E. B. ....Lawton
FOX, FRED ....Lawton
FERGUSON, L. W. ....Lawton
GOOCH, L. T. ....Lawton
HAMMOND, F. W. ....Lawton
HATHAWAY, E. P. ....Lawton
JOYCE, CHAS. W. ....Fletcher
KERR, GEO. E. ....Chattanooga
KNEE, L. C. ....Lawton
LUTNER, THOS. R. ....Lawton
MARTIN, CHAS. M. ....Elgin
MITCHELL, E. BRENT ....Lawton
PARSONS, O. L. ....Lawton
VAN MATRE, REBER M. ....Lawton

COTTON

BAKER, G. W. ....Walters
COTTON, W. W. ....Walters
HALSTEAD, A. B. ....Temple
JONES, M. A. ....Walters
SCISM, MOLLIE F. ....Walters

CRAIG

ADAMS, F. M. ....Vinita
BAGBY, LOUIS ....Vinita
BRADSHAW, J. O. ....Welch
DARROUGH, J. B. ....Vinita
GASTINEAU, F. T. ....Vinita
HAYS, P. L. ....Vinita
HERRON, A. W. ....Vinita
LEHMER, ELIZABETH ....Vinita
MARKS, W. R. ....Vinita
McMILLAN, J. M. ....Vinita
McPIKE, LLOYD H. ....Vinita
MITCHELL, R. L. ....Veterans Hospital, Muskogee
SANGER, PAUL G. ....Vinita
STAPLES, J. H. L. ....Bluejacket
STOUGH, D. B. ....Vinita
WALKER, C. F. ....Grove

CREEK

BISBEE, W. G. ....Bristow
COPPEDGE, O. S. ....Depew
COWART, O. H. ....Bristow
CROSTON, GEO. C. ....Sapulpa
CURRY, J. F. ....Sapulpa
HAAS, H. R. ....Sapulpa
HOLLIS, J. E. ....Bristow
JONES, ELLIS ....Sapulpa
KING, E. W. ....Bristow
LAMPTON, J. B. ....Sapulpa
LEWIS, P. K. ....Sapulpa
LONGMIRE, W. P. ....Sapulpa
McDONALD, C. R. ....Mannford
MOTE, PAUL ....Sapulpa
NEAL, WM. J. ....Drumright
REESE, C. B. ....Sapulpa
REYNOLDS, E. W. ....Bristow
REYNOLDS, S. W. ....Drumright
SCHRADER, CHAS. T. ....Bristow
SCHWAB, B. C. ....Sapulpa
SISLER, FRANK H. ....Bristow
SMITH, WENDELL L. ....Drumright
STARR, O. W. ....Drumright
WILLIAMS, J. CLAY ....Neosho, Mo.
ZAMPETTI, H. A. ....Drumright

CUSTER

ALEXANDER, C. J. ....Clinton
BOYD, T. A. ....Weatherford
CUNNINGHAM, CURTIS B. ....Custer City
CUSHMAN, HARRY R. ....Clinton
DEPUTY, ROSS ....Clinton
DOLER, C. ....Clinton
FRIZZELL, J. T. ....Clinton
GOSSOM, K. D. ....Custer City
HINSHAW, J. R. ....Butler
LAMB, ELLIS ....Clinton
LEWIS, R. W. ....Clinton
LINGENFELTER, PAUL ....Clinton
LOYD, E. M. ....Taloga
McBURNEY, C. H. ....Clinton
PAULSON, A. W. ....Clinton
PIERSON, DWIGHT ....Clinton
ROGERS, McLAIN ....Clinton
RUHL, N. E. ....Weatherford
SPEED, Jr., H. K. ....Clinton
STOLL, A. A. ....Clinton
ST. PETER, M. A. ....Custer City
TISDAL, WM. ....Clinton
TUTTLE, A. D. ....Portalis, N. Mex.
VIEREGG, FRANK R. ....Clinton
WOOD, J. G. ....Weatherford

GARFIELD

BAGBY, E. L. ....Enid
BAKER, R. C. ....Enid
BITTING, B. T. ....Enid
BRADY, J. H. ....Fairview
CHAMPLIN, PAUL B. ....Enid
DUFFY, FRANCIS M. ....Enid
GREGG, O. R. ....Enid
FEILD, JULIAN ....Enid
HARRIS, D. S. ....Drummond
HAMBLE, V. R. ....Enid
HINSON, BRUCE R. ....Enid
HOPKINS, P. W. ....Enid
HUDSON, F. A. ....Enid
HUDSON, H. H. ....Enid
HYER, J. V. ....Garber
JACOBS, R. G. ....Enid
MAYBERRY, S. N. ....Enid
McCROSKIE, M. R. ....Fairview
McEVOY, S. H. ....Enid
MERCER, J. WENDALL ....Enid
METSCHER, ALFRED JOHN ....Enid
MILES, G. O. ....Enid
NEILSON, W. P. ....Enid
NEWELL, JR., WALDO B. ....Enid
NEWELL, W. B. ....Enid
REMPEL, PAUL H. ....Enid
RHODES, W. H. ....Enid
ROBERTS, C. J ....Enid
ROBERTS, D. D. ....Enid
ROSS, GEORGE ....Enid
ROSS, HOPE ....Enid
RUDE, EVELYN ....Enid
SHANNON, H. R. ....Enid
SHAVER, S. R. ....Fairview
SHEETS, MARION E. ....Enid
TALLEY, EVANS E. ....Enid
VANDEVER, H. F. ....Enid
WALKER, JOHN R. ....Enid
WATSON, J. M. ....Enid
WILKINS, A. E. ....Covington
WILSON, GEO. S. ....Enid
WOLF, E. J. ....Waukomis

GARVIN

ALEXANDER, ROBT. M. ....Paoli
CALLAWAY, JOHN R. ....Pauls Valley
GREENING, W. P. ....Pauls Valley
GROSS, T. F. ....Lindsay
JOHNSON, G. L. ....Pauls Valley
LINDSEY, RAY H. ....Pauls Valley
MONROE, HUGH H. ....Lindsay
PRATT, CHAS. M. ....Lindsay
ROBBERSON, JR., MARVIN E. ....Wynnewood
ROBBERSON, M. E. ....Wynnewood
SHI, A. H. ....Stratford
SHIRLEY, EDWARD ....Pauls Valley
SULLIVAN, C. L. ....Elmore City

GRADY

BAZE, ROY E. ....Chickasha
BAZE, W. J. ....Chickasha
BONNELL, W. L. ....Chickasha
BOON, U. C. ....Chickasha
BYNUM, TURNER ....Chickasha
COOK, W. H. ....Chickasha
DOWNEY D. S. ....Chickasha
EMANUEL, ROY ....Chickasha
LEEDS, A. B. ....Chickasha
LITTLE, AARON ....Minco
MARRS, S. O. ....Chickasha
MASON, REBECCA H. ....Chickasha
McCLURE, H. M. ....Chickasha
MITCHELL, C. P. ....Chickasha
PYLE, OSCAR S. ....Chickasha
RENEGAR, J. F. ....Tuttle
WOODS, L. E. ....Chickasha

GRANT

HARDY, I. V. ....Medford
LAWSON, E. E. ....Medford
LIVELY, S. A. ....Wakita

GREER

BORDER, G. F. ....Mangum
BROWN, F. R. ....Mangum
HOLLIS, J. B. ....Mangum
LANSDEN, J. B. ....Granite
LOWE, J. T. ....Mangum
MEREDITH, J. S. ....Duke
OLIVER, W. D. ....Mangum
PEARSON, LEB. E. ....Mangum
POER, E. M. ....Mangum
RUDE, JOE C. ....Collis P. Huntington Memorial
                                        Hosp., Boston, Mass.

HARMON

HOLLIS, L. E. ....Hollis
HOPKINS, S. W. ....Hollis
HUSBAND, W. G. ....Hollis
JONES, J. E. ....Hollis
LYNCH, R. H. ....Hollis
RAY, W. T. ....Gould
STREET, O. J. ....Gould
YEARGAN, W. M. ....Hollis

HASKELL

CARSON, WM. S. ....Keota
HILL, A. T. ....Stigler
RUMLEY, J. C. ....Stigler
WILLIAMS, N. K. ....McCurtain

HUGHES

BENTLEY, J. A. ....Allen
BUTTS, A. M. ....Holdenville
DAVENPORT, A. L. ....Holdenville
MAYFIELD, IMOGENE BUTTS ....Holdenville
FORD, R. B. ....Holdenville
HICKS, C. A. ....Wetumka
HOWELL, H. A. ....Holdenville
KIES, B. B. ....Wetumka
MORRIS, R. D. ....Allen
MUNAL, JOHN ....Holdenville
PRYOR, V. W. ....Holdenville
TAYLOR, W. L. ....Holdenville
WALLACE, C. S. ....Holdenville

JACKSON

ABERNETHY, EDW. A. ....Altus
ALLGOOD, JOHN M. ....Altus
BERRY, THOS. W. ....Hugo, Colorado
BIRD, JESSE ....1545 N. W. 44th, Oklahoma City
BROWN, R. F. ....Altus
CROW, E. S. ....Olustee
ENSEY, J. E. ....Altus
FOX, RAYMOND H. ....Altus
HIX, JOSEPH B. ....Altus
MABRY, EARL W. ....Altus
McCONNELL, L. H. ....Altus
REID, JOHN R. ....Altus
SPEARS, C. G. ....Altus
STARKEY, WAYNE ....Altus
STULTS, J. S. ....Altus
TAYLOR, ROBT. Z. ....Blair

JEFFERSON

ANDRESKOSKI, W. T. ....Ryan
BROWNING, W. M. ....Waurika
COLLINS, D. B. ....Waurika
DERR, J. I. ....Waurika
EDWARDS, F. M. ....Ringling
HOLLINGSWORTH, J. I. ....Waurika
MAUPIN, C. M. ....Waurika
McCALIB, D. C. ....Ringling
WADE, L. L. ....Ryan

JOHNSTON

LOONEY, J. T. ....Tishomingo

KAY

ARMSTRONG, W. O. ....Ponca City
ARRENDELL, C. W. ....Ponca City
BARKER, W. JACKSON ....Ponca City
BEATTY, J. H. ....Tonkawa
CLIFT, M. C. ....Blackwell
CURRY, JOHN R. ....Blackwell
GARDNER, C. C. ....Ponca City
GHORMLEY, J. G. ....Blackwell
GIBSON, R. B. ....Ponca City
GORDON, D. M. ....Ponca City
GOWEY, H. O. ....Newkirk
HOWE, J. H. ....Ponca City
HUDSON, J. O. ....Braman
KENSINGER, R. R. ....Blackwell
KREGER, G. S. ....Tonkawa
MALL, W. W. ....Ponca City
MATTHEWS, DEWEY ....Tonkawa
McELROY, THOMAS ....Ponca City
MILLER, D. W. ....Blackwell
MOORE, G. C. ....Ponca City
MORGAN, L. S. ....Ponca City
NEAL, L. G. ....Ponca City
NIEMANN, G. H. ....Ponca City
NORTHCUTT, C. E. ....Ponca City
NUCKOLS, A. S. ....Ponca City
OBERMILLER, R. G. ....Ponca City
PETERS, M. L. ....Blackwell
RISSER, A. S. ....Blackwell
SANGER, W. W. ....Ponca City
VANCE, L. C. ....Ponca City
WAGGONER, E. E. ....Tonkawa
WAGNER, J. C. ....Ponca City
WALKER, I. D. ....Tonkawa
WHITE, M. S. ....Blackwell
WRIGHT, L. I. ....Blackwell
YANDELL, HAYS R. ....Ponca City
YEARY, G. H. ....Newkirk

KINGFISHER

DIXON, A. ....Hennessey
HODGSON, C. M. ....Kingfisher
LATTIMORE, F. C. ....Kingfisher
TAYLOR, JOHN R. ....Kingfisher

KIOWA

ADAMS, J. L. ....Hobart
ADAMS, RICHARD ....Hobart
ANDERSON, H. R. ....Mountain View
BONHAM, J. M. ....Hobart
BRAUN, J. P. ....Hobart
FINCH, J. WM. ....Hobart
FREEMAN, W. H. ....Sentinel
HATHAWAY, A. H. ....Mountain View
MOORE, J. H. ....Hobart
RITTER, J. M. ....Roosevelt
WALKER, F. E. ....Lone Wolf
WATKINS, B. H. ....Hobart

LE FLORE

BAKER, F. P. ....Talihina
BEVILL, S. D. ....Poteau
BOOTH, G. R. ....LeFlore
BRADLEY, FRANK ....Talihina
COLLINS, E. L. ....Panama
DEAN, S. C. ....Howe
FAIR, E. N. ....Heavener
HARTSHORNE, G. E. ....Spiro
LOWREY, R. W. ....Poteau
MINOR, R. W. ....Williams
ROGERS, G. A. ....Talihina
ROLLE, NEESON ....Poteau
SHIPPEY, W. L. ....Poteau
WOODSON, O. M. ....Poteau
WRIGHT, R. L. ....Poteau

LINCOLN

ADAMS, J. W. ....Chandler
BAILEY, C. H. ....Stroud
BAUGH, HAROLD ....Meeker
BROWN, BYRON B. ....Davis
BROWN, F. C. ....Sparks
BURLESON, NED ....Prague
ERWIN, PARA ....Wellston
HURLBUT, E. F. ....Meeker
MARSHALL, A. M. ....Chandler
NICKELL, U. E. ....Davenport
NORWOOD, F. H. ....Prague
ROBERTSON, C. W. ....Chandler
ROLLINS, J. S. ....Prague

LOGAN

*BARKER, C. B. ....Guthrie
BARKER, PAULINE ....Guthrie
CORNWELL, N. L. ....Coyle
DRESBACH, H. V. ....Mulhall
FIRST, F. R. ....Crescent
GARDNER, P. B. ....Guthrie
HAHN, L. A. ....Guthrie
HILL, C. B. ....Guthrie
LARKIN, W. H. ....Minco
LE HEW, Jr., J. L. ....Guthrie
MEAD, W. W. ....Guthrie
MILLER, WM. C. ....Guthrie
PETTY, C. S. ....Guthrie
PETTY, JAMES ....Guthrie
RINGROSE, R. F. ....Guthrie
RITZHAUPT, L. H. ....Guthrie
SOUTER, J. E. ....Guthrie
*Deceased

MAJOR

SPECHT, ELSIE ....Fairview

MARSHALL

HOLLAND, J. L. ....Madill
RAFF, JOS. S. ....Madill
YORK, J. F. ....Madill

MAYES

ADAMS, SYLBA ....Hayward, Wis.
HERRINGTON, V. D. ....Pryor
MORROW, B. L. ....Salina
PUCKETT, CARL ....22 W. Sixth, Oklahoma City
WERLING, E. H. ....Pryor
WHITAKER, W. J. ....Pryor
WHITE, L. C. ....Adair

McCLAIN

COCHRANE, J. E. ....Byars
DAWSON, O. O. ....Wayne
KOLB, I. N. ....Blanchard
McCURDY, W. C. ....Purcell
ROYSTER, R. L. ....Purcell

McCURTAIN

BARKER, N. L. ....Broken Bow
CLARKSON, A. W. ....Valliant
LOKEY, J. P. ....Idabel
McBRAYER, W. H. ....Haworth
McCASKILL, W. B. ....Idabel
MORELAND, J. T. ....Idabel
MORELAND, W. A. ....Idabel
OLIVER, R. B. ....Idabel
SHERRILL, R. H. ....Broken Bow
SIZEMORE, PAUL ....Broken Bow
WILLIAMS, R. D. ....Idabel

McINTOSH

JACOBS, L. I. ....Hanna
LITTLE, D. E. ....Eufaula
ROY, EMILE ....Checotah

STONER, RAYMOND WARD ....Checotah
TOLLESON, W. A. ....Eufaula
WOOD, JAS. L. ....Eufaula

MURRAY

ANADOWN, P. V. ....Sulphur
BALL, ERNEST ....Sulphur
BROWN, BYRON B. ....Davis
BURKE, RICHARD M. ....Sulphur
DeLAY, W. D. ....Sulphur
FOWLER, Jr., A. ....Sulphur
LUSTER, J. C. ....Davis
PARKER, WARREN E. ....Davis
POWELL, W. H. ....Sulphur
ROSE, ERNEST ....Sulphur
SADLER, F. E. ....Sulphur
SLOVER, GEO. ....Sulphur

MUSKOGEE

BALLANTINE, H. T. ....Surety Bldg.
BERRY, W. D. ....Barnes Bldg.
BRUTON, L. D. ....Commercial Natl. Bldg.
COACHMAN, E. H. ....Manhattan Bldg.
DIVINE, DUKE G. ....Wagoner
DORWART, F. G. ....Barnes Bldg.
EWING, F. W. ....Surety Bldg.
FITE, E. H. ....Barnes Bldg.
FITE, W. P. ....Barnes Bldg.
FRYER, S. J. ....Surety Bldg.
FULLENWIDER, C. M. ....Barnes Bldg.
HAMM, S. G. ....Haskell
HOLCOMB, R. N. ....Surety Bldg.
JOBLIN, W. R. ....Porter
KAISER, GEO. L. ....562 No. Sixth
KLASS, O. C. ....Surety Bldg.
KUPKA, J. F. ....Haskell
McALISTER, L. S. ....Barnes Bldg.
MOBLEY, A. L., Vets. Facility, Albuquerque, N. M.
NEWHAUSER, MAYER ....Vet. Administration
NEELY, S. D. ....Commercial Natl. Bldg.
OGLESBEE, C. L. .... County Health Unit
OLDHAM, Jr., I. B. ....426 North Sixth
OLDHAM, Sr., I. B. ....426 North Sixth
PUGH, ROBT. E. ....17th & W. Bdwy.
SAUNDERS, H. V. ....437 Post Office Bldg.
SCOTT, H. A. ....Commercial Natl. Bldg.
THOMPSON, M. K. ....Surety Bldg.
TILTON, W. B. ....Vet. Hospital, Muskogee
WARTERFIELD, F. E. ....Commercial Natl. Bldg.
WEAVER, W. N. ....Barnes Bldg.
WHITE, CHAS. ED ....2430 Boston
WHITE, J. H. ....Surety Bldg.
WOLFE, I. C. ....426 North Sixth
WOODBURN, JOEL T. ....Surety Bldg.

NOBLE

COLDIRON, D. F. ....Perry
COOKE, C. H. ....Perry
EVANS, A. M. ....Perry
FRANCIS, J. W. ....Perry
HEISS, J. E. ....Perry
RENFROW, T. F. ....Billings
WIGNER, R. H. ....Marland

NOWATA

KURTZ, R. L. ....Nowata
LANG, S. A. ....Nowata
PRENTISS, H. M. ....Nowata
ROBERTS, S. P. ....Nowata
SCOTT, M. B. ....Delaware

OKFUSKEE

BLOSS, JR., C. M. ....Okemah
BOMBARGER, C. C. ....Paden
BRICE, M. O. ....Okemah
COCHRAN, C. M. ....Okemah
JENKINS, W. P. ....Okemah

LUCAS, A. C. ....Castle
MELTON, A. S. ....Okemah
PEMBERTON, J. M. ....Okemah
PRESTON, J. R. ....Weleetka
SPICKARD, L. J. ....Okemah
WRIGHT, H. L. ....Okemah

OKLAHOMA

ADAMS, ROBT. H. ....501 Ramsey Tower
AKIN, R. H. ....400 West Tenth St.
ALFORD, J. M. ....Medical Arts Bldg.
ALLEN, E. P. ....1200 North Walker
ALLEN, GEO. T. ....1200 North Walker
ANDREWS, LELIA E. ....1200 North Walker
ARRINGTON, C. T. .... 715½ North Walnut
BAILEY, F. M. ....CCC Camp, High Rolls, N. M.
BAILEY, WILLIAM H. ....301 West Twelfth St.
BAIRD, Jr., W. D. ....2519½ S. Robinson
BALYEAT, RAY M. ....1200 North Walker
BARB, THOS. J. .... 240 West Commerce
BARKER, CHAS. E. ....505-13 Osler Bldg.
BARRY, G. N. .... 801 N.E. 13th
BATCHELOR, J. J. ....Medical Arts Bldg.
BATES, C. E. ....Vet. Admin., Dearborn, Mich.
BAUM, E. ELDON ....Medical Arts Bldg.
BELL, A. H. ....300 West 12th St.
BERRY, CHAS. N. ....Medical Arts Bldg.
BEYER, M. R. .... 2006 N.W. 39th
BINKLEY, J. G. ....Medical Arts Bldg.
BINKLEY, J. SAM ....Medical Arts Bldg.
BIRGE, JACK P. ....Ramsey Tower
BOATRIGHT, LLOYD C. ....Perrine Bldg.
BOGGS, NATHAN ....Perrine Bldg.
BOLEND, REX ....Medical Arts Bldg.
BONDURANT, C. P. ....Medical Arts Bldg.
BONHAM, WM. L. ....Medical Arts Bldg.
BORECKY, GEORGE L. ....Ramsey Tower
BORDER, C. L. .... American Nat'l. Bldg.
BOWEN, RALPH ....1200 North Walker
BRADLEY, H. C. ....Perrine Bldg.
BRANHAM, D. W. ....Medical Arts Bldg.
BREWER, A. M. ....Perrine Bldg.
BROWN, G. W. ....Medical Arts Bldg.
BRUNDAGE, C. L. ....1200 North Walker
BURTON, JOHN F. ....Osler Bldg.
BUTLER, H. W. ....1200 North Walker
CAILEY, LEO F. ....Medical Arts Bldg.
CAMPBELL, COYNE H. ....719 No. Robinson
CATES, ALBERT ....Medical Arts Bldg.
CAVINESS, J. J. ....Medical Arts Bldg.
CHARNEY, L. H. ....Medical Arts Bldg.
CLARK, ANSON L. ....Medical Arts Bldg.
CLOUDMAN, H. H. ....Medical Arts Bldg.
CLYMER, CYRIL E. ....Medical Arts Bldg.
COLEY, A. J. ....Hightower Bldg.
COLEY, JOE. H. ....Hightower Bldg.
COLLINS, H. D. ....Medical Arts Bldg.
COLLOPY, PAUL J .... State Health Dept.
COLONNA, PAUL C. ....800 E. 13th
COOPER, F. M. ....Medical Arts Bldg.
COSTON, TULLOS O. ....Medical Arts Bldg.
CUNNINGHAM, JOHN A. .... 209 N.W. 13th
DAILY, H. J. ....Medical Arts Bldg.
DANIELS, HARRY A. ....610 N.W. 9th St.
DEMAND, F. A. ....1200 North Walker
DERSCH, WALTER H. ....Medical Arts Bldg.
DICKSON, GREEN K. ....1200 North Walker
DILL, FRANCIS E. .... Medical Arts Bldg.
DOUDNA, HUBERT E. .... 800 N.E. 13th
DOUGHERTY, VIRGIL F. .... Sudan, Africa
DOWDY, THOS. W. ....Medical Arts Bldg.
EARLY, R. O. ....Medical Arts Bldg.
EASTLAND, WM. E. ....Medical Arts Bldg.
ELEY, N. P. ....400 West Tenth St.
EMENHISER, Jr., LEE K. .....Medical Arts Bldg.
ERWIN, F. B. ....Medical Arts Bldg.
ESKRIDGE, J. B. ....1200 North Walker
FAGAN, HERMAN ....400 N.W. 10th
FARIS, BRUNEL D. ....Medical Arts Bldg.

FELTS, GEO. R. ....Osler Bldg.
FERGUSON, E. G. ....Medical Arts Bldg.
FERGUSON, E. S. ....Medical Arts Bldg.
FISHMAN, C. J. ....132 West Fourth St.
FITZ, R. G., Taming Fu Hoppi, Prov. No. China
FLESHER, THOS. H. ....Edmond
FOERSTER, HERVEY A. ..... Medical Arts Bldg.
FORD, HARRY C. ....Medical Arts Bldg.
FRIERSON, S. E. ....Medical Arts Bldg.
FULTON, CLIFFORD C. ....Medical Arts Bldg.
FULTON, GEO. S. ....American Natl. Bldg.
GALLAGHER, C. A. .... 610 N.W. 9th
GARRISON, GEO. H. ....1200 North Walker
GEE, O. J. ....Medical Arts Bldg.
GIBBS, ALLEN G. ....Ramsey Tower Bldg.
GLOMSET, JOHN L. ....621 Osler Bldg.
GOLDFAIN, E. ....Medical Arts Bldg.
GOODWIN, R. Q. .... Medical Arts Bldg.
GRAHAM, ALLISON T. ....26 S.W. 25th
GRAY, FLOYD ....1200 N. Walker
GRAY, J. WORTH ....1315 South Agnew
HALL, CLARK H. ....Medical Arts Bldg.
HAMMONDS, O. O. ....623 North East 18th St.
HARBISON, FRANK ....Terminal Bldg.
HARBISON, J. E. ....Terminal Bldg.
HARRIS, HENRY W. ....1200 N. Walker
HASKETT, PAUL E. ....Hales Bldg.
HASSLER, GRACE CLAUSE ....Med. Arts Bldg.
HATCHETT, J. A. ....Medical Arts Bldg.
HAYES, BASIL A. ....625 North West 10th St.
HAZEL, O. G. ....1200 N. Walker
HEATLEY, JOHN E. ....Medical Arts Bldg.
HERRMANN, JESS .... Medical Arts Bldg.
HETHERINGTON, A. J. ....2014 Gatewood Ave.
HICKS, F. B. ....Medical Arts Bldg.
HIRSHFIELD, A. C. ....Medical Arts Bldg.
HOLLIDAY, J. R. ....1200 N. Walker
HOOD, F. REDDING ....1200 North Walker
HOOT, M. P. ....Bartlesville, Okla.
HOWARD, R M. ....Osler Bldg.
HUGGINS, J. R. ....Medical Arts Bldg.
HULL, WAYNE M. ....800 N.E. 13th
HUNTER, GEO. ....State Health Dept.
HYROOP, GILBERT L. .... Medical Arts Bldg.
ISHMAEL, WM. K. .... 605 N.W. 10th
JACKSON, A. R. ....2528½ South Robinson
JACOBS, MINARD F. ....Medical Arts Bldg.
JANCO, LEON ....10 West Park Place
JETER, HUGH ....1200 North Walker
JOLLY, W. J. ....615 West 14th St.
JONES, HUGH ....Medical Arts Bldg.
KELLER, W. F. ....Medical Arts Bldg.
KELSO, JOSEPH W. .... Medical Arts Bldg.
KELTZ, BERT F. ....Medical Arts Bldg.
KERNODLE, S. E. ....First Natl. Bldg.
KIMBALL, G. N. ....Medical Arts Bldg.
KUHN, JOHN F. ....Medical Arts Bldg.
KUHN, Jr., JOHN F. ....Medical Arts Bldg.
LACHMANN, ERNST ....801 East 13th St.
LAMB, JOHN H. ....Medical Arts Bldg.
LAMBKE, PHIL M. ....605 North East 28th St.
LaMOTTE, GEORGE A. ....Colcord Bldg.
LANGSTON, WANN ....Medical Arts Bldg.
LAWSON, PAT .... 818 N.W. 11th
LEMON, C. W. ....Medical Arts Bldg.
LENNY, FANNIE LOU ....400 N.W. 10th
LEONARD, C. E. ....Supply, Okla.
LINDSTROM, W. C. ....Medical Arts Bldg.
LINGENFELTER, F. M. ....1200 North Walker
LITTLE, JOHN R. ....Ramsey Tower
LONG, LEROY ....Medical Arts Bldg.
LONG, LEROY D. ....Medical Arts Bldg.
LONG, WENDELL ....Medical Arts Bldg.
LOVE, ROBT. S. ....Perrine Bldg.
LOWRY, DICK ....1200 North Walker
LOWRY, TOM ....1200 North Walker
LOY, C. F. ....Perrine Bldg.
LUTON, JAMES P. ....Medical Arts Bldg.

McCABE, R. S. ....Medical Arts Bldg.
MacDONALD, J. C. ....300 N.W. Twelfth St.
MARGO, E. ....605 N.W. 10th
MARIL, JOS. J. ....Medical Arts Bldg.
MARTIN, HOWARD C. ....Ramsey Tower
MARTIN, J. T. ....1200 N. Walker
MASTERSON, MAUD M. ....Medical Arts Bldg.
McBRIDE, EARL D. ....605 N.W. 10th
McGEE, J. P. ....1200 N. Walker
McHENRY, D. D. ....Skirvin Tower
McHENRY, L. C. ....Medical Arts Bldg.
McKINNEY, MILAM F. ....Medical Arts Bldg.
McNEILL, PHIL M. ....Medical Arts Bldg.
MECHLING, GEO. S. ....Osler Bldg.
MELVIN, JAMES H. ....Perrine Bldg.
MESSENBAUGH, J. F. ....Colcord Bldg.
MILES, W. H. ....Municipal Bldg.
MILLER, NESBITT L. .... Medical Arts Bldg.
MILLS, R. C. ....Hightower Bldg.
MOORE, C. D. ....Perrine Bldg.
MOORE, ELLIS ....Medical Arts Bldg.
MOOR, H. D. ....800 N.E. Thirteenth St.
MOORMAN, FLOYD ....1200 North Walker
MOORMAN, L. J. ....1200 North Walker
MORGAN, C. A. ....First Natl. Bldg.
MORGAN, VANCE F. ...... State Health Dept.
MORLEDGE, WALKER ....Osler Bldg.
MORRISON, H. C. ....807 North West 23rd St.
MULVEY, BERT M. ....Medical Arts Bldg.
MURDOCH, RAYMOND L. ......Medical Arts Bldg.
MUSICK, ELMER R. ....Medical Arts Bldg.
MUSICK, V. H. ....Medical Arts Bldg.
MUSSILL, W. M. ....Medical Arts Bldg.
MYERS, RALPH E. ....1200 North Walker
NAGLE, PATRICK S. ....1021 No. Lee
NEFF, EVERETT B. ....1200 No. Walker
NICHOLSON, B. H. ....301 N.W. 12th
NOELL, ROBT. L. ....Medical Arts Bldg.
O'DONOGHUE, D. H. ....Medical Arts Bldg.
O'LEARY, CHAS. M. ....Medical Arts Bldg.
OWEN, CANNON A. .... 1200 N. Walker
PATTERSON, ROBT. U. ...... 700 N.W. 18th
PAULUS, D. D. ....301 West Twelfth St.
PAYTE, J. I. ....2429 Aurora Court
PENICK, GRIDER ....Colcord Bldg.
PHELPS, S. ....Medical Arts Bldg.
PINE, JOHN S. ....Medical Arts Bldg.
POSTELLE, J. M. ....Medical Arts Bldg.
POUNDERS, CARROLL M. ....1200 North Walker
PRICE, J. S. ....1200 North Walker
RECK, J. A. ....Colcord Bldg.
REED, HORACE. ....Osler Bldg.
REED, JAMES ROBERT ....Medical Arts Bldg.
REICHMANN, RUTH S. ....124 North West 15th St.
RIELY, LEA A. ....Medical Arts Bldg.
RILEY, J. W. ....119 West Fifth St.
ROBINSON, J. H. ....301 West Twelfth St.
RODDY, JOHN A. ....Ramsey Tower
ROGERS, GERALD ....Osler Bldg.
ROSENBERGER, F. E. ....Perrine Bldg.
ROUNTREE, C. R. ....1200 North Walker
RUCKS, Jr., W. W. .... 301 West Twelfth St.
RUCKS, W. W. ....301 West Twelfth St.
SADLER, LEROY H. ....Osler Bldg.
SALOMON, A. L. ....1200 N. Walker
SANGER, F. A. ....Key Bldg.
SANGER, F. M. ....Key Bldg.
SANGER, WINNIE M. ....Key Bldg.
SARGENT, J. FRANK ....320 N.W. 10th
SEIBOLD, GEO. J. ....Wichita Falls, Texas
SERWER, MILTON J. ...... 1200 North Walker
SEWELL, DAN R. ....400 North West Tenth St.
SHELTON, J. W. .... Medical Arts Bldg.
SHEPPARD, MARY V. S. ....1200 North Walker
SHORBE, HOWARD B. ....Medical Arts Bldg.
SIMON, BETTY HARRIS .... 1000 N.W. 41st
SMITH, CHAS. A. ....719 No. Robinson
SMITH, D. G. ....First National Bldg.
SMITH, EDW. N. ....217 Plaza Court
SMITH, RALPH A. ....443½ North West 23rd St.

SNOW, J. B. ....1200 North Walker
STANBRO, GREGORY E. .... Medical Arts Bldg.
STARRY, L. J. ....1200 North Walker
STONE, S. N. ....Edmond
STOUT, M. E. ....209 West Thirteenth St.
STRADER, S. ERNEST ....Hightower Bldg.
STRECKER, W. E. ....Medical Arts Bldg.
SULLIVAN, ELIJAH S. ....Medical Arts Bldg.
TABOR, GEO. R. ....First National Bldg.
TAYLOR, C. B. ....Medical Arts Bldg.
THOMPSON, W. J. ....1200 N. Walker
TOOL, DONOVAN ....Edmond
TOWNSEND, CARY W. ....Medical Arts Bldg.
TRENT, ROBT. I. ....Medical Arts Bldg.
TURNER, HENRY H. ....1200 North Walker
UNDERWOOD, E. L. ....Somerset, Texas
VAHLBERG, E. R. ....Perrine Bldg.
VON WEDEL, CURT ....610 N. W. 9th St.
WAILS, T. G. ....Medical Arts Bldg.
WAINWRIGHT, TOM L. ....Medical Arts Bldg.
WARMACK, J. C. ....200 N.W. 16th
WATSON, I. N. ....Edmond
WATSON, O. ALTON ....1200 N. Walker
WATSON, R. D. ....Britton
WEIR, MARSHALL W. ....Ramsey Tower
WELLS, EVA ....Medical Arts Bldg.
WELLS, WALTER W. ....Medical Arts Bldg.
WEST, W. K. ....1200 North Walker
WESTFALL, L. M. ....Medical Arts Bldg.
WHITE, ARTHUR W. ....Medical Arts Bldg.
WHITE, OSCAR ....1200 North Walker
WHITE, PHIL E. ....Perrine Bldg.
WILDMAN, S. F. ....Medical Arts Bldg.
WILKINS, HARRY ....Medical Arts Bldg.
WILLIAMS, L. C. ....1200 N. Walker
WILLIAMSON, W. H. ....128 N.W. 14th
WILLIE, JAS. A. ....Medical Arts Bldg.
WILSON, KENNETH J. ....Medical Arts Bldg.
WOLFF, J. P. ....1200 N. Walker
WOODWARD, NEIL W. ....1200 North Walker
WRIGHT, HARPER ....240 West Commerce
YOUNG, A. M. ....Medical Arts Bldg.
YOUNG, 3rd, A. M. ....Medical Arts Bldg.

OKMULGEE

ALEXANDER, LIN ....Okmulgee
ALEXANDER, ROBT. L. ....Okmulgee
BOLLINGER, I. W. ....Henryetta
BOSWELL, H. D. ....Henryetta
CARLOSS, T. C. ....Morris
CARNELL, M. D. ....Okmulgee
COTTERAL, J. R. ....Henryetta
EDWARDS, J. G. ....Okmulgee
GLISMANN, M. B. ....Okmulgee
HOLMES, A. R. ....Henryetta
HUBBARD, RALPH ....1501 E. 11th, Okla. City
HUDSON, W. S. ....Okmulgee
KILPATRICK, G. A. ....Henryetta
LESLIE, S. B. ....Okmulgee
MABEN, CHAS. S. ....Okmulgee
MATHENEY, J. C. ....Okmulgee
McKINNEY, G. Y. ....Henryetta
MING, C. M. ....Okmulgee
MITCHENER, W. C. ....Okmulgee
NELSON, J. P. ....Beggs
RAINS, H. L. ....Okmulgee
RODDA, E. D. ....Okmulgee
SIMPSON, N. N. ....Henryetta
SMITH, C. E. ....Henryetta
TRACEWELL, GEO. L. ....Okmulgee
VERNON, W. C. ....Okmulgee
WALLACE, V M. ....Morris
WATSON, F. S. ....Okmulgee

OSAGE

AARON, W. H. ....Pawhuska
BAYLOR, R. A. ....Fairfax
DALY, J. F. ....Pawhuska

DOZIER, B. E. ....Snidler
ETHERTON, MONTE C.....C.C.C. Camp, Pawhuska
GOVAN, T. P. ....Pawhuska
GUILD, C. H. ....Shidler
HEMPHILL, G. K. ....Pawhuska
HEMPHILL, P. H. ....Pawnuska
KARASEK, M. ....Shidler
KIMBALL, M. C. ....Webb City
LIPE, E. N. ....Fairfax
LOGAN, C. K. ....Hominy
RAGAN, T. A. ....Fairfax
RUST, M. E. ....Pawhuska
SMITH, R. O. ....Hominy
WALKER, G. I. ....Hominy
WALKER, ROSCOE ....Pawnuska
WEIRICH, C. R. ....Pawhuska
WILLIAMS, CLAUDE W. ....Pawhuska
WORTEN, D. ....Pawhuska

OTTAWA

AISENSTADT, E. ALBERT ....Picher
BARRY, J. R. ....Picher
CANNON, R. F. ....Miami
CHESNUT, W. G. ....Miami
CONNELL, M. A. ....Picher
CUNNINGHAM, P. J. ....Miami
DeARMAN, M. M. ....Miami
DeTAR, G. A. ....Miami
DOLAN, W. M. ....Picher
HAMPTON, J. B. ....Commerce
HETHERINGTON, L. P. ....Miami
HUGHES, A. R. ....Afton
KERR, W. C. ....Picher
LANNING, J. M. ....Picher
McNAUGHTON, G. P. ....Miami
MILLER, H. K. ....Fairland
PURSLEY, TURNER ....Picher
RALSTON, B. W. ....Commerce
RITCHEY, H. C.
RUSSELL, RICHARD ....Picher
SAYLES, W. JACKSON ....Miami
SHELTON, B. W. ....Miami
SIEVERS, CHAS. M.
SMITH, W. B. ....Fairland
WORMINGTON, F. L. ....Miami

PAWNEE

BERNSTEIN, MAXWELL ....Pawnee
BROWNING, R. L. ....Pawnee
HADDOX, C. H. ....Pawnee
JONES, R. E. ....Pawnee
LeHEW, ELTON W. ....Pawnee
LeHEW, J. L. ....Pawnee
ROBINSON, E. T. ....Cleveland
SADDORIS, M. L. ....Cleveland
SPAULDING, H. B. ....Ralston

PAYNE

BASSETT, C. M. ....Cushing
CLEVERDON, L. A. ....Stillwater
DAVIS, BENJ. ....Cushing
DAVIDSON, W. N. ....Cushing
FRIEDEMANN, PAUL W. ....Stillwater
FRY, POWELL E. ....Stillwater
HACKLER, JOHN F. ....Stillwater
HARRIS, E. M. ....Cushing
HERRINGTON, D. J ....Cushing
HOLBROOK, R. W. ....Perkins
LEATHEROCK, R. E. ....Cushing
MANNING, H. C. ....Cushing
MARTIN, JOHN F. ....Stillwater
MARTIN, J. W. ....Cushing
MITCHELL, L. A. ....Stillwater
PERRY, D. L. ....Cushing
PUCKETT, HOWARD L. ....Stillwater
RICHARDSON, P. M. ....Cushing
ROBERTS, R. E. ....Stillwater

SMITH, A. B. ....Stillwater
SMITH, HASKELL ....Stillwater
STRAHN, EVA ....Stillwater
THOMPSON, W. C. ....Stillwater
WAGGONER, ROY E. ....Stillwater
WALTRIP, J. R. ....Yale
WILHITE, L. R. ....Perkins
WRIGHT, J. M. ....Stillwater

PITTSBURG

BARTHELD, F. T. ....McAlester
BAUM, F. J. ....McAlester
COLLINS, GLENN J. ....McAlester
COOPER, FRED B. ....McAlester
DORROUGH, JOE ....Haileyville
GEORGE, L. J. ....Stuart
GREENBERGER, E. D. ....McAlester
HARRIS, J. M. ....Wilburton
KAISER, WM. H. ....McAlester
KILPATRICK, G. A. ....McAlester
KLOTZ, W. F. ....McAlester
KUYRKENDALL, L. C. ....McAlester
LIVELY, CLAUDE E. ....McAlester
McCARLEY, T. H. ....McAlester
MILLER, F. A. ....Hartshorne
MUNN, J. A. ....McAlester
NORRIS, T. T. ....Krebs
PARK, J. F. ....McAlester
PEMBERTON, R. K. ....McAlester
RAMSAY, W. G. ....Quinton
RICE, O. W. ....McAlester
RUSSELL, ALLEN R. ....McAlester
SAMES, W. W. ....Hartshorne
SHULLER, E. H. ....McAlester
WAIT, WILL C. ....McAlester
WELCH, A. J. ....McAlester
WILLIAMS, C. O. ....McAlester
WILLOUR, L. S. ....McAlester
WILSON, HERBERT A. ....McAlester
WILSON, McCLELLAND ....McAlester

PONTOTOC

BRECO, J. G. ....Ada
BRYDIA, CATHERINE ....Ada
BURROWS, L. I. ....Ada
CANADA, E. A. ....Ada
CRAIG, JOHN R. ....Ada
COWLING, ROBT. E. ....Ada
CUMMINGS, ISHAM L. ....Ada
DEAN, W. F. ....Ada
EVANS, R. ERLE ....Ada
GULLATT, E. M. ....Ada
LEWIS, E. F. ....Ada
LEWIS, MILES L. ....Ada
McDONALD, GLEN W. ....Ada
McKEEL, SAM A. ....Ada
MILLER, OSCAR H. ....Ada
MOREY, JOHN B. ....Ada
MUNTZ, E. R. ....Ada
NEEDHAM, C. F. ....Ada
PETERSON, WM. G. ....Ada
ROSS, SAMUEL P. ....Ada
RUTLEDGE, JAS. A. ....Ada
SUGG, ALFRED R. ....Ada
WEBSTER, M. M. ....Ada
WELBORN, ORANGE E. ....Ada

POTTAWATOMIE

ANDERSON, R. M. ....Shawnee
APPLEWHITE, G. H. ....Shawnee
BAKER, M. A. ....Shawnee
BALL, W. A. ....Wanette
BAXTER, GEO. S. ....Shawnee
BLOUNT, W. T. ....Durant
BROWN, R. A. ....Prague
BYRUM, J. M. ....Shawnee
CAMPBELL, H. G. ....St. Louis, Okla.

CARSON, F. L. ....Shawnee
CARSON, JOHN ....Shawnee
CORDELL, U. S. ....McComb
CULLUM, J. E. ....Earlsboro
FORTSON, J. L. ....Tecumseh
GALLAHER, F. C. ....Shawnee
GALLAHER, PAUL ....Shawnee
GALLAHER, W. M. ....Shawnee
GASTON, JOHN I. ....Shawnee
GILLICK, D. W. ....Shawnee
HUGHES, H. E. ....Shawnee
HUGHES, J. E. ....Shawnee
IRBY, J. P. ....Maud
KAYLOR, R. C. ....McCloud
KEEN, FRANK M. ....Shawnee
MATTHEWS, W. F. ....Tecumseh
McADAMS-WILLIAMS, ALPHA ....Shawnee
McFARLING, A. C. ....Shawnee
McFARLING, JOHN ....Shawnee
NEWLIN, FRANCES P. ....Shawnee
PARAMORE, C. F. ....Shawnee
RICE, E. E. ....Shawnee
ROWLAND, T. D. ....Shawnee
STEVENS, WALTER S., 315 P. O. Bldg., Okla. City
WALKER, J. A. ....Shawnee
WILLIAMS, A. J. ....McLoud
STOUGH, A. R. ....Tecumseh
YOUNG, C. C. ....Shawnee

PUSHMATAHA

CONNALLY, D. W. ....Antlers
HUCKABAY, B. M. ....Antlers
KIRKPATRICK, J. ....Tuskahoma
LAWSON, JOHN S. ....Antlers
PATTERSON, E. S. ....Antlers

ROGERS

ANDERSON, F. A. ....Claremore
ANDERSON, P. S. ....Claremore
ANDERSON, W. D. ....Claremore
BASSMAN, CAROLINE ....Claremore
BIGLER, EARL E. ....Claremore
CALDWELL, C. I. ....Chelsea
COLLINS, B. F. ....Claremore
HOWARD, W. A. ....Chelsea
JENNINGS, K. D. ....Chelsea
MELOY, R. C. ....Claremore
NELSON, D. C. ....Claremore

SEMINOLE

CHAMBERS, CLAUDE S. ....Seminole
DEATON, A. N. ....Wewoka
GIESEN, A. F. ....Konawa
HUDDLESTON, W. T. ....Konawa
LYTLE, WM. R. ....Seminole
MOSHER, D. D. ....Seminole
PACE, L. R. ....Seminole
REEDER, H. M. ....Konowa
STEVENS, C. ....Seminole
SHANHOLTZ, MACK I. ....Wewoka
VAN SANDT, GUY B. ....Wewoka
VAN SANDT, MAX M. ....Wewoka

SEQUOYAH

MORROW, J. A. ....Sallisaw

STEPHENS

COKER, JOHN K. ....Duncan
GARRETT, S. S. ....Duncan
HARGROVE, FRED T. ....Duncan
IVY, W. S. ....Duncan
KING, E. G. ....Duncan
LINDLEY, E. C. ....Duncan
McCLAIN, W. Z. ....Marlow
McMAHAN, A. M. ....Duncan
PATTERSON, J. L. ....Duncan

RICHARDSON, R. W. ....Duncan
TALLEY, C. N. ....Marlow
THOMASSON, E. B. ....Duncan
WALKER, W. K. ....Marlow
WATERS, CLAUDE B. ....Duncan
WEEDN, Jr., A. J. ....Duncan
WILLIAMSON, S. H. ....Duncan

TEXAS

BLUE, JOHNNY A. ....Lawton
HAYES, R. B. ....Guymon
LEE, DANIEL S. ....Guymon
SMITH, MORRIS ....Guymon
THURSTON, H. E. ....Texhoma

TILLMAN

ALLEN, C. C. ....Frederick
ARRINGTON, J. E. ....Frederick
BACON, O. G. ....Frederick
BOX, O. H. ....Grandfield
CHILDERS, J. E. ....Tipton
COLLIER, E. K. ....Tipton
DAVIS, W. W. ....Davidson
FISHER, R. L. ....Frederick
FRY, F. P. ....Frederick
FUQUE, W. A. ....Grandfield
OSBORN, JR., JAMES D. ....Frederick
SPURGEON, T. F. ....Frederick

TULSA

ALLEN, V. K. ....1001 Medical Arts Bldg.
ALLISON, T. P. ....Sand Springs
ARMSTRONG, O. C. ....915 Medical Arts Bldg.
AMENT, C. M. ....305 Ritz Bldg.
ATCHLEY, R. Q. ....507 Medical Arts Bldg.
ATKINS, P. N. .... Medical Arts Bldg.
BARHAM, J. H. ....314 New Daniel Bldg.
BEESLEY, W. W. ....501 Medical Arts Bldg.
BEYER, J. W. ....621 McBirney Bldg.
BLACK, HAROLD J. ....209 Medical Arts Bldg.
BOLTON, J. F. ....211 Medical Arts Bldg.
BRADFIELD, S. J. ....607 Medical Arts Bldg.
BRADLEY, C. E. ....202 Medical Arts Bldg.
BRANLEY, B. L. ....315 Med. Arts Bldg.
BRASWELL, JAS. C. ....1109 Medical Arts Bldg.
BROGDEN, J. C. ....414-15 Medical Arts Bldg.
BROOKSHIRE, J. E. ....313 Ritz Bldg.
BROWNE, HENRY S. ....615 Medical Arts Bldg.
BRYAN, Jr., W. J. ....801 Medical Arts Bldg.
CALHOUN, C. E. ....Sand Springs
CALHOUN, WALTER H. ....405 Daniels Bldg.
CAMERON, PAUL B. ....604 S. Cincinnati
CARNEY, A. B. ....402 Atlas Life Bldg.
CHALMERS, J. S. ....Sand Springs
CHILDS, D. B. ....1226 South Boston
CHILDS, HENRY C. ....1226 South Boston
CHILDS, J. W. ....1226 South Boston
CLINTON, FRED S. ....823 Wright Bldg.
CLULOW, GEO. H. ....410 McBirney Bldg.
COHENOUR, E. L. ....1102 Medical Arts Bldg.
COOK, W. ALBERT ....1006 Medical Rrts Bldg.
COULTER, T. B. ....1011 Medical Arts Bldg.
CRAWFORD, WM. S. ...1228 Exchange Bank Bldg.
CRONK, FRED Y. ....801-05 Medical Arts Bldg.
DAILY, R. E. .... .Bixby
DAVIS, B. J. ....Sand Springs
DAVIS, G. M. ....Bixby
DAVIS, T. H. ....404 Medical Arts Bldg.
DEAN, W. A. ....610 Medical Arts Bldg.
DENNY, E. R. ....1105 Medical Arts Bldg.
DIEFFENBACH, N. J. ....708 Medical Arts Bldg.
DUNLAP, ROY W. ....808 Medical Arts Bldg.
EADS, CHAS H. ....607 Medical Arts Bldg.
EASON, K. K. ....401 Atlas Life Bldg.
EDWARDS, D. L. ....203 Philcade Bldg.
EVANS, HUGH J. ....303 Medical Arts Bldg.
EWELL, WM. C. ....1307 S. Main

FARRIS, H. LEE ....303 Medical Arts Bldg.
FLACK, F. L. ....Natl. Bank of Tulsa Bldg.
FLANAGAN, O. A. ....214 Braniff Bldg.
FORD, H. W. ....417 Oklahoma Natl. Bank Bldg.
FOREY, W. W. ....Bixby
FRANKLIN, S. E. ....Broken Arrow
FULCHER, JOSEPH ....417 Medical Arts Bldg.
GARRETT, D. L. ....701 Medical Arts Bldg.
GLASS, FRED A. ....404 Medical Arts Bldg.
GODDARD, R. K. ....Skiatook
GOODWIN, SAMUEL ....603 Medical Arts Bldg.
GORRELL, J. FRANKLIN, 610 Medical Arts Bldg.
GRAHAM, HUGH C. ....1307 So. Main St.
GREEN, HARRY ....1116 Medical Arts Bldg.
GROSSHART, PAUL ....302 Medical Arts Bldg.
HARALSON, CHAS. H. ....816 Medical Arts Bldg.
HARRIS, BUNN, ...Box 356, Jenks
HART, M. M. ....1232 South Boulder
HART, M. O. ....1232 South Boulder
HAYS, LUVERN ....Med. Arts Bldg.
HENDERSON, F. W. ....304 Medical Arts Bldg.
HENLEY, MARVIN D. .... Medical Arts Bldg.
HENRY, G. H. ....801 Medical Arts Bldg.
HOKE, C. C. ....207 Philtower Bldg.
HOOPER, J. S. ....Woodward
HOOVER, W. D. ....201 Philcade Bldg.
HOUSER, M. A. ....628 McBurney Bldg.
HOTZ, CARL J. ....604 South Cincinnati
HUBER, WALTER A. ...1113-14 Medical Arts Bldg.
HUDSON, MARGARET G., 411 Medical Arts Bldg.
HUDSON, DAVID V. ....215 Medical Arts Bldg.
HUMPHREY, B. H. ....Sperry
HUTCHISON, A. ....Bixby
HYATT, EMRY G. ....604 South Cincinnaui
JOHNSON, CHAS. D. ....1117 Medical Arts Bldg.
JOHNSON, E. O. ....206 Medical Arts Bldg.
JOHNSON, R. R. ....Sand Springs
JONES, W. M. ....204 Medical Arts Bldg.
KEMMERLY, H. P. ....902 Medical Arts Bldg.
KRAMER, A. C. ....415 Medical Arts Bldg.
LARRABEE, W. S. ....411 Medical Arts Bldg.
LAYTON, O. E. ....Collinsville
LeMASTER, D. W. ....902 Medical Arts Bldg.
LHEVINE, MORRIS B. ....1007 Medical Arts Bldg.
LONEY, W. R. R. ....301 Medical Arts Bldg.
LOWE, J. O. ....402 Atlas Bldg.
MacDONALD, D. M. ....1739 South Utica
MacKENZIE, IAN ....511 Medical Arts Bldg.
MARKLAND, JAMES D. ....Medical Arts Bldg.
MARGOLIN, BERTHA ....214 Medical Arts Bldg.
MAYGINNIS, P. H. ....505 Palace Bldg.
McCOMB, L. A. ....801 Medical Arts Bldg.
McDONALD, J. E. ....310 Medical Arts Bldg.
McGILL, RALPH A. ....1010 Medical Arts Bldg.
McKELLAR, MALCOLM ....604 South Cincinnati
McQUAKER, MOLLY ....1648 East 13th St.
MILLER, GEORGE H. ....206 Atlas Bldg.
MISHLER, D. L. ....604 S. Cincinnati
MOHRMAN, S. S. ....604 Daniels Bldg.
MUNDING, L. A. ....516 Medical Arts Bldg.
MURDOCK, H. D. ....1011 Medical Arts Bldg.
MURRAY, P. G. ....506 Medical Arts Bldg.
MURRAY, SILAS ....501 Medical Arts Bldg.
MYERS, F. C. ....502 Daniels Bldg.
NEAL, JAMES H. ....1944 North Denver Place
NELSON, I. A. ....1107 Medical Arts Bldg.
NELSON, F. J. ....603 Medical Arts Bldg.
NELSON, F. L. ....Atlas Life Bldg.
NELSON, M. O. ....307 Medical Arts Bldg.
NESBITT, E. P. ....917 Medical Arts Bldg.
NESBITT, P. P. ....917 Medical Arts Bldg.
NORMAN, G. R. ....17½ North Lewis
NORTHRUP, L. C. ....410 McBirney Bldg.
OSBORN, GEO. R. ....1105 Medical Arts Bldg.
PAVY, C. A. ....801 Medical Arts Bldg.
PERRY, FRED ....804 Atlas Life Bldg.
PERRY, HUGH ....804 Atlas Life Bldg.
PERRY, JOHN C. ....618 McBirney Bldg.
PIATT, A. D. ....Medical Arts Bldg.

PIGFORD, A. W. ....1001 Medical Arts Bldg.
PIGFORD, CHARLES ....Medical Arts Bldg.
PIGFORD, R. C. ....1001 Medical Arts Bldg.
PITTMAN, COLE D. ....1009 Medical Arts Bldg.
PORTER, H. H. ....510 Medical Arts Bldg.
PRICE, HARRY ....407 Medical Arts Bldg.
RAMEY, CLYDE ....612 Palace Bldg.
RAY, R. G. ....401 Atlas Bldg.
REECE, K. C. ....1101 Medical Arts Bldg.
REYNOLDS, J. L. ....305 Palace Bldg.
RHODES, R. E. LEE ....509 Medical Arts Bldg.
RICHEY, S. M. ....3830 West 44th St.
RILLER, L. E. ....Mercy Hospital
ROGERS, J. W. ....407 Medical Arts Bldg.
ROTH, A. W. ....607 Medical Arts Bldg.
RUPRECHT, H. A. ....604 South Cincinnati
RUPRECHT, MARCELIA ....604 South Cincinnati
RUSHING, F. E. ....505 Medical Arts Bldg.
RUSSELL, G. R. ....604 South Cincinnati
SCHRECK, PHILIP M. ....603 Medical Arts Bldg.
SEARLE, M. J. ....202 Medical Arts Bldg.
SHEPARD, R. M. ....306 Medical Arts Bldg.
SHEPARD, S. C. ....706 Medical Arts Bldg.
SHERWOOD, R. G. ....412 Wright Bldg.
SHIPP, J. D. ....Sisler Clinic
SHOWMAN, W. A. ....409 Medical Arts Bldg.
SIMPSON, CARL F. ....502 Medical Arts Bldg.
SINCLAIR, F. D. ....Springer Clinic
SIPPEL, M. E. ....1542 East 15th St.
SISLER, WADE ....807 South Elgin
SMITH, D. O. ....604 South Cincinnati St.
SMITH, N. R. ....703 Medical Arts Bldg.
SMITH, ROY L. ....809 Medical Arts Bldg.
SMITH, R. N. ....1017 Medical Arts Bldg.
SMITH, W. O. ....203 Philcade Bldg.
SPANN, L. A. ....305 Roberts Bldg.
SPRINGER, M. P. ....604 South Cincinnati
STALLINGS, T. W. ....724 South Elgin
STEVENSON, JAS. ....615 Medical Arts Bldg.
STEWART, H. B. ....3500 East 27th Place
STUART, FRANK A. ....311 Medical Arts Bldg.
STUART, L. H. ....1107 Medical Arts Bldg.
SUMMERS, C. S. ....611 Daniels Bldg.
SWANSON, K. F. ....Springer Clinic
TRAINOR, W. J. ....1011 Medical Arts Bldg.
TURNBOW, W. R. ....908 Medical Arts Bldg.
UNDERWOOD, D. J. ....414-15 Medical Arts Bldg.
UNDERWOOD, F. L. ....1001 Medical Arts Bldg.
UNGERMAN, ARNOLD H. ....902 Med. Arts Bldg.
VENABLE, S. C. ....1135 South Quaker
WALKER, W. A. ....322 Kennedy Bldg.
WALLACE, J. E. ....914 Medical Arts Bldg.
WALL, G. A. ....902 Medical Arts Bldg.
WARD, B. W. ....823 Wright Bldg.
WEST, T. H. ....612 Medical Arts Bldg.
WHITE, ERIC M. ....Medical Arts Bldg.
WHITE, N. STUART ....416 Medical Arts Bldg.
WHITE, P. C. ....312 Medical Arts Bldg.
WILEY, A. RAY ....812 Medical Arts Bldg.
WITCHER, R. B. ....910 Medical Arts Bldg.
WOODSON, FRED E. ....908 Medical Arts Bldg.
ZINK, ROY ....807 Daniels Bldg.

WAGONER

BATES, S. R. ....Wagoner
CRANE, FRANCIS S. ....Wagoner
PLUNKETT, J. H. ....Wagoner
RIDDLE, H. K. ....Coweta

WASHINGTON

ATHEY, J. V. ....Bartlesville
BEECHWOOD, E. E. ....Bartlesville
CHAMBERLIN, E. M. ....Bartlesville
CRAWFORD, H. G. ....Bartlesville
CRAWFORD, J. E. ....Bartlesville

DORSHEIMER, G. V. ....Dewey
ETTER, F. S. ....Bartlesville
GENTRY, RAYMOND C. ....Bartlesville
GREEN, O. I. ....Bartlesville
HUDSON, L. D. ....Dewey
KINGMAN, W. H. ....Bartlesville
LeBLANC, WM. ....Ochelata
PARKS, S. M. ....Bartlesville
REWERTS, F. C. ....Bartlesville
SHIPMAN, W. H. ....Bartlesville
SMITH, J. G. ....Bartlesville
SOMERVILLE, O. S. ....Bartlesville
STAVER, B. F. ....Bartlesville
TORREY, J. P. ....Bartlesville
VANSANT, J. P. ....Dewey
WEBER, H C. ....Bartlesville
WEBER, S. G. ....Bartlesville
WELLS, C. J. ....Bartlesville
WORD, L. B. ....Bartlesville

WASHITA

BENNETT, D. W. ....Sentinel
BUNGARDT, A. H. ....Cordell
DARNELL, E. E. ....Colony
HARMS, J. H. ....Cordell
LIVINGSTON, L. G. ....Cordell
McMURRY, J. F. ....Sentinel
NEAL, A. S. ....Cordell
TRACY, C. M. ....Sentinel
WEAVER, E. S. ....Cordell
WEBER, A. ....Bessie

WOODS

BENJEGERDES, THEODORE D. ....Beaver
CLAPPER, E. P. ....Waynoka
DOUGAN, A. L. ....Amorita
ENSOR, D. B. ....Hopeton
HALL, RAY L. ....Waynoka
McGREW, EDWIN A. ....Beaver
ROGERS, CHAS. L. ....Carmen
ROYER, CHAS. A. ....Alva
SIMON, JOHN F. ....Alva
SIMON, WM. E. ....Alva
STEPHENSON, ISHMEL F. ....Alva
STEPHENSON, WALTER LOGAN ....Aline
TEMPLIN, OSCAR E. ....Alva
TRAVERSE, CLIFFORD A. ....Alva

WOODWARD

BEAM, J. P. ....Arnett
BELL, J. T. ....Woodward
CAMP, E. F. ....Buffalo
CHUMLEY, C. P. ....Supply
DARWIN, D. W. ....Woodward
DAY, J. L. ....Supply
DUER, JOE L. ....Taloga
DUNCAN, J. C. ....Forgan
ENGLAND, MYRON ....Woodward
FORNEY, C. J. ....Woodward
HILL, T. A. ....Seiling
JOHNSON, H. L. ....Supply
LEACHMAN, T. C. ....Woodward
NEWMAN, FLOYD ....Shattuck
NEWMAN, MESHECH HASKELL ....Shattuck
NEWMAN, O. C. ....Shattuck
NEWMAN, ROY ....Shattuck
RUTHERFORD, V. M. ....Woodward
SILVERTHORNE, C. R. ....Woodward
TEDROWE, C. W. ....Woodward
TRIPLETT, T. B. ....Mooreland
VINCENT, DUKE W. Vici
WALKER, HARDIN ....Rosston
WILLIAMS, C. E. ....Woodward

THE JOURNAL
OF THE
OKLAHOMA STATE MEDICAL ASSOCIATION

VOLUME XXXII	McALESTER, OKLAHOMA, JULY, 1939	Number 7

The Anatomy of Operative Incisions*

E. EUGENE RICE, M.D., F.A.C.S.
SHAWNEE, OKLAHOMA

Operative incisions have as their objects the exposure of the underlying structures in order that diseased or injured organs or structures may be removed, repaired, or treated.

In planning the incision for any operative procedure five desiderata have to be kept in view:

1. Access should be suitable and adequate to the part to be exposed or explored. Small incisions, if adequate, are to be recommended, but should give a good visual field and sufficient room to accomplish the surgery anticipated. Incisions should not be placed too near bony or cartilaginous boundaries.

2. The blood supply should be effective and thereby avoid as much as possible the risk of defective union or post-operative hernia. The best incisions from this point of view are those which pass through the muscular fibers, splitting and separating them, but not dividing them.

3. The nerve supply should be carefully preserved, especially avoiding division of the motor nerves as paralysis of the muscles will c a u s e considerable discomfort with loss of tone of the muscle which may be permanent. The superficial s e n s o r y nerves will usually regenerate and sensation will return to normal within a reasonable time.

4. Prevention of injury to the muscles and aponeuroses is very important and as

*Read before the Section on General Surgery, Annual Meeting, Oklahoma State Medical Association, Oklahoma City, May, 1939.

far as possible when the fibers are to be cut and not separated they s h o u l d be cleanly divided. Hemostasis should be accomplished without undue trauma to the fibers themselves.

5. The cosmetic results of exposed incisions are very important. Undesirable and unsightly scars can be reduced to a minimum by following the natural folds of the skin, accurate approximation of the skin edges with the use of subcuticular or fine dermal sutures, reducing the length of the incision as much as possible with good surgery, and placing the scar where it may be covered with jewelry or clothing.

The site of the incision contemplated depends upon the underlying s t r u c t u r e s which are to be exposed. It should be planned so that it will cause the least t r a u m a to the protecting or overlying structures.

The direction of the incision is usually determined by the direction of the fibers of the underlying m u s c u l a r structures. This rule may be varied for the sake of better exposure, in extensive surgery, or for cosmetic reasons.

The specific anatomy of surgical incisions depends upon the definite portion of the body needing surgical attention and may be considered under the headings:

ABDOMINAL incisions are probably the most frequently used and the more common may be considered as:

1. Paramedian celiotomy incision, which may be either high or low, should be made

slightly to the side of the linea alba, the skin first being incised, the panniculus adiposis separated, the anterior fascia of the rectus abdominus m u s c l e cut, the muscle fibers pushed aside or the fibers separated, the posterior fascia and the peritoneum incised.

2. Lateral celiotomy incision is the same except it is made along the outer border of the rectus muscle, the fascia divided close to the linea semilunaris and the outer border of the rectus retracted toward the midline.

3. The gridiron, often called McBurney's incision, has the advantage of leaving the strength of the abdominal wall unimpaired. After the diagonal incision of the skin is made, the external oblique fascia is incised, the fibers of the internal oblique are separated, then the fibers of the transversalis fascia with the peritoneum is incised.

4. Inguinal incision for the repair of inguinal hernia exposes the external oblique fascia which, after incision, exposes the internal oblique muscle and the conjoined tendon with Poupart's ligament exposed laterally to which usually the transversalis fascia is sutured. Care should be taken to avoid injury to the ilio-inguinal nerve which is exposed. The extension of the peritoneum forms the hernial sac.

5. Femoral hernia incision o p e n s the skin, exposes the aponeurosis of the external oblique and the internal oblique muscle, the ilioinguinal nerve and the deep epigastric vessels, Poupart's, Cooper's and Gimbernat's ligaments, and the pectineal fascia. Repair is made by suturing Poupart's ligament to the pectineal fascia after removal of the sac.

KIDNEY i n c i s i o n s depend upon the amount of exposure desired, the most useful of which are:

1. Kelley's incision through the superior lumbar triangle the boundaries of which are the posterior margins of the oblique muscles of the abdominal wall, the quadratus lumborum, and the 12th rib, its floor is the aponeurosis of the oblique muscles and the latissimus covers it, separates the fibers of the latissimus and enlarges the triangle by blunt force, careful not to injure the 12th dorsal or the 1st lumbar nerve.

2. Mayo's incision is a longitudinal S-shaped incision through the skin, superficial fascia and the posterior layer of the lumbodorsal fascia exposing the posterior s u p e r i o r l u m b a r triangle by cutting through the external and internal obliques and the latissimus dorsi muscles, exposing the transversalis which is opened freely.

3. Israel's incision is an oblique opening from the j u n c t i o n of the 12th rib and erector spinae muscle downward to anterior to the anterior superior spine of the illium, separating the fibers of the external oblique and cutting the fibers of the internal oblique.

4. Robson's incision has the advantage of exposing the kidney without dividing the muscle fibers or weakening the abdominal wall and without w o u n d i n g the blood vessels or nerves. This begins at the anterior superior spine of the illium and extends backward toward the tip of the last rib. The fibers of the external oblique are cut and its aponeurosis are separated and retracted, the m u s c u l a r fibers of the internal oblique separated and the transversus split and separated forming a diamond shaped space in which the transverse fascia is exposed and incised.

THORACIC incisions depend upon the operation contemplated. The site and length and position is determined which is most often used posteriorly. The most common operations upon the chest wall is for rib resection and thoracoplasty. The skin is incised following either the course of the bone underneath or the direction of the muscle fibers. The posterior incision involves the trapezius with cutting or separation of the muscle fibers, the romboidus major and minor and the vertebral fascia.

BREAST incisions for benign g r o w t h s usually follow the skin folds while for malignant lesions from the anterior axillary fold to the epigastrium. The pectoralis major and minor are exposed and the exertions of the serratus anticus after removal of the breast tissue. In radical amputation the structures of the axillary space are exposed including the axillary artery and vein and the lower portion of the brachial plexus.

NECK incisions follow the skin folds for

cosmetic reasons or the muscular borders for proper exposure. The most common operation in the neck is upon the thyroid gland, where, after incision of the skin, the platysma lies directly under the superficial fascia and is reflected with it. The omohyoid, sternohyoid, and the sternothyroid muscles are retracted after longitudinal incision in the midline. For more exposure these strap muscles may be divided laterally between forceps, exposing the anterior fascia of the thyroid gland.

HEAD incisions are usually semi-circular to facilitate the raising of a bone flap for intracranial work in which after incision of the skin, with the base of the flap downward to preserve the nerve and blood supply, and superficial fascia, the aponeurosis of the occipito-frontal muscle is incised and the percramium reflected.

EXTREMITY incisions are made in the direction of the muscle fibers for practically all operative work except for amputations which must necessarily cut these structures transversely.

In summarizing it is necessary to remember that in making operative incisions to do as little trauma to the underlying structures as possible, not to injure the nerve supply and maintain adequate blood supply to all the parts involved.

BIBLIOGRAPHY

1. Gray's anatomy: Numerous references.
2. Rose and Careless: Manual of Surgery, X Edition, PP 1071-2.
3. Anspach: Gynecology, pp 624-636.
4. Lewis: Practice of Surgery, Vol. VII, Chap. 9, pp 14-39.

———————o———————

Preliminary Report on the Use of Histidine in the Treatment of Hunner's Ulcer*

K. F. SWANSON, M.D.   MALCOLM McKELLAR, M.D.
TULSA, OKLAHOMA

This is offered with apologies for its incompleteness. No claims are made and no conclusions drawn, due to admixture of other therapy and lack of optimum control. We do not believe Histidine to be a miracle worker in this condition, but do think that, added to other therapy, it has benefited some difficult and long standing cases of Hunner's ulcer.

Histidine is an amino acid necessary for the maintenance of life. It is found most abundantly in hemoglobin and to a lesser extent in various fish proteins. Chemically it is described as alpha-amino beta imidazole propionic acid.

As the hydrochloride, it has been used in the treatment of gastroduodenal ulcer alone with debatable benefit. In combination with other therapy histidine has been beneficial, though no one knows how it acts in relieving pain. H. Kohl has found occult bleeding is controlled even if the ulcer shows no tendency toward healing. This is produced by reduction of the coagulation time. In hemophilia, the coagulation time may be reduced to normal by the continuous administration of histidine. This process can not be duplicated in vitro and evidently the amino acid must mobilize factors of coagulation.

A four per cent aqueous solution of histidine hydrochloride was given intramuscularly to a series of cases of so-called Hunner's ulcer of the urinary bladder over varying periods of time in doses of 5 c.c. each.

H. Kohn has observed the action of histidine is prolonged and intensified if given with calcium and vitamin C therapy and in our cases at present we are using this combined treatment for interstitial cystitis.

Localized submucous fibrosis, the elusive ulcer of Hunner or interstitial cystitis occurs mostly in adult females. The eti-

*Read before the Section on Genito-Urinary Diseases and Syphiiology, Annual Meeting, Oklahoma State Medical Association, Oklahoma City, May 2, 1939.

ology is obscure and whether focal infection (as stressed by Hunner) in the tonsils, teeth, sinuses and female cervix, etc., play any important role, is questionable. Often none exist and removal of such foci when they do exist, usually seem of no benefit. Meads considers previous urinary infection, neglected pyelitis or cystitis a contributing. factor and Hunner emphasized ureteral stricture, finding it in about one-half his cases. Other authors do not concur in these findings and characteristically, the urine is sterile and the involved tissue negative on bacteriological cultivation.

Pathologically this is not an ulcer simply of the mucous membrane, but an involvement of the underlying structures—some-·times the entire thickness of the bladder wall. The epithelium is flattened or denuded, but the basement m e m b r a n e is usually intact. There is edema of the submucous and muscular coats with engorgement of the vessels and lymphatics and round cell infiltration. Fibrous tissue replacement occurs, and with healing a dense fibrous stellate scar persists. The lesion may be single or multiple and clasically it is in the dome of the bladder.

Symptoms are frequency and pain, day and night, with varying periods of intensity. The pain is knifelike, usually suprapubic or may be referred to rectum, vulva, buttocks or thighs. Burning and terminal tenesmus may be present and associated with hematuria. Orman had a case in whom eating caused pain in the left lower quadrant due to peristalsis in the neighborhood of the ulcer. Hematuria, usually microscopic, is present in 70 per cent of cases. Bladder capacity is 150 c.c. or less.

Cystoscopically, the condition may be overlooked. Characteristically, one finds a reddened or necrotic appearing area surrounded by a pale mucous membrane. Or a stellate fissure may be seen surmounting congested tissue. Bleeding occurs on distention and may designate the site of an otherwise obscure lesion.

Standard features of treatment consist of—

1. General care of patient and any attending ailments, such as associated granular urethritis and removal of foci of infection.

2. Fulguration of the entire pathological area under anesthesia and repetition at intervals.

3. Hydraulic distention of the bladder.

Resection of the ulcer and presacral sympathectomy have been largely discontinued.

The following cases were given histidine alone and in conjunction with some of the above therapy. Most of them had many months or years of standard therapy without lasting improvement.

1. J. T., single, white, female, 37, with a typical lesion in the dome, was treated by fulguration and distention, 1934 to 1937, without marked or lasting improvement. Histidine was then given in daily doses for eight days. The patient did not return then for one month at which time an exacerbation occurred during the menses. Fulguration was repeated and followed with hydraulic distention and histidine therapy, with more improvement than before seen. During the past two months Dr. McKellar had added ca Gluconate 10 c.c.—10 per cent intravenously at the time of her other treatment. She has now a bladder c a p a c i t y of 13 ounces and shows objective as well as subjective improvement.

2. E. L., single, white, female, 50, was first seen by Dr. McKellar in 1935, with cystitis, bladder neck obstruction and a 600 c.c. residual of p u r u l e n t urine. The bladder neck was resected and she did well until July, 1937, at which time she returned with a marked cystitis. Sulfanilamide q u i c k l y took care of the infection but a typical Hunner's ulcer was discovered in the dome extending to the right ureteral orifice. Vesical distention plus histidine was instituted once weekly for three months. Her improvement was marked. She stayed away for three and a half months and returned with another attack of cystitis and another area of interstitial cystitis. Treatment was repeated as before and after six months, no ulcer can be found, though she has recurring attacks of cystitis. This case is unusual because of association of grossly infected urine.

3. W. A. M., white, male, 68, whose symptoms began in 1916 consisting of fre-

quency and pain. In 1925, he was scoped and an elusive ulcer was found in dome of bladder. Later the same year he had a punch operation of the bladder neck by Dr. Caulk. His relief was short. In 1930 the bladder was opened at the Mayo Clinic. Resection had been intended but the lesion was too extensive so open fulguration was carried out. Relief was short. Later the same year—in fact d u r i n g the same hospital stay, pre-sacral sympathectomy was carried out. Relief was more lasting but his symptoms returned in a matter of months.

January, 1938, the bladder capacity was 150 c.c. urine clear and he was suffering from p a i n and frequency. Cystoscopy showed a small ulcer in the left dome. He was given histidine alone every third day for two months. His capacity increased to 300 c.c. and the specific gravity of the urine which was usually 1,003 to 1,008 increased to 1,020. Pain and frequency was considerably diminished. He did not want to be scoped for a follow up, so objectively we can only guess what the cystoscopic picture would be.

4. Mrs. H. Mc., white, female, 55, with a grown child of 20 years, had pain and frequency for eight years. Urine contained microscopic blood and a few pus cells. Cystoscopy showed a typical lesion anteriorly and close to bladder neck. Bladder capacity was 100 c.c. The bladder was fulgurated on three different occasions and hydraulic distention carried out over a period of four months. Improvement was slight and objectively the lesion showed extension. Histidine therapy was then b e g u n — given bi-weekly for two months. Improvement was marked and bladder capacity increased to 300 c.c. She disappeared then and we believed she had sought solace elsewhere. However, seven m o n t h s later, she dropped in before office hours, told the nurse she was 90 per cent better and had had no treatment in the interim. However, she also added that she had become a Christian Scientist in the meantime and gave Mary Baker Eddy most if not all the credit for her improved condition.

5. Mrs. M. O., white, female, 44, married with several grown children, was seen October 4, 1937, with complaints of frequency and pelvic pain. Cystoscopy showed a linear lesion in the left dome which bled on distention. Bladder capacity was 120 c.c. During the year previous, she had had a hysterectomy, appendectomy, anterior and posterior colporrhaphy and a hemorrhoidectomy. Hydraulic distention and histidine therapy were begun and some improvement noted after four months. However, it was not marked so the lesion was fulgurated and the former procedure was repeated. At the end of f o u r months more, improvement was marked and bladder capacity was nine ounces. She has not been seen since that time.

6. Mr. C. E. H., white, male of 40, with symptoms of frequency and pain in right lower quadrant and bladder for 10 years. He had had a chronic vesiculitis and numerous attacks of epididymitis during this time, as well as gonorrhea and syphilis. The u r i n e was clear with microscopic b l o o d. Cystoscopy revealed t h r e e distinct patches of interstitial cystitis. He was fulgurated and not seen then again for six months when he returned with an epididymitis. When this subsided he was again fulgurated, the bladder appearing unimproved. After some six months of distention, he was given a course of histidine, after which the symptoms considerably lessened. He has not returned since that time, but on communication, he writes that he is able to work again selling insurance which was impossible before, because of frequency and pain.

7. C. P. H., white, male, 50, with a history of pain and frequency for many years. Numerous long standing urethral strictures, a perineal-scrotal urinary fistula and a purulent urine complicated the picture. He had had a prostatic resection elsewhere t h r e e years before without relief. After a period of urethral dilatations, he was scoped and an interstitial c y s t i t i s found near the right dome. This was fulgurated and distention and histidine

therapy carried out for four months. At this time pain was gone, bladder capacity 11 ounces and cystoscopically the area showed healing.

8. Mrs. S., white, f e m a l e of 68, with grown children. Her complaints were pain and frequency for past five or six years. Urine was n e g a t i v e during that time and she had never been scoped. Bladder capacity was eight ounces but distention past that point caused bleeding and a typical single linear lesion, was seen in the anterior wall of the bladder. Histidine was given once a week for six weeks with hydraulic distention. Improvement was marked and the symptoms practically disappeared. However, before we could scope her again, she contracted pneumonia and nearly died. While convalescing at home during

this past week, she informed us by phone that she had no further bladder trouble.

9. P. M., single, white female of 45. (This is not a case of Hunner's ulcer, but is included because of histidine which was given.) She had severe frequency, burning and pain extending over several years. Cystoscopy revealed small cysts and inflammatory plaques scattered over the trigone plus a granular urethritis. After two years of much and varied treatment and wishing the patient elsewhere, her symptoms had improved little, though cystoscopically little remained except some excrescences at the b l a d d e r neck. Three months of histidine was instituted and the symptoms left. When last heard of, she was concerned mainly with a menopausal syndrome.

————o————

Management of a Maternity Service with Nurse Attendance at Delivery in a Rural Area*

A Preliminary Report

ISADORE DYER, B.S., M.D.
Consultant Obstetrician
Director Maternity Program
Cooperative District No. 1
Oklahoma State Health Department

There have been many methods devised during the last five years to develop the use of Public Health nurses and Public Health Administration in a more comprehensive sense in maternity services. These programs have developed into a number of different manners in the method used to cope with rural maternity needs. Much progress therefore has been accomplished, and in those areas wherein such services are offered, the a n n u a l mortality rates have been reduced.

Of course, we all know the problems confronting the progress of maternity care in general. Of these, perhaps the problem of education of the patient and coping with

the manner of living in rural communities as well as contending with the existing superstitions is the greatest.

There does not seem to be any set rules or policies with which one could establish such a service in any one community without adapting them to the peculiarities of the given district, so one finds variations in the manner in which maternity programs are directed.

Realizing the need of intensive maternity care in the northeastern section of Oklahoma, the Childrens' Bureau has cooperated with the State Health Department in establishing a program in District No. 1. This district comprises the five counties: namely, Adair, Cherokee, Delaware, Mayes and Sequoyah. Now, the one important

*Read before the Section of Public Health, Annual Meeting, Oklahoma State Medical Association, Oklahoma City, May 1, 1939.

point which I should wish to stress is that this program was established in a district wherein a full-time health service has been in existence for two years. The ice was already broken; the public was already conscious of public health work, and most important of all there were no administrative problems. By this is meant the same personnel, office and otherwise, were employed to assist in the maternity program.

May first of this year marks the completion of a full year of this service. It is significant in many ways and when we look back the year has been filled with many experiences both in the field and in the unit office, and there have been numerous changes that have had to be made often at the expense of progress in a rapidly developing program. However, even with the changes made from time to time, it is felt that for the most part they were to the betterment of the program as it exists today.

Not having any set policies with which to fall back upon for support, an attempt was made to formulate a service which would fit into this given community. Early, it was realized that to establish nurse attendance at delivery in all of the five counties would be folly. This would not have been possible until the administrative problems could have been worked out in a smaller community. Still, it was felt that the five counties should have a maternity program to aid the work done in the field by the public health nurses in the respective areas.

In short, maternity clinics were established in each of the five counties. The clinic sites were picked in strategic areas where the attendance would justify their presence. In all of the five counties, the county seats have been one of the clinic sites. These are centrally located and oftentimes a patient will "come to town," even at the preference of attending a clinic closer to her home. Seventeen to 19 such clinics are held each month.

These clinics are open to anyone whom the nurse deems eligible. Emphasis is placed on those patients who have no family physician, those who are determined to be delivered by midwives and those who are eligible for the Indian hospitals. On the other hand, they are also open to patients who are referred by local physicians

in consultation. The general routine consists of complete physical examinations with pelvimetry, Wassermann and vaginal smear. Every attempt is made to stress the necessity of medical care at delivery, and many patients are thus referred to physicians who otherwise would not consider it essential. Maternal hygiene is stressed, and these clinic visits, together with the nursing field visit, set the stage as it were for an uneventful, clean delivery.

One of the most convincing results of this service is the increased attendance in the outlying counties, with not a great increase in the field load of the nurse. Further, they have found that it is far easier to complete their maternity care if they can get a patient to come into a clinic to have a physician r e i t e r a t e and back their teaching with c o n c r e t e care. It teaches the patient the value of measurements, and introduces a pelvimeter into areas wherein it was unknown. It backs the efforts of any practicing physician in the area who might be ambitious enough to give adequate care. On the other hand, no attempt has ever been made to belittle any physician regardless of his teaching. Should such an occasion arise, attempts are made to convince the physician of the value of different teaching, but whatever he might tell a patient remains law as far as we are concerned. Many patients have been thus aided. Abnormalities have been d i s c o v e r e d and treatment arranged through the private physician. Barriers have been broken down and from month to month we saw less restraint on the part of patients to be completely examined. Many very interesting stories could be told of these clinics. Mothers have presented themselves, self-referred, after a life of six and s e v e n pregnancies unattended medically. They often state that for years they have been going through pregnancy with the dread of something being wrong. Not having had the financial means to enlist the services of a physician, they went on and took their own chances. These are the most cooperative of all patients. It is remarkable how interested they are to have a complete examination and with what complete consent they s u b m i t to antepartum care. In one of the clinics in Cookson Hills, I saw one little girl wade the Illinois river last summer to get to the clinic site. She did it all summer because it saved her 10 miles going the way of the bridge. To my horror this winter on one of those cold, bleak, rainy days, she presented herself. On questioning, she announced that a friend had agreed to paddle her across the river in a flat-bottomed boat for a small sum and if it were possible she would like to get back as soon as possible because he was waiting to paddle her across to her home. Here, the value of prenatal care had been brought home with optimum success.

In Cherokee county a different facility was organized. Here, in addition to the clinics outlined, a larger staff was available (five nurses), and nurse attendance was offered at time of delivery. This delivery service was available to any patient in Cherokee county who was delivered by a physician who in turn was in good standing with his State and County Medical Society. Here, even further attempts were made to continue care through the whole problem of maternity care. Here, further, there was available a means to keep in close contact with patient and physician so that when referrals were made to physicians, he gave adequate prenatal and postpartum care. This one important phase of the program helped to make it a success. Nurses in this county were not confronted with the disappointment in referring a patient after teaching prenatal care and have the physician tell her to call him when the baby was on its way and be sure to have the $25. So often without the support of the practicing physician, nothing constructive can be accomplished in the field.

In managing the delivery service, problems galore presented themselves. There was the difficulty of a call schedule and d i f f i c u l t y in not overworking any one nurse beyond her ability. There was the problem of adapting a uniform method of technique for the physicians to use in this area so that equipment could be uniform.

Unlike any other State Health Department Maternity Service I know of, we are using a wet technique for delivery. This is by no means original. It is precisely the technique employed at the Chicago Maternity Center and at DeLee's, without any added equipment or changes so often seen in like services. This technique is simple

and in teaching such care, it is felt that a physician does not become accustomed to an elaborate sterile linen technique, to feel lost should later he be confronted without the nursing aid. This wet technique employs only water, a few pans found in any home, and a hot stove to produce a clean, sterile field. Gloves are b o i l e d in the home as well as instruments. It seems very unadvisable to establish an elaborate sterile linen technique when very few if any rural practitioners have access to an autoclave, or more so, have the time or help to prepare such supplies. This technique has proved very successful in that we have yet to report a puerperal infection of any importance.

It is agreed that public health nursing, medical care, teaching of the patient to observe the value and demand such care and nurse attendance at delivery are all essentials for maternity care, which would lower the mortality rate in a given area. This is all possible when the given patient can afford to buy medical care. However, in this particular district, the economic status is such that half of the pregnant mothers are unable to afford such service, even if they desire same. Realizing such a status in northeastern Oklahoma, $5,000 was set aside to purchase this care for indigent patients. Indigency was determined by the patient's statement together with the investigation of a trained Medical Social Welfare Worker allotted the program by the Child Welfare Division of the Oklahoma Department of Public Welfare, and the statement by the private physician. This was afforded those eligible and the private physicians received fees in direct proportion to the amount of care given the patient. $25.00 was the top fee for care prior to the fifth month; $20.00 after the fifth month and prior to the seventh month; $17.50 the last two months, and $15 for delivery. These fees included a postpartum examination. The patient had sole right to choose her physician, and no attempt has ever been made to recommend. With these funds available, that group who needed maternity care foremost, have been cared for.

In addition to all the mentioned facts concerning the service, consultation is offered any physician in the five counties at any p e r i o d during a given pregnancy.

Intrapartum help is available. This renders a rural physician a service at a time when it is most needed.

In establishing such a service in conjunction with a Public Health A g e n c y, there are two important aspects to consider. This, in short, specialized service versus generalized service. In a pure unprejudiced view, I think it well to consider the value of each. This is pertinent to the Oklahoma program because of the fact that in our limited experience we have tried both methods of management. I do not feel that there is any other method to match a specialized service from the pure standpoint of the thoroughness of a maternity program in a given area. Nurses well trained in maternity can concentrate on the one phase, unhampered by the daily distractions of a generalized p r o g r a m. Their interest is mirrored in the quality of their work, the enthusiasm and thoroughness of the patient contact, the willingness to accept delivery call and the interest shown, and the freedom from contact with infectious and contagious diseases.

Four well trained nurses c o u l d work with minimum supervision, and the irregularities attenuating this type of service would not disrupt the daily routine of a generalized program. This was our experience.

The generalized program, on the other hand, affords a balanced public health program. The quality of the work done in maternity is in direct proportion to the disposition of the nurse. The quality of the service in general will vary with the amount of extraneous work a given nurse might be called upon to perform in a given area. Delivery call with a few nurses on the staff as we have, oftentimes disrupts clinic schedules regardless of how well a nurse might plan her work in advance. She becomes acquainted with a family as a whole, it is true, but she cannot possibly attain the home visit number required together with the other phases of her program and attain a high degree of quality. Again, in an a c t i v e maternity program wherein postpartum calls are to be made promptly, one or the other part of her work will suffer. A generalized program still remains ideal, in an utopian sense. It is necessary if, from the standpoint of

actual expense, we are to utilize the services of public health nurses to develop maternity care as we have shown. The one great fact which always determines the value of a service, rests with the individual nurse. If we were f o r t u n a t e enough to obtain women who were proficient in public health, and on the other hand were trained sufficiently in obstetrics and liked the art, the problem would be simple. But although a Public Health Certificate may be obtained in nine months, four months in obstetrics in a postgraduate sense, does not qualify a nurse in obstetrics to the same degree. A good obstetrical nurse is comparatively rarer than a public health nurse, and obstetrical nurses if well trained, have had little time to develop t h e m s e l v e s in the whole public health field. The same is very true for supervision. One can obtain a good obstetrical supervisor, but one cannot make a public health nurse proficient as an obstetrical supervisor in four months.

The development of this program has been stimulating from every degree. The cooperation from the medical profession has been foremost in its success. During the year, 480 mothers were given prenatal care. Many of these registered will deliver later on. Of this number, 250-odd have received medical aid at delivery including nurse attendance. Approximately 50 per cent of all patients carried were declared indigent and from all standpoints would have been without medical care other than that given at the p r e n a t a l clinics. These f i g u r e s apply only to Cherokee county.

There was one maternal death which, much to our disappointment, occurred at the eleventh month of the service. This patient, a 16-year-old primipara, was unknown to our r e c o r d s. She developed eclampsia the morning she went into labor and since the husband was unfamiliar with the aid offered, he was ignorant of any source of help. After two attempts to arouse the interest of physicians in this county and in an adjoining county, and having been refused because of lack of funds, a sympathetic physician was contacted. He arrived after the patient had had eight hours of eclamptic convulsions. She was hospitalized and died the next day of pulmonary edema and the usual sequelae of severe untreated eclampsia.

This one case serves as an example for the need of further education of rural women; it further stresses the need for care in an indigent group which are largely responsible for the abnormal maternal mortality in rural areas.

———————o———————

Temporo-Mandibular Syndrome (Costen's Syndrome)*

Lee K. Emenhiser, M.D.
OKLAHOMA CITY, OKLAHOMA

This is a clinical syndrome of neuralgias and ear symptoms associated with disturbed function of the temporo-mandibular joint on one or both sides. Although the dental profession has studied, treated, and recognized symptoms and signs of this pathological joint for many years, it was Costen[1] of St. Louis who, in 1934, established this condition before the medical profession as a definite clinical syndrome entity. Many cases of headache, catarrhal deafness, glossopharyngeal neuralgia, "burning tongue" and trismus are allowed to exist because we do not recognize the abnormal excursion of the mandibular condyle in its glenoid fossa.

Abnormal excursion of the mandibular condyle can be the result of malocclusion of natural teeth, absence of molar teeth on one or both sides, edentulous mouths, ill-fitting dentures, shrinkage of the alveolar ridges beneath dental plates, etc. This leads to a decrease in the vertical dimension of the jaw, and to a "loose joint" with permanently stretched capsule allowing extreme excursion or subluxation of condyle. This "wandering condyle" can press abnormally on surrounding structures, blocking the Eustachian tubes, causing destructive changes in the joint itself, and producing various symptoms by impingement on the auriculo-temporal and chorda-tympani nerves.

*Read before the Eye, Ear, Nose and Throat Section, Annual Meeting, Oklahoma State Medical Association, May 2, 1939.

SYMPTOMS

Ear Symptoms:

1. Intermittent or continuously impaired hearing.
2. Stopping or "stuffy" sensation in the ears, marked about meal time.
3. Tinnitus, usually "low buzz" in type, less often a snapping noise while chewing.
4. Dull or "drawing" pain within the ears.
5. Dizziness and nystagmus.

Pain and Irritative Symptoms:

1. Pain and aching around temporo-mandibular joint and over side of head, mostly in temporal region.
2. Headache about the vertex and occiput and behind the ears (typical site of posterior sinus pain) increasing toward the end of the day (atypical sinus history suggestive of eye headache).
3. Burning or aching sensation in the throat (glossopharyngeal neuralgia).
4. Burning tongue (glossodynia).
5. Dry mouth with almost total absence of saliva and, rarely, excessive saliva.
6. Occasional herpes of the external ear canal and buccal mucosa, most marked on the edentulous side.
7. Pain attacks after movement of jaw or chewing tough substances.
8. Trismus.

Signs:

1. Maloccluding original teeth, lack of

molar teeth on one side or badly fitting dental plates, permitting over-closure.

2. Mild catarrhal deafness, improved at once by inflation of Eustachian tubes.

3. Dizzy spells, relieved by inflation of tubes.

4. Tenderness to palpation of one or both mandibular joints.

5. Looseness of condyles within the joint capsule, and weaving of condyles from side to side on opening or closing jaw.

6. Marked comfort to patient from inter-posing a flat object between the jaws.

7. The presence of the typical headache when sinuses or eyes are found to be negative.

8. X-ray study s h o w i n g destructive changes or abnormal excursion of condyle in temporo-mandibular joint.

Let's briefly review the anatomy and physiology of this joint according to Cunningham[6].

"This j o i n t is the articulation of the head of the mandible with the articular fossa and articular eminence of the temporal bone. It is a synovial joint; and its cavity is separated into an upper and a lower part by an articular disc.

"The capsular ligament is attached superiorly to the temporal bone around the margins of the articular fossa and eminence, and inferiorly to the neck of the mandible. Its lateral part is thickened to form a triangular band called the temporó-mandibular ligament. That ligament is attached by its base to the zygoma and the tubercle of the root of the zygoma, and by its apex to the lateral side of the neck of the mandible.

"The articular disc is an oval plate of fibro-cartilage whose periphery is fused with the capsular ligament, and it therefore divides the joint cavity completely into an upper and a lower compartment. The upper is the large compartment, since the upper articular surface is the wider.

"The synovial membrane is in two separate parts. It lines the capsular ligament around each chamber, and is reflected on to the disc.

"The only ligaments proper to the joint are the capsular and temporo-mandibular.

Two other ligaments—the spheno-mandibular and stylo-mandibular—are described with the joint because they connect the mandible with the cranium; but they are not closely related to the joint, and add but little to its strength. For that matter, the joint does not rely on any of its ligaments: it is chiefly the muscles of mastication that keep the mandible in its place.

"The movements of the mandible at the joint are the following: 1. depression; 2. elevation; 3 protraction; 4. retraction;- 5. side to side or chewing movements.

"When the mandible is depressed the articular disc and the head of the mandible moves forward in the articular fossa, and the head finally takes up a position below the articular eminence. The f o r w a r d gliding of the disc and head in the upper compartment of the joint is accompanied by another movement in the lower compartment—a rotation of the head of the mandible on the lower surface of the articular disc. Elevation of the mandible or closure of the mouth is brought about by a reverse series of changes in both compartments of the j o i n t. There is some doubt about the position of the transverse axis around which the movements of elevation and depression take place, but it is generally supposed to be situated at the level of the mandibular foramen. The movements are therefore least at that level, and consequently the inferior dental vessels and nerves are not unduly stretched when the mouth is opened and shut. In protraction and retraction the movement is confined chiefly to the upper compartment of the j o i n t, and the head of the mandible, with the articular disc, glides forwards and backwards upon the temporal articular surface. In the chewing movements of the jaw, the mandible is carried alternately from one to the other side.

"The muscles on each side which are chiefly engaged in producing these movements are the following: 1. depressors—the platysma, the mylo-hyoid, and the anterior belly of the digastric; 2. elevators—the masseter, medial pterygoid, temporal; 3. protractors—the lateral pterygoid, and to some extent the medial pterygoid and the superficial fibres of the masseter; 4. retractors—the posterior fibres of the temporal and the deep fibres of the masseter;

5. side to side movement is produced by the muscles of opposite sides acting alternately."

The ear symptoms of impaired hearing, stopping or stuffy sensation in the ears, tinnitus, dull or "drawing" pain within the ears, dizziness and nystagmus are due to blockage of the Eustachian tube with derangement of intratympanic pressure. Costen[3] showed on a cadaver section how this comes about and I quote him as follows:

"In all cases except those in which the catarrhal deafness was due to chronic nasal infection or those h a v i n g a coincident nerve deafness, the hearing improved at once after inflation. Finding it difficult to reconcile this prompt change with the previous theories as to concussion of the internal ear structures, which if correct would require months for recovery, anatomical study was made by serial sections through the joint and ear structures. A plane was found in which, when the jaw of the soft tissue specimen was overclosed manually (to imitate similar overclosure in life), all soft tissues next to the Eustachian tube, including the tensor veli palatini muscle bordering the membranous anterior edge of the tube and the adjacent sphenomeniscus m u s c l e, were seen to wrinkle and close the tube firmly. This coincided with the fundamental studies of Prentiss who demonstrated relaxation of the spheno-mandibular ligament when the mandible is closed and the fact that the ligament is a part of the general fascia which encloses the external and internal pterygoid muscles. These functions explain the improvement in condition of the Eustachian tubes when the "bite' 'is opened, whether the ears are treated or not, accounts for the habit of the deafened person dropping the mouth open when intently listening, and explains the comfort afforded the miner who opens his Eustachian tubes just before the concussion of a blast, by dropping his mouth open—all dependent upon tensing the spheno-mandibular ligament.

"The symptoms of tinnitus was accounted for by the buzzing sensation which occurs in typical catarrhal deafness, and the less frequent snapping noises, attributed to perforations of the meniscus of the joint, as originally described by Prentiss.

"Dizziness which could be relieved by

inflation of the Eustachian t u b e s, and therefore distinguished from that of toxic labyrinthitis, was found in 14 of the 52 ear cases."

Headache and pain around the temporomandibular joint is explained by Costen[3] as follows: "1. erosion of the bone of the glenoid or mandibular fossa, and impaction of the condyles against the thin bone separating them from the dura and its rich nerve supply; 2. irritation by the uncontrolled movement of the condyles backward or mesially, of the auriculotemporal nerve, which passes intimate to the mesial side of the capsule between the condyle and the tympanic plate to distribute over the temporal and vertex regions; 3. production of reflex pain and sensory disturbance in the various connections of the chordatympani nerve, the condyle irritating it where it emerges from the tympanic plate at the mesial edge of the glenoid fossa through the petrotympanic fissure.

"Reasoning from the fact that the mandibular joint capsule is weaker on the mesial side, and the glenoid fossa is protected laterally by the zygoma, it, was assumed that in the jaw with unilateral loss of teeth the joint on the unsupported side would suffer most destruction. Observation of the jaw movements of this type of case showed that the patient attempts to occlude the remaining teeth by weaving the jaw laterally toward them. The mandibular teeth slip beyond the maxillary on occlusion, and the condyle on the unsupported side is pulled mesially and upward by the chewing muscles. Exactly the same thing happens when the natural teeth are worn or badly occluding and fail to take the impact of the chewing movement. The joint on the poorly supported side is destroyed. Its condyle slips mesially on closure, impacts the nerve and initiates pain on the same side. Twenty-one cases fall into this group, and the various pains invariably occur on the side on which proper molar support is entirely lost. The joint on the same side is usually quite tender to palpation internally, and functions with a crunch when palpated externally. Ear symptoms, as stopping and deafness, are notably absent in these unilateral neuralgia cases. Each case showing stoppage of the ear or dizziness was at once relieved."

Burning or aching sensation in throat, u s u a l l y unilateral, stimulating glosso-pharyngeal neuralgia, may be due to the c o n d y l e irritating the auriculotemporal nerve and through its connections with the otic ganglion and glossopharyngeal nerve cause referred pain over the glossopharyngeal nerve sensory distribution.

Burning tongue (glossodynia) without local lesions, usually unilateral, may be explained by the condyle irritating the auriculotemporal nerve (which is a branch of the mandibular nerve) and then referred pain over the lingual nerve (which is also a branch of the mandibular nerve). The lingual nerve supplies sensory function to the anterior 2/3 of tongue and "burning" may be limited to this area but the whole tongue may burn on the affected side due to r e f e r r e d pain also over the glosso-pharyngeal nerve which supplies the posterior 1/3 of the tongue.

Disturbance of salivary secretion, either excessive dryness of the mouth or excessive salivation (slobbering) may be explained by condyle irritating the chorda tympani nerve which supplies the motor fibers for innervation of the submaxillary and sublingual salivary glands and by condyle irritating the auriculotemporal nerve which contains, in addition to the sensory fibers to joint and over side of head, the motor fibers for innervation of the parotid salivary gland. Taste may be disturbed through the irritation of the chorda-tympani nerve.

Vesicular eruptions or herpes about the external canals, corners of mouth, hard palate or the buccal mucosa which cleared up after repositioning the jaw is proof that their source is pressure irritation by the c o n d y l e on the auriculotemporal and chorda-tympani nerves. Costen[4] s t a t e s about 20 per cent of his cases show herpes.

Many patients will give history of pain or f a t i g u e in the mandibular joints or headache or pain in face after chewing tough substances or after talking a while, anything that causes abnormal movements of condyle in the worn joint.

Recently Costen[5] has described trismus as being a cause of temporo-mandibular joint disfunction in patients with normal occlusion. Any irritation of any of the sensory branches of the trigeminal nerve can cause trismus or spastic contraction of

the muscles of mastication which are supplied by the mandibular division of the trigeminal nerve, through reflex pain. On attempting to open the mouth, the trismus tends to hold or limit the excursion of that condyle, resulting in excessive stress or compression of the condyle on the meniscus and mandibular joint structures, producing more pain again, which causes more trismus—thus a vicious cycle is established, f i n a l l y resulting in destructive changes within the joint. One 16-year-old patient of Costen's had trismus for a year, with beginning destruction and symptoms in the temporo-mandibular joint on same side. X-ray s h o w e d an impacted unerupted third molar on that side, presumably the source of trismus. Extraction of offending tooth relieved the trismus, consequently repositioning the condyle normally.

Careful h i s t o r y of symptoms and the signs as noted in first part of this paper should be sought for and X-rays taken of both temporo - mandibular j o i n t s with mouth open and closed in the Sproull position as d e s c r i b e d by Drs. Sherwood Moore and Wendell Scott in Costen's article[4] or the technique used by Dr. Edwin C. Ernst[7]. Points to be seen by X-ray study are: 1. erosion of condyle and articular tubercle; 2. abnormal excursion of condyle; 3. impaction of condyle; 4. bone destruction; 5. ankylosis; 6. fibrosis of joint capsule.

All of the above symptoms and signs will not be present in any one case, and it will be noticed that the ear symptoms predominate in the bilateral cases or edentulous mouths as a pressure effect producing "catarrhal deafness" and the pain and irritative symptoms predominate in cases with loss of molar support on one side only, or with malocclusion sufficient to cause pathology of one or both temporo-mandibular joints.

Treatment: Repositioning of condyle or condyles to near as possible normal relationship in the joint by dental reconstruction. Increasing the vertical dimension of jaw only a small amount to remove condyle from range of impinging upon the nerves can relieve many cases of pain and irritative symptoms. "Opening the bite" too much will exaggerate the symptoms.

Approximate testing before permanent dentures advised to prove the presence or absence of these factors is done by the use of one millimeter thickness cork d i s c s, which are placed within the patient's jaw for a short test at the time of the examination, and when not conclusive the patient is given the discs and instructed to carry them within the jaws for a few days, several hours a day. The patient can talk and carry on ordinary duties with these cork discs between jaws in molar regions. Changes in the nature of the symptoms are reported on his return. The prognosis in a given case depends on these factors: (a) the accuracy with which refitted dentures relieve abnormal pressure on the joint, the increase of vertical dimension keeping the moving condyles out of range of dura, c h o r d a - tympani and auriculotemporal nerves; (b) the extent of injury to the Eustachian tube and to the condyle, the meniscus and the joint capsule.

Schultz[8] has described a m e t h o d of shortening and strengthening the capsule of the joint by injecting into the joint a fibrosing agent, sodium psylliate. I have never done this but it sounds reasonable and he reports good results.

COMMENTS

1. Neuralgias about the head and ear symptoms f o r m a definite clinical syndrome associated with temporo-mandibular joint pathology.

2. Relief can be obtained after proper dental reconstruction to reestablish the normal relationship of the condyle within the glenoid fossa.

3. The neuralgias and deafness associated with this syndrome simulate disorders of eyes, ears, and sinuses and must be carefully differentiated.

4. It is necessary for the physician to cooperate with the dentist in reconstruction of jaw—some cases can be relieved by merely putting on an overlay in molar region, placing in a bridge, or constructing a new set of dentures, properly fitted, in edentulous patients. Cases of malocclusion of natural teeth present the greatest difficulty.

5. In all cases of headache, neuralgias about the head and ear trouble, the teeth and absence of teeth should be examined as well as the temporo-mandibular joints for this syndrome.

BIBLIOGRAPHY

1. Costen, J. B.: A Syndrome of Ear and Sinus Symptoms Dependent Upon Disturbed Function of the Temporomandibular Joint; Ann. Otol., Rhin. and Laryng., 43:1, March, 1934.
2. Costen, J. B.: Summary of the Neuralgias and Ear Symptoms Associated With the Mandibular Joint; The Mississippi Doctor, August, 1937, pp. 33-42.
3. Costen, J. B.: Some Features of the Mandibular Articulation as it Pertains to Otolaryngology; International Journal of Orthodontia and Oral Surgery, Vol. 22, No. 10, page 1,011, October, 1936.
4. Costen, J. B.: Neuralgias and Ear Symptoms Associated with Disturbed Function of the Temporomandibular Joint; The Journal of the American Medical Association, July 25, 1936, Vol. 107, pp. 252-255.
5. Costen, J. B.: Personal Communication.
6. Cunningham's Manual of Practical Anatomy, Vol. 3, 9th Edition, 1935.
7. Ernst, Edwin C.: X-ray Study in Relation to the Mandibular Joint Syndrome. Radiology, Vol. 30, No. 1, pp. 68-75, January, 1938.
8. Schultz, Louis W.: A Treatment for Subluxation of the Temporomandibular Joint; Journal of the American Medical Association, Vol. 109, pp. 1,032-1,035, September 25, 1937.

---O---

Extrapleural Pneumothorax Operation*

PAUL B. LINGENFELTER, M.D.
CLINTON, OKLAHOMA

Extrapleural pneumothorax, contrary to the usual belief in this country, is a very old procedure. According to p a s t records the first operation was performed by Tuffier in 1891 and the collapse was maintained by refills of air. The operation was probably discarded as the result

*Read before the Section on Surgery, Annual Meeting, Oklahoma State Medical Association, Oklahoma City, May 3, 1939.

of unsatisfactory facilities for the continuation of pneumothorax in the m o d e r n way. The previous n a m e for this procedure was the Plombage operation and the materials used were numerous varying from rubber bags, to the different types of foreign material such as wax, vaseline, the combination of same, gauze packs, fat and muscle transplants. The result of all of these was somewhat disheartening; however, there was an occasional successful case.

Graf deserves credit for the present revival of interest in the procedure. He, like many others, had many basal complications following the well known thoracoplasty, for which this operation offers some benefit.

TECHNIQUE OF OPERATION

Present operative medication consists of rather heavy doses of opiates and barbiturates. The operation is carried out under local and intercostal block anesthesia.

Patient is placed in a horizontal and lateral position with face and upper side tilted downward and forward. A 10 to 14 centimeter incision is made parallel to the rib selected for approach into the thoracic cavity. A split muscle incision is made down through the trapezius and rhomboid muscles thus exposing the posterior thoracic cage. A six to eight centimeter segment of the rib is removed. We have found it better to identify the extrapleural plane using curved forceps for blunt dissection along the upper periosteal margin at the junction of the intercostal muscle attachments. Great care must be taken to secure the line of cleavage along the intrathoracic fascia. Quite frequently the tendency is to err and find one's self either intrapleural or outside the endothoracic fascia. The latter will promptly be noted by the presence of intercostal nerves and soft tissues torn loose from the intercostal beds and found lying in the freed lung portion.

The line of cleavage along the intrathoracic plane once having been made the remaining separation is carried out by blunt dissection with fingers and small sponges mounted on curved sponge sticks and using either lighted retractors or sponge sticks to retract the lung from the lateral chest wall. Dissection is carried from back to front over the apex and last around the mediastinal border partly by feel and partly by direct vision. The extent of dissection depends upon the extent of the disease. We have found it best to carry dissection two or three interspaces below the diseased area posterior. The operative area is irrigated with saline and the solution removed. If there is any question of postoperative oozing, the area is partially filled with saline; this is removed within 24 hours.

In the closure lies an important step in the success of the operation. The first layer varies in the individual case; in some cases it is possible to approximate the thickened periosteum over the resected rib area, in others the first layer will be the intercostal muscle and in still other cases the first closing layer will be the posterior serratus muscles and the overlying posterior thoracic aponeurosis or the intercostal muscles and lumbo-dorsalis fascia followed by outer layers. Entire closure is made with interrupted figure of 8, number 2 black silk suture, each layer being sutured to the previous one.

INDICATIONS FOR EXTRAPLEURAL PNEUMOTHORAX OPERATION

1. In cases with unsatisfactory intrapleural pneumothorax, where the lung tissue is plastered to the chest wall, resulting in unsatisfactory closure of cavities.

2. Where there is no space whatsoever as a result of attempted intrapleural pneumothorax.

3. In cases where there is fairly extensive cavitation accompanied by either unilateral or bilateral lesions, in which cases there is too much activity to warrant thoracoplasty.

4. Very young individuals, where the thoracic cage has not reached maturity, and in old people too old for the more extensive procedure.

5. Cases with large adhesions containing lung tissue which cannot be successfully treated by closed pneumonolysis.

CONTRAINDICATIONS AND COMPLICATIONS

1. In cases with extensive thin walled cavities located along the chest wall with very little reaction, such are likely to be perforated. One such unavoidable opening occurred in our series after some 40 odd cases had been done.

2. In cases with extensive apical cavitations in which the blood supply to the outer wall has been destroyed, the freeing of such cavitation from the chest wall has produced a gangrenous sluff of the outer surface. Such occurred in one of our cases 10 days postoperative.

3. The operation should not be used in preference to intrapleural pneumothorax.

4. Other complications have been the interruption of the parietal pleura giving localized pneumothorax.

5. We have had frequent hemorrhages along the costochondral border anteriorly at the level of the first, second and third ribs where there are several nutrient arteries extending to the parietal plural surface; all of these have been controlled by high frequency coagulating current.

6. Serous effusion invariably follows, and the formation of a thickened fibrinous capsule results.

7. One case was complicated by rather extensive blood clots, which were removed by re-operation for further collapse.

8. One incision has opened giving a complete communication with the extrapleural space.

9. We have also had a spread to the contralateral side and spreads to the base of the so-called good portion of the lung on the operative side.

9-a. Postoperative dyspnea due to a mediastinal shift and cardiac embarrassment.

10. One case of partial superior vena-cava obstruction on the right relieved by reducing the extraplural pneumothorax pressure.

11. The effusion in two of our cases thus far has developed into tuberculous empyema of the extraplural space.

12. Several of our cases were operatively prepared for a partial thoracoplasty (two ribs) before the procedure, so that in the event the extrapleural dissection had been impossible, the partial thoracoplasty could be performed.

Such cases are:

a. In cases having very adherent pleura and underlying thin-walled cavities, the cavities are very likely to be perforated.

b. Cases with dense, heavy fibrosis and thickened pleura, as such cases will do better with relaxation by thoracoplasty and destruction of the periosteum.

CONCLUSIONS

1. Extrapleural pneumothorax is one of the most outstanding operative additions to the treatment of pulmonary tuberculosis since the a d v e n t of thoracoplasty.

2. The operation will partially supplant thoracoplasty for the following reasons:

(a). Cosmetic reasons. There is no mutilation visible as in thoracoplasty.

(b). Comparatively speaking, there is a very small amount of shock in proportion to the extent of the collapse as compared with thoracoplasty.

(c). Operation is possible on patients too sick for thoracoplasty and will be of g r e a t e r assistance in such cases.

(d). There will be fewer thoracoplasties because patients will have had the indications f o r t h e extrapleural pneumothorax operation b e f o r e their c o n d i t i o n would warrant thoracoplasty.

3. At a later date when it is deemed advisable to discontinue the collapse such has been done by refilling the space with oil or by thoracoplasty.

4. Many cases will undoubtedly take air refills the rest of their lives.

5. Some cases may be allowed to develop obliterative pneumothorax by discontinuing air refills.

6. It is very unlikely that the average lung will re-expand, due to a very thick, fibrous c a p s u l e lining the extrapleural space.

7. We have done 48 operations on 44 patients with one fatality, 10 days post-operative, giving us at this time a 2.3 per cent mortality.

8. It is too soon to make any final conclusions in respect to this operation as our oldest cases are not yet a year old.

REFERENCES

Belsey, R.: Journal of Thoracic Surgery, August, 1938.

Overholt and Tubbs: Journal of Thoracic Surgery, August, 1938.

Roberts, J. E. H.: British Journal of Tuberculosis, April, 1938.

Monod, Oliver: Journal of Thoracic Surgery, December, 1938.

Tendon Transplantation in Ocular Muscle Paralysis*

HARVEY O. RANDEL, M.D.

OKLAHOMA CITY, OKLAHOMA

In cases of permanent paresis and diplopia, except in certain position of the head and eyes, putting the eyes in a more convenient or comfortable p o s i t i o n by advancement with or without recession, or tenotomy, separate or combined with advancement, will often be sufficient to relieve the diplopia phobia manifested in this type of case. This procedure has been practiced for years, and seems more adapted to concomitant squint or where a paralyzed lateral rectus has recovered power and structural as well as innervational changes have resulted in contracture of the apponent, thereby perpetuating the existing deformity. It may also be used to advantage as in tenotomy of the yoke or conjugate L inf. oblique in cases of sup. rectus paralysis or weakening of sup. oblique in inf. rectus paralysis due to overaction.

Dr. Brittan F. Payne, in the Archives of Ophthalmology, July, 1938, reports a case of abducens paresis successfully operated by this method. (Advancement Recession.) However, the patient was able to abduct the eye to the primary position, demonstrating some lateral rotation. The end result in this case was particularly gratifying in that no diplopia was found in any direction of the gaze. He states, however, that the case was specific in type, and the paralysis of relatively r e c e n t origin. Where there is complete paralysis of the Ext. Rectus muscle, which is the most common of all individual muscle palsies, the sixth cranial nerve being more vulnerable to attack, due to its exposed course, tendon transplantation offers the most, although no operation will relieve the diplopia in every position of the eyes. This operation would seem to be the proper application in all of the Recti extra ocular muscles unless it be the sup. rectus.

O'Connor has summarized in his article on tendon transplantation that this might be an incorrect application because of a possible interference with downward rotation. This operation is credited with being the most extensive of muscle operations, although I find that it is much easier than I anticipated. The advancement is less complicated, the eye ball being held by the sup. and inf. recti. This also eliminates tension on the stitch. I follow the technique as o u t l i n e d by Lancaster in Berens Text of Ophthalmology, transplanting half of the sup. and inf. rectus to act for the lateral or medial rectus. I divide the operation into two stages, doing a recession of the apponent one month later in order to determine more accurately the amount or distance I wish to recede the attachment. This also shortens the time of the first operation, which is time consuming under the most favorable circumstances. I use general anaesthesia for the first stage and local for the second. O'Connor uses local, and advises that the inner three-fourths of the tendons be transplanted, calling attention to the lessening of apponent and restraining effect as compared to transplanting the outer halves. He formerly in five cases transplanted the entire tendons of the vertical recti but abandoned the operation because of marked vertical deviation in two cases.

Peter, in his recent text advocates a recession of the internus reattaching the muscle about 5 mm. back of the stump. He also recommends that this be performed at the same time of the tendon transplantation.

Report of a case:

Mrs. B., age 68. This was a case of complete abducens palsy from fracture of the skull of four years duration. Transplantation of the outer halves combined with advancement of the externus permitted

*Read before the Section on Eye, Ear, Nose and Throat, Annual Meeting, Oklahoma State Medical Association, Oklahoma City, May 2, 1939.

her to abduct the eyes to the primary position. One month later a recession of 2 mm. of the internus increased the ext. rotation seven degrees, and left the internus adequate for convergence. Five degrees or left hyperphoria was c o r r e c t e d with prisms. The cosmetic result was excellent and she experiences no difficulty in the primary position (eyes front).

BIBLIOGRAPHY

1. Payne, Brittan F.: Archives of Ophthalmology, July, 1938.
2. O'Connor, Roderic: Ocular Tendon Transplantations; Archives of Ophthalmology, February, 1931.
3. Lancaster in Berens: The Eye and Its Disease; W. B. Saunders Company, 1936.
4. Peter, Luther C.: Extra Ocular Muscles, Philadelphia, Lea & Febiger, 1936.

———————o———————

New Books

CANCER HANDBOOK of the Tumor Clinic, Stanford University School of Medicine. Edited by Eric Liljencrantz, M.D., Chief of Tumor Clinic, Stanford University School of Medicine, Consultant in Neoplastic Disease, United States Naval Hospital, Mare Island, and United States Marine Hospital, San Francisco. Stanford University Press, Stanford University, California. London, Humphrey Milford, Oxford University Press.

The material presented in this book was assembled for postgraduate instruction at the Stanford University School of Medicine. The methods outlined are those used in their Tumor Clinic. It is divided into 12 chapters, the first being the Cancer Problem with discussion of the inherent and extrinsic factors in the causation of cancer. It is classified both clinically and microscopically.

The next chapter gives a complete discussion as to radiation therapy. Other chapters are devoted to cancer from a regional standpoint; Leukemias and Lymphoblastomata and Bone Tumors are discussed in separate chapters. There are 50 illustrations and charts making this a very complete and concise discussion of the Cancer Problem and the arrangement is ideal for students.

———————

TEXTBOOK OF OBSTETRICS WITH SPECIAL REFERENCE TO NURSING CARE: by Dr. Charles B. Reed and Bess I. Cooley, R. N. of the Wesley Memorial Hospital, Chicago. Published by The C. V. Mosby Company, St. Louis. Price $3.00.

———————

AN INTRODUCTION TO SOCIOLOGY AND SOCIAL PROBLEMS: by Deborah Machurg Jensen, R. N., B. Sc. Published by The C. V. Mosby Company, St. Louis, Missouri. Price $2.75.

VARICOSE VEINS. By Alton Achsner and Howard Mahorner, School of Medicine, Tulane University. Publishers, The C. V. Mosby Company, St. Louis, Missouri. Price, $3.00.

This book is dedicated to Rudolph Matas, universally acclaimed Father of Modern Vascular Surgery, and the foreword is from his pen.

The publishers have made this a beautiful production and the text is systematically arranged in nine chapters, covering history, anatomy, pathology, physiology, etiology, clinical aspects, examination, treatment of varicose veins and ulcers.

There are 50 illustrations and two color plates. In all this is a most comprehensive discussion of the subject with the results of the investigation of the disturbed physiology, the use of appropriate diagnostic tests and the evaluation of methods of treatment.

———————

A TEXTBOOK OF SURGERY (Second Edition): By American Authors, Edited by Frederick Christopher, B.S., M.D., F.A.C.S., Associate Professor of Surgery at Northwestern University Medical School; Chief Surgeon, Evanston (Illinois) Hospital. Second Edition, Revised. 1,695 pages with 1,381 illustrations on 752 figures. Philadelphia and London: W. B. Saunders Company, 1939. Cloth, $10.00 net.

The first edition of this book was universally accepted as one of the most complete one volume works on the subject of surgery. Its thorough indexing makes reference easy and its completeness recommends it as the ideal desk reference.

Every subject is covered by some known authority and one consequently feels that they have the last word on any particular subject in this compilation.

This second edition brings the book distinctly up to date and can be assured of an enthusiastic reception.

———————

TREATMENT BY DIET. By Clifford J. Barborka. Published by J. B. Lippincott Company, Philadelphia. Price, $5.00.

This work now in its fourth edition since 1934 has successfully met the demand for such a book both by the general practitioner and the specialist.

There is no reason to be confused in reading this book and prescribing the proper diet as it is arranged so that one may easily determine the caloric value, carbohydrate, protein and fat content and the quantities in household measurements.

Convenient tables as to percentage of carbohydrates in vegetables and fruits, comparative servings of cereals, bread stuffs, dairy products, meats, vegetables and fruits simplify the arrangement of the indicated diet.

All diseases in which diet is of paramount importance are discussed including diabetes mellitus, gout, obesity, underweight, nephritis, anemia, diseases of the digestive tract, deficiency diseases, et cetera.

Ketogenic diet and food allergy are liberally discussed.

In all this is a presentation of the subject that can be well adapted to any physicians' needs.

———————

PRACTICE OF ALLERGY: By Warren T. Vaughan, M.D., Richmond, Va. Published by C. V. Mosby Company, 3525 Pine Blvd., St. Louis, Mo. Price, $11.50.

This third edition differs from previous editions as it is a thorough treatise on the subject and written for the medical profession only. It deals with botany, bacteriology and mycology. Skin, gastro-intestinal, eye, nose, throat and nervous findings are discussed as to symptoms.

The reading matter is divided into 80 chapters so classified as to make easy reference.

The book is profusely illustrated with original photographs and charts.

Symptoms, diagnosis, treatment and prophylaxis are all covered in a very complete manner. There is much original work and in a bibliography covering 30 pages credit is given to any authorities quoted.

This is a complete and valuable work and will be very useful to any physician interested in the subject.

THE JOURNAL

OF THE

Oklahoma State Medical Association

Issued Monthly at McAlester, Oklahoma, under direction of the Council.

Copyright, 1939, by Oklahoma State Medical Association, McAlester, Oklahoma.

Vol. XXXII	JULY	Number 7

This is the official Journal of the Oklahoma State Medical Association. All communications should be addressed to The Journal of the Oklahoma State Medical Association, McAlester Clinic, McAlester, Oklahoma. $4.00 per year; 40c per copy.

The editorial department is not responsible for the opinions expressed in the original articles of contributors.

Reprints of original articles will be supplied at actual cost provided request for them is attached to manuscripts or made in sufficient time before publication.

Articles sent this Journal for publication and all those read at the annual meetings of the State Association are the sole property of this Journal. The Journal relies on each individual contributor's strict adherence to this well-known rule of medical journalism. In the event an article sent this Journal for publication is published before appearance in The Journal the manuscript will be returned to the writer.

Failure to receive The Journal should call for immediate notification of the Editor, McAlester Clinic, McAlester, Oklahoma.

Local news of possible interest to the medical profession, notes on removals, changes of addresses, births, deaths and weddings will be gratefully received.

Advertising of articles, drugs or compounds unapproved by the Council on Pharmacy of the A. M. A., will not be accepted.

Advertising rates will be supplied on application.

It is suggested that wherever possible members of the State Association should patronize our advertisers in preference to others as a matter of fair reciprocity.

Printed by News-Capital Company, McAlester.

EDITORIAL

THE POWER OF PERSONAL APPEAL

By
LEWIS J. MOORMAN, M.D., Oklahoma City

We are living in an age of relative unrest and instability; an age in which scientific and mechanistic advances have run far ahead of our comprehension and our power of equable integration. The resulting confusion has initiated political, industrial, economic and sociological concepts which threaten the very foundations of personal freedom. Individualistic prerogatives are rapidly succumbing to socialistic trends.

Fortunately human nature is a constant factor. Like the golden thread of truth, it runs unbroken and unchanged throughout the ages. If we search diligently in the mud-tinged current of modern life, we find it, the same genuine human entity, lamenting past failures and losses and anxiously contemplating an uncertain future.

Inherent in human nature, and interwoven with the golden thread of truth, stand religious freedom and the unhampered choice of a physician. Not long ago James Whitcomb Riley wrote: "Why not idealize the doctor some." Riley was the people's poet; he touched the average heart with a broad h u m a n thrust. Beginning with Socrates, this sentiment has been expressed by many of the world's greatest philosophers. It still occupies a fallow spot in the hearts of all people who are fortunate to have the services of a worthy physician.

The average doctor and the average citizen have much in common. . Chief among their common interests, are the freedom of choice and the personal relationship between doctor and patient. To many patients, t h e s e fundamental principles are quite obvious, and, in their opinion, worthy of preservation even at the point of the sword. To others, though equally precious, they may remain as latent or subconscious rights and privileges.

As physicians, it is not only our privilege, but our duty to inform the latter group as to the evils of socialized medicine, and to warn both groups whenever danger threatens and to encourage intelligent opposition to political schemes which, inevitably, lead to the deadening influences of bureaucratic control.

The frequent contact, the vital relationship, and the unselfish mutual interests between doctor and patient result in opportunities for education which should be accepted by every physician as a grave responsibility. It is not only the family physician's duty to give his patients the best available medical care, but it is his duty to preserve and safeguard the system of practice through which the best may always be made available. .

We have reason to believe that in the near f u t u r e, every reputable physician may be supplied with suitable educational material which he may pass on to the patient with the stamp of his approval and the influence of his personal appeal. In the meantime, we should make use of every opportunity to have a heart to heart talk with our patients about our mutual interests which are being seriously threatened by unwarranted paternalism.

---o---

ACTIVITIES OF THE A.M.A.

Feeling that it is important for the members of the State Association to be familiar with some of the major projects of the American Medical Association we are going to publish some extracts from the report of the Board of Trustees and some Standing Committees.

"The total income in 1938 was larger than in 1937, but the increase in total expenditures was considerably larger than the increase in income. Income from interest on investments was slightly larger in 1938 than in the preceding year. Total expenditures were larger than income by the sum of $11,401.51."

It has been the earnest purpose of the Board of Trustees and of the Editorial Department to maintain the Journal of the American Medical Association in its established position of leadership in the field of medical journalism and to increase its usefulness both as a scientific periodical and as a defender of the public interest.

Among the new features developed during the past year has been the Student Section, which appears once each month, dealing with matters pertaining especially to student activities and to medical schools. It is proposed to continue the development of this department of the Journal so as to meet the apparent need for contact between the student, the intern, the resident and the practicing physician.

The activities of the Library have been continued along the same lines previously followed. There was a considerable increase in the number of periodicals lent to subscribers, and the Package Library has continued to supply material largely for the use of members of the Association who do not have ready access to medical libraries. Approximately 5,000 individual inquiries on medicobibliographic subjects were answered during the past year, and more than 1,500 persons visited the Library in search of such material. The Quarterly Cumulative Index Medicus constitutes the major project of the Library Department.

The earnings of the Cooperative Medical Advertising Bureau, through which we obtain most of our national advertising, in 1938 were $33,392.45, of which amount the sum of $17,500 was distributed among the state journals after the operating costs of the Bureau had been deducted. The total amount of the value of advertising contracts secured through the Bureau for the State medical journals was $166,704.57.

Briefly, the important work of the Council on Physical Therapy for 1938 has been directed toward the consideration of radium and radon seeds, artificial l i m b s, audiometers, hearing aids, roentgen ray apparatus, the study of radio interference caused by electromedical equipment, the r e v i s i o n of the Handbook of Physical Therapy and of the booklet "Apparatus Accepted," and the examination of other therapeutic apparatus.

Consultants on audiometers and hearing aids, on artificial limbs, on roentgen ray apparatus and on radium and radon products have cooperated with the Council in connection with the formulation of standards, the preparation of articles and the consideration of apparatus in the respective fields.

The interference with radio communications by electromedical equipment was one of the important subjects coming before the Council. A joint meeting was held at which members of the Medical profession, representatives of the manufacturers of electromedical equipment, of radio manufacturers and o t h e r interested bodies, and officials of the Federal Communications Commission were p r e s e n t. Ways and means of solving the problems were considered but no definite a c t i o n taken.

The Council on Physical Therapy has revised the Handbook of Physical Therapy and brought it up to date. The booklet "Apparatus Accepted" has been revised and reprinted.

The Council has continued its investigation of and reporting on apparatus submitted and in some instances has investigated and reported on products not submitted.

The Council on Industrial H e a l t h has completed its first year of organized activity and much attention has been directed to internal organization and scope. The establishment of headquarters office and a bulletin have greatly facilitated the conduct of its affairs. Preliminary work designed to introduce order into the chaotic field of industrial medical nomenclature is approaching completion. P l a n s are under way to create an abundance of opportunities for sound instruction in the fundamentals of industrial hygiene designed for the undergraduate medical student and for the postgraduate education of physicians. Contacts have been established with all the constituent associations, and committees of industrial health have been established in most of the states where the degree of industrialization seems to warrant it. Steps have been taken to make available authoritative information on clinical and administrative phases of industrial health. Ramifications of medical relationships under workmen's compensation are realized and the Council will work toward uniformity of administration and elevation of medical standards. The Council has instituted an investigation into the relationship between trauma and appendicitis. Its cooperation has been invited to determine the degree of medical interest involved in vocational rehabilitation. Independent agencies interested in industrial health have been investigated and activities of those which have important contributions to make to the health of the worker will be brought to the attention of the medical profession."

The following is a summary of the report of the Bureau of Legal Medicine and Legislation: *"Federal Legislation*—Seventy-Fifth Congress: The new Federal Food, Drug and Cosmetic Act was approved by the President June 16, 1938, and the provisions of it relating to new drugs became effective immediately. The other provisions will become effective June 25, 1939. Under the provision of a law enacted by the Seventy-Fifth Congress, osteopaths are given the same status as doctors of medicine under the United States Employees' Compensation Act.

Seventy-Sixth Congress: The Wagner bill to amend the Social Security Act proposes to give life to the recommendations of the Interdepartmental Committee to Coordinate Health and Welfare Activities. Essentially the bill proposes to provide federal subsidies to induce the states to under-

take new activities and to enlarge activities already under way in certain economic, health and medical service fields named in the bill. The Capper sickness insurance bill contemplates a federal appropriation of $200,000,000 annually to i n d u c e the states to develop and maintain systems of health insurance.

Other federal subsidies are proposed in pending bills to enable states to provide hospital beds for tuberculous persons, medical care for transients or nonresidents, financial aid to the disabled, and to improve measures for the diagnosis, treatment and control of cancer.

A survey of narcotic conditions is proposed in a pending measure, and the creation of a National Institute of Epilepsy similar to the National Cancer Institute is contemplated by another bill. Other federal proposals would authorize federal income taxpayers to deduct the amount expended for medical services, and would amend the Federal Food, Drug and Cosmetic Act for the relief of a nostrum exploited for the relief of asthma.

A proposal to bring under the old-age and unemployment provisions of the Social Security Act organizations operated exclusively for religious, charitable, scientific, literary or educational purposes has been indefinitely postponed by the House Committee on Ways and Means.

The House Committee on World War Veterans' Legislation has filed a report of its investigation of veterans' hospitals but recommended no increase in beds. The present building program is being carried out with the aid of more than $13,000,000 obtained by the Veterans' Administration from PWA. Proposals continue to be made to Congress for the construction of new hospitals. The injustice that has been done to contract surgeons of the Spanish-American War continues.

Three bills propose the reorganization of the civil administrative agencies of the executive branch of the government but none provide for the establishment of a federal department of health or contain any authorization whereby such a department may be created. A pending bill, however, does propose the establishment of such an executive department with a secretary of health at its head. Another bill proposed the establishment of a United

States Medical and Surgical College to be located in the District of Columbia, in which graduates of accredited medical and surgical colleges will be trained for army, navy or public health work.

The incorporation and the legalization of cooperative medical service organizations in the District of Columbia is contemplated by a pending bill.

State Legislation—During the year, as it has done in prior years, the Bureau kept constantly in touch with state legislation of medical interest, promptly advising state associations of legislative proposals that seemed to be of particular importance. Compulsory health insurance proposals were defeated in Massachusetts, New York and Rhode Island, but a commission was created in New York to study the matter and to report back to the legislature. Hospital service corporations were authorized in Kentucky, Louisiana and New Jersey. Other Legislation enacted in one or more states related to osteopathy, chiropractic, venereal diseases, narcotic drugs, vaccination, pneumonia control, educational qualifications of applicants for licenses to practice medicine and the causes for which such licenses may be revoked.

State Legislation by Initiative—Initiative measures in California and Colorado that would have jeopardized the public health and welfare in those states were decisively rejected by the people. Proposed initiative measures in Oklahoma and Ohio did not appear on the ballot."

The Bureau of Health Education, during the past year has done much which will be of interest, not only to the doctors but to the laity as well, as is evidenced by the following summary of their activities:

"The Bureau handled 5,474 communications from doctors, medical societies and cooperating agencies, 8,220 inquiries from the lay public and 1,145 pieces of radio audience mail. The Bureau broadcast 37 dramatized radio programs in cooperation with the National Broadcasting Company. The radio library furnished scripts to 128 county medical societies and 21 state medical associations, distributing a total of 5,540 scripts covering 876 titles. Special radio broadcasts were arranged in connection with the annual session at San Francisco and the special session of the House of Delegates at Chicago. The Bureau cooperated with the Committee for the Protection of Medical Research and distributed 5,430 copies of pamphlets on protection of medical research to senior medical students; these were accompanied by an equal number of pamphlets on medical economics. Cooperation was given to five major departments of the United States government. The Bureau represented the American Medical Association in cooperative projects with the National Congress of Parents and Teachers, the General Federation of Women's Clubs, the National Committee for Boys and Girls 4-H Club Work, the National Education, the American Public Health Association, State and Territorial Health Authorities, National Organization for Public Health Nursing and the Federal Communication Commission's Committee on Evaluation of School Broadcasts. Public addresses were given to 157 audiences in 20 states, requiring 42,-859 miles of travel; these audiences numbered 45,786 persons. Clipping loan collections from Hygeia were furnished to 095 doctors in 46 states to aid them in preparing addresses for the public. The Bureau issued 12 new pamphlets and revised five old pamphlets. Eighty-two items were contributed to the Journal and 34 to Hygeia. Revision of the periodic health examination blank and manual was begun. The Joint Committee on Health Problems in Education of the National Education Association and the American Medical Association was completely reorganized."

The Bureau of Medical Economics has undertaken several important studies during the past year, the report of these studies is summarized in the following:

"*Studies of Medical Care*—Medical societies in 45 states and the District of Columbia are participating in the Study of Medical Care. Already 416 county medical societies in 36 states with the cooperation of other agencies and organizations interested in medical services have completed a study of the need and supply of medical care in their communities.

A special study of free medical services rendered by physicians and dentists throughout the United States has been made by having records of free medical services kept for three representative periods of seven days each.

A supplementary report will summarize the results of the Study of Medical Care and the special study of free medical services.

Medical Service Plans— Medical societies throughout the country have taken a very active part in the study and development of medical service plans. A supplementary report, "Organized Payments for Medical Services," has been prepared which describes practically all the various methods of organizing payments for medical services.

The prepayment of group payment medical service plans w h i c h have received consideration from medical societies can be classified into two main types: (1) unit service plans, which provide medical services through participating physicians who agree to accept a prorated division of whatever funds are available after administrative and other expenses are paid; (2) cash indemnity plans, which provide a designated amount of cash to assist members in meeting their medical bills. Experience gained under each of these types of medical service plans will, no doubt, produce much helpful information.

Group Hospitalization — Hospital insurance plans organized by hospital administrators and physicians have continued to receive widespread attention. One major problem in connection with these plans is concerned with the question of including or excluding special medical services, such as anesthesia, pathology and radiology. The experience gained in the operation of these plans emphasized the importance of the recommendations of the House of Delegates that such special medical services be omitted from a hospital service contract or included only on the basis that cash benefits be payable directly to the member.

The development of medical s e r v i c e plans raises a further question as to the relation between hospital service p l a n s and other medical services in the hospital-surgical and general medical services. The concensus seems to be that a medical service plan should be kept separate in its organization and administration f r o m a hospital service plan.

Relations Between Physicians and Hospitals — Various organized arrangements for the payment of medical services in hos-

pitals brought into sharp focus the necessity for establishing a clearer understanding of relationships between the hospital departments of anesthesia, radiology, pathology and physical therapy and physicians practicing in these departments.

Medical Fee Schedules—An exhaustive survey of county medical society fee schedules has been completed. All the county fee schedules that could be obtained were classified and tabulated into a composite fee table, which includes a t o t a l of 606 items and the "average" minimum and maximum fees for each item.

A supplementary report, "Medical Fee Schedules," has been completed in accordance with the r e q u e s t of the House of Delegates that a study be made of the advisability and necessity of fee schedules.

Collecting Medical Fees—A significant development in medical economics during recent years has been the organization of credit and collection bureaus by county medical societies or by groups of physicians. The movement toward professional control of agencies for the collection of medical accounts has been reported in a special study, "Collecting Medical Fees." This report also outlines and discusses the various systems used by commercial collection agencies and gives particular emphasis to the practices that tend to defraud the u n w a r y physician. Physicians are urged to familiarize themselves with the preferable procedure to follow in the use of a third party agency to collect medical accounts.

Sickness Finance Companies — Recently interest has been evinced in the development of special medical finance plans under the auspices of medical societies or groups of physicians. Patients now have access to a variety of lending agencies and careful study should be given to the development of financing arrangements under the sponsorship of medical societies.

Malpractice Insurance — Policy provisions and rates for malpractice insurance have been s u b j e c t e d to considerable changes in the past few years. Increasing underwriting losses have caused insurance companies to become concerned over the selection of malpractice risks. The present unsettled situation in the underwriting of malpractice i n s u r a n c e is due to many causes, not the least of which has been the recent attempts to discredit the medical profession.

National Health Program—Analysis and statements pertaining to the N a t i o n a l H e a l t h Survey were prepared for the Board of Trustees and the committee appointed by the House of Delegates to confer and consult with proper federal representatives.

Department of Justice Investigation — Every possible assistance was given to the investigator from the Department of Justice to examine all the source files and correspondence of the Bureau which might have a bearing on the mission for which he was sent."

These are but a few of many activities of the Parent organization but should be sufficient evidence that every physician in Oklahoma who is legally practicing medicine should become a Fellow of the American Medical Association; and give both his moral and financial support to the organization without which there would be chaos in the practice of medicine, from which not only would the individual physician suffer but also the health of the community which he serves. As we remarked in a recent editorial "every physician should pay his way by supporting Organized Medicine and not be a *hitch-hiker* along the highway of medical progress."

———————o———————

TRANSACTIONS OF THE FORTY-SEVENTH ANNUAL SESSION OF THE OKLAHOMA STATE MEDICAL ASSOCIATION, OKLAHOMA CITY, MAY 1, 2, 3, 1939.

Council

The Council met in regular session at the Skirvin Hotel, Oklahoma City, May 1, 1939, 3:30 p.m., with the President, Dr. H. K. Speed, presiding, with all members present.

The minutes of the last two meetings of the Council, February 3rd and April 14th, 1939, were read and without correction adopted.

The Secretary-Treasurer-Editor then requested the appointment of an Auditing Committee and the following were appointed: Doctors James Stevenson, V. C. Tisdal and Phil McNeill.

Dr. Finis W. Ewing gave the report of the Committee on Public Policy and Legislation. He expressed the Committee's appreciation to the members of the Council and other members of the Association for their support, mentioning particularly special work done by Doctors McLain Rogers, J. D. Osborn, Jr., and Louis H. Ritzhaupt.

Dr. Risser made a motion that the report of the Committee be accepted and that thanks be extended to the members of the Committee and to those who so ably assisted during the session of the Legislature. Seconded by Dr. Aisenstadt and unanimously carried.

On motion by Dr. Aisenstadt it was agreed that a copy of this be sent to Dr. Ewing and members of his Committee. Seconded by Dr. Tisdal and carried.

Dr. Templin made a motion, seconded by Dr. Kuyrkendall, that subscription to the Journal be made co-existent with membership and that memberships were to become delinquent as of April 1st. Carried.

The following budget was submitted and approved by the Council, to be presented in their report to the House of Delegates:

Salaries:

Secretary-Treasurer-Editor	$ 1,200.00
Executive-Secretary	3,000.00
Stenographer	1,500.00
Travel expense, Executive-Secretary	400.00
Social Security Tax	115.00
Rent	300.00
Telegraph and Telephone	125.00
Postage	250.00
Stationery and Printing	350.00
Bonds and Audit	100.00
Publication of Journal	5,000.00
Expense, Annual Meeting	650.00
Expense, Council and Delegates	300.00
Expense, Public Policy & Legislation	2,250.00
Interest	300.00
Sundry (Misc. office supplies)	100.00
Post Graduate Fund	1,500.00
Cancer Committee	750.00
Payment on Note	2,000.00
TOTAL	**$20,190.00**

Estimated Income

Advertising	$ 5,500.00
Memberships	17,000.00
Interest on Bonds	227.50
Exhibits	350.00
TOTAL	**$23,077.50**

Dr. McNeill discussed the budget and accepted a copy of the contract, under which the Journal is published, in order to compare it with other proposed contracts.

On motion of Dr. Willour, seconded by Dr. Aisenstadt, it was recommended that the House of Delegates reduce the dues of the Association to $10.00 per year.

Dr. Kuyrkendall then presented a letter from Dr. T. H. McCarley offering his resignation from the Editorial Staff of the Journal and on motion of Dr. Kuyrkendall, seconded by Dr. Stevenson, the resignation was accepted.

Dr. Stevenson discussed the merger of the Nowata and Washington County Medical Societies, stating that it was his opinion that this would be of marked advantage to both Societies; he also presented a written petition from these Societies requesting this merger.

On motion of Dr. Stevenson, seconded by Dr. Risser, the merger was authorized by unanimous vote.

Dr. Speed spoke briefly about the excellence of the Public Health Program and Dr. Fulton moved that the House of Delegates be requested to create a Section on Public Health as part of the regular meeting of the State Association. Carried unanimously.

The Auditing Committee submitted the following report, unanimously adopted:

Dr. H. K. Speed, President   May 1, 1939
Oklahoma State Medical Association,
Oklahoma City, Okla.

We, the Auditing Committee of the Council, have the following report to make: Each item of receipts and disbursements have been checked from the auditor's report and the Secretary-Treasurer's statement of same, and found to be correct.

Respectfully submitted,
V. C. Tisdal,
James Stevenson,
Philip M. McNeill.

On motion of Dr. Willour, duly seconded, the Council adjourned to meet on call of the President.

L. S. Willour,
Secretary-Treasurer-Editor.

Council

Oklahoma City, May 2, 1939, 5:30 p.m.
Meeting called to order by the President, Dr. H. K. Speed.

Members present: Doctors H. K. Speed, E. Albert Aisenstadt, Walter Hardy, O. E. Templin, V. C. Tisdal, A. S. Risser, Phil M. McNeill, James Stevenson, J. A. Walker, W. A. Howard, L. C. Kurykendall, J. S. Fulton, L. S. Willour.

The question of the membership of Dr. Ralph Hubbard, Okmulgee County Medical Society, was brought before the Council. This was discussed by Dr. Phil McNeill and Dr. J. A. Walker. Dr. Willour then addressed the Chair and stated he had just left a meeting of the Okmulgee County Medical Society and it was requested that no action be taken by the Council, as they (Okmulgee County Society) preferred to handle the matter in their own way, and that it would be done to the satisfaction of the Association.

On motion of Dr. Walker, seconded by Dr. McNeill, and unanimously carried, no action was taken at this time.

Dr. McNeill then presented to Dr. Willour a proposed contract for publication of the Journal which was discussed, by the Council. However, no official action was taken by the Council.

Dr. Walker made a motion that the Council express to Dr. Speed its respect and high esteem, appreciating his services as President. Seconded by Dr. Aisenstadt and carried.

On motion, duly seconded, the Council adjourned, to meet on call of the President.

L. S. Willour,
Secretary-Treasurer-Editor.

Council

Oklahoma City, May 3, 1939, 10:45 a.m.
Meeting called to order by the President, Dr. W. A. Howard.

Members present: Doctors W. A. Howard, J. S. Fulton, L. C. Kuyrkendall, Phil M. McNeill, E. Albert Aisenstadt, A. S. Risser, O. E. Templin, V. C. Tisdal, James Stevenson, J. A. Walker, Henry H. Turner, J. D. Osborn, Jr., L. S. Willour, and the Executive-Secretary, Mr. R. H. Graham, by invitation.

Dr. Willour requested authority to pay the bills incident to the Annual Meeting and on motion of Dr. Fulton, seconded by Dr. Risser this authority was granted.

The Council next proceeded to elect an Editorial Board of the Journal and the following were nominated: Drs. Ned Smith, Tulsa, Basil A. Hayes, and L. J. Moorman, Oklahoma City, and L. S. Willour, McAlester. Ballot was cast and resulted in the election of Drs. Smith, Moorman and Willour.

On motion of Dr. Stevenson, seconded by Dr. Risser, and unanimously carrying, the Secretary's salary was named at $100 per month with stenographic hire not to exceed $25 in any one month.

On motion of Dr. McNeill, seconded by Dr. Risser, the Executive-Secretary was authorized to move his office to Oklahoma City and spend what time he might think advisable with Dr. Willour before the move is made.

On motion of Dr. Willour, seconded by Dr. Turner, the budget was increased $300, for the purpose of secretarial hire to the Executive-Secretary.

On motion of Dr. Fulton, seconded by Dr. Kuyrkendall, and carried, the Secretary and Executive Secretary were authorized to attend the American Medical Association meeting in St. Louis with expenses paid by the State Association.

Dr. Walker made a motion that the Council express themselves as appreciating the services of Dr. Aisenstadt as Councilor from his district and commend him for the efforts expressed.

On motion, duly seconded and carried, the Council adjourned.

L. S. Willour,
Secretary-Treasurer-Editor.

---o---

Editorial Notes—Personal and General

DR. FRED WEIDMAN, who is head of the Post-Graduate Division of the Department of Dermatology of the University of Pennsylvania, was entertained Wednesday evening, June 21, at the Oklahoma Club by members of the Oklahoma State Dermatology Association. Dr. Weidman with his wife and two children are on their way to the west coast.

DR. GERALD ROGERS, Oklahoma City, was principal speaker at the annual banquet of Alpha Epsilon Delta Honorary Pre-Medical Fraternity at the University of Oklahoma recently. Mr. Jay McCormack, senior medical student in the University of Oklahoma School of Medicine, spoke on some of his experiences in medical school.

DR. G. F. MATHEWS, Commissioner of Health, has recently announced the appointment of the following doctors as county health superintendents.

Dr. Polk Fry, Jr., Frederick, Tillman county.
Dr. J. C. Rumley, Stigler, Haskell county.
Dr. J. I. Derr, Waurika, Jefferson county.
Dr. S. S. Garrett, Duncan, Stephens county.
Dr. L. T. Lancaster, Cherokee, Alfalfa county.
Dr. L. V. Baker, Elk City, Beckham county.
Dr. W. F. Griffin, Watonga, Blaine county.
Dr. R. K. McIntosh, Jr., Tahlequah, Cherokee county.
Dr. J. P. Beam, Arnett, Ellis county.
Dr. W. S. Cary, Reydon, Roger Mills County.
Dr. Walter R. Toblin, Porter, Wagner county.

---o---

Summer Diarrhea In Babies

Casec (calcium caseinate), which is almost wholly a combination of protein and calcium, offers a quickly effective method of treating all types of diarrhea, both in bottle-fed and breast-fed infants. For the former, the carbohydrate is temporarily omitted from the 24-hour formula and replaced with eight level tablespoonfuls of Casec. Within a day or two the diarrhea will usually be arrested, and carbohydrate in the form of Dextri-Maltose may safely be added to the formula and the Casec gradually eliminated. Three to six teaspoonfuls of a thin paste of Casec and water, given before each nursing, is well indicated for loose stools in breast-fed babies. Please send for samples to Mead Johnson & Company, Evansville, Indiana.

ABSTRACTS : REVIEWS : COMMENTS
and CORRESPONDENCE

SURGERY AND GYNECOLOGY
Abstracts, Reviews and Comments from
LeRoy Long Clinic
714 Medical Arts Building, Oklahoma City

The Surgical Treatment of Gastric and Duodenal Ulcers in the Obese Patient: Waltman Walters, M.D., and O. T. Clagett, M.D.; Staff Meetings of the Mayo Clinic, April 26, 1939, Vol. 14, No. 17.

Obesity may add considerably to the technical difficulties and hence to the risk of surgical procedures on the stomach especially if partial gastrectomy is performed. Because of this the obese patient who has a gastric or duodenal lesion may be denied operation.

In the surgical treatment of peptic ulcer anastomosis of the stomach to the jejunum without entero-anastomosis between the afferent and efferent loops is assumed to be preferable to anastomosis with entero-anastomosis since the former results in a more satisfactory dilution and neutralization of acid gastric contents. Posterior and anterior anastomoses seem to be equally effective if entero-anastomosis is not performed. However, the most frequent indication for the anterior type of anastomosis is an obese patient who has a thick, heavy, fat mesocolon. In such a case the chance that postoperative edema of the mesocolon may produce an obstruction at the anastomosis is considerable. Anterior anastomosis is indicated likewise in those few cases in which the mesocolon is so short that sufficient space does not exist between the arcades of the transverse colic vessels to make the anastomosis. In the obese patients it may be necessary to use such a long proximal loop of jejunum for the anastomosis that entero-anastomosis between the afferent and efferent loops of the anastomosis is required to prevent stasis of duodenal secretions in the proximal jejunal loop. This entero-anastomosis drains off the alkaline duodenal secretions and prevents in part their regurgitation into the stomach, hence the neutralizing and diluting effect on the acid gastric secretions is partially lost. That there are other important factors in the problem is apparent since excellent clinical results are frequently obtained with an anterior anastomosis and entero-anastomosis even though the level of the acid in the stomach is not significantly reduced.

The authors report a series of patients where it seems likely that the obesity of the patients might complicate the operative procedure and perhaps determine the type of operation to be performd. At operation, however, they found in all but one case in spite of the obesity, the mesocolon itself was not found to be as thick and fat as was expected and it was possible to establish anastomoses posterior to the colon without difficulty. Their results were satisfactory showing that obesity is not necessarily a contra-indication to surgical procedure in cases of duodenal and gastric lesions.

Dr. Walters, in discussing the paper, called attention to the fact that he had previously presented a discussion of advanced age and cardio-vascular disease as factors influencing the risk of surgical procedure. He pointed out that he had called attention to the fact that patients in the older age group seemed to stand necesesary surgical procedures with little higher operative mortality than patients in the younger age group. He also showed that cardio-vascular disease in relation to surgical procedures did not cause prohibitive risks and that these patients could be operated upon with reasonable safety if cardiac decompensation or auricular flutter was not present.

The present report has to do with the obese patients, most of whom had been operated on during the past month before this report was made for benign ulcers of the stomach or duodenum. In most of these cases partial gastrectomy was performed and it was possible to make an anastomosis posterior to the colon without an entero-anastomosis.

It is known that this procedure in cases of duodenal ulcer is followed by a maximal degree of reduction of gastric acidity due in part to the dilution of the gastric acids by the alkaline secretion from the pancreas, biliary tract, and the duodenum brought into the stomach through the stoma made at the time of the partial gastrectomy or the gastro-enterostomy stoma. An entero-anastomosis in such cases would allow part of these alkaline intestinal secretions to pass through the proximal into the distal loop of jejunum without entrance into the stomach and hence as great a reduction of gastric acidity would not be obtained. Walters says, however, that it does not always seem necessary to gain a maximal reduction of acidity to obtain a good result in the surgical treatment of gastric or duodenal ulcer.

Tomoda and Aramaki, after considerable experimental work, concluded that the success or failure of an operative procedure on the stomach does not have a clear relation either to the lowering or to the increasing of the acid values. The consideration of the acid values alone in a stomach that has been operated on has no value in determination of the success or failure of a given operation.

One may not entirely agree (believing that when a relative achlorhydria is obtained, there is less likelihood of recurring ulceration) yet it does not always seem necessary to get a maximum degree of reduction in gastric acidity to secure satisfactory result.

If the transverse mesocolon of the obese patient who has a gastric or duodenal ulcer is so fat that proper emptying of the stomach cannot be obtained by an anastomosis to the jejunum posterior to the colon, a longer loop of jejunum may be used and the anastomosis may be made more easily anterior to the colon. In perhaps a third of these cases an entero-anastomosis will be necessary to prevent accumulation of fluid and gastric retention in the long proximal loop of jejunum. Occasionally an obese patient upon whom an anastomosis has been made posterior to the colon may develop gastric retention which continues for a considerable period. In such cases even though the patient's fluids and blood electrolytes are maintained by intravenous injection of normal saline and glucose solutions and occasionally by administration of blood, Walters has felt that it is unwise to allow the condition to continue beyond the fourteenth or fifteenth day without providing a method of introducing nourishment into the intestinal tract. This he has accomplished by means of a temporary jejunostomy tube. The jejunal tubes are kept in long enough to allow the inflammation at the anastomosis or in the transverse mesocolon to subside and the gastro-intestinal anastomosis to empty the stomach satisfactorily.

The author's conclusion is that obesity is not a contra-indication to necessary surgical procedures in a case of gastric or duodenal ulcer.

Comment: We believe with Abbott and Rawson (Journal American Medical Association, June 20, 1939, page 2,414) that the use of their double lumen tube in the postoperative care of gastro-enterostomy patients is preferable to the temporary enterostomy tubes as used above. However, the important consideration is that one with an obese patient or with an anastomosis where gastric retention is anticipated should provide beforehand for the introduction of nourishment into the small intestinal tract, at the same time, if possible, keeping the stomach itself cleaned out with suction.

LeRoy D. Long.

Pituitary Gonadotropic Extracts for Treatment of Amenorrhea, Menorrhagia, and Sterility: Ralph E. Campbell, M.D., and Elmer L. Sevringhaus, M.D.; American Journal of Obstetrics and Gynecology, June, 1939, Vol. 37, No. 6, page 913.

The authors have presented syndromes, with examples by case histories of each, which are considered to be the result of underactivity of ovarian hormones and they feel dependent upon underactivity of the anterior pituitary gland in supplying gonadotropic hormone. It is their feeling that the endocrine responsibility for amenorrhea, oligomenorrhea, menorrhagia, irregular cycles, and sterility with anovulatory bleeding lies in pituitary hypofunction in most instances.

It is with this thought in mind that they present several cases of each of these syndromes which have been treated by gonadotropic anterior pituitary extract. The timing of the therapy is considered of especial importance and in accordance with their concept of the time of increasing activity in the pituitary gland, they have employed a long series of repeated daily doses extending from five to 15 days beginning at the onset of menstrual flow. They, however, condemn continuous injections of a potent gonadotropic substance and feel that it should be withdrawn after the first 15 days of a menstrual cycle. They have used several preparations which have not been standardized by a single method and, therefore, the unit strength is not consistent. They have employed Prephysin, marketed by Chappel Bros. Laboratory, Gonadogen, produced by the Upjohn Laboratory, and gonadotropic antuitrin, made by Parke-Davis.

They present cases demonstrating the use of gonadotropic anterior pituitary hormone in each of the following syndromes: secondary amenorrhea; menorrhagia; sterility; and primary amenorrhea. They have attempted to use patients studied for a sufficiently long time to make possible sound judgment as to the adequacy of therapy. Many of the patients demonstrate marked success while others are partial failures.

They emphasize the importance of all means for accurate diagnosis and are enthusiastic about the advantages of endometrial punch biopsies, vaginal epithelial samples secured by pipette as well as of pregnandiol determinations in the urine. The endometrial biopsy reflects in at least a qualitative sense the activity of the ovary. The epithelial sample examined by the technique of Papanicolaou and Shorr, they feel, gives an excellent idea of the estrin activity of the ovary. The pregnandiol determinations in the urine give a qualitative and quantitative estimation of the progestinal activity.

It is their opinion that, if these aids fail to show definite response, treatment may well be increased or abandoned whether or not the menstrual flows are occurring at regular intervals. They likewise feel that results are not obtained in a single month and should be continued over a considerable time.

They feel that the use of long series of daily repeated doses at the beginning of each menstrual cycle is necessary and have been demonstrated to be safe.

It is their further conclusion that the preparations now available are not well enough standardized and potent enough.

Comment: This is an extremely interesting study since the authors have attacked various syndromes of ovarian dysfunction by the use of anterior pituitary extract in an attempt to thereby stimulate the ovary into adequate activity for correction of the symptomatology. This conception that most of the ovarian dysfunctions rest primarily upon anterior pituitary dysfunction can hardly be substantiated with our present knowledge, yet we all well understand that there are many instances of so-called ovarian dysfunction in which the ovaries are entirely normal in their response to pituitary influence but the anterior pituitary influence is not properly regulated or sufficiently potent to produce the average activity in the ovary. It is in these instances that the employment of a sufficiently potent gonadotropic anterior pituitary hormone will be of tremendous advantage. Their conception of the timing of the gonadotropic administration is also interesting in that they feel it must be given with the onset of menstrual flow in order to produce ovulation at the average midmenstrual time.

This article, as well as practical experience, well demonstrates the fact that the results of therapy depend upon the most careful and comprehensive investigation. The additional aids, such as endometrial punch biopsies, epithelial smear examinations, and pregnandiol determinations are to be strongly endorsed in this direction. Of the three the endometrial examination is probably to be considered of more reliable assistance than is the epithelial smear and can be done with considerably less effort than can repeated pregnandiol urine determinations.

Wendell Long.

Treatment of Vulvovaginitis With Estrogen: Charles Mazer, M.D., and Fred R. Schechter, M.D.; The Journal of the American Medical Association; May 13, 1939, Vol. 112, No. 19, page 1925.

This is a rather long article reviewing etiology, diagnosis, and pathology of gonococcic vaginitis in children as well as the basis of treatment of this disease with estrogen.

They report a series of 118 patients of gonorrheal vulvovaginitis treated principally by hypodermic administration of estrogen and by vaginal suppositories of estrogen. In this study as well as in others, the oral administration has been a dismal failure.

In those treated with hypodermic injections, there was a clinical and bacteriological cure in 78 of 81 children with a 10 per cent incidence of recurrence.

In those treated with vaginal suppositories, there was a clinical and bacteriological cure in 33 of 34 children.

All patients received treatment for eight weeks regardless of earlier clinical and bacteriological cures which was considered a safeguard against recurrence of the infection.

Comment: This article is essentially a substantiation of the work of Te Linde which has been abstracted in these columns and which has shown a greater success in cure by the use of vaginal suppositories than by hypodermic or oral administration and has also shown less influence upon the breasts and secondary sex characteristics.

In this series the vaginal suppositories employed contained 200 rat units of estradiol benzoate (progynon-B). These were inserted nightly upon retiring for a period of eight weeks.

The vaginal suppositories employed by Te Linde were amniotin, 1,000 international units each night.

There seems little question but that the vaginal therapy is much more effective in the treatment of vulvovaginitis in children and it is certainly a safe as well as an effective therapy.

Wendell Long.

Adeno-Myo-Sarcoma of the Kidney: Tumor of Wilms (L'Adeno-Myo-Sarcome du Rein: Tumeur de Wilms). By Eugene Gaulin, F.R.C.S. (Canada), Chef du Service d'Urologie a l'hopital General d'Ottawa, Consultant a l'hopital du Sacre-Coeur de Hull; L'Union Medicale du Canada, May, 1939, Vol. 68, No. 5, page 470.

In order to show the general conception of the author with reference to the subject under discussion, I quote the first paragraph of his contribution: "Known universally under the name of tumors of Wilms, the mixed tumors of the renal parenchyma in the infant have been the subject of numerous and serious studies for several years." There is a reference to many authors, all of them concluding that sarcoma of the kidney, adeno-sarcoma, myo-sarcoma, rhabdo-myo-sarcoma are but histological varieties of embryonic tumors of the kidney, all of them possessing certain common histological characteristics not found in adeno-carcinoma; that all of them develop rapidly, silently, and nearly always in young children—most often in infants.

The author reports the cases of four little patients, indicating that his sole purpose is to make an inventory of clinical, pathologic and therapeutic knowledge touching the subject. The ages of the four patients were 12 months, 15 months, 30 months, and 37 months.

In the case of each patient the child had been brought because of an enormous swelling of the abdomen on one side. In each there was striking emaciation.

There was an enormous, firm, painless, partially movable mass in the case of each child.

In one patient there was blood in the urine; none in either of the other three.

In the average patient an intravenous pyelogram did not show evidences of function on the affected side.

There was a pronounced hemoglobinemia in all, ranging from 40 per cent to 60 per cent. In one there was an R.B.C. of 2,787,500. In two others the R.B.C. was 4,000,000 and 4,100,000 respectively, and in a fourth patient the R.B.C. was 4,137,000. Even with these (the last three) fairly good R.B.C. reports, it is striking that the hemoglobin percentage was uniformly low.

There was fever in every patient, sometimes as high as 103° F. The author suggests that the fever is due to absorption from necrotic areas.

In the cases of all the patients reported, there were investigations including X-ray examinations of the bones, before management was undertaken, in order to try to determine, if possible, if there were evidences of metastases. In none of the patients was there any evidence of metastasis before treatment.

In the case of the first child, an infant one year of age, a nephrectomy was done under nitrous-oxygen anesthesia without any preliminary roentgenotherapy. There was no particular difficulty, from a technical point of view, in connection with the operation, which was completed within about half an hour. The child did badly after the operation, the author mentioning particularly vesperal elevation of temperature. Death occurred 38 days after the operation.

The final diagnosis, based upon a histological examination of the removed tissue, was embryonic adeno-carcinoma of the kidney ("adenomyosarcome embryonnaire due rein").

The second patient was a child of three years who was brought to the hospital by the father because of swelling of one side of the abdomen and blood in the urine. In all other respects the history was very much like that of the first child, with the exception of the profound anemia present in the first child. A nephrectomy under nitrous oxide gas anesthesia was done, the preoperative diagnosis being a left hypernephroma. The patient did well until between three and four months after the operation, when it was discovered that there was an invasion of the operative scar in the abdomen. In this case, the histologic examination after the nephrectomy presented the characteristics of Wilms tumor.

In the third child there was a mass the size of two fists filling the right side of the abdomen in a child two years and five months of age. The mass was firm, painless, and mobile. The clinical diagnosis was Wilms tumor. A nephrectomy was done under cyclopropane anesthesia. The histological examination after operation confirmed the clinical diagnosis. The child died six months after the operation.

The fourth patient, 15 months of age, was brought to the hospital because of an enlargement of the right side of the abdomen. In all other respects the history was very much like that of the three preceding children.

It was decided to give the child deep X-ray therapy before undertaking a surgical operation. During the course of the X-ray treatment, there was a sudden leukopenia, with great weakness. In order to nourish the child gavage was undertaken and there were two transfusions of blood. After the forced feeding and the transfusions of blood there was rapid improvement with a hemoglobin of 63 per cent and a red count of 5,000,000. The white blood count was 5,700.

Following the X-ray treatments, there had been great reduction in the size of the tumor which could scarcely be palpated. Following the technique of Dean and others, nephrectomy was deferred for about three weeks. At that time operation was done under nitrous oxide anesthesia. The operation was not at all difficult. There was no evidence of perinephritis or of thrombosis of the vena cava or renal veins.

The histological examination confirmed the diagnosis of Wilms tumor.

The child was discharged from hospital February 12, 1938, and at the time of this report, May, 1939, appeared to be perfectly well.

It will be observed that in the case of these four children reported by the author, nephrectomy was done in each of three of them, none of them living longer than about six months. In the case of the fourth child, nephrectomy was done three weeks after deep X-ray therapy, and for longer than a year the child has been well. I have neglected to remark that X-ray therapy had not been employed in the first three children reported.

The mortality of Wilms tumor in infants is discouragingly high. Cabot is quoted as having set the mortality at about 95 per cent, but with improved methods of treatment, the average mortality, according to the author, is around 86 per cent to 90 per cent. In the series reported by the author, the mortality was 75 per cent, and it is strikingly important to recall that the only child who has lived longer than a few months after the operation had deep preoperative roentgenotherapy.

According to the author, there are no grounds for believing that radiotherapy alone would be of any lasting benefit in the case of a patient suffering of Wilms tumor. He quotes Priestley and Broders to the effect that radiotherapy alone has not cured a single patient. In this connection, the author expresses himself as having considerable confidence in a combination of preoperative radiotherapy, followed by nephrectomy. He suggests that the preoperative radiotherapy be given according to the technique of Coutard.

The author indicates that the diagnosis of Wilms tumor is not difficult. He believes that, in principal, all renal tumors of the infant are adenomyo-sarcomas. Palpation reveals a mass that apparently has its origin in one of the hypochondria. This mass is firm, painless, very often mobile. One of the striking characteristics of the mass is that it is much more prominent on the abdominal side than it is in the loin—a mass "qui ne bombe pas dans les fosses lombaires, mais qui plutot pousse en avant et lateralement."

A pyelogram should be made in the case of every patient. If it is not possible to do a retrograde pyelography, one should have recourse to an intravenous pyelography. While not giving information as definite as a retrograde pyelography, the information, in connection with the clinical picture, is usually confirmatory.

In connection with the differential diagnosis, one must consider suprarenal tumors (tumors of Grawitz), polycystic kidneys (always bilateral), massive hydronephrosis, splenomegaly, intestinal tumors, and peritoneal tuberculosis. As a rule, it is not difficult to make a differential diagnosis.

Notes: While the consideration of Wilms tumor is of particular interest to the urologist, this article is reviewed here because the tumor appears to occupy a position in one side of the abdomen, and for that reason a differential diagnosis is of extreme importance. ·

LeRoy Long.

———o———

EYE, EAR, NOSE AND THROAT

Edited by Marvin D. Henley, M.D.
· 911 Medical Arts Building, Tulsa

Certain Postoperative Complications of Cataract Operations. Carl Berens, M.D., and Donald Bogart, M.D., New York, N. Y. Digested from Sec. Ophth., A.M.A., 1938, and published in Digest of Ophthalmology and Otolaryngology, June, 1939.

"This is a report of a total of 1,004 clinic patients which were operated on for cataract by surgeons, assistant surgeons and house surgeons at the New York Eye and Ear Infirmary during the past two years. Of this number there were 702 extracapsular extractions (70 per cent) performed and 302 intracapsular extractions (30 per cent). In evaluating the results, it must be remembered that the extracapsular as well as the intracapsular extractions were often performed by inexperienced surgeons, and that frequently preoperative complications were present.

"Striate Opacity of the Cornea.—It is believed that striate keratitis may be caused by (1) folding of the deeper layers of the cornea, especially Descemet's membrane, (2) difference in tension in the vertical and horizontal diameters of the cornea, resulting from incision near the corneal margin,

(3) injury to Descemet's membrane during delivery of the lens, and (4) trauma of the endothelial cells covering Descemet's membrane.

"Prevention.—A large section, care in employing instruments, and the use of half-normal physiologic solution of sodium chloride, warmed to body temperature, apparently are aids in preventing the development of traumatic striate opacity.

"Treatment.—Hot applications and the instillation of ethyl morphine hydrochloride seem to be beneficial.

"Incarceration and Prolapse of the Iris.—Prolapse of the iris, which usually occurs within three or four days after operation, may be heralded by the fact that the patient complains of slight pain.

"Cause.—Prolapse of the iris in unsutured wounds may be caused by (a) trauma, (b) defective incisions or (c) omission of iridectomy. Prolapse of the iris alone was observed in six of our patients on whom extracapsular extraction had been performed and in two of the intracapsular cases. In one of these patients the herniated iris was noted five days after the operation, and the eyes were irritated for several weeks postoperatively, final vision was 20/40.

"Prevention.—If the incarceration is slight, usually no serious difficulty results, especially if the iris is covered by conjunctiva. If the sutures are holding, it may be safe to apply physostigmine ointment and allow a few days to elapse before operation. The application of trichloracetic acid is valuable for the treatment of certain types of prolapse of the iris.

"If prolapse is extensive and not covered by conjunctiva, a small iridectomy should be performed and the wound closed with sutures. If prolapse is extreme a conjunctival flap should be made by dissection upward from the cornea; after the protruding iris has been excised the flap is drawn downward over the cornea and sutured below. However, if sutures are in place, the wound should be gently opened, the iris grasped with iris forceps and iridectomy performed.

"Hemorrhage into the Anterior Chamber.—Postoperative hemorrhages may appear in the anterior chamber with or without pain; they usually originate from the sclera or from the iris, rarely from the conjunctiva. Hyphemia developed at 12 (4 per cent) of the intracapsular extractions and in 10 (1.4 per cent) of the extracapsular extractions. Vail found that hyphemia occurred in 7.59 per cent of all cases of cataract extraction.

"To prevent the occurrence of hemorrhages careful preliminary studies are necessary in order to eliminate foci of infection or to raise resistance to them. Coagulation and bleeding time should be normal. Diabetes and high blood pressure should be controlled and syphilis should be excluded. The patient should not be permitted to cough or strain. At the time of dressing, the eyes, while closed, should be gradually adapted to light; the healthy eye should be opened first. After the eyelashes of the eye that has been operated on are free from secretion, the patient should be instructed to open both eyes and the lower eyelids should be drawn down gently.

"Treatment.—Large hemorrhages may protrude between the lips of the wound. It may be necessary to remove part of the clot in order to permit the wound to close. If repeated hemorrhages occur, coagulation, bleeding time and the number of platelets should be studied. Calcium gluconate injected intravenously, normal horse serum, snake venom and brain extract may be administered.

"Detachment of the Choroid. — Subchoroidal exudates, which occur quite frequently, may be seen as dark grayish round masses, usually extending into the vitreous from the anterior part of the choroid. These exudates often absorb with surprising rapidity. In our practice these cases have not been accompanied by serious visual disturbances. Although the choroid seemed to be completely detached in a girl, aged 18 years, after 10 days no ophthalmoscopic evidence of detachment was observable.

"Detachment of the choroid was observed in only one case in which intracapsular extraction had been performed. However, in this series of 1,004 extractions, routine ophthalmoscopic examinations were not made for several weeks postoperatively. Detachment of the choroid occurs at the time of operation in almost all cases, according to O'Brien. Hill found detachment of the choroid in 75 per cent of the cases within 24 hours after intracapsular extraction. He does not feel justified in using the ophthalmoscope immediately after operation; therefore, as a result of examining 24 hours later, he believes that the percentage probably is considerably less than it actually is.

"Expulsive Intra-Ocular Hemorrhages. — Fortunately, expulsive intra-ocular hemorrhage is a rare complication. It is recognized by the sudden and profuse flow of blood, which forces out the contents of the eyeball, replacing them with clotted blood. The choroid and retina are torn from the sclera. Postoperative histologic examination seems to indicate that the hemorrhage is caused by ruptured choroidal veins. Following expulsive intra-ocular hemorrhages, the eye is usually destroyed.

"Detachment of the Retina.—According to Woodruff, retinal detachment following extraction of a cataract is practically incurable. He obtained cures in only 18 per cent of the cases subjected to operation.

"Cause.—Retinal detachment is not necessarily a complication of the operation but may be caused by anterior choroiditis of tuberculous or focal infectious origin. Myopia and loss of vitreous were the important factors in 30 cases of retinal detachment reported by Shapland. Of our series of 1,004 patients, retinal detachment occurred in three cases in which extracapsular extractions were performed and in one case in the intracapsular series.

"Treatment.—Cruise reported successful results following the Safar operation. A cure by the same method is also reported by Hine in a case in which detachment occurred after a needling operation. One of our most successful results was obtained in a case of retinal detachment following extraction of a cataract. The Gonin method, combined with aspiration of the subretinal fluid, results in closure of a tear hole, complete reattachment and final visual acuity of 20/30.

"Glaucoma After Extraction of a Cataract. — Hypertension immediately following operation on a cataract is observed infrequently, even though glaucoma may have been present before operation, as it was in nine (3 per cent) of the intracapsular cases and in 27 (3.9 per cent) of the extracapsular cases.

"When the lens swells rapidly—for example, in cataract caused by dinitrophenol or dinitrocresol—removal of the lens apparently cures the glaucomatous condition. Tension is likely to be increased if the cataract is immature and soft lens matter remains, especially in congenital and juvenile cataracts in which complete discission of the lens has been attempted and only the anterior capsule has been incised.

"Of the 1,004 extractions performed at the New York Eye and Ear Infirmary, secondary glaucoma occurred in two of the intracapsular extractions and in seven of the extracapsular extractions.

"Treatment.—In glaucoma caused by swelling of the lens or by lens matter, removal of the lens or lens particles improves the condition. If chronic simple glaucoma, which is not caused by swelling of the lens, is present, a filtering cicatrix may de-

velop. This tendency should be favored by massage if there is a satisfactory conjunctival flap, and by excision of some of the scleral lip of the wound, which should be made with a keratome at the time of operation. Hypertension caused by iridocyelitis may respond to the use of mydriatics and paracentesis or aspiration of the anterior chamber. Hypertension, produced by chronic iridocyelitis and wounds in which the vitreous, lens capsule and iris are incarcerated, may be extremely rebellious to treatment.

"If hypertension persists in spite of the use of miotics, mydriatics, aspiration, or paracentesis and no cause in the nature of a focal infection or other disease can be found, operation must be performed. If a simple extraction has been performed, we usually prefer iridocorneosclerectomy. If there is a coloboma of the iris, we perform corneosclerectomy over one pillar combined with iridencleisis. If this does not suffice, the operation is performed on the other pillar. The wound may be reopened under a conjunctival flap with a cataract knife or special sclerotomy scissors. If these measures fail the trephine may be used or a seton operation may be employed.

"After-Cataract.—It is estimated that prior to the present trend to substitute capsulotomy forceps for the cystotome in extracting senile lenses, approximately 25 per cent of operations on cataracts were followed by secondary cataracts of appreciable opaqueness. Of the series of 1,004 patients, secondary membranes formed in 38 cases in which extracapsular extraction had been performed; 38 discission operations were performed and it was necessary to repeat the operation in three cases. Dense secondary membranes followed five intracapsular operations.

"In performing an extracapsular extraction of a cataract there can be no argument concerning the use of the multiple sharp-toothed capsule forceps, taking care to remove as large a segment of the anterior capsule as is possible. If this procedure is followed it will rarely be necessary to perform a discission operation. Removal of blood and all lens matter with the aid of a Hildreth lamp assists in preventing dense secondary membranes.

"Treatment.—Most of these secondary cataracts are of slight or moderate thickness and respond favorably to a well selected discission. The choice of operation for secondary cataract is important. Lyster advocates freeing the iris from the secondary membrane by a sawing movement with a short knife. The more experience one has, the more one is likely to agree with Fox that they should be carefully cut with scissors. Dense membranes are cut with less traumatism with long thin-bladed iridocapsulotomy scissors after a small subconjunctival incision has been made at the limbus with a narrow (3 mm.) hollow ground keratome; the keratome also punctures the membrane. In making these incisions, it is well to avoid the area of the wound, especially if extensive scar tissue is present. To maintain dilation after the anterior chamber is opened in operations for secondary membrane, atropine combined with a 1:1,000 solution of epinephrine may be used preoperatively.

"Intra-Ocular Inflammation.—Mild inflammation with a slight tendency to the formation of posterior synechiae is commonly observed. Focal infections, as probable etiologic factors, have been discovered in some cases. Of our series of 1,004 patients, iridocyclitis occurred in seven on whom extracapsular extraction was performed.

"In some cases, toxic lens substance, that is, so-called endophthalmitis phacogenetica, may be a factor. Straub was convinced that this type of inflammation was caused by the presence of lens matter in the eye. In other cases, there seems to be a definite sensitiveness to lens antigen, so-called endophthalmitis phaco - allergica. Frankling and

Cordes believe that this condition may be mistaken for infection. It is especially important to perform intradermal tests with lens antigen in all patients who have had one eye removed in which the lens was injured or one eye has been operated on for cataract, especially if marked chronic inflammation followed an extracapsular extraction.

"Sympathetic Ophthalmitis.—Sympathetic ophthalmitis, which tends to affect the second eye, is fortunately a rare complication of an operation for cataract. Our impression is that the best treatment of these cases is the removal of or raising the patient's resistance to foci of infection, combined with the use of nonspecific therapy, especially typhoid vaccine, followed by aspiration of the anterior chamber or paracentesis.

"In sympathetic ophthalmitis, operation to improve vision should be delayed until all signs of inflammation have been absent for at least a year.

"Suppurative Postoperative Infection. — Fortunately suppurative postoperative infection is rare when rigorous methods of asepsis have been employed. Suppurative intraocular infection occurred in one patient in our entire series of 1,004. Extracapsular extraction was performed on this patient and the eye was lost. The causative organism was not determined.

"Prevention.—A speculum with solid blades should be used to keep the eyelashes as well as the border of the eyelid and meibomian glands out of the field of operation. We have used 1 per cent silver nitrate as suggested by Bell.

"Treatment.—The wound should be opened immediately with a spatula and smears and cultures should be taken and prompt antiseptic treatment instituted. If any organism which responds to any particular therapeutic measure is found, this treatment should be employed: for example, ethylhydrocupreine hydrochloride in the presence of pneumococcic infection. When the cornea is invaded, the anterior chamber is usually involved; the anterior chamber may be irrigated with 1:4,000 solution of hexylresorcinol. If the pneumococcus, which may be typed, is found, pneumococcus serum should be employed. However, if no special organisms are found, it is well to prescribe intravenous typhoid vaccine or typhoid H antigen. As soon as it is apparent that the eyeball cannot be saved, a horizontal incision should be made in the cornea; the intra-ocular contents should be allowed to drain for a day or so or the contents may be immediately evacuated.

"Loss of Vitreous.—Subchoroidal hemorrhage may be the exciting factor in the loss of vitreous, but injury to the eye, vomiting, straining or traumatism are more common causes. It is stated that tying the sutures involves a real risk, for in the short period of time necessary for this procedure a considerable amount of vitreous may be lost. However, this criticism does not seem to apply to the untied sutures and conjunctival bridge.

"Loss of vitreous occurred in 30 of the 302 intracapsular extractions (9.9 per cent), whereas this complication was observed in 63 (9 per cent) of the extracapsular extractions. These figures possibly are significant in regard to the greater danger from loss of vitreous following intracapsular extraction in the hands of the average surgeon when one realizes that extraction in capsule usually was not attempted in patients with complicated cataracts.

"Prevention.—A wound thoroughly closed, as soon as the lens is expressed, by a complete conjunctival flap held by sutures, which include the episcleral tissue and the presence of the iris are safeguards. Careful nursing to see that the patient avoids strain or injury is important. Coughing should be controlled by sedatives, posture and local nasal treatments. Vomiting caused by drugs should be

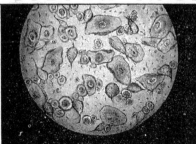
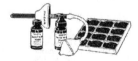

prevented by preoperative trial of the drugs to be employed postoperatively. If cataract is present in only one eye, the vitreous in this eye is usually liquid. A flap should be prepared and sutures should be put in place so that the lens may be extracted with a spoon.

"Treatment.—If much solid vitreous is incarcerated and the conjunctival flap is not wide and complete, excision of the protruding vitreous is indicated after the eye has been carefully anesthetized. Before the vitreous is excised, the conjunctiva above the cornea should be undermined and two double-armed sutures placed so that the flap may be made to cover the cornea immediately. If a good conjunctival flap is present sutures should be placed in this."

Management of Glaucoma Following Cataract Operation. B. Y. Alvis, M.D., St. Louis. American Journal of Ophthalmology, May, 1939.

The term postoperative glaucoma includes cases which have pain, congestive symptoms, have to do with the time of onset relative to operation, effect on vision, etc., but they all have one common condition, i.e., increased intraocular pressure. The author divides his cases into two groups: one, including those that arise soon after the cataract extraction or needling and, second, those that appear long, half a year or more, after the operation. The first he terms acute congestive glaucoma, the second chronic or simple glaucoma.

Etiology is obstruction of the drainage angle. There are many causes, operative and postoperative for this condition.

The pathology is discussed and characteristic findings are given in eyes that have been enucleated.

Under "Prevention" the following are given by the author:

1. The incision is the most important feature of the operation. It should follow the corneoscleral junction and should have a conjunctival flap above to aid in coaptation of the margins. It must be ample in size.

2. Avoid loss of vitreous. One cannot secure a neatly closed wound free of capsule, iris, cortex, and vitreous if the latter is protruding through the wound. The actual vitreous substance lost is much less important than the complications of wound closure.

3. The question of iridectomy, complete, peripheral, preliminary, or simple extraction has been argued pro and con. Statistics of large reported series are not definitely favorable to any one method. Without question an intact iris with the angle free offers the best protection against entanglement of vitreous, capsule, and cortex in the wound. The difficulties of delivering the lens through a round pupil and of avoiding iris adhesions or even prolapse often more than outweigh these advantages. Unless the pupil dilates freely and well, I believe the complete iridectomy the safer procedure.

4. Intracapsular or extracapsular extraction presents another field of argument. Again it seems obvious that the complete removal of the lens favors an open angle and a wound free from adhesions, but if such a delivery can be accomplished only by an undue traction on the zonula, excessive pressure, and danger of vitreous loss, the gain is too dearly bought.

5. The toilet of the wound is a step of great importance in avoiding postoperative glaucoma. Great care in freeing the wound of all debris of capsule, iris, cortex, and clots in order to secure quick and accurate wound closure is entirely worth while. A large bubble of air injected into the anterior chamber at the close of the toilet is sometimes helpful in freeing the angle.

6. In capsulotomy a single, small vertical cut through the membrane or a small inverted V opening made with a narrow knife needle with a tapered shank, so that vitreous will not be drawn into the corneal wound, should be made. The pitfalls here are the flooding of the anterior chamber with vitreous and the anterior synechia of hyaloid or capsule. A vitreous tag in the wound that easily escapes notice may lead to low-grade infection and congestion causing glaucoma.

The discussion should be postponed until the eye is quiet. Use no atropine after needling unless iritis develops and the eye is soft.

7. The tension should be taken frequently in postoperative cases, and these should be kept under observation for some months if possible.

Under "Treatment" he gives the following:

1. Local medicaments are the miotics, the mydiatics, and the epinephrine preparations.

(a) The miotics, pilocarpine and eserine, approximately head the list of local therapeutic agents. These are, after all, our most dependable agents. It is our practice to begin with pilocarpine 1 per cent. Some cases respond at once with lowered tension. In most this response is only temporary and soon increasing strengths of pilocarpine (up to 5 per cent) are necessary. If these do not aid, eserine is used, beginning with 0.5 per cent solution. If eserine maintains lowered tension but must be used for a long period, an eserine sensitization develops. Eserine alkaloid in castor oil or in an ointment base may then be used. Even after surgical measures, one often must continue the miotics.

(b) The mydriatics-homatropine and atropine. In an occasional case with frank iritis these may reduce tension and lead to a cure, but must be handled with great caution.

(c) Epinephrine preparations-glaucosan, suprarenin bitartrate (a 2 per cent solution or in ointment form) epinephrine 1/100, epinephrine 1/1,000 as a pack are useful in certain cases of postcataract glaucoma. As a rule, in the acute or congested stage, the epinephrine preparations are not helpful. They may even cause severe pain and a further rise of tension. After the miotics have been used for some time, perhaps even after surgery and if the case has reached a stage with little congestion, when the tension remains up in spite of treatment, one may find this concentrated epinephrine surprisingly effective. One must be cautious at the beginning. Give the first treatment at the office or hospital where the tension can be measured after an hour or so. If the tension rises abruptly, a paracentesis should be done at once and eserine instilled. Even when epinephrine is helpful epinephrine is best used in conjunction with a miotic. I can, however, think of three patients who use only epinephrine 2 per cent in water-soluble base, and only when they feel pain or blurring vision, indicating a rise of tension.

2. Local physical therapy includes heat, cold, and massage.

(a) Hot fomentations. Frequent and prolonged, this is the most useful of all nursing measures.

(b) Radiant heat. The infrared lamp, a simple 16 c.p. carbon filament bulb, any electric heating device may be the source. On ward service the infrared lamp is more apt to be applied as much and as often as ordered than moist heat which requires constant attendance of the nurse. Also radiant heat seems to penetrate deeper.

(c) Ice-cold applications. In occasional congestive cases cold may give greater relief from pain than heat, and should not be forgotten. Heat is more often useful.

(d) Massage of the eyeball may help to keep open an operative drain.

3. Constitutional medication.

(a) Ergotamine tartrate-intramuscular or oral administration of 1 mg. (1/60 gr.) doses has been recommended and seems to have been useful in some of our own cases.

(b) Calcium, gluconate or chloride. Both these medications are used for their effect on the sympathetic nervous system.

(c) Intravenous hypertonic solutions serve to withdraw fluid from the tissues and actually reduce intraocular tension. This effect is transitory lasting at most a few hours. This is useful as a preoperative measure.

(d) Purging and sweating fall in the category and have not seemed worth while in our observation.

(e) Fever therapy may be useful where tension is secondary to uveitis. Typhoid bacilli are our choice, but milk or the hypertherm or hot baths may be used.

4. Surgical measures.

In the great majority of cases surgery is necessary. No one operation has found favor with any convincing majority of eye surgeons, but the following have the most success to their credit:

(a) Iridectomy. H. Knapp reported marked success in an early series of cases, following similar experience has not been so favorable especially in recent years.

(b) Cyclodialysis is considered the operation of choice in this particular type of glaucoma by Elschnig, Fuchs, Gradle, and others. It does serve to break up anterior synechiae of iris and capsule and doubtless is successful in many instances. It also is easy to do and does not mutilate the eye nor preclude subsequent operations by the same or other methods. Our own experience with this operation is not so satisfactory.

(c) Iris inclusion. This operation has grown largely in favor in recent years. Its simplicity and safety in execution and the permanency of drainage secured make it a valuable measure. Even when the immediate reduction of pressure may be insignificant or nil, the ultimate result may be good.

(d) Trephining, especially if done in an area where the iris has been undisturbed previously is successful in a fair proportion of cases.

(e) Sclerectomy or iridosclerectomy (Lagrange) or Berens irido-corneo-sclerectomy are operations to be considered.

A few case reports are included in this article.

----------------o----------------

PLASTIC SURGERY
Edited by
GEO. H. KIMBALL, M.D., F.A.C.S.
404 Medical Arts Building, Oklahoma City

Utilization of the Temporal Muscle and Fascia in Facial Paralysis. James Barrett Brown, M.D., St. Louis, Mo. Annals of Surgery, June, 1939.

The author has brought out an operation which utilizes the temporal muscle and fascia to give anchorage for fascial strips and to gain some emotional expression of the face afflicted by paralysis. This is different from previous operations in that the muscle is utilized for facial action, being innervated by the fifth nerve.

Previous operations have been done for congenital paralysis especially. Among these operations are anastomosis of motor nerve. Some of these have been very successful.

Eden, in 1911, and Gillies in 1917, used strips of temporal fascia turned downward over the zygoma to support the face. J. S. Davis in 1911 and Gallie and Le Mesieur, in 1923, published the results of extensive work on the free transplantation of fascia, and the first report of free fascial strips to support the paralyzed face was made by Blair in 1926.

In this article the author outlines the method for the combination operation in which fascial strips are anchored directly into the temporal muscle and fascia. The technique of anchoring the fascia is outlined. The operation is described in detail as to the incision, the manner of inserting the fascia and the manner of fixation. It is necessary and important to attach the fascia on the muscle nerve to the coronoid attachment.

The author states that the secondary operation may be needed where there is an excess of skin where there is an extremely drooped cheek.

Post-operative course: Large pressure dressing is used held with adhesive. Chewing is prohibited. After several days a collodion dressing and fine mesh gauze is used for support. This dressing is continued for two to three weeks before activity is allowed. After some weeks a conscious muscle activity comes into play resulting in some emotional expression.

Facial Muscle and Speech Training: One of the most important points, for a successful outcome, is that the patient should train his facial movements. This included the use of the newly attached fifth nerve which will produce a slight smile and a nasolabial fold on a slight setting action of this closing muscle; and of equal importance is learning not to overact on the sound side. It seems that many people with facial paralysis, in speech and laughter, throw about twice as much movement into the sound side of the face as they probably would if both sides were working. Therefore, a fundamental of the training might be for these patients to try to become rather "glum," and work from this point towards a limited movement on the sound side and an involuntary or subconscious setting of the fifth nerve muscles on the repaired side, in smiling. Of course, sudden emotions will always register mainly on the sound side; there is probably no way of controlling this, and it would be the same even with a successful nerve anastomosis.

If there are other speech defects, such as lisping, training by a professional should be of great value, because everything that will help overcome other persons noticing the face of one of these patients is desirable.

Eye Involvements: As has been mentioned before some elevation of the sagged lower lid is obtained by the operation on the face. If it needs further support, a single fascial loop can be put through the lid and held on each end, above in the opposite frontalis—which may give some slight emotional expression—and on the outside in the temporal fascia.

Heavy drooping brows may be raised by extending the skin incision over the forehead, undermining down to the brow, elevating and excising the excess skin, and reattaching it to the scalp. For the apparent exophthalmos a small external canthoplasty can be performed to narrow the opening. Cervical sympathectomy has been recommended to produce the enophthalmos of a Horner's syndrome, but this procedure would be contraindicated if there were already a heavy overcast eyebrow.

When ptosis of the upper lid exists with seventh nerve paralysis, the problem of getting the lid elevated becomes very acute. If an extra-ocular muscle operation will not suffice, the lid can be elevated with a single loop of fascia from the temporal fascia, through the tarsal border of the lid, across to the opposite frontalis. An extra loop may be necessary to help in the elevation and may be attached to the inert tissue in the forehead. This implies that the lid will be held open all the time, and trouble with the cornea will result if it is not kept protected carefully.

The use of the fifth nerve muscles is not recommended in trying to get elevation of the upper lid because of giving movements that would appear too gross and too conscious.

Comment: The author contributes an advance in the treatment of cases with paralysis of the face as well as those involving the eyelid (traumatic). The results appear to be good. Special significance of this operation is that it outlines muscular action for facial expression in contrast to other operations where there is a permanent fixation of the part by fascial strip fascia.

One might choose between motor nerve anastomosis, fascial strip embedded in muscle or a combination of fascial strip and frontalis masseter muscle support.

The author is to be complimented on the clear cut manner in which he presents this technique. It seems more direct and simple to perform this operation than either the nerve anastomosis or the so-called masseter and temporal fascia operation.

---o---

CARDIOLOGY

Edited by F. Redding Hood, M.D.
1200 N. Walker St., Oklahoma City

The Action of Parahydroxyphenylisopropylamine (Paredrine) On the Heart; A Clinical Study of a New Epinephrine-Like Compound. Morris H. Nathanson, M.D., F.A.C.P., Los Angeles, California. (Annals of Internal Medicine, May, 1939, Vol. 12, No. 11.)

It is well established that epinephrine is the most valuable therapeutic agent in the prevention and treatment of cardiac standstill. Its action increasing ventricular excitability is variable and at times minimal. Ephedrine has been the only substance available which was effective when administered by mouth and its therapeutic value has been limited due to its comparative weakness and its unpleasant side actions due to central nervous stimulation. This paper advances paredrine which stands between epinephrine and ephedrine in chemical structure. In a series of cases treated by these three drugs, it is generally found that in their effect on cardiac standstill ephedrine and paredrine produced the same qualitative effects but that the effect of paredrine was observed earlier and that the duration was longer. Of special interest was the fact that the symptoms due to central nervous system stimulation such as nervousness, tremor, and apprehension were not observed in any case following paredrine. Headache of moderate severity was noted in two cases and was promptly relieved by nitroglycerine. The effect of epinephrine on heart block is variable and may have the following results in auriculo-ventricular

block: (1) the ventricular rate may be increased and the block remain unaffected; (2) there may be a variable degree of lessening of the block; (3) beneficial effects as indicated by the prevention of syncopal attacks may occur without acceleration of the ventricular rate or the modification of the block. The author gives a summary of six case histories showing the effect of paredrine as being similar to that of epinephrine but producing a more constant action and without central nervous system effects. The similarity in the modification of the electrocardiogram following the administration of epinephrine and paredrine is further evidence of the epinephrine on the heart.

Comment:

The effect of paredrine is less intense but more prolonged than that of epinephrine. The chief advantage of paredrine lies in this respect so that the drug is effective on oral administration. The superiority over ephedrine is its greater intensity of action and the absence of unpleasant side effects. Therapeutic indication for paredrine in cardiac disease is therefore the same as for epinephrine and ephedrine, which is primarily the prevention and treatment of cardiac standstill. A dose of 40 to 60 mg. three or four times a day appears to be sufficient to raise ventricular rhythmicity to a degree so that the tendency to ventricular standstill is definitely lessened.

Summary:

1. Parahydroxyphenylisopropylamine (paredrine) is a drug related in chemical structure to epinephrine and ephedrine.

2. The substance is effective on oral administration.

3. Paredrine effectively prevents the c a r d i a c standstill induced by pressure on the carotid sinus and is at least twice as effective as ephedrine in this action.

4. When administered in dosage effective in preventing cardiac standstill, paredrine does not produce unpleasant side effects due to central nervous stimulation.

5. Paredrine has an epinephrine-like action in auriculo-ventricular block.

6. Paredrine produces changes in the ventricular complex of the electrocardiogram similar to those which follow the administration of epinephrine.

7. Paredrine has certain advantages over epinephrine and ephedrine in the therapy of cardiac and ventricular standstill.

General Medicine. A Slowly Absorbed Gelatine-Epinephrine Mixture. W. C. Spain, M.M., M. B. Strauss, B. A., and A. M. Fuchs, M.D. (Modern Medicine.) (The Journal of Medical Progress, June, 1939, Vol. 7, No. 6.)

Impressed by the need for a slow-acting epinephrine, Keeney of Baltimore last year reported the successful use of peanut oil as a dispersion medium for the drug. But a possibly more convenient method of preparing a slow-acting epinephrine by mixing it with gelatine, sodium chloride, chlorbutanol, sodium bisulfite, glycerine and water, is reported by the authors. This mixture is nontoxic, nonantigenic, reasonably stable, and can be easily self-administered with a regular needle and syringe, this last being an advantage over the peanut oil method. The principal disadvantage of this new mixture is that it must be warmed before administration.

Although the gelatine-epinephrine preparation is a 1:500 solution, containing twice as much epinephrine as the ordinary 1:1000 solution, pallor, palpitation and tremor are both infrequent and delayed. It is possible that the risk occurring with other therapeutic agents administered by injection (diphtheritic, scarlatinal and streptococcic toxoids, pollen extract, horse serum) might be minimized by the addition of gelatine. The gelatine-epinephrine mixture is prepared as follows:

To a solution containing 40 cc. of glycerine and 130 cc. of distilled water are added 1.8 Gm. of sodium chloride, 1.0 Gm. of chlorbutanol, 0.2 Gm. of sodium bisulfite and, last, 40 Gm. of gelatine. This preparation is placed in a one-liter pyrex Florence flask and mixed vigorously by rotation, then sterilized by autoclaving for 30 minutes at 20 pounds pressure. The 1:500 epinephrine solution is made by adding one part of a 1:100 solution to four parts of the sterile gelatine mixture.

———————o———————

INTERNAL MEDICINE
Edited by Hugh Jeter, M.D., 1200 North Walker, Oklahoma City

Sterile Motile Spermatozoa, Proved by Clinical Experimentation. Frances I. Seymour, M.D. The Journal of the American Medical Association, Vol. 112, No. 18, May 6, 1939.

In this case the author describes a case in which he seems to have proven conclusively that the usual test for sterility in male has proven unreliable. The spermatazoa count in this patient was 94,000,-000 per cubic centimeter of fluid, the motility good and pus absent. His wife's examination was entirely negative and there appeared to be no reason why she should not conceive. The only debilitating influence of the husband seems to be the fact that he was "constantly subject to grueling effects of university routine," he being a professor in a university. Cross insemination later proved the husband incapable of fertilizing his wife and also incapable of fertilizing other subjects, whereas both his wife and the other females were satisfactorily impregnated by insemination from other males.

Comment: It is hardly conceivable that spermatazoa normal in number and quality could have given such results, but "proof of the pudding is in the eating," and therefore we must accept this report.

A Bedside Method for Detecting Dextrose in the Urine. Herman L. Jacobius, New York. The Journal of The American Medical Association, Vol. 112, No. 18, May 6, 1939.

In this the author describes a simple method for the determination of dextrose in the urine, which

he calls a bedside test. It has the advantage of being quickly executed and also inexpensive as compared with other tests in as much as very little reagent is used for each test.

The principle of the test is simply the saturation of asbestos with Benedict's solution, add a drop or two of urine and heat over a noncharring flame such as Bunsen burner, stove range or alcohol lamp. Various colors are obtained in the course of one minute's heating, orange being interpreted as 3 per cent or more, canary yellow 1 to 3 per cent, greenish yellow 0.5 to 1 per cent, faint yellow on a green background 0.1 to 0.5 per cent and no change 0.07 per cent.

Tests of diabetic urine of known dextrose concentration, determined by more elaborate quantitative methods, showed an agreement with the results obtained with the asbestos applicators close enough for ordinary clinical purposes.

One hundred samples of normal urine were tested and none gave a false positive reaction.

———————o———————

UROLOGY
Edited by D. W. Branham, M.D.
514 Medical Arts Building, Oklahoma City

Urologic Hypertension. Chauncey C. Maher and Paul H. Wosika. **And—Unilateral Chronic Pyelonephritis with Arterial Hypertension.** D. W. McIntyre. Journal of Urology, June, 1939.

These two articles are of importance as they represent a trend of investigation hither-to somewhat neglected that may explain in many instances of high blood pressure the etiologic factor responsible.

The first article by Doctors Maher and Wosika, details the study of 101 patients who had both hypertension and urologic defects and their potential relationship. The majority of these, so far as their urologic pathology is concerned includes chiefly, infection and obstruction of the tract. The trend of these two factors, as far as could be determined by autopsy of cases, is kidney damage of a variable degree.

These authors are convinced that hypertension would appear to be associated with urologic pathology more often than is ordinarily believed and they suggest that before a patient may be classified as having hypertension of unknown origin, the entire urinary tract must be proved to be normal from an urologic standpoint.

The second article is a case record that illustrates this point. A relatively young white male adult suffered from hypertension for a number of years. A medical diagnosis of early malignant arteriolar hypertension was made on a previous admission to the hospital. He returned later having had an attack of renal colic. A hydronephrosis complicated with infection was found on cystoscopic investigation. Removal of the affected kidney was followed by a marked drop in blood pressure which on further observation has remained within normal limits. Apparently arterial diseases associated with unilateral pyelonephritis was responsible for the

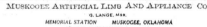
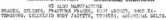

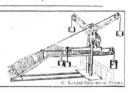

hypertension and a cure by nephrectomy was obtained.

Comment: Because renal pathology of a so-called urologic character is often of a silent nature it is well, before the physician condemns an individual to what might be called an early death, some attention should be paid to the urinary tract for urologic pathology.

Undoubtedly there are many instances of chronic nephritis and hypertension of undetermined origin that rests on an urologic basis.

Rupture of the Urinary Bladder. Leon M. Bogart, M.D. The Urologic and Cutaneous Review, May, 1939.

The percentage of rupture of the urinary bladder runs about 15 per cent in the authors series of 51 cases of fractured pelvis. This is in accord with similar series hitherto reported in the literature.

Because this complication far over shadows in immediate importance the injury done to the bones the attending physician must be continually on his guard in order to diagnose its presence early and apply appropriate surgical treatment.

The diagnosis is not only made on the symptoms and signs referable to the urinary bladder but must be corroborated by X-ray examination. The author suggests the making of a retrograde cystogram using a urethral catheter and instilling 2 per cent sodium iodide as a contrast agent.

The treatment is immediate exploratory laparotomy with drainage of the bladder and surrounding tissues when the extravasation is pronounced.

Comment: In this day and age of frequent automobile accidents fractured pelves are a common occurrence and because the bladder is so frequently injured the physician who sees these cases early must make the diagnosis. Procrastination in the treatment of bladder rupture means the chances for the patients' ultimate recovery is lessened.

I somewhat disagree with the method of diagnosis by X-ray where it was suggested a catheter be inserted in the bladder in order to make a cystogram. Catheters and cystoscopes undoubtedly increase the liability of infection and should not be used unless absolutely necessary. The administration of the intravenous dyes to visualize the tract obviates this possibility. Not only may the rupture be demonstrated by the excretion cystogram but the type of rupture, whether it be intraperitoneal or extraperitoneal may be shown. Intraperitoneal rupture shows the dye collecting in the inferior abdominal cavity in a mass and extraperitoneal rupture reveals the contrast substance extravasating up along the fascial planes of the pelvis.

———o———

Physicians As Artists

"From time immemorial, medicine and art have been closely associated. The same skill that makes the surgeon's fingers deft with scalpel and ligature is at work in the beautiful examples of sculpture and carving shown in this book. The eye that so quickly and accurately evaluates the gradations in color and texture between normal and pathologic tissue coordinates the hand that wields the painter's brush. The man who chooses medicine as his life's work is largely motivated by a love for his fellow man, else he would select a vocation offering greater monetary reward. From the beginning, he is trained to exercise his powers of observation, and in time develops imagination, sympathy, understanding, philosophy and reverence, all of which are the very essence of art. Moreover, he deals with that most exquisite form of divine art and beauty, the human body.

"An artist-physician has said: 'The tendency of most persons is to regard the artist with awe as a superman endowed with talents not vouchsafed to the ordinary mortal. Most doctors have a latent artistic sense which may be developed to a remarkable degree by constant practice. When opportunity affords, slip away to the park or country, sit down on a camp-stool and practice sketching from nature. At first the results may not be satisfying, but in course of time you will be gratified to notice a marked improvement. An ample sketching kit may be purchased for a small sum and any local artist will be glad to give you instruction.'

"At the least, every physician is able to develop a sensitiveness to and an appreciation for fine art. He can also cultivate a hobby which if not one of the fine arts, is in the class of 'work by the side of work.' Dr. Charles A. Dana, who has always stressed the value of cultural medicine, has advised: 'Be a collector, for example, of stamps or automobiles, or old books, or neckties or pins; or find diversion in some collateral branch of science; the lore of birds, of fishing and shooting. Make a garden or cultivate shrubs and flowers. These kinds of activities will make your life happier and your professional character more attractive and effective.'"

—Quoted from "Parergon," published by Mead Johnson & Company, Evansville, Ind. Free copy available on request.

———o———

THE JOURNAL
OF THE
OKLAHOMA STATE MEDICAL ASSOCIATION

| VOLUME XXXII | McALESTER, OKLAHOMA, AUGUST, 1939 | Number 8 |

Stricture of the Urethra*

J. W. ROGERS, M.D.
407 Medical Arts Building
TULSA, OKLAHOMA

I think, due to the fact that we see fewer and less complicated strictures during the past few years, that we may be inclined to forget that people are still subject to strictures and that they may suffer in numerous ways on account of them. There has been little written on the subject in recent years and aside from one important form of treatment there has been no radical change in the care of this condition during the past 25 years.

Strictures have been treated by dilatation for many centuries. Movitt, in the Urological and Cutaneous Review, in March, 1937, states that "When Pompeii, destroyed and buried in 30 B.C., was unearthed, there were found, among other utensils in the houses, metal instruments quite similar to the metal sounds and catheters we are now using."

Due to the modern use of milder drugs, the more enlightened patients suffering from gonorrhoea and the more gentle manner in which such infections are treated, we see fewer and fewer strictures, and we see them and treat them earlier and more proficiently than was the case a quarter of a century ago.

It was quite a common thing to see patients, 25 years ago who had had internal urethrotomies done and were often in a sad state as a result.

There are innumerable classifications of strictures and I will call your attention to a few of them.

I.—As to Etiology.

A. Congenital, in which there are certain malformations of the urethra due to faulty developments.

B. Inflammatory, usually caused by gonorrhoea but occasionally by other infections.

C. Traumatic, these strictures may be caused by direct blows to the perineum, as in falling astride some object, by pelvic fractures, instrumentation, as sometimes occurs following transurethral operations and sometimes caused by patients using foreign bodies in the urethra. Chemical irritations, such as bichloride of mercury, lysol, etc., may come under this heading.

The vast majority of strictures are caused by a gonorrhoeal infection and, as I said previously, we are seeing fewer each year.

II.—Classification as to Size, Peterson classifies them as——

A. Open, when a No. 19F, or large sound can be passed.

B. Close, those from 10 F to 19 F.

C. Tight, those from filliform size to 10 F.

D. Impassable, those in which a filliform cannot be passed. But an impassable stricture is only relatively impassable, depending on one's perseverence, patience, and tools at hand.

*Read before the Section on Genito-Urinary and Syphilology, Annual Meeting, Oklahoma State Medical Association, May 2, 1939, Oklahoma City.

I recall a case that was sent into the hospital suffering severely, his abdomen was distended and I thought I could feel the distended bladder, he was able to void only a drop of urine at a time and this had been going on for two or three days. The urethra was anesthetized and we worked for 30 minutes trying to get by a stricture in the bulbous portion of the urethra. I was about r e a d y to make a supra-puncture when a filliform passed and with a follower catheter I obtained only about an ounce of urine. I was very much surprised and shuddered to think of what would have happened had I used a trocar. I don't recall of ever having a case of inflammatory stricture that I was unable to finally get a filliform through.

III.—Clinical classification.

  A. Organic.
    1. Congenital.
    2. Acquired.
      a. Inflammatory, mostly caused by gonorrhoea.
      b. Traumatic.
  B. Spasmodic, those caused by spasm of the urethral muscles. It isn't always easy to be sure with which type one is dealing.

I was called to see a patient who had been operated on for appendicitis 24 hours previously, he had been unable to void and unsuccessful attempts at catheterization had been made. He gave no history of any previous urinary trouble. After injecting a local anesthetic I tried to pass soft rubber catheters, wax c a t h e t e r s, straight and curved, and finally filliforms, I was unable to engage a filliform or pass the obstruction in any way. Under general anaesthesia, a 27 sound was passed without difficulty and he had no further difficulty in voiding.

IV.—Classification According to Pathology.

  1. According to the d i r e c t i o n of the formation.
    a. The annular type in w h i c h the scar tissue encircles the lumen of the urethra.
    b. Irregular, in which a portion of the urethra is involved in its circumference and then distally or proximally the remaining circumference is involved.
    c. Nodular, in which the lumen is obstructed by two or more scar formations.
  2. According to consistency.
    a. Soft, granular variety in which the stricture is of recent origin, bleeds easily and yields readily to treatment.
    b. The resilient type, this is more difficult to dilate and following d i l a t a t i o n, complications may arise. This type of stricture might be better treated with the electrotome than by simple dilatation.
    c. Indurated type, this type is extremely hard to dilate and electrourethrotomy is the treatment of choice.

Pathology: An organic stricture in a fibrous tissue formation which takes place gradually and on urethroscopic examination one will find a r i g i d t u b e in the scarred portion, with slight contractility of the walls and the normally pink walls are replaced by a white lining, often with fissures, ulcerations, and minute abscesses.

Symptoms: The most common symptom of stricture, is a periodic u r e t h r a l discharge following a protracted gonorrheal infection. There is a chronic urethritis with p e r i o d s of quiescence followed by active inflammation. Other c o m m o n symptoms are of an obstructive nature, the stream is small, there is a tendency to dribbling, there may be lack of force to the stream, frequency is often complained of, dysuria and the most distressing of all symptoms, c o m p l e t e retention. Other s y m p t o m s sometimes encountered are bleeding from the urethra itself, cystitis, terminal bleeding, pyuria, incontinence, diminished or complete loss of s e x u a l power, pain in the perineum and in complicated cases, loss of general health.

Complications are numerous and varied. Epididymitis, prostatitis, prostatic and urethral calculi, periurethritis, cystitis, and even pyelitis, periurethral abscess, and urinary extravasation.

Diagnosis: Given a suspicious history, the diagnosis is made by instrumentation. I think the flexible bulbous bougie is the instrument of choice and these may be had in all sizes and one may have to use several sizes to find two or more strictures of different caliber in the same urethra.

Anesthetize the urethra, I prefer 1:500 nupercain, inject liquid petrolatum without very much pressure and then begin to test out the urethra with the bougie. It is often necessary to do a meatotomy, as it would be foolish to try to find a size 27 stricture through a size 20 meatus. The bulb may pass through a strictured area without one being able to detect it, if it is nearly the same size as the instrument, but on removing it one will often feel the pull as the bulb comes through the strictured area. One should locate the size and position of all the strictures at one sitting.

Treatment: The majority of strictures r e s p o n d to urethral dilatation and this should be carried out gradually and gently. The large caliber s t r i c t u r e s are often smoothed out in three or four treatments, using two or three different sized sounds at each treatment. The small caliber, soft granular strictures respond almost equally well to treatment t h o u g h one may be alarmed at the bleeding that sometimes follows instrumentation in these cases.

About a year ago I had a patient whose chief complaint was bleeding from the urethra. On examination, I found a slight bloody discharge, after he voided there was some terminal bleeding. Massaging the seminal vesicles and prostate more blood was expressed from the urethra. I concluded that the bleeding was from the prostate and seminal vesicles, injected neosilvol into the bladder and asked him to report the next day. He was no better and on examination of the urethra with bulbs I found numerous strictures of various sizes. I passed a size 20F sound and the bleeding was quite profuse, this continued off and on for several days. I examined the urethra through a urethroscope and used silver nitrate on a bleeding point to no avail, the bleeding was almost alarming, to say nothing of being most distressing to the patient. In my search for help I ran across a statement by Cabot, that such bleeding could usually be controlled by the passage of an oversized sound. I was able to pass a size 26 F sound without much difficulty and to my amazement the bleeding stopped at once. I saw the patient again about a year afterwards and this time he was suffering from a periurethral

abscess that I opened and advised some more treatments for the strictures but he hasn't shown up again and likely won't until he has some other distressing complication.

The treatment of the small c a l i b e r resilient strictures may require the patience of a Job on the part of both operator and patient but with care and not trying to hurry the cure one can do wonders. Anesthetize the urethra, inject oil and pass a filliform, and after trying for a time with no success, if one is not dealing with acute retention, allow the patient to rest a few days, using frequent hot sitz baths and then try again, sometimes one can fill the canal with filliforms and get one to pass by pushing on each one separately. Sometimes it is said to be possible to use a urethroscope and visualize the opening. I have never used this method successfully. If the filliform is tight, it is well to leave it in place an hour or two or even for 12 to 24 hours, at the next treatment one can usually use a follower, size 10 to possibly 12F or 14 F. If one uses an oral urinary antiseptic for a day or two before the dilatation is attempted there will likely be no urethral chill or other complications following instrumentation. I like for the patient to be on sulfanilamide or neoprontosil for at least 24 hours before and after the instrumentation. One can often gradually work these strictures up to the place where a 19 or 20 F metal sound can be p a s s e d and then the dilatation is more rapid. I hesitate to use a metal sound smaller than an 18F. The effect of the sound is not only mechanical dilatation but increased vascularization of the affected area, causing absorption of the fibrosis.

Gradual dilatation has been considered the treatment of choice in most cases for at least 25 years, for most strictures. For a time before that, internal urethrotomy with a cutting blade was a common practice and the final result was usually bad. We have all seen those fibrotic, tough strictures that were very difficult to dilate and those patients that dreaded the sight or thought of a sound, and it seems to me that we may have a fairly simple solution to these cases in the use of the urethroelectrotome.

In June, 1936, Riba of Chicago, published in the Journal of the American Medical

Association, a report of the use of electro-urethratome in the treatment of a variety of strictures. In all the cases he reported, he did only one electrourethrotomy on each patient and over a three-year period had only one known recurrence out of 49 patients. The operation is usually an office procedure, under local anaesthesia, there is little bleeding and it seems likely that there is little resultant scar forma-tion. It is well in all stricture cases to have them report at intervals of a few months to a few years for an examination, but getting an apparently well patient to report is a problem that I have never solved.

REFERENCES

Movitt, Solomon O. The Urologic Cutaneous Review.
Riba, L. W. J.A.M.A., June 6, 1936, P. 1971.
Koll, Irvin S. Medical Urology, 1937.
Herman, Leon. The Practice of Urology, 1938.

---O---

The Post-Operative Management of Tonsillectomies*

G. E. HASLAM, M.D.
ANADARKO, OKLAHOMA

The subject of this paper deals with a problem of such common knowledge to the otolaryngologist that I feel an apology is due for my selection, however, tonsillectomy has become so lightly regarded by the average layman as a minor office procedure, in many instances as a result of advice from their family physician; and the operation is being performed by physicians other than specialists, and even cultists of all ranks—with frequent poor r e s u l t s and recollections of harrowing post-operative days; that I feel a few remarks along this line may not be amiss.

Taking for granted that the patient has been adequately examined pre-operatively, and sufficient reason found to subject him to this operation; and that the operation has been thoroughly done; what shall we do with him for the ten days to two weeks during his recovery?

First: the advisability of hospitalization. There can be no question that the proper place for the performance of tonsillectomies is in an equipped hospital, and that the patient should remain there under the observation of his physician and nurse for at least 24 hours in the case of children, and l o n g e r if advisable in the case of adults, especially so if any interruption in the normal postoperative course occurs.

For the first day they should be kept quiet and as comfortable as possible. This may be attained by the use of the ice collar and opiates — particularly codeine which may produce less nausea — and sedatives when they will suffice. This will suffice in the average or normal case. It is probably advisable to restrain all food until late afternoon, or at least six to eight hours following operation, when liquids and very soft solids may be taken if desired. Little discomfort is complained of in eating ice cream or cold milk drinks.

Those cases operated in the office should be done fairly early in the morning and held over under observation u n t i l late afternoon, especially so before being permitted to drive any distance to their homes. If any untoward circumstances arise during the course of the day it is far safer to transfer them to a hospital for the night at least.

Upon dismissal from the hospital or office certain specific instructions should be given the patient for his own comfort and safety, and the simplest way of impressing your orders is in written or printed form. I have used typewritten instructions for several years which are handed and explained to him before he leaves the hos-

*Read before the Section on Eye, Ear, Nose and Throat, Annual Meeting, Oklahoma State Medical Association, Oklahoma City, May 2, 1939.

pital, and have found he will come much nearer following my orders in such form, and less often break over. It seems to reduce the post-operative complaints and unfortunate complications often met with.

First of all he is instructed as to his diet. I realize that it is common practice with some men to permit their patients to eat what they wish, and "can," beginning with the second day, but after having been called upon several occasions to control hemorrhage from the eating of dry crackers and "corn bread" for the first two or three days post-operative, and there are many patients who will do just this unless otherwise instructed, has impressed upon my mind the fact that the denuded surface we leave in the throat should be protected from as much trauma as possible. The first three or four days are best limited to liquid diet, with soft solids which require little or no chewing. The following four to six days the diet may be increased to include the softer vegetables which should be well chewed before swallowing. The majority of the patients should be able to resume their regular diet on the ninth or tenth day, at which time all pain and discomfort is usually past. The diet list in addition to being soft should be simple as possible and one easily prepared and available to the average family.

Rest in bed should be insisted upon for at least two to three days, afterwards sitting up and moving around the home for several days longer — always avoiding exertion and exercise. C h i l d r e n will usually go about their indoor playing with no untoward circumstances. The laborer, and those engaged in strenuous occupations, along with those who use their voice to a large extent should arrange before hand to absent themselves from their work for at l e a s t ten days. Occasionally it might become necessary for some office workers and like occupations to return to work within five to six days, but more often this class of worker is glad to remain away for at least one week.

The use of gargles and sprays following tonsillectomy still remains a moot question, with about as many favoring their use as those against such procedures. In the child gargling is usually unnecessary, and frequently they have n e v e r been taught to do so. The adult will often insist upon using a gargle of some form, particularly to combat the foul breath present for several days, and to relieve as much as possible the discomfort in swallowing. The type of gargle to be used depends upon the choice of the physician or patient. In the main it is perhaps best to use here the simplest and most common used, and I doubt always if any specific gargle is of more value than another.

For the relief of pain, and particularly while swallowing, aspirin or Dobels will usually suffice, though there are a number of solutions, tablets, lozenges and gums on the market, and many of them good and effective, but most of them no more so than the simplest. Ten grains of aspirin to one-half glass of water will more often give good r e s u l t s than any other one gargle I know of. For the relief of the foul breath so many complain of any of the more deodorant mixtures suffice, and the best of them are none too effective until nature has finished her work in the healing of the denuded surface.

The use of laxatives is best confined to mild types, since we are dealing here with a loss of strength and dehydration from a disturbance of diet and decreased fluid intake, as a result of which purging will only exaggerate. The matter of the coated tongue frequently seen is one in which a few will attempt to relieve by the frequent use of laxatives and purgatives unnecessarily, and which if left alone will correct itself when healing has taken place.

Regarding the complications following tonsillectomy probably the one most frequently met with, and the most troublesome as a rule is that of hemorrhage. Hemorrhage may be classified in two types: primary, which occurs very early, within a few hours after operation, and secondary, which develops anywhere from the second day on, but usually on the fifth to eighth day. Of the two types the primary is the most difficult to handle, and may at times be of serious nature. The secondary hemorrhage is usually of less severity, and much more easily controlled.

Primary hemorrhage as above stated, will occur within a few hours following operation, and it is for this reason best to keep the patient hospitalized until all danger from this source has passed. Under hospitalization such hemorrhages can be detected more readily and properly taken care of before any extensive loss of blood can occur. They are also controlled with the minimum amount of discomfort to the patient. If all bleeding and oozing is stopped completely before the patient leaves the operating room the frequency of primary hemorrhages will be greatly diminished. There are several methods of controlling such hemorrhage, and the one to be used is preferably that type with which the operator is most familiar. Following local anaesthetics we are often able to carry out the necessary procedures without any further anaesthetic, though the injection of procaine and epinephrine may be necessary. Following the general anaesthetic it may be advisable to place the patient under anaesthesia again to completely and satisfactorily control the bleeding. All clots should be removed from the fossa, as they seldom offer any aid in the control of bleeding, and often appear to produce a certain amount of suction themselves which may actually aggravate such a condition. After the removal of clots the actual bleeding point, or points are located if possible, and clamped with the tonsil hemostat. After c l a m p i n g two methods of choice may be used to tie off the bleeder. A s u t u r e may be placed, preferably, the figure of eight, going into the musculature both above and below the bleeding point, with fine catgut — or a purse string suture may be used, taking in several points surrounding the clamp. In suturing I prefer a stout full curved round needle, with any ordinary needle-holder. The second m e t h o d, and one which I much prefer, is the simple placing of a slip-knot ligature around the bleeding point. With a slip-knot tied before hand, the short end is firmly clamped with a second hemostat as near the end as possible and cut short. The long slip-end is placed over the end of the hemostat holding the bleeding point, and passed down being gradually tightened until the end of the hemostat is reached. The noose can easily be slipped over the point of the hemostat and tightened fairly tight, then removing the hemostat on the bleeder, and the one holding the short end of the ligature. The long end is then cut with the scissors. This type ligature will re-

main in place for several hours, and often for two to three days. They practically always remain long enough to permit the vessel to retract into the musculature.

Occasionally where well formed anterior and posterior pillars have been preserved it is possible to snugly fit a sponge into the fossa, to which tape has been anchored, and by allowing it to remain in place for several hours adequately control the milder types of hemorrhage. The tape should always be held with a clamp, or fastened to the face or ear with adhesive tape. The suturing of pillars over sponge, or the suturing of the pillars together is not desirable, and should not be attempted unless considered absolutely necessary, since it predisposes to infection, requires subsequent removal, and tends to produce adhesions and scar tissue. Hemorrhage deep down near the base may require suturing of the pillars near the bleeding point.

Secondary hemorrhage as stated before usually occurs on the fifth or sixth day. The latest one I have any recollection of in my own experience occurred on the fifteenth day, however in the presence of severe infections they may occur on even later days. Examination almost invariably will reveal a clot within the fossa, the removal of which by a cotton sponge, or sponge forceps will often alone stop the bleeding. Here again the presence of a clot appears to exert a suction action upon the bleeding point. This type hemorrhage is usually less severe, and more easily handled. Again several methods of control are available. Pressure by a soft cotton sponge, held in the fossa for a few minutes will often suffice. The sponge may be dipped in various solutions according to the desire of the individual physician, the most frequently used solutions being hydrogen peroxide, chloride of iron, tincture of benzoin, and others.

I particularly like the application of a caustic, such as 50 per cent silver nitrate, on a small tipped applicator directly to the bleeding point, and have found it most effective, and easily used in the average case. The injection of procain and epinephrine, two to three drops at several points surrounding the bleeding point will also work effectively in many cases, due to the action of the epinephrine and the edema of the tissue produced by the fluid. It has been found that the simple injection of physiological salt solution will give the same results. However, the procain will relieve the pain if further procedures must be resorted to. There are numerous other methods of controlling hemorrhage, all of them being good in the hands of the physician accustomed to using them. The use of ligatures or sutures is rarely if ever necessary.

True sepsis following tonsillectomy is seldom seen, and if properly examined pre-operatively, and a history of too recent throat infection ruled out will very rarely cause us any worry. Too hasty operation following attacks of acute follicular tonsillitis; or low grade streptococci infections; or in the presence of infection of the gums or mouth may cause us to regret this lack of precaution. However, in the event of such an infection post-operatively they should be handled in the same manner as if operation had never occurred. The streptococcic organism is probably the most frequent offender, and the one causing the greatest concern when present in a fossa. In the past they have been difficult to handle, but today by the use of sulfanilamide the fear of such infections has been greatly reduced. Infections from the Vincents' organism may be treated locally with the various remedies in use, and generally by the use of arsenicals and bismuth.

Edema makes swallowing more difficult and uncomfortable but does not often require treatment. If relief becomes necessary astringent sprays or applications should suffice.

Infections of the lungs have been considered as rare complications in the past, however more recent figures seem to indicate that they are not so rare as formerly thought. It is quite likely they occur and recovery follows without our being aware of such conditions being present. The method by which these infections reach the lungs is still in dispute. It is generally thought to be by one of two most common routes: tracheobronchial or venous. The periphery of the lung is the most common site of the lesion though no portion is safe from infection. The size may vary from a centimeter in diameter to involvement of an entire lobe.

Treatment of these cases calls for the close cooperation of the otolaryngologist, internist and bronchoscopist, together with the surgeon on occasion. From the medical aspect, rest in bed, fresh air and sunshine, nourishing diet with vitamin tonics are essential, together with postural drainage. Many cases will r e c o v e r through such handling.

From the aspect of the bronchoscopist aspiration, irrigation and medication of the diseased area is effective in the hands of a competent man. Together with the assistance of the internist the large majority of cases may be well managed and complete recovery result.

The surgeon has found good results follow artificial pneumothorax in those cases of central abscesses, and from thoracotomy where the area can be reached without disturbance of healthy tissue.

The choice of treatment to be used will depend largely upon the location of the lesion, the severity of the attack, and the facilities available at hand. With proper precaution, this complication can be often guarded against, and weeks of convalescence avoided.

TWO DOCTORS DESCRIBE METHOD OF COMBATING SERUM SICKNESS

A ray of hope for those who suffer untoward reactions from the administration of serum for such conditions as tetanus, diphtheria, scarlet fever and pneumonia, is contained in a paper by Lee Foshay, M.D., Cincinnati, and O. E. Hagebusch, M.D., St. Louis, in The Journal of the American Medical Association for June 10, which describes a method of combating serum sickness.

A preparation known as histaminase was given by mouth or intramuscular injection to 22 patients with unfavorable reactions to serum, the authors report. Twenty of these experienced definite relief in from one to 36 hours after taking the preparation.

While only rarely fatal, serum sickness is frequent and often severe. Its symptoms, which include intolerable itching, nausea, vomiting, redness of the skin, wheals, headache, chills and the like, may follow any time from a few hours to as much as seven days after the administration of serum.

One of the most common experiences with serum sickness involves those taken to hospitals for treatment of various types of wounds. One of the first steps in the treatment of such victims is the injection of anti-tetanus serum to prevent possible tetanus infection as the result of contamination of open wounds.

As to the possibilities of the substance serving as a prevention for serum reactions, the authors say: "It is possible that the use of the substance before the injection of serum will prevent the occurrence of serum sickness in some instances and ameliorate the severity in others. The treatment appears to be rational, highly effective, safe and devoid of untoward effects."

Bladder Infections in the Female*

D. W. BRANHAM, M.D.
OKLAHOMA CITY, OKLAHOMA

The female bladder is particularly vulnerable to bacterial invasion and subsequent inflammatory processes. Primary non-specific cystitis, an uncommon condition in the male, occurs so frequently in the female that few women reach the age of menopause without suffering from one or more attacks. Cystitis in the male is more often associated with either an upper urinary tract infection or inflammatory disease of the prostate.

This undue susceptibility to infection is doubtless dependent upon the female anatomy, i.e. a short patent urethra located in intimate relation to structures that normally harbor a multitude of organisms both pathogenic and non-pathogenic. These organisms under certain conditions may pass with comparative ease to the bladder. In addition secondary etiologic factors that tend to produce cystitis may include trauma to the urethra at intercourse and lack of careful personal hygiene following defecation.

In the past considerable emphasis has been placed on malposition of the uterus as a factor in producing bladder irritability. Because insufficient attention has been directed to the role of infection in the urethra and bladder as a cause for such symptoms, ill advised operative procedures have been recommended in the hope that relief may follow such surgery. In most instances bladder irritability in the female is due to infectious lesions either at the bladder neck or within the bladder itself and is not due to pressure on the bladder by diseased or displaced pelvic structures. Certainly no patient should be submitted to a gynecologic operation for the relief of frequency and pain at urination until a thorough examination has been made of the lower urinary tract to exclude chronic infectious processes or such pathologic changes as the so-called elusive or Hunner's ulcer of the bladder.

Acute cystitis presents comparatively few diagnostic difficulties. It is important to emphasize that only the simplest diagnostic measures should be performed during an acute phase of cystitis. The physician should take a careful history in order to determine whether complicating factors such as: stones, tumors and hydronephroses which predispose to such infection, may be present. A careful inspection and examination should be made of the urethra as well as any expressed secretion in order to rule out the presence of an acute gonococcal infection. If there is no apparent contraindication a catheterized specimen of urine should be obtained and the centrifuged urinary sediment examined both as a wet smear and after it has been stained by Gram's method. As a rule no instrumental manipulation and especially no ureteral catheterization is advisable during the early acute phase of such an infection.

Under ideal conditions an X-ray plate of the patient's kidneys, ureters and bladder should be taken at this time but frequently financial reasons dictate a less expensive diagnostic course. One should not lose sight of the fact that the patient consults the physicians primarily for relief of the unpleasant symptoms and has a considerably lessened interest in possible complicating factors at that moment. Thus if a financial hardship is entailed by the correct diagnostic X-ray procedure it may be expedient to empirically rule out possible upper tract complications by observing the improvement obtained by standard therapeutic procedures.

Of paramount importance in the management of acute cystitis is the identification of the type of organism present in the urine. Stained smears by the Gram method of the well centrifuged urine sediment will ordinarily suffice for this purpose. Culture of the urine is desirable but in the majority of instances a carefully stained smear will be all that is necessary. The

*Read before the Section on Genito-Urinary Diseases & Syphilology, Annual Meeting, Oklahoma State Medical Association, Oklahoma City, May 2, 1939.

method of making a Gram stain easily and rapidly is clearly described by Pelouze in his book. In making smears for bacteriologic diagnosis from urine the addition of a small amount of acetic acid will clarify those specimens cloudy with phosphates, without changing the morphology of the cellular elements other than to hemolyze the red blood cells.

In approximately 75 per cent of nonspecific urinary tract infections the offending organism will be the colon bacillus. In the properly stained smear these bacilli are short thick rods which take the Gram counter stain. A small percentage of these infections will be due to the proteus bacillus, an urea-splitting organism. Strongly alkaline urine with an ammoniacal odor is sugggestive of such infection. Gram positive b a c i l l i are occasionally found and when discovered are due usually to contamination from the vulva and vaginal areas. The remaining 25 per cent of bladder infections will be caused by the staphlococcus and streptococcus group of organisms. Gram negative or Gram positive cocci in clumps or chains are not identified as easily as the colon group of organisms as they may be fewer in number and may be incorporated with the mucous and cellular debris of the smear. A type of coccus not infrequently found is the streptococcus fecalis. This is a r a t h e r large lancet shaped Gram positive diplococcus w h i c h has the peculiar clinical characteristic of producing an i r r i t a b l e bladder causing frequent and painful urination without an inflammatory reaction commensurate with the distress. As this particular type of infection necessitates a specific type of therapy, a cystitis which is due to both the streptococcus fecalis and a bacillus may require additional careful attention. Usual treatment may be followed by a r a p i d disappearance of the Bacilli in the urine but b e c a u s e of the Gram positive coccus there may be little or no improvement in the patient's symptoms.

A certain small percentage of bladder infections are due to the tubercle bacilli from an open tuberculosis of the kidney. Urinary tract tuberculosis should be suspected in every instance where the symptoms of cystitis are severe, constant and unresponsive to the ordinary therapeutic measures.

In the large majority of instances, bladder infections in the female present a satisfactory therapeutic r e s p o n s e to our modern medication. Important, today, in combating this frequently found condition are four drugs: sulfanilamide, methenamine, mandelic acid and neosalvarsan. Sulfanilamide administered in doses of 30 to 80 grains daily rapidly produces satisfactory results in most of the bacillary infections. However, it is apparently less effective in inhibiting the growth of coccal infections. Sulfanilamide has the additional advantage of being non-irritating to the bladder wall and, therefore, may be prescribed in hyperacute inflammatory conditions. This is in contrast to the effect produced by methenamine which liberates formalin in an acid medium and in the bladder may cause irritation even to the point of producing a hematuria. Because of this methenamine has more therapeutic value in the more chronic phases of bladder infections.

Mandelic acid administered in appropriate doses and with careful attention paid to the hydrogen in concentration of the urine is an effective medication in bacillary infections. With the exception of the streptococcus fecalis mandelic acid is not an effective agent in the coccal infections. When used to combat the organisms for which they are indicated, both sulfanilamide and mandelic acid produce rapid amelioration of symptoms in practically all acute urinary tract infections. Examination of the urine microscopically or culturally will determine the length of time medication must be maintained.

Neoarsphenamine is i n d i c a t e d in the treatment of urinary tract infections when the offending organism is of the coccal type. Four to six doses of 0.3 Gms. to 0.45 Gms. of this drug intravenously five days apart will be followed by a high percentage of satisfactory results. In combating infections due to the streptococcus fecalis there are two effective therapeutic measures, namely, neoarsphenamine and mandelic acid.

For the sake of brevity no complete discussion is possible as to the various general indications and contraindications in the use of these drugs. The toxic reaction of sulfanilamide on the blood, the irritating effect of mandelic acid on the renal parenchyma and the toxic systemic reactions due to neosalvarsan are factors that should be kept in mind. Judgement should always be exercised in any choice of medication and one important criterion to guide the physician is this—if the age, condition of the patient, urinalysis, or blood pressure indicates renal insufficiency reduce the usual dosage until it is possible to observe how. the patient tolerates the medication.

Therapeutic adjuncts other than urinary antiseptics in the treatment of acute infections of the bladder are the use of antispasmodics and sedatives. A prescription that has proven of palliative value is a mixture of Tr. opium and Tr. Bellodonna in an elixir of phenobarbital. Bed rest, if possible, is always advisable and in obstinate cases it may be an imperative measure. Irrigation and instillation of medicaments into the bladder for bactericidal effect, in general have been followed by disappointing results. In the past this was a common therapeutic procedure but with the advent of more potent bactericidal drugs this type of treatment has been found unnecessary.

Despite the short course of many acute infections of the bladder a chronic bacteruria frequently follows. Although evidence of a chronic inflammatory condition, such as pus cells in the urine may be absent and the patient may be free of symptoms, bacteria may still be present and will only be discovered if the careful routine examination includes a Gram stain of the centrifuged urine sediment. It is important for the physician to realize this and to persist in his treatment until all bacteria are completely eliminated as proven by either several microscopic examinations of the urinary sediment or by culture of the urine itself.

Unless such a completely satisfactory result is obtained and unless the possible contributing causes or foci are removed not only recurrences may be expected but more dangerous sequelae due to extension of the infecting organisms to adjacent and contiguous structures may result.

Examination of Contacts—A Factor in Syphilis Control

MACK I. SHANHOLTZ, M.D., C.P.H.
Director, Seminole County Health Unit
WEWOKA, OKLAHOMA

Since the time public health was in its infancy, the control of communicable disease has been recognized as a basic principle for the protection of a community. The health officer and his staff have been greatly interested in the isolation and quarantine of the infectious person. Epidemiological ingestigation as to the cause or the source of the disease and the prevention of further spread or the occurence of secondary cases have been stressed. This has been a factor in bringing about the great reduction over the past 20 years in many of our common communicable diseases.

Needless to say, these procedures and investigations have been used very sparingly in the control of syphilis. And still syphilis is one of the communicable diseases and perhaps our No. 1 health problem today. It is amenable to treatment and public health management.

We fully realize that the community should be protected against the early infectious case himself, as well as his source and his contacts. Why, then, hasn't there been more stress put on the practical epidemiology and the control of syphilis? Many obstacles peculiar to the disease itself must be overcome. In general, there has been and still is gross neglect on the part of the practicing physicians in reporting the disease to health authorities. The disease has been so camouflaged in secrecy and taboos that the doctors have not felt justified in even divulging its whereabouts to health departments. In the early stages of the disease, the patient feels so well generally that quarantine other than by confinement in an institution is impossible. We know from the estimated prevalence of the disease today that an institutional quarantine of all early cases would be impracticable. How, then, can the spread of the infection be checked?

We have one available effective method and that is "chemical quarantine," or regular and adequate treatment of the early infectious case. If these cases are found and put under adequate and regular treatment, they are no l o n g e r a menace or source of spread. One excellent method of uncovering these early cases is to examine all antecedent and subsequent contacts of every known early case of syphilis which is under supervision. This has been recognized as a sound method of practical epidemiology in syphilis ever since the pioneer work in 1933 as carried out by Smith and Brumfield.

This work was carried out at the University of Virginia Hospital and published in the J. A. M. A. Their original 119 cases named 196 contacts, of whom 93 were examined. Seventy-four of these 93 were found to be syphilitic. You will notice that only 47 per cent of the contacts named were brought in for examination. Although this work was remarkable from the standpoint of its being one of the first practical approaches to the problem as well as the actual accomplishments, the percentage of the named contacts examined is not high according to present day standards. The reason for this was a lack of sufficient field workers at that time to carry out the follow up work, and in their place letters were substituted for the most part. Today, this same clinic is working on a cooperative basis with a special United States Public Health Syphilis Unit, which should make follow up work on contacts more efficient.

A similar study to that of Smith and Brumfield was carried out by Clark in Brooklyn. Recently, Levinson of the New York Health Department made an investigation of selected cases for determining the efficiency of contact examination as a means of finding early cases. Although

his figures were not large enough to be significant, the results were favorable.

The follow up work and examination of contacts is recognized by syphilologists and public health people alike as one of our most effective weapons in control. It is the keystone in the syphilis control program which is usually given under three heads: 1. education; 2. investigation; 3. treatment.

Due to the nation wide publicity campaign, put on for the most part through the efforts of Surgeon General Parran, the educational program is, in my opinion, far ahead of the other two. The effect it has had on the public in general is quite evident to those doing work in syphilis. It used to be startling to a new patient to hear about the serious after-effects the disease was capable of producing and the long course of treatment required for a cure. Today, this is not news to many patients because they have already been enlightened. The doctor who still believes six treatments sufficient for cure (we still have a few remaining) can expect his patients soon to come back with some such answer as "Quit your kidding, doc! I know it takes 70 treatments to cure me." If he fails to take a blood test on one of his prenatal cases, he can expect her to remind him that she wants one.

The a d v a n c e made in treatment is greater than that in epidemiology or case investigation. Practicing physicians are taking more interest in treating more patients, many of whom are reporting for treatment on account of the above mentioned educational drive. Numerous clinics conducted by health departments are springing up all over the country for treatment of indigent cases, but they are too few in number in most localities to cope with the problem. In my opinion, there never will be any noticeable reduction in the prevalence of syphilis until there is a coordination and a marked advance made in both treatment and investigating facilities, since one is useless without the other. Free clinics for those who can not pay, and enough field workers to carry out case investigation for the clinic as well as for the practicing physicians in the community are essential. The family doctor does not have a field worker or the time, and perhaps the inclination, to do this himself.

However, the majority of them would welcome a competent worker to do this for him.

I believe that for the effective control of syphilis there should be some government agency responsible for treating indigent cases and for doing follow up work on patients of p r i v a t e physicians. The most logical organization to carry out this work is the county or city health department. Some reorganization of p r e s e n t health departments, and the establishment of many new ones would be necessary for efficient handling of the problem. The health officers and nurses in the departments understand syphilis and the means of preventing its spread.

Much tact and ingenuity is required to get a patient to name all his contacts in many instances, and health officers become very adept at this procedure. The public health nurse is the logical one to do the follow up work because she already knows many of the families in her district and has gained their confidence. For the most part, she would have little or no trouble in getting family contacts in for examination because she can go about this in the same manner she would in getting a child in for toxoid or other routine procedures. This, I believe, is much better than sending a contact worker who depends on force or fear as a means of getting people in. Force or fear can be used occasionally when it becomes absolutely necessary, but shouldn't have to be used often.

Anyone doing contact work should have a basic knowledge of the disease itself such as its incubation period, the time interval between the three stages, its mode of spread, and treatment methods. With the knowledge any registered nurse has of disease in general, a little special training which could be r e c e i v e d in short courses or conferences would make it possible for her to develop into a very efficient field worker for syphilis contacts.

It will be necessary to have every town and county s e r v e d by some organized agency responsible for the control of syphilis, and these organizations must cooperate with each other. The contacts of a patient in one county may live in another district, and if the workers in one area will notify other organizations of contacts in their district, all contacts can be f o u n d and

brought in for examination and treatment if necessary. This has worked out well in Seminole, Pontotoc, and Okfuskee counties. When a patient under treatment moves from one of these counties to another, the record of his treatment is sent to the county health department where he has moved, and treatment can be continued without a lapse. Such organizations and cooperation are necessary if there is to be any marked reduction in the disease in general.

SUMMARY

1. Contact investigation is an important procedure in the control of syhpilis.

2. The county and city health departments are the logical organizations to take responsibility for the control of syphilis.

3. There is a need for an expansion or development of more health departments so as to cover the spread completely.

4. We can't hope to see any marked reduction in the prevalence of syphilis until such organizations are established. They can co-ordinate education, investigation, and treatment of the disease.

* * * *

DISCUSSION

Dr. G. W. McDonald, Ada: I greatly enjoyed Dr. Shanholtz's presentation of this paper, and I feel that it touches on a subject which is very important to the Public Health control of syphilis.

It is surprising that a program so well founded and productive of such great good has not received its just share in the annals of Medical Literature. As to the relative importance of the three points in the control of syphilis mentioned by Dr. Shanholtz, namely, education, treatment and investigation, I feel no more emphasis can be placed on one than the others. It would be as wise to ask which of the legs of a three-legged stool is most important. As with the stools, no two are effective without the third. The f i r m foundation of syphilis control must rest with equal burden on each of its three components. Yet as Dr. Shanholtz says investigation has been the m o s t greatly neglected of the three. All of you who have treated syphilis, have, I feel, sooner or later, come to realize that even the most complete care is bound to be in many cases fraught with dangers and disappointments. When we see these patients, even those who have been very religious in their regularity, and on whom we have spent many hours of study and labor, develop, in spite of our most valiant efforts, muco-cutaneous relapse, neurological symptoms, etc., it occurs to us beyond all doubt the greatest tribute we can make to the health of our communities is the prevention of syphilis rather than its treatment. Here, if ever, an ounce of prevention is w o r t h many pounds of cure.

The treatment of syphilis at best is a patch-up job and the prevention of one case t h r o u g h epidemiological investigation of source and spread contacts is worth more than ten so-called cures.

I feel that these investigations can be made and definite r e s u l t s secured even with a minimum staff. To illustrate this may I present a small series which has come to light in Pontotoc county.

On routine visits to the county jail we found a man then in active secondary stage and a healing chancre. He was being held for performing an abortion on a young lady. His previous occupation had been that of fortune teller and had probably done abortions on numerous occasions. On inquiry into his sexual history for the past three months he gave a history of sexual contact with eight women. These women were contacted as soon as possible, and it was found, on examination immediately, that three had positive blood and were in early primary stage. They had had no other sexual contacts. Another refused examination but it was found later that she had gone to her private physician who reported to us that she was found to have primary sores and was being treated by him. Another was found to have had irregular treatment d u r i n g the past six months from her private physician. Since this was the only case whose duration was longer than that of the fortune teller's it is surmised that this is the source of his infection.

Three other girls were found negative, both on physical examination and blood Wassermans. Several times s i n c e that time attempts have been made to get these girls for re-examination but it was found that two of them had been out of the county.

Recently there came to our office a man with an early chancre who gave as his only contact one of the girls who had been negative on her first examination. She was immediately sent for but was at that time living in Fort Smith, Ark. Being acquainted with the health officer in Fort Smith I wrote to him telling of the circumstances of the case. A few days later I received a reply saying the girl had been located, Wasserman taken and that she had early secondaries, for which treatment was instituted. Since then she has returned to us for continued treatment.

The interesting thing about this is that this girl is the only one of this series known to have transmitted the disease to a third person, all other contacts having treatment instituted before other sexual c o n t a c t s were made.

We are making an attempt at this time to locate the two remaining contacts who were negative on their first examination, to determine whether subsequently they have shown evidence of the disease.

This series, while shorter than some I have seen, demonstrates several factors:

First—t h a t epidemiological investigations are productive of good results even when carried on by health units of minimum staffs.

Second—it is not at all difficult to stimulate patients to give their contacts.

Third—contacts can be rounded up, examined and put under treatment before a g r e a t number of other healthy persons have been exposed. Thus cutting down the case load in any given community.

Fourth—it demonstrates to a great degree the necessity of such control measures in all surrounding areas. Many t i m e s contacts are given which, because of their geographical location are beyond jurisdiction of the local health unit, or because of the distance, travel to such contacts by the personnel of the local unit is economically unsound. In these cases it is of distinct value to both communities that a liason may be established with other health units to the end that names and addresses of contacts may be referred from one to the other.

It is my sincere hope that this paper of Dr. Shanholtz's will stimulate greater efforts in the investigation work a m o n̄g those health units already in the field and t h a t the possibilities of productive, co-operative effort of several health units may stimulate the formation of new units.

I feel that a complete coverage of Oklahoma with active health units is the greatest hope for the effective control of syphilis in the state.

———————————0———————————

The Emergency Treatment of Airplane Injuries

ROY L. FISHER, B.S., M.D., F.A.C.S.
FREDERICK, OKLAHOMA

I have nothing new or spectacular to offer in this paper. After all, a major fracture presents the same problems regardless of the manner in which it occurs. Airplane injuries probably differ from injuries received in other modes of transportation in that they are more apt to be multiple and extremely serious in nature. I might add that head injuries and fractures of the spine are probably more frequent also.

Airplane crashes, when they occur, may be in out of the way places in rough terrain or close to airports and thickly populated centers, all of which have a direct bearing on the emergency treatment of the injured occupants. Without reservation it may be stated, that it is better to transport the doctor to the patient instead of transporting the patient to the doctor for the emergency treatment of these injuries. In the Military Service medical officers travel to the scene of the accident by air whenever it is possible to do so. In this manner a Flight Surgeon can often reach a crash within 15 or 20 minutes, whereas, if he depended on ground transportation an hour and s o m e t i m e s much longer periods of time would be required. In general it may be said that every two hours delay means an extra week in the hospital. In the San Antonio area we have more accidents than any other section in the United States because this is our Air Corps training center. Flight Surgeons and well equipped ambulances are kept on the flying line during all training periods. The importance of a Flight Surgeon's presence at the scene of a crash as soon as it is humanly possible to get there cannot be over-emphasized. Army ambulances lo-cated in the training area are equipped with radio receivers. When a crash occurs some distance from one of the fields, it is first located by airplane. When the pilot or observer locates the crash they guide the ambulance to the scene by radio instructions via the shortest possible route. This is especially helpful and time saving in sections of the country where section lines are not laid out and terrain is rough and thickly wooded. In the event of the failure of a radio set, the pilot can still guide the ambulance to its destination by pre-arranged signals such as dropping a left wing for left turn and right wing for a turn to the right, etc. The ambulances are easily distinguishable from the air by the O. D. coloring and markings.

In the new metal ships in use today, both commercial and service types, crashes are very often fatal. Gross weights are much greater due to the increase in the size of the s h i p s and engines. They are well streamlined and wing loading is h e a v y, with the result that when they do crash they hit hard and fast as compared to the older fabric type, with large wing span and much less gross weight. A metal ship falling any distance at all is almost sure to prove fatal to its occupants. Accidents are much less frequent, however, because the equipment and engines of today are highly efficient.

The fire hazard is less also. Engines are improved. Magnetos have replaced batteries doing away with battery sparks from broken terminals and short exhaust stacks have replaced the old long type which has reduced fire hazard 50 per cent alone. When fire does o c c u r it is in practically an explosive manner and will usually be at intense heat within 30 seconds, before even close observers can get near the ship. To combat this factor army airdromes have fire t r u c k s, chemicals, asbestos suits and crash kits, all manned by trained personnel. However, because of the fact that the fire is a gasoline type, and extremely explosive, even these precautions have proven of very little value.

If the accident has been of a non-fatal nature and the victim is unable to get out himself, the first problem and a most important one, is to extricate him from the p l a n e without inflicting further injury. This is where the average layman falls down and may acutally do more injury to the victim than the crash itself. To get the occupant out of the plane it is often necessary to cut away parts of the fuselage. This is done with heavy wire cutters, hacksaws and ordinary axes.

Experiments at W r i g h t Field on old ships have proven that an axe is probably the best tool to cut through supporting members when it can be used w i t h o u t danger of striking the injured occupant. The crash kit carried by all army ambulances and kept in readiness at all Air Corps stations consists of the following pieces of equipment:

Flash lights, fire extinguishers, grappling hook with steel cable, bolt cutters, wire cutters, pipe cutters, hacksaws, axe, sledge hammer, crowbar, metal snips and dirk knife.

When ships nose over, trenching beneath the ship with picks and shovels is sometimes necessary in order to reach the occupants. If ordinary cutting away of parts or trenching beneath the airplane will not extricate the injured, it is better to wait until a wrecking crew arrives with the necessary tripods and block and tackle equipment with which to raise the ship or to move its position so that successful removal of the occupants can be accomplished.

The emergency treatment of airplane injuries consists of five factors which are as follows:

1. Shock treatment.
2. Control of hemorrhage.
3. Proper splinting of all fractures.
4. Dressing of all wounds.
5. Proper transportation to hospitals.

TREATMENT OF SHOCK

Shock is always present in these injuries varying in degree depending on the type of injury and upon the individual. Certain people are more likely to be shocked than others. They seem to react more readily to the causes of shock. Conditions that may produce profound s h o c k in some people may cause but little disturbance in others. The army believes in the administration of morphine in adequate dosage as the first procedure in the treatment of shock. All army ambulances carry morphine, thermal pads of the chemical type, to provide heat, plenty of woolen blankets and all other accepted stimulants. Morphine in sufficient dosage to control pain and insure rest, plenty of blankets and thermal pads to maintain body heat and warmth is probably the best emergency treatment.

CONTROL OF HEMORRHAGE

Hemorrhage and shock are often closely allied, and the t r i n i t y of hemorrhage, shock and infection is a formidable combination. The liability of hemorrhage to emerge into shock must always be borne in mind. Any hemorrhage, unless it be internal, can be controlled in the vast majority of cases by keeping cool and using common sense. If the bleeding is coming from one point, pressure can be made with a sterile pledget of gauze and gradually withdrawn until the bleeding point is located, clamped and then secured by ligature if possible. If the bleeding comes from several points and if sudden and profuse, pack with sterile gauze and make adequate pressure until it is checked. If the packing can be slowly removed and the individual bleeding points picked up and sutured do so, if not, leave the packing alone. Avoid always the blind application of a clamp. If necessary, in severe b l e e d i n g from an extremity, apply a tourniquet to control the vessel until it can be picked up and ligated. In badly mangled limbs tissue resistance is always low and a tourniquet should not be left on any longer than absolutely necessary. Depriving these t i s s u e s of blood for a period of an hour or more is a s e r i o u s handicap in the healing of the wound and if a careful clamping of the individual vessels can be done, the eventual results will be much better.

Proper Splinting of All Fractures

Major fractures of the extremities which will require immobilization for transportation are usually obvious and determination of the details of the fracture does not fall under the head of emergency treatment and should be deferred until the patient is hospitalized where definite treatment is instituted.

Major fractures must be properly splinted before a patient is transported because the movement of the fragments causes severe pain, damages surrounding tissues, may convert closed fractures into open ones, increases hemorrhage and shock and causes death. It was for these reasons that the wounded were first splinted on the battlefields by the various armies during the World War. It has been stated by Army Surgeons that the routine application of the Thomas splint on the field reduced the mortality from 80 per cent to 20 per cent in gunshot fractures of the femur. Today the Thomas splint is still ideal for immobilization of fractures of the extremities and if available should always be used. All army ambulances carry a supply of these splints as well as a wire litter which is also ideal.

As is usually the case in commercial or civilian plane crashes, Thomas splints are not available. This does not justify the prevailing tendency to dump a patient into an automobile and rush him several miles to the nearest doctor's office, drugstore or farmhouse adding insult to injury when the patient may be dying of shock. It is much better to cover severely injured patients with blankets allowing them to lie on the ground until they can be splinted properly and moved in a suitable ambulance. All major fractures can be sufficiently immobilized for emergency transportation by means of simple board splints and boards are always available somewhere nearby.

In fractures of the spine or pelvis the ladder splint is very efficient. It consists of two long boards which are fastened together by three cross pieces. If hammer and nails are not available the cross pieces can be tied on. The splint is padded with any material available and the patient is bound to it. This also serves as a litter and is useful for patients with internal injuries. In simple fractures of the clavicle all that is necessary is to place the arm in a triangular sling. In severe injuries in the region of the shoulder a pad should be placed in the axilla and the arm immobilized against the chest with the forearm and hand in a sling. Fractures of the lower humerus and elbow region can be immobilized by two boards, the one on the inside extending from the axilla to the finger tips and the one on the outer aspect from the shoulder to the finger tips. Further immobilization can be secured by binding the arm to the side. Forearm fractures and fractures of the wrist can be immobilized in dorsal and volar splints extending beyond the elbow to prevent rotation and the forearm placed in a triangular sling.

In fractures of the hip, shaft of the femur and knee it is necessary to immobilize the lower extremity and the trunk. A certain amount of immobilization can be secured by binding the two lower extremities together but it is best to use two b o a r d splints, a short one extending from the crotch to the foot and a long board extending on the outside from the axilla to the foot. Rotation is prevented by tying the foot to the splint. In fractures below the knee it is desirable to include the thigh, using two boards long enough for this purpose in the usual manner. A pillow also makes a comfortable and efficient splint.

In fractures of the skull the best emergency treatment is the treatment for shock, that is morphine and plenty of blankets. Here again waiting for a properly equipped ambulance, r a t h e r than using the first passing automobile will often be a life saving procedure. No attempt should be made to reduce fractures of the nose at the scene of the accident. Bleeding can be controlled by packing the nose and this should suffice until the patient is hospitalized. Fractures of the mandible are equally important. Immobilizing the mandible against the upper jaw with adhesive or a bandage is all that is necessary for a temporary splint.

Dressing of Wounds

In facial injuries the hasty "emergency care" usually given these victims often jeopardizes the possibility of a good end result. Hurried closure of wounds with skin clips and heavy suture material is to be condemned. Hemostasis and a sterile dressing at the scene of the accident is sufficient. Surgical repair should not be attempted until it can be done properly under conditions that will leave a minimal scar. Facial disfigurements are a source of great mental anguish and not infrequently engender psychologic handicaps that ruin social and business careers, so let's prevent them whenever possible. In severe bleeding from the mouth be sure to examine the tongue because the source very often is a deep laceration of this organ requiring immediate suture.

The emergency treatment of lacerations regardless of location is hemostasis and sterile dressings, to prevent further entrance of dirt. The treatment of compound fractures begins at the scene of the accident with hemostasis, sterile dressings and proper splinting. In the emergency treatment of burns, morphine for the control of pain, sterile dressings applied to the burned areas and blankets to keep the patient warm will probably be all you can do. I shall make no attempt to discuss the various methods advocated for the treatment of burns except to condemn the use of grease base ointments as an emergency dressing applied on a denuded area already potentially infected.

Proper Transportation

It is much better to leave the patient at the scene of the crash under improvised s h e l t e r, after emergency treatment has been given than to improperly transport him to a hospital in a poor conveyance. Whenever possible wait for a good ambulance with l i t t e r s, plenty of s p l i n t s, blankets, thermal pads and other necessary equipment. Don't put him hastily into any kind of a car and rush him madly at breakneck speeds over any kind of roads to the hospital. In observing this precaution you may save a life. The army has proven beyond a doubt the value of the airplane ambulance. It has saved many lives because of the speed and ease in which injured patients can be transported long distances. Airplane ambulances are kept in readiness today at strategic points throughout the United States by the Air Corps.

An interesting story in connection with the development of the airplane ambulance by the army was related to me recently by Major T. L. Gilbert, the Commanding Officer of the Air Corps Reserve Unit located in this city, which was as follows: Several years ago when engines lacked the reliability of present day power plants, forced landings were not at all uncommon. If engine failure occurred over rough country the pilot could not jump and leave his p a t i e n t in the ship so a method had to be developed to parachute the patient safely to earth in order that both their lives would be spared. Major Gilbert was one of the officers assigned to work out a successful method that would take care of such a situation. They constructed a litter similar to the one shown you with heavy straps fastening the patient securely on the inside.

They next devised a parachute that was attached to the litter and that would open automatically when it cleared the ship, a drop of about 10 feet. They strapped a dummy weighing 150 pounds in the litter and made many drop tests. In each test the dummy strapped securely in the litter floated lightly to earth. The litter was pushed out feet first and as soon as the chute opened the litter floated to the earth in a horizontal position, landing lightly.

Summary

1. Injuries are usually m u l t i p l e and serious and our main concern is to save a life.

2. Start first-aid immediately on reaching the patient. Morphine can be given, hemorrhage o f t e n controlled and sometimes splints can be applied while help is working to extricate the patient from the plane.

3. Use all supportive measures at hand.

4. Control hemorrhage.

5. Cover all wounds with sterile dressings to prevent further contamination.

6. Splint them where they lie.

7. Provide proper transportation.

For their h e l p f u l suggestions in the preparation of this paper I wish to express my appreciation and thanks to:

Lt. Col. N. C. Mashburn, Commandant of the School of Aviation Medicine, Randolph Field, Texas.

Major T. L. Gilbert, Commanding Officer, Air Reserve Unit, Oklahoma City, Oklahoma.

Capt. Chas. L. Leedham, Flight Surgeon, Randolph Field, Texas.

THE JOURNAL
OF THE
Oklahoma State Medical Association

Issued Monthly at McAlester, Oklahoma, under direction of the Council.

Copyright, 1939, by Oklahoma State Medical Association, McAlester, Oklahoma.

Vol. XXXII	AUGUST	Number 8

Entered at the Post Office at McAlester, Oklahoma, as second-class matter under the act of March 3rd, 1879.

This is the official Journal of the Oklahoma State Medical Association. All communications should be addressed to The Journal of the Oklahoma State Medical Association, McAlester Clinic, McAlester, Oklahoma. $4.00 per year; 40c per copy.

The editorial department is not responsible for the opinions expressed in the original articles of contributors.

Reprints of original articles will be supplied at actual cost provided request for them is attached to manuscripts or made in sufficient time before publication.

Articles sent this Journal for publication and all those read at the annual meetings of the State Association are the sole property of this Journal. The Journal relies on each individual contributor's strict adherence to this well-known rule of medical journalism. In the event an article sent this Journal for publication is published before appearance in The Journal the manuscript will be returned to the writer.

Failure to receive The Journal should call for immediate notification of the Editor, McAlester Clinic, McAlester, Oklahoma.

Local news of possible interest to the medical profession, notes on removals, changes of addresses, births, deaths and weddings will be gratefully received.

Advertising of articles, drugs or compounds unapproved by the Council on Pharmacy of the A. M. A., will not be accepted.

Advertising rates will be supplied on application.

It is suggested that wherever possible members of the State Association should patronize our advertisers in preference to others as a matter of fair reciprocity.

Printed by News-Capital Company, McAlester.

EDITORIAL

HOSPITAL INSURANCE

In many localities throughout the state there have been organized companies for the purpose of furnishing hospitalization. These companies have been of various sorts, some organized on a non-profit basis, some as mutuals and others incorporated for profit to the stock holders.

There has been some controversy as to the attitude of organized medicine toward the whole program and in certain localities where physicians have been interested in the organization there has been some question as to ethics.

It appears to the editor that the solution of the problem is very simple and that a few general principles can govern these organizations making them acceptable so far as organized medicine is concerned.

First: There should be a free choice of hospital. If this is not the case, in privately operated hospitals or those with a closed staff the selling of hospital insurance would amount to the selling of the professional service of the physician or surgeon connected with the hospital. In all policies no hospital should be given the preference as to rate or service furnished, each must have the same status and receive the same compensation.

Second: No professional service should be covered by the policy. Hospital service only, this to include room, board, nursing service, operating room service, medicines, dressings, et cetera. No professional service, this should include laboratory, X-ray and anesthetic service. This to conform to the action of our House of Delegates.

There are advantages to the Doctors of the State in Hospitalization Insurance and it would be well for the physicians to encourage such a movement if the above mentioned principles are carefully kept in mind.

---o---

INSURANCE PROGRAM

Life insurance is thoroughly recognized as the most rapid and safest method of developing an estate, especially is this true with the physician who, all too often, has poor business judgment and lacks the time to make the necessary investigation of financial investment. Old Line Insurance Companies (those financially sound) offer to us their facilities for investing and all pay a reasonable rate of interest and in most instances more than can be secured at the banks on time deposit or from the Government on bonds.

The one feature is the rapidity of developing an estate for as soon as one premium is paid and the policy delivered the estate is i n c r e a s e d, in case of death, by the amount of the face of the policy and by the end of the second policy year there has developed a real money value besides the protection afforded.

The problem before the insured after acquiring the insurance is the development of an Insurance Program.

Money left in a lump sum to your beneficiary is apt to be poorly invested or foolishly expended and this leaves your family without financial security which you may think has been provided.

The money for maintainence or perhaps education of your children has been squandered and the result you felt sure of can not be attained.

The method of avoiding this disaster is to so develop a program that the lump sum will be sufficient to meet the obligations of one's last illness, burial and other debts, the balance of the policy to be paid in annuities at stated intervals and if there are children to educate, separate allowance can be made for such a purpose.

All the details of a good insurance program cannot be considered here; however, your insurance agent should be a specialist in this subject and can suggest to you all the necessary details so that the money you are now investing in premiums may come back to your beneficiaries so distributed as to accomplish the most good and thus fulfill your ambitions in an effort to properly protect and care for your loved ones after you are gone.

ON THE QUESTION OF ADVISING THE YOUTH ABOUT THE PRACTICE OF MEDICINE AS A VOCATION

There has been a tendency, and for very good reasons, to discourage young men from studying medicine. Many doctors who have sons have advised them against medicine as a career. This has largely been brought about by the spector of socialization of medicine. The marked trend toward state medicine has painted the picture of the future doctor as one with a lower income, a lack of individual privileges in his practice and a lowering of the standards of living for the future. There is plenty evidence to support such a picture. Also discouraging is the fact that approximately one-third to one-fourth of the men completing their pre-medic course can not be admitted to medical schools on account of the limited admitted number in the class and lack of facilities of caring for more and the over crowding of the profession.

However, to offset this, is one bright star on the horizon which shows that all of the future is not gloomy. Two hundred and forty-three leading foundations now give annually a total of $38,500,000 toward medicine and public health education, outranking all other educational benefits. During 1937, last year for which figures are available, purposes relating to medicine and public health benefitted to the extent of $13,495,898, while education, in second place, received $9,170,318. These figures reveal more than appears on the surface. In the first place it would indicate that vast funds are available for properly conducted research work and for more advanced training in the study of medicine. What is more important is that the American public is sufficiently health conscious to make these funds available and are sufficiently interested that it is doubtful the public will ever permit any lowering of standards of medical practice by accepting compulsory socialization of medicine.

—A. RAY WILEY, M.D.

USE OF LAXATIVES

Nearly every 15 minutes there comes over the radio some misinformation relative to the use of cathartics. This is so constantly kept before the lay public that our population is rapidly developing the cathartic habit which of course is increasing the sales of the numerous products advertised thus fulfilling the purpose of the vast expenditures by the purveyors of such preparations.

The harm that is being done can be seen by the family physician of the country. One never hears the dangers spoken of, it is never mentioned that cathartics should never be administered in the presence of abdominal pain, the listening public is never told of the dangers and complications in acute appendicitis when laxatives are taken.

Now you may ask, what can be done about it? And the answer is that the medical profession must make a campaign in an effort to overcome the terrible effects of this malignant advertising, bring to our people the truth relative to the danger of cathartics under certain circumstances.

In the State of Pennsylvania the Medical Association made a very strenuous campaign in an effort to lower the mortality from appendicitis and the principal note was avoidance of the use of cathartics in the presence of abdominal pain. Stickers were prepared to be used on m o n t h l y statements and letters telling of this danger. Perhaps something could be done by us to offset the misinformation placed before the public both in print and over the radio.

———————o———————

A.M.A. INDICTMENT QUASHED!

———————

Justice James M. Proctor, upholding a defense demurrer to indictments, ruled on July 26 that the American Medical Association and its fellow defendants were not engaged in a trade as defined by the antimonopoly statutes. Counsel for the doctors had contended their activities could not be governed by the Antitrust Law, that they were engaged in a "learned profession" rather than a trade. On December 20, 1938, a District of Columbia Grand Jury, acting on evidence presented by the Justice Department, indicted the American Medical Association, the Medical Society of the District of Columbia, the Washington Academy of Surgery, the Harris County (Texas) Medical Society and 21 individual physicians for violation of the Sherman Antitrust Law. These organizations and individuals, the indictment read, were "engaged in a continuing combination in conspiracy in restraint" of trade in hampering the activities of Group Health Association, Inc., for the District of Columbia, an organization established in 1937 to hire physicians and nurses and provide hospital care on a cooperative basis to government employees. Defense attorneys had contended that all their clients' activities were directed solely at the maintenance of the ethics and standards of the profession.

At the headquarters of the Association, officials, including Dr. Olin West, Secretary, and Dr. Morris Fishbein, Editor, said:

"The principles and policies of the American Medical Association do not forbid nor have they ever contemplated any opposition to a well considered expanded program of medical service, when the need can be established; neither is there any fundamental principle or policy which in any manner opposes aid to the indigent when indigence can be established.

"The American Medical Association has a l w a y s welcomed investigation by any authorized agency of the nature of its organization or of the conduct of its work or of its activities, firmly reliant in the belief that every action taken by the Association has been in accordance with its constitutional organization in the interests of the public welfare for advancing standards and quality of medical service for the American people; and that at no time has it violated the established law of the federal, state, or municipal governments of this country. Moreover, by the very nature of its organization, it has preserved constantly the democratic principles on which the Government of the United States is founded and maintained."

———————o———————

Editorial Notes—Personal and General

The Fite Clinic, Muskogee, will be located, after September 1, 1939, on the seventh floor of the Commercial National building. Dr. William Henry Doyle is added to the staff in the department of dermatology and syphilology and associated radium and X-ray therapy.

———————

DR. J. F. PARK, McAlester, is in England. He will attend clinics in London and in Edinburgh during his absence of some six weeks.

———————

DR. HUGH H. MONROE of Lindsay has been appointed as county health superintendent of Garvin county. Dr. Monroe's appointment was effective as of June 28.

———————

DR. GRADY MATHEWS has announced the appointment of DR. F. R. HASSLER as county health superintendent of Pottawatomie county. Dr. Hassler took over his new position July 15.

———————

DR. N. ROBERT DRUMMOND has recently become an associate with DR. GEORGE H. KIMBALL of Oklahoma City. Dr. Drummond's internship was served at University Hospital and for the past year he has served as resident at St. Anthony Hospital.

———————

DR. W. B. DAVIS of Stroud who recently underwent an appendix operation is convalescing at the Rollins Hospital, Prague, Oklahoma.

———————

DR. JAS. L. SCHULER of Durant has formed a partnership with DR. P. B. RICE formerly of Oklahoma City. The new firm will be known as the "Schuler-Rice Clinic." Dr. Rice is a graduate of the University of Oklahoma Medical School and recently completed his internship at the Oklahoma City General Hospital.

———————

DR. JAMES S. PETTY of Guthrie has been elected the new Chairman of the Medical Staff of the Cimarron Valley Wesley Hospital. Other elected officers are: Dr. Wm. C. Miller and Dr. P. B. Gardner.

DR. NED BURLESON of Prague is busily studying the Manual of Arms having recently enlisted in the Medical Corps of the National Guard.

The Valley View Hospital of Ada recently celebrated its first anniversary. Since its opening the hospital has treated patients from 17 states outside of Oklahoma and many other counties outside of Pontotoc county. Valley View Hospital is to be complimented on the fine service it has rendered during its first year of operation.

DR. C. P. BONDURANT of Oklahoma City was one of the winners in the contest sponsored by the Daily Oklahoman & Times for amateur photographers. Dr. Bondurant won first in the Facial Study Class.

DR. and MRS. F. T. BARTHELD, of McAlester, have returned from an eastern trip, including a visit to the World's Fair.

DR. and MRS. J. B. LAMPTON and their daughter, Judith, of Sapulpa spent the month of June in Philadelphia where Dr. Lampton did post-graduate work at the Pennsylvania Hospital.

DR. W. C. TISDAL who until recently was superintendent of the Western Tuberculosis Sanatorium at Clinton, has entered private practice in that city and will be associated with DR. PAUL LINGENFELTER.

DR. T. W. PRATT, who recently completed his internship at University Hospital, has established his practice in Cheyenne, Oklahoma.

Oklahoma Doctor Honored

DR. L. J. MOORMAN of Oklahoma City has recently been honored by the American Trudeau Society by being selected as its President-Elect. Dr. Moorman will serve during 1940-41. He has, in the past, served organized medicine as President of the Oklahoma State Medical Association, the Southern Medical Association and is at the present time a member of the Editorial Board of the Oklahoma State Medical Journal.

Iron Lung for Western Oklahoma

Western Oklahoma is fortunate, indeed, in having in that part of the state an American Legion group progressive and farseeing enough to give to the communities they serve the facilities of the latest advancement in modern medical science. The American Legion units of the 6th, 7th and 8th Districts have recently purchased two new type iron lungs, one for adult use and one for infant use. The lungs will be placed in the Western Oklahoma Charity Hospital at Clinton. Governor Leon C. Phillips and Lieut. Governor James E. Berry were present at the dedication ceremonies.

The Package Library

The Library of the American Medical Association has collected published material, in the form of reprints and pages from periodicals, on many phases of medicine and surgery. This material will be loaned to members of the Association or to **individual** subscribers to its publications for a small charge. The collection does not contain articles in foreign languages, or articles on highly specialized topics, but these may be supplied when especially requested.

Following is the list of rules governing the package library:

1. The service is supplied only to members of the Association and to **individual** subscribers to its periodicals.

2. Requests for packages must be in writing and should be addressed "Library, American Medical Association."

3. Only one package may be borrowed at one time.

4. Twenty-five cents in stamps must be enclosed to cover postage and part of expense of collecting the material. THIS SHOULD NOT BE ENCLOSED IN THE PACKAGE BUT SHOULD BE SENT UNDER SEPARATE COVER.

5. Packages must not be kept longer than six days.

6. Packages, or items contained therein, that are lost can be replaced, if at all, only by the purchase of some or all of the lost items. The actual cost of replacing such items must be borne by the borrower.

7. When returning the package, tear off the slip sent with package and paste on wrapper. Please notify The Library, American Medical Association, 535 N. Dearborn St.—postal card is sufficient—when the package is mailed back.

Examinations American Board of Obstetrics and Gynecology

The next written examination and review of case histories (Part I) for Group B candidates will be held in various cities of the United States and Canada on Saturday, January 6, 1940, at 2:00 P.M. The Board announces that it will hold only one Group B, Part I, examination this year prior to the final general examination (Part II), instead of two as in former years. Candidates who successfully complete the Part I examination proceed automatically to the Part II examination held in June, 1940.

Applications for admission to Group B, Part I, examinations must be on file in the Secretary's office not later than October 4, 1939.

The general oral and pathological examinations (Part II) for all candidates (Groups A and B) will be conducted by the entire Board, meeting in Atlantic City, N. J., on June 8, 9, 10, and 11, 1940, immediately prior to the annual meeting of the American Medical Association in New York City.

Applications for admission to Group A, Part II examinations must be on file in the Secretary's office not later than March 15, 1940.

After January 1, 1942, there will be only one classification of candidates, and all will be required to take the Part I examinations (written paper and case records) and the Part II examinations (pathological and oral).

For further information and application blanks, address Dr. Paul Titus, Secretary, 1015 Highland Building, Pittsburgh (6), Pennsylvania.

The American Can Company has available to the physicians of Oklahoma their recent publication "The Canned Food Reference Manual." This manual was compiled by the Nutrition Research Laboratory of the American Can Company and presents interesting data on conservation of food essentials, dietary requirements, nutritional and public health aspects of canned foods, canning procedure as well as a wealth of other authoritative material. Should you care to receive this manual correspond with the American Can Company, 230 Park Avenue, New York City, N. Y.

Oklahoma City Clinical Society, 1939 Meeting

The time is now appropriate to call attention to the forthcoming meeting of the Oklahoma City Clinical Society. As every Oklahoma physician knows, this meeting was omitted last fall in deference to the Southern Medical Association. The committees have been busy however, and are all set to put on a program this fall second to none. From far and near have come compliments and congratulations to the Oklahoma City group for the splendid organization they have maintained through the lean years of the depression. Each succeeding year the meeting has grown greater and better, and from the plans which have been made known to us thus far, the program for 1939 will be the best yet.

Speakers who will appear on the program are as follows:

Dr. Rock Sleyster, Wauwatosa, Wisconsin—President of American Medical Association; psychiatrist.

Dr. Albert H. Aldridge, New York, New York; obstetrics.

Dr. Edgar G. Ballenger, Atlanta, Georgia; urology.

Dr. Lewellys F. Barker, Baltimore, Maryland, internal medicine.

Dr. Lowell S. Goin, Los Angeles, California; roentgenology.

Dr. Harry S. Gradle, Chicago, Illinois; ophthalmology.

Dr. John A. Kolmer, Philadelphia, Pennsylvania; pathology.

Dr. Frank H. Lahey, Boston, Massachusetts; surgery.

Dr. Joe V. Meigs, Boston, Massachusetts; gynecology.

Dr. A. Graeme Mitchell, Cincinnati, Ohio; pediatrics.

Dr. Emil Novak, Baltimore, Maryland; endocrinology-gynecology.

Dr. Hobart A. Reimann, Philadelphia, Pennsylvania; internal medicine.

Dr. Erwin R. Schmidt, Madison, Wisconsin; surgery.

Dr. Herman C. Schumm, Milwaukee, Wisconsin; orthopedics.

Dr. Marion B. Sulzberger, New York, New York; dermatology.

Dr. William A. Wagner, New Orleans, Louisiana; otolaryngology.

Every practitioner in Oklahoma should make his plans to attend all or part of a program featuring such a magnificent array of talent. Don't forget the dates, October 30, 31 and November 1 and 2.

--------o--------

Try Pablum On Your Vacation

Vacations are too often a vacation from protective foods. For optimum benefits a vacation should furnish optimum nutrition as well as relaxation, yet actually this is the time when many persons go on a spree of refined carbohydrates. Pablum is a food that "goes good" on camping trips and at the same time supplies an abundance of calcium, phosphorus, iron, and vitamins B and G. It can be prepared in a minute, without cooking, as a breakfast dish or used as a flour to increase the mineral and vitamin values of staple recipes. Packed dry, Pablum is light to carry, requires no refrigeration. Easy-to-fix Pablum recipes and samples are available to physicians who request them from Mead Johnson & Company, Evansville, Ind.

New Books

DISEASES OF THE NOSE AND THROAT; by Dr. Charles J. Imperatori and Dr. Herman J. Burman. Published by J. B. Lippincott Company, Philadelphia. Price, $7.00.

The second edition of this work follows the same instructive plan as in the first edition. The material in this book is arranged somewhat differently than the ordinary manner. The book is written in more or less of outline form. The symptoms, diagnosis and treatment is considered first followed by the pathology. The treatment is considered in its infinite detail and I believe it is well presented. The illustrations of the methods of procedure of the examination and operative t r e a t m e n t are numerous and fine as to detail.

The second edition contains newer phases of allergy related to otolaryngology as well as a discussion of many other diseases not included in the previous edition.

"OPERATIVE ORTHOPEDICS" (First Edition): by Willis C. Campbell, M.D., Memphis, Tenn. Publishers, C. V. Mosby Company, 3525 Pine Bvld., St. Louis, Missouri. Price $12.50.

One has to but look at the name of the author to be sure of the worth of this publication. The reviewer has spent many hours with Dr. Campbell in his Clinic and watched the methods of examination, preparation, operation and after care and it is fortunate that he has been able to explain these methods in this exhaustive and detailed manner.

This work of over 1,100 pages is systematically divided into 23 chapters with the material in each chapter sub-divided in such a manner as to make handy reference.

The completeness with which each subject is covered is one outstanding feature, not only is the text complete but the illustrations demonstrate in detail the subject matter and leave nothing to the imagination. There are 845 of these illustrations, nearly all original drawings and X-rays. The drawings illustrate the various steps in operative procedures and are not only artistic but show distinctly every detail.

Anatomy, physiology, pathology, mechanics, operative procedure, pre and post operative care all receive due attention by the author.

Many of the surgical procedures are original and each operation advocated is backed by the long experience of Dr. Campbell and his corps of able associates and the ultimate result is based on the observation of the patient at the conclusion of treatment in all cases where possible.

This book is indispensable to the orthopedic surgeon and as many of the procedures are applicable to the practice of general surgery it will find an important place in every surgical library.

MEDICAL STATE BOARD EXAMINATIONS: by Harold Rypins, A.B., M.D., F.A.C.P. Published by J. B. Lippincott Company, Philadelphia. Price $4.50.

This is the fourth edition of a book that has given fine service to the candidate for examination before the State or National Boards as he is given a classification of questions and answers that relieve him of much reading and directs his thoughts along the lines of the usual questions asked.

The material is treated concisely and collateral material is omitted. In this manner the applicant finds the essential facts covered in 448 pages.

Only by studying this book can one be convinced of its value and the amount of time and energy conserved.

THE OKLAHOMA PRENATAL EXAMINATION LAW

G. F. Mathews, M.D., Commissioner
Oklahoma State Health Department

The Prenatal Examination Law prepared by the American Social Hygiene Association under the direction of Bascom Johnson was introduced in the last session of the legislature by Senator Ritzhaupt and co-authors, amended and passed. The state-wide interest and support of the medical societies did much to assure the passage of this bill and is greatly appreciated.

The attention of physicians engaged in obstetrics is called to the provisions under section 2 requiring a statement on the birth certificate showing whether a blood test for syphilis was made and the date of the test and if not made the reason why the test was not made. In no case shall the result (positive, negative, etc.) of the test be stated on the birth certificate.

On the new 1939 birth certificates space has been provided for the above data on line 23 (b). If the old form is used the data may be written on the margin.

Examples: 23 (b) Blood test taken 1-15-39
or
23 (b) Blood test not taken, patient refused, etc.

The text of the law is as follows:

Senate Bill No. 92

AN ACT RELATING TO SEROLOGICAL BLOOD TESTS FOR SYPHILIS DURING PREGNANCY AND REPORTS THEREOF.

BE IT ENACTED BY THE PEOPLE OF THE STATE OF OKLAHOMA:

SECTION 1. Every physician attending a pregnant woman in the State during gestation shall, in the case of each woman so attended, at her request or with her consent, take or cause to be taken a sample of blood of such woman at the time of first examination, and submit such sample to an approved laboratory for a standard serological test for syphilis. Every other person permitted by law to attend upon pregnant women in the State, but not permitted by law to take blood tests, shall cause the blood of such pregnant woman to be taken by a duly licensed physician and submitted to an approved laboratory for a standard serological test for syphilis. The term "approved laboratory" means a laboratory approved for this purpose by the State Commissioner of Health. A standard serological test for syphilis is one recognized as such by the State Commissioner of Health. Such laboratory tests as are required by this Act shall be made on request without charge by the State Department of Public Health.

SECTION 2. In reporting every birth and stillbirth, physicians and others permitted to attend pregnancy cases and required to report births and stillbirths shall state on the certificate of birth whether a blood test for syphilis has been made during such pregnancy upon a specimen of blood taken from the woman who bore the child for which a birth or stillbirth certificate is filed and, if made, the date when such test was made, and, if not made, the reason why such test was not made. Such information shall be in addition to that required to be included in certificates of birth by Section 4509, Oklahoma Statutes 1931. In no event, however, shall the certificate of birth state the result of the test herein required.

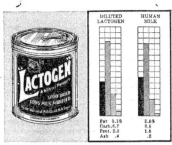

Additions To Roster

Atoka:
Cody, R. D._____Coalgate

Beckham:
Lester, J. A._____Elk City

Cherokee:
Deutsch, Harry L._____Tahlequah

Cleveland:
Petway, Aileen_____1716 N. Phillips, Oklahoma City

Garvin:
Wilson, H. P._____Wynnewood

Grady:
Hammond, James H._____Minco

Kiowa:
McIllwain, Wm. H._____Roosevelt

LeFlore:
Jones, L. D._____Talihina
Woodson, E. M._____Poteau

Logan:
Gray, Dan_____Guthrie

Muskogee:
Earnest, A. N._____Barnes Building
Rafter, J. G._____Manhattan Building

Okfuskee:
Carroll, W. B._____Okemah

Oklahoma:
Clark, Ralph O._____1706 S.E. 29th St.
Crick, L. E._____Edmond
Deupree, Harry L._____Medical Arts Bldg.
Howard, Robt. B._____1200 No. Walker
Lain, Everett S._____Medical Arts Bldg.
Randel, Harvey O._____Medical Arts Bldg.
Stillwell, Robt. J._____American Nat'l Bldg.
Weir, Marshall W._____Ramsey Tower Bldg.
Wells, Lois Lyon_____800 N.E. 13th St.
Witten, Harold B._____Harrah

Ottawa:
Jacoby, J. S._____Commerce

Payne:
Oehlschlager, F. Keith_____Yale

Rogers:
Beson, C. W._____Claremore

Seminole:
Price, J. T._____Seminole
Stephens, A. B._____Seminole
Walker, A. A._____Seminole
Ware, T. H._____Seminole

Sequoyah:
Newlin, W. H._____Sallisaw

Stephens:
Carmichael, J. B._____Duncan
Smith, L. P._____Marlow

Tulsa:
Roberts, T. R._____417 Wright Bldg.

Woods:
Cheatwood, W. R._____Alva

---o---

Swelling of Joint Due to Allergy

The first case in which recurrent swelling of a joint was definitely traced to allergic factors is cited by Herbert Berger, M.D., Tottenville, Staten Island, N. Y., in The Journal of the American Medical Association for June 10.

Elimination of the foods causing the allergy, he states, not only relieved the other allergic manifestations—gastrointestinal disturbances and hay fever—but also stopped the recurring collection of joint fluid responsible for the swelling and caused a general puffiness of the skin entirely to disappear.

He concludes from a review of the incidence and cause of the condition that all these symptoms do not constitute a disease but are due to a variety of general and local factors.

USUAL DREAD OF PROSTATECTOMY IS UNFOUNDED, PHYSICIAN SAYS

Reduction of Operating Hazards Lowered Mortality Rate to Only 2.4 Per Cent Among Omaha Doctor's Patients

There is little reason for the dread by the average person of prostatectomy (surgical removal of the prostate or of a part of it), Edwin Davis, M.D., Omaha, Neb., declares in The Journal of the American Medical Association for June 17 in an article which discusses the factors tending to minimize the hazards from this operation.

Pointing out that in a series of his cases totaling 741 the mortality rate was only 2.7 per cent, Dr. Davis enumerates and discusses briefly "the various factors which are responsible for this conspicuously low mortality rate and which have placed this operation in the category of so-called finished operations. This term seems permissible because the mortality rate so closely approximates the 'normal' death rate for the age of 70 and because questionnaire records show that, of aged persons, many of whom have unrelated ailments and symptoms which might readily be confused, 82.3 per cent voluntarily classified themselves as 'well' and 98.8 per cent as 'well or improved.' The lowering of the mortality rate has been essentially a process of elimination of the various hazards one by one."

Elaborating on the mortality rate, the author says that "according to the American experience tables of mortality, of 100 persons alive at the age of 70, six may be expected to die before reaching 71. Carrying this comparison to its extreme in absurdity, if the period of hospitalization for prostatectomy was one year, the 'normal' death rate might be said to be more than twice the postprostatectomy death rate."

The various hazards of prostatectomy listed by Dr. Davis include retention or insufficient secretion of urine, infection, hemorrhage (immediate and delayed), complications due to the anesthesia, inflammation of the epididymis and vascular "accidents," that is blood clots in the heart, lung or brain arteries. He asserts that "all but the last named are controllable and have been reduced to a negligible minimum.

"There is no reason why the mortality rate of prostatectomy in the aged and debilitated should not be made to compare favorably with that of operations for hernia in the young and robust."

---o---

X-Ray Pictures Aid Obstetricians

X-ray pictures of the pelvis in pregnancy are a valuable auxiliary to clinical studies in indicating the probable course of labor and in determining the best method of delivery, Emanuel M. Rappaport, M.D., Jamaica, N. Y., and Samuel J. Scadron, M.D., New York, declare in The Journal of the American Medical Association for June 17.

Greatest accuracy is attained, they point out, when both the clinical and X-ray methods are combined, that is when obstetricians familiar with pelvic X-rays examine the films as well as the patient. "We do not believe," they state, "that the roentgenologist (X-ray specialist) alone can render a more accurate opinion (except academically) than the experienced obstetrician. For the inexperienced clinician, however, the X-ray record should be a valuable guide. Moreover, both the obstetrician and the roentgenologist must know their limitations."

The use of X-rays is especially important in those cases in which cesarean operation or instrumental aid will be necessary because of a contracted pelvis or some other pelvic abnormality.

Normal delivery may be expected in the great majority of instances when clinical and X-ray studies agree that the pelvis is large enough for the fetus.

ABSTRACTS : REVIEWS : COMMENTS
and CORRESPONDENCE

SURGERY AND GYNECOLOGY
Abstracts, Reviews and Comments from
LeRoy Long Clinic
714 Medical Arts Building, Oklahoma City

Recurrent Perforations of Gastro-Duodenal Ulcers (Les Perforations Iterapives des Ulceres Gastro-Duodenaux). By Henri Grizaud, Chirugien des Hopitaux Coloniaux, Medecin-Chef de l'Hopidal d'Abijou. ("Cote d'Inoire.") La Presse Medicale, January 11, 1939.

There is a reference by the author to a recent article by J. Gosset, Jouneau and Allamand, published in La Presse Medicale, October 22, 1938, upon the subject of "Recurrent Perforations of Gastro-Duodenal Ulcers." It was the general conclusion of the authors quoted that such ulcers have a distinct tendency to recur. The author reports the case of a medical officer in the Colonial Service who had had a perforation of a gastric ulcer in 1935, at which time there was an emergency operation, the suture being closed by sutures placed in such a way that there was inversion of the margins. No other operation was attempted at that time.

After the operation the patient did well for several years, having returned to active service in the Colonial army following a rather long period of rest and appropriate management.

In August (presumably August, 1938) there was an attack of dysentery at which time the ulcer symptoms reappeared. About the time that the dysentery was controlled there was sudden, agonizing abdominal pain, short and rapid breathing, much sweating, but no distinct board-like abdomen (mais pas de ventre de bois). There were all the classical evidences of perforation, with the exception of a board-like abdomen. However, there was some rigidity, and notwithstanding the absence of this classical sign it was believed that there had been a perforation.

The patient was seen two hours after the symptoms appeared. He was 36 kilometers from a well equipped military hospital. The confrere who was in attendance, and who is the author of the article under consideration, gravely and logically discusses the question as to whether the patient should be subjected to an operation in the field, where there was only meagre equipment and facilities, or be transported the 36 kilometers to the well equipped military hospital. Taking into consideration the early diagnosis, in connection with inadequate facilities for a major operation in the field, the patient was transmitted to the hospital where he arrived in a condition apparently as good as before the journey was undertaken.

After arriving at the hospital where there were X-ray facilities, a radiogram of the upper abdomen, showing a line of what appeared to be air or gas between the liver and the diaphragm, confirmed the diagnosis.

Operation was done at once under ether anesthesia. There were adhesions of the omentum to the surrounding structures, and after they were separated much dirty fluid was found in the right upper abdomen. With some difficulty, a perforation the size of a lentil, circular in shape, clean cut borders, and surrounded by scar tissue, was disclosed in the distal portion of the stomach. It was sutured, and the suture line was reinforced by suturing over it surrounding available tissue, it being possible to draw the same omentum over it. A drain was placed in the subhepatic area, and it remained in place for three days. There was satisfactory recovery, and, with proper management, the patient did well after the operation. It is quite apparent that the author who was treating the patient had two distinct convictions: The first was not to undertake a major operation with inadequate facilities in the field in the early hours after a perforation; the second was that he did not believe it wise to do more than to close the perforation and provide for drainage.

In the same number of La Presse Medicale there is another interesting and instructive article on practically the same subject, the title of the article being:

Recurring Perforations of the Duodenum (Les Perforations Iterapives des Ulceres Duodenaux), by J. Bottin, of Liege, Belgium.

In this article by Bottin there is a general discussion of the proper procedure in the presence of symptoms and signs of perforation, the author mentioning, incidentally, the proper procedure in connection, not only with recurrent perforations, but in connection, also, with primary perforations of the stomach and duodenum. It appears that it is the custom in the clinic that he represents to be very conservative, particularly in the presence of symptoms and signs of perforation that is primary—that is, in the case of an individual who had not had an operation before. In such a case the advice is to simply close the perforation, without any attempt to do a gastro-enterostomy or a resection. It appears that he believes that that simple procedure, with necessary drainage, is all that should be done in the case of such a patient.

The author reports the cases of several patients in which there were recurrent perforations, and, notwithstanding that the title of his communication is "Recurring Perforations of the Duodenum," in the cases that he reports there was, without exception, a recurrent perforation of the stomach. It is assumed that there is a typographical error in connection with the title of the communication.

The author is distinctly inclined to be conservative in connection with perforations of any character, whether they are primary or recurrent.

In one of the patients reported by Bottin there were both gross and histological evidences of carcinoma of the stomach, but the statement is made that it was impossible to determine whether the carcinoma of the stomach had arisen from a previous ulcer. Such pathology requires more radical surgery.

There is a significant statement that when there is simple closure, with drainage, if necessary, after a primary perforation, it has been shown that about 40 per cent of the patients were apparently cured—that is, they did not have any subsequent symptoms and signs indicative of ulcer of the stomach or duodenum.

Comments: 1. It appears from both of the above articles that the authors are of the distinct opinion that after a primary perforation of stomach or duodenum the operation should be conservative— that is, proper closure of the perforation, with drainage, if necessary. 2. In the case of recurrent perforations of stomach or duodenum the surgeon ought to be inclined to conservatism, radical operations, like resection, being reserved for certain patients in which there is definite evidence of malignancy. 3. It should be noted that in the first article drainage was employed for only three days. Knowing something about the technic of the average French surgeon, this is a surprising statement. It has been our experience that if a drain is employed it should be left in place for a much longer time—even 10 days in the case of some patients. We believe that removal of drainage after only three days might be disastrous. 4. The discussion by the military surgeon about the advisability of transporting the patient to hospital rather than undertake an abdominal operation in the field, or in any place where there are not good facilities, is valuable, and we endorse it fully. We believe that the transportation of a patient is much less hazardous than to undertake an intra-abdominal operation without reasonably adequate facilities.

LeRoy Long.

Recent Advances in the More Common Problems of Minor Anorectal Surgery: Robert A. Scarborough, M.D., San Francisco, California; Surgery, June, 1939, Vol. 5, No. 6, page 952.

The treatment of anorectal disease too long remained in the hands of the charlatan, who glibly promised cures without surgery and dispensed "painless pile dissolvents."

It is important to realize that the vast majority of pathologic conditions occurring in this region must be approached and treated by the special application of general surgical principles.

Hemorrhoids: It is, unfortunately, still true that from 26 to 50 per cent of patients with carcinoma of the rectum, within easy reach of the examining finger, still receive treatment for some other supposed rectal condition (usually hemorrhoids) for weeks and months before the correct diagnosis is made.

There has been increasing recognition of the fact that true appreciation of the presence and size of hemorrhoids cannot be gained by mere external inspection, nor is digital examination of particular value because of the softness and easy compressibility of internal hemorrhoids. Internal inspection is of prime importance, preferably with an anoscope which has an oblique internal orifice. In the determination of treatment it is important to recognize internal and external hemorrhoids as such. Most surgeons now realize that patients do not actually suffer from hemorrhoids but from the complications of hemorrhoids, and proper treatment must depend upon what those complications are. Those situated above the mucocutaneous or pectinate line and covered with mucous membrane are always internal hemorrhoids and those situated below this line and covered by skin are always external hemorrhoids regardless of their relative position inside or outside of the anal canal at the time of examination. Too often a doctor as well as a patient attempts by main force to "reduce" an acutely thrombosed external hemorrhoid, inflicting more harm than good upon the unhappy patient. It is to be remembered that the mucocutaneous line is also the landmark for the upward extent of sensory innervation. When the patient's chief complaint is pain, the cause of this pain must be at or distal to this line and regardless of how big or how vascular or how eroded are his internal hemorrhoids it must be realized that this pain is not going to be relieved by treatment directed solely to the internal hemorrhoids. Regardless of size, the patient's symptoms may not be from the hemorrhoids at all but may be due to a great variety of other causes, including cancer. In evaluating the recommended methods of treatment for hemorrhoids, it must be realized that the only satisfactory application of any of these methods will depend upon the surgeon's complete understanding of the true pathologic condition present and the correct application of the proper method of treatment to the particular condition existing.

Thrombosis of external hemorrhoids is usually due to multisacculated intraluminar thromboses rather than from the result of a mechanical rupture of an anal varicosity with formation of an extraluminar hematoma. Conservative treatment of the small thrombosed external hemorrhoid by rest, hot Sitz baths, and stool lubrication will be followed by gradual resolution and fibrosis in the course of from a few days to a week or more. Incision and expression of the clot are to be discouraged as this rarely shortens the natural course of the disease. Block excision of the multisacculated clots should be done through an elliptical incision in the overlying skin so devised that the edges of the incision will fall accurately together at the end of the operation. If properly accomplished, with no sutures or ties employed, relief is complete in a short time. There is some debate as to the advisability of immediate operation in cases of diffuse thrombosis of external and internal hemorrhoids, but the majority of surgeons prefer immediate operation, discounting the danger of embolism, liver abscess, or stenosis (resulting from inability to judge the amount of tissue necessary to remove).

Careful perusal of the literature of the last few years does not lead to the impression that the operation of hemorrhoidectomy has yet escaped from its unenviable reputation for postoperative pain. The various types of operation in vogue a hundred years ago still have their proponents. This situation encourages the charlatan who glibly promises cures without surgery. It also has led to the popularity of so-called "ambulant methods." And yet, in actual fact perhaps the greatest advance in minor anorectal surgery has been in the operative treatment of hemorrhoids. This has not occurred as a result of a new type of operation, but by awakening recognition of the fact that hemorrhoidectomy is fundamentally a plastic operation performed upon tissues of peculiar anatomic characteristics in a region incapable of complete physiologic rest and inevitably subject to infection. Merar, in 1939, laid down certain rules for hemorrhoidectomy: (1) Avoidance of every form of injury, mechanical, thermal, chemical; (2) application of that expert and particular care to which this area, as one of the most sensitive regions in the body, is entitled; (3) utilization of a tried and tested routine preoperative and postoperative regime; (4) selection of an open, nonburning, nontraumatizing method of operation.

In plastic surgery great emphasis is placed on preoperative preparation and particularly on postoperative care of wounds. This is of vital importance in hemorrhoidectomy and upon this depends in considerable part the postoperative comfort of the patient. There are two noteworthy omissions in present-day postoperative routine; the large retention rectal tube routinely employed a few years ago, and the practice of "tying up the bowels" for a week or more after operation. The retention rectal tube was a constant source of irritation to the wound and elicited a reflex spasmodic contraction of the sphincters which was harmful to healing and most uncomfortable to the patient. The early passage of a soft but formed stool will accomplish the desired effect in so far as postoperative dilatation is concerned with the minimum of discomfort to the patient. This is accomplished by giving food immediately after operation together with some agar, mineral oil or tragacanth preparation to assure a formed but soft stool. Spontaneous defecation usually occurs on the third or possibly fourth postoperative day and is far more desirable than the use of enemas or more drastic catharsis.

The importance of complete muscular relaxation for correct plastic surgery on the rectum cannot be overstressed. The position on the table is important. (The author prefers the prone ventral position). The object of the operation is to make a thorough removal of the groups of varicose veins underlying the mucous membrane of the distal portion of the rectum and the skin of the anal canal with satisfactory functional result and a minimal deformity. It is important to recognize the fact that sterilization of the operative field is impossible. Sutures placed distal to the mucocutaneous line will increase postoperative discomfort. Divulsion of the sphincters is generally disapproved. The idea of c a u s i n g temporary paralysis by stretching of the sphincters is based on a false premise.

Injection Treatment of Hemorrhoids: This method of treatment was originated in 1866 by Blackwood and exploited by charlatans and ignorant practitioners for many years causing it to fall in disrepute because of the many unfortunate complications incurred. Today, it is realized to be of some value, but it is universally conceded and emphasized that injection therapy is restricted to the treatment of internal hemorrhoids and should never be used for external hemorrhoids. Injection of sclerosing solution below the mucocutaneous line produces severe pain and is usually followed by extensive painful necrosis and sloughing of tissue. Perhaps sufficient stress has not been laid upon its contraindications in the treatment of internal hemorrhoids which are complicated by inflammation, thrombosis, marked ulceration, or strangulation, or in the presence of associated conditions, such as cryptitis, fissure, or fistula.

For practical purposes one may say that the injection method is suited and should be confined to the treatment of uncomplicated, superficially eroded, internal hemorrhoids in the patient whose only symptom is bleeding. Any patient who has pain as a primary complaint necessarily has some pathologic condition at or below the level of the mucocutaneous line and will not be relieved of his pain by injection treatment. One sees many claims of permanent cure with injection treatment, but the majority of surgeons believe that this form of treatment exceptionally produces permanent cure. If one is to employ injection treatment, patient should be told that the effect may not be expected to be permanent, but may give satisfactory temporary relief from bleeding and that further treatment may eventually be required.

Of the sclerosing solutions the two most popular at the present time are: (1) quinine and urea hydrochloride (5 per cent) and (2) phenol, 5 per cent in vegetable oil.

Prolapse: It is probable that injection treatment has a place in the treatment of prolapse, incomplete or partial. A number of surgeons now believe that all degrees of prolapse should be treated by injection, and only if failure results should operation be considered.

LeRoy D. Long.

Experience with Surgical and Radiation Therapy in Carcinoma of the Corpus Uteri. William P. Healy, M.D., and Robert L. Brown, M.D., New York, N. Y. American Journal of Obstetrics and Gynecology, July, 1939, Vol. 38, Page 1.

This is an extremely valuable report giving the latest statistical information upon the treatment of carcinoma of the body of the uterus at Memorial Hospital in the 15-year period 1918 to 1932. The subject material is a group of 197 patients who received primary treatment during that interval. Of this 197, 93 were treated by a combination of surgery and radiation, 96 by radiation therapy alone and eight by surgery alone.

The symptoms of carcinoma of the uterine body begin usually after the menopause and in this series 78 per cent of the patients stated that the onset of symptoms occurred after menstruation had ceased. The most important and frequent symptom of carcinoma of the uterine body is uterine bleeding and it was found in 98 per cent of this group of 197 patients. In 97 per cent the bleeding was postmenopausal or intermenstrual while in one per cent menorrhagia only was noticed.

Pain was present in 27 per cent of the cases and these authors feel it is a symptom of some prognostic significance. Of the 53 patients complaining of pain 66 per cent later died of carcinoma, whereas of the 144 patients without pain only 37 per cent died of carcinoma. They also point out that in 43 per cent of the patients complaining of pain when their history was taken, and who later died of carcinoma, there was no palpable evidence of extension beyond the uterus at initial examination. They feel, therefore, that pain in some cases at least indicates the extension beyond the uterus before such extension can be verified by examination.

Vaginal discharge was noted in their histories in only 35 per cent of the patients and in the patient's minds was not as important as the presence of blood.

In 101 patients who were subjected to abdominal operation 38 per cent were found to have both fibromyoma and carcinoma of the uterus. The authors emphasize the fact that the source of bleeding cannot be considered as non-malignant just because of palpable fibroids and that examination of endometrial tissue is a prerequisite to an accurate diagnosis.

The entire series of 197 patients was divided into clinical groups according to the extent of the carcinoma as evidenced by observation and palpation. It appeared worthwhile from both a prognostic and therapeutic standpoint to so sub-divide the patients into clinical groups according to the size of the uterus and palpable extent of disease. "If the uterus is not larger than the size of a 2½ months gestation, and if there is no evidence of extension of carcinoma beyond the uterus (Group II), the five-year survival rate is 60 per cent if based upon the entire series of 197 cases without regard to treatment, and 88 per cent if based upon results in a smaller series of cases treated according to what is considered by us as the preferred method of treatment. If the uterus is larger than a 2½ months gestation (Group 11-A) our findings indicate that the chance for cure from radiation alone is extremely low. If there is palpable extension of carcinoma beyond the uterus (Group III) the chance for five-year survival is approximately 10 per cent." In group I they have placed all patients in whom there is no palpable enlargement of the uterus. It is also interesting that when the uterus was larger than a 2½ months gestation, the five-year survivals were only 35 per cent regardless of method of treatment.

All patients were likewise grouped upon a histological basis. Approximately half of all cases were adenoma malignum, one-fourth were adenocarcinoma grade II and approximately one-fourth adenoma grade III or IV. They believe that the histological type has a direct relation to chance for cure and is of a definite prognostic importance. The five-year survival rate for adenoma malignum grades I and II was 60 per cent, for adenocarcinoma grade II it was 42 per cent, for adenocarcinoma grade III and IV it was 20 per cent and for adenoacanthoma 60 per cent. By histological grouping they also demonstrated a definite difference in methods of treatment particularly in the adenoma malignum group where radiation alone yielded 39 per cent five-year survival, whereas 78 per cent of the patients with the same lesion treated by radiation followed by hysterectomy were well five years later. The difference was far less in adenocarcinoma grade II with percentages 41 and 44 per cent respectively. The results in their 10 cases of adenoacanthoma were 60 per cent with no significant difference between the two methods of treatment.

"Radiation alone has definite curative value in cases which for one reason or another cannot be subjected to subsequent panhysterectomy, the five-year survival rate for the group of 96 patients treated by radiation alone being 39 per cent. When only clinical Groups I and II are considered the five-year survival is 56 per cent and the five-year cure (free from all evidence of carcinoma five years or more) is 47 per cent."

These authors believe that the ideal treatment based upon their present experience is intra-uterine radon, usually not less than 3,600 millicurie hours, supplemented by roentgen ray and followed by hysterectomy. In their group of 28 cases so treated there were 79 per cent five-year survivals. They have found the risk of any major complication under this plean of treatment very slight. In considering the five-year survival rate for all patients treated by any combination of radiation and therapy in this series of 179 regardless of the particular technic employed 55 per cent were found to have survived five years or more.

The authors feel that their greater survival rate with their present method of treatment is due to the fact that a slightly larger dosage of radium emanation is being employed followed by hysterectomy.

It is entirely noteworthy that in 25 cases where a dosage of 3,000 to 3,300 millicurie hours was employed there was complete disappearance of carcinoma in 52 per cent and in 20 patients receiving 3,400 to 4,000 millicurie hours 60 per cent showed residual carcinoma. However, the remainder or 40 per cent of those receiving 3,400 to 4,000 milligram hours did have residual carcinoma and therein lies the principal reason for including hysterectomy as a part of the treatment of carcinoma of the body of the uterus. The advantages given for the combination of preoperative radiation and subsequent hysterectomy as seen by these authors are: 1. "It is conceivable that radiated carcinoma even if not completely destroyed is somewhat less likely to enter blood or lymph channels or to remain as viable implants in the pelvis at the time of hysterectomy than is carcinoma which has not been subjected to radiation." 2. "Second and far more significant is the fact that the results of the combined method of treatment as now employed is definitely better than those obtained by surgery alone." This is especially true considering the group of 28 patients receiving 3,000 to 4,000 millicurie hours of intrauterine radiation followed by hysterectomy where the survival rate at the end of five years was 79 per cent.

These authors quote Arneson who recently reviewed the literature on the surgical treatment of corpus cancer and found that of 927 reported cases 57 per cent of the patients were living five years or more afterwards.

Comment: This article has been reviewed more completely than is my usual practice because it contains certain information that should be in the hands of every doctor and other material which should be added to the fund of knowledge of one who is attempting to treat this disease.

In the first place, any post-menopausal bleeding must be considered a symptom of malignancy until the diagnosis is disproved. It is likewise true that intermenstrual bleeding must be looked upon with almost equal suspicion and that with intermenstrual bleeding or post-menopausal bleeding, whether or not fibroid tumors are present, the only accurate means of diagnosis is diagnostic curettage and microscopic examination.

This article has also emphasized the prognostic value of clinical grouping and the immediate lesson to be derived from this information is the all important advantage of early diagnosis and treatment before the disease has advanced to the later clinical groups.

In the rather small group of 28 cases in which 3,000 to 4,000 millicurie hours of radon were employed in the uterus followed by hysterectomy with 79 per cent survival rate there is good statistical evidence for the employment of preoperative irradiation.

This combined with the report of Arneson is convincing argument in favor of preoperative irradiation in sufficient dosages from 3,000 to 4,000 milligram hours of radium, with hysterectomy following in about eight weeks.

There is sound reason in this article both from the pathological findings and the ultimate survival rates for including hysterectomy in the treatment of carcinoma of the body of the uterus whether or not radiation has been employed.

Wendell Long.

————————o————————

EYE, EAR, NOSE AND THROAT
Edited by Marvin D. Henley, M.D.
911 Medical Arts Building, Tulsa

Significance of Venous Pulsation of the Eye Ground. Paul Weinstein, M.D., Report of the Eye Department of the Albert Apponyi Polyclinic at Budapest. British Journal of Ophthalmology, June, 1938.

The fact that there is a pulsation of the eye-ground has been an established fact since 1853. Arterial pulsation is pathological. In contradistinction venous pulsation is physiological.

The origin of arterial pulsation is still an unknown phenomenon. There are two theories in regard to venous pulsation. One is that spontaneous venous pulsation is caused by the wave of arterial pulsation transpiring through the capillaries, into the vein and thus inducing it to pulsate. The theory generally accepted is that the pressure of the central retina vein is higher than the tension of the eye; if the difference between ocular tension and venous pressure is absent, an increased amount of blood enters the eye at every systole, ocular tension is increased, becomes greater than the venous pressure, and the circulation being obstructed, causes the vein to pulsate. Therefore the logical conclusion is that the venous pulsation of the eyeground is chiefly dependent on ocular tension. This is also shown by the fact that under mydriatics, the spontaneous venous pulsation increases.

Baurmann says the pressure of the central retinal vein is also dependent on intracranial pressure (i.c.p). The author has observed previously that the blood-pressure of the eyeground is generally diminished in pregnant women as is also the ocular tension. He found that in 38 per cent of the pregnant women examined in the clinic, spontaneous venous pulsation was apparent. The average systolic blood pressure of this group was 123 mm. systolic. Where the venous pulsation was not present the blood pressure was lower. From examinations in this clinic it was determined that venous pulsation is more commonly present in individuals, who have a disposition to hypotonia, complaining about headache and giddiness. There is a discussion of the relationship of i.c.p. and cysternal puncture, pressure of the retinal vein and spontaneous pulsation.

The author closes with the following paragraph: "According to my researches spontaneous venous pulsation of the eyeground therefore originates by two mechanisms. One of them consists of a transpiring of the arterial capillary pulsewave at high blood-pressure, towards the vein. The other works by the i.c.p. being eventually diminished, the pressure within the central retinal vein being reduced to the level of ocular tension, and thus inducing pulsation. There can be of course no discussion about the validity of Pines' opinion published in the August number of the Brit. Jl. Ophthal., 1938, according to which local anatomical conditions, namely, an angular bend of the central retinal vein within the physiological excavation of the papilla influences pulsation, the less so, as in a given case the one, or other, or both eyes display venous pulsation.

The Treatment of Hysphonia and Allied Condition. Cortlandt Macmahon, London. The Journal of Laryngology and Otology, June, 1939.

Some of the causes of dysphonia mentioned are: after operation on throat and larynx; infection of the vocal cords from antra, teeth, tonsils and nasopharynx; certain affections of the heart; a general asthenia from any severe illness may affect the internal tensors and adductors of the larynx; it may accompany neurasthenia; gross misuse of the voice; it may be a sequela of functional aphonia.

Instruction on production of voice is an important factor in the writer's treatment of this condition. He says: "For acquiring a good voice a healthy condition of the nose is essential." Correct breathing, especially nasal breathing exercises, are helpful.

Difficulty in speaking following the removal of the thyroid gland is one of the most severe conditions that one has to deal with. The first thing is to get the patient to acquire gentle lower costal breathing and get rid of the upper costal breathing. This produces a deeper pitch of voice and this is helped by pressing the tongue down 100 times night and morning on the sound of "ah." This encourages the adductor muscles to relax and the abduction muscles to function better. In case of impairment of voice following an operation for intrinsic carcinoma of the larynx, the treatment is exactly the same. Voice training may cause nodes on the cords to disappear entirely; if nodes are present the voice is seriously impaired. Lupus of the larynx has been observed only once in the experience of the writer. This was in a young girl who was given two years complete vocal rest and voice training.

Misuse of the voice causes the most common types of dysphonia. Medical examination is necessary before voice training is started. Some of these patients are cured by altering the pitch of the voice, stretching the throat muscles by means of the tongue depressor, and getting correct breathing. Overbreathing and tensing of the throat muscles may produce a dysphonia by putting a strain on the cords. Functional aphonia in connection with dysphonia is discussed—the technique being given to bring back the voice.

The most difficult to treat of all affections of the voice is spastic dysphonia. Sir St. Clair Thomson and Mr. Negus compare this affliction to that of writer's cramp. It usually occurs from overwork, consequent exhaustion and talking along

in normal voice for several sentences when suddenly a voice is produced with a very high pitch. The voice comes and goes in this strange manner. Exercises for voice training are given, these help in getting emotional control. The Eunuchoid voice is calamity to its possessor. The cause of this according to the author: "At puberty when the larynx grows in size and the cords increase in length, the ary-vocales muscles have not as is usual at this stage of life ceased to exercise their function of shortening the vibrating surfaces of the cords like the fingers on a violin string." The treatment is highly successful.

In laryngectomy cases the new voice should be tried as soon as the leakage from the pharynx has ceased. The patient should not attempt to acquire the pharyngeal voice and at the same time use an artificial larynx. There is not any bibliography.

X-Ray Treatment of Infections: A Review of the Literature and Report of Cases of Mastoiditis and Sinusitis. B. R. Dysart, M.D., Pasadena. The Annals of Otology, Rhinology, and Laryngology, June, 1939.

The author's attention was first called to improvement following X-rays of what is considered probably o p e r a t i v e mastoiditis. Following the taking of the picture, there was decided improvement in about 24 hours. A review of the literature shows over 200 published articles with many favorable comments and little or none unfavorable on X-ray treatment of inflammatory conditions. Too large doses may aggravate the condition—small doses do not do any harm.

Arthur U. Desjardins of the Mayo Clinic says: "It seems likely that the infecting organism also plays a part in the effect of irradiation. The fact that streptococcus infection often causes little or no leucocytic infiltration may explain why, except in erysipelas, inflammatory lesions of this character do not respond so well, on the whole, as lesions caused by the staphylococcus."

His opinion is that the X-ray causes a disintegration of lymphocytes and causes the protective substances (antibodies, etc.) of these to be freed and made more readily available for the defense of the invading organism than when they were in the lymphocytes. Among lesions benefited by this form of treatment he mentions furuncle, carbuncle, acute simple adenitis, acute parotitis, complicating operations on the colon and other abdominal structures, abscesses and cellulitis of soft tissues, onychia and paronychia, mastitis, sinusitis and mastoiditis in selected cases.

Experimental reports show no effect of X-ray on organisms in culture media. To get the best results treatment should be instituted early, before suppuration. Charles Goosmann uses this treatment in postoperative mastoiditis with continued suppuration with good results. Wagner reported three cases with fatal results following large doses of X-ray in purulent pelvic infections. Diphtheria carriers are said to respond well to X-ray. Twelve cases were treated with X-ray, with a picture that showed an acute mastoiditis with enough haziness to consider operation. One to four doses were given at intervals of five days. These cases are reported in detail. According to the author treatment of sinusitis has not been as satisfactory as otitis media and mastoiditis.

A bibliography is appended to this article.

Perforated Peptic Ulcer from an Abscess of the Brain of Otitic Origin. Shirley Harold Baron, M.D., New London, Conn. Archives of Otolaryngology, June, 1939.

This is a case report of unusual interest. There is a two-page discussion of the clinical reports of similar cases. The author believes this ulcer to be of neurogenic origin. As early as 1845 there are recorded experiments on the neurogenic origin of peptic lesions. His discussion of the experimental reports brings this data up to date (Metler and co-workers, 1936).

I will give as brief a summary of the case as possible to retain the important points. A woman, age 26, was admitted to the hospital; chief complaint was pain in and around the left ear accompanied by a foul-smelling discharge; the ear had been discharging for the past 12 years following influenza; three and a half years before admittance to the hospital she had been advised that she should have an operation on her left mastoid; she refused operation then because of cessation of pain; the discharge was the only untoward sign until two weeks before coming into the hospital she complained of a dizziness and an unsteady gait; four days before coming into the hospital she had pain in the left mastoid region, temporal and occipital headache, nausea and vomiting; in the hospital examination showed much foul-smelling pus, perforated drum, swelling of the posterior superior wall, slight tenderness in the left mastoid region, absence of air conduction, inactive left labyrinth, ocular movements normal, pupils normal in appearance and reaction, fundi negative; neck flaccid, knee jerks and abdominal reflexes active, ankle jerks not elicited, Kernig's and Babinski's absent; abdomen negative; temperature on admission 98° F., pulse 70 and respiration 20; W.B.C. 10,140, 84 polys, 15 small lumphs, 1 monocyte, 85 per cent hemoglobin; X-ray showed a sclerotic left mastoid; a radical left mastoid was done; cholesteatoma were found in the antrum; the dural and sinal plates were removed—no perisinal or epidrual abscesses present; middle ear culture showed Bacillus mucous capsulatus; for five days the postoperative course was uneventful and then began a fluctuation of temperature that became greater daily (97.4° to 105.4°); blood cultures were negative; there was no rigidity or very little; ophthalmoscopic examination showed superior and nasal borders of the nerve head indistinct—no definite swelling; the temperature being characteristic of a lateral sinus thrombophlebitis (eleventh day postoperative) it was decided to explore further on the following day; at this time the general condition of the patient seemed good—pulse 80-130 —no nausea or vomiting—no particular complaints except a feeling of mild discomfort in the left side of the head; the night before the second operation was to be done the next morning the patient died suddenly. The autopsy showed: abscess of the brain, thrombosed lateral sinus, mastoiditis, perforated gastric ulcer, s e p t i c spleen and acute glomerular nephritis.

The author feels that the perforated gastric ulcer was caused by the abscess of the brain. Abscess of the brain·was considered from the first but exploration was not done because of lack of physical findings.

---o---

PLASTIC SURGERY
Edited by
GEO. H. KIMBALL, M.D., F.A.C.S.
404 Medical Arts Building, Oklahoma City

Gastrointestinal Ulcerations Following Burns: by John L. Kelley, M.D., Boston, Massachusetts. From the American Journal of Surgery, July, 1939.

The author calls attention to the fact that ulcerations of the gastrointestinal tract which occur as complications of cutaneous burns are commonly called Curling's ulcerations, but two articles appeared in literature 10 years prior to Curling's series describing similar lesions. The fact that Curling's paper described a lesion specifically of the duodenum, and his series is the largest series yet published attaches his name to this condition.

Perry and Shaw report five cases in 149 fatal burns in a period of 50 years, 1843-1892. Other series show much lower incidence. No incidence of gastrointestinal ulceration was reported in the Peter Brigham Hospital, 1913-1937, with 17 fatal burns.

The etiology is given consideration with no definite conclusions reached. The most probable cause would seem to be concentration of the blood stream with its attenuate slowing of circulation and thrombosis in the mucosal vessels. Other factors considered are adrenal damage, neurogenic etiological factors, and toxic absorption. The pathology of these lesions is similar to other acute ulcerations. These lesions may be single or multiple, the former usually occurring in the duodenum between the pylorus and ampulla of Vater, the latter usually along the lesser curvature of the stomach. These ulcers are usually acute and terminate in either perforation or healing, although at least one case has been demonstrable in X-ray 13 years after original burn.

Symptoms are usually pain of an ulcer type, hematemesis and usually occur between 18 hours and 100 days. This complication of burns is more frequent in children than in adults, although lately more cases have been reported in adults. "To conclude that hematemesis or melena in burned patients is due to ulceration is justified in a large majority of instances."

Prophylactic treatment for gastrointestinal ulceration following burns would appear to be the modern treatment of burns. This is generally supportive, and dilution of the blood stream with normal saline and glucose. Also the control of pain with opiates is an important factor. Local treatment with eschar producing agents such as tannic acid and gentian violet is conducive to the conservation of blood serum and proteins. The active treatment of the ulcer is the same as medical treatment of ordinary peptic ulcer. The indication of surgical intervention is the same as peptic ulcer, that is, perforation and hemorrhage.

Conclusion: The author has reviewed the literature carefully. It is to be noted that gastrointestinal ulcerations, as a sequelae of burns, is rather uncommon.

The author outlines the treatment for such cases. The modern treatment of extensive burns has apparently lessened the incidence of this condition.

Surgery of the Cleft Palate: by Arthur E. Smith, M.D., D.D.S., and James B. Johnson, M.D., Los Angeles, Calif. From the American Journal of Surgery, July, 1939.

The authors call attention to the fact that cleft palate is not due to mal-development of the parts, but non-fusion of the component parts of the face. This non-fusion may exist in any fusion line, but is most common in the lip and palate regions. "Of the congenital facial anomalies, none has commanded more attention than the cleft palate, and probably none has proved more difficult or baffling from the surgical standpoint." The mental hazards of the unoperated or unsuccessful operated cleft palate are hardly accountable to the normal individual. The deformity should be corrected early in life because of the endless chain of mental and physical sequelae. It is usually thought that an inferiority complex develops from a chain of events begun early in the life of an individual, and especially at the beginning of school age. For this reason, the palate should be corrected before the time of beginning school.

In outlining the treatment of a condition, a definite objective must be established. This is usually the removal of the handicap or handicaps which accompany the deformity. These are stated by the author to be not only mechanical closure of the cleft, but the establishment of a long flexible non-scarred normal functioning soft palate which forms velum hanging from the hard palate. "It is only optimism or ego on the part of the surgeon to feel that satisfactory results have been obtained when merely closure of the cleft has been accomplished."

Further correction of the deformity includes the second operation on the cleft palate and reconstruction of nasal deformity usually accompanying these defects. The chief factor in the correction of the cleft palate is restoration of normal speech.

The etiology of cleft palate and hare lip is discussed, but no new theories are brought forth, and no definite etiology is assigned.

The incidence is reported from one large series of births in which there is one cleft to 100,000 births in white children, and one cleft to 1,,800 births in colored children. The occurrence is relatively higher in boys than in girls.

A relatively simple classification of the type of cleft palate is given. Closure of the cleft by mechanical appliances is discussed and condemned except as a temporary measure to prepare for plastic reconstruction in advanced age, and advanced diseases as cancer, tuberculosis, and syphilis.

Surgical treatment of closure of the lip is best done as soon as the patient's condition permits, possibly within the first three or four weeks of life. The authors believe that the ideal age for the closure of cleft palate is three or four years. A two-stage procedure is given for the closure of the cleft palate with "push-back" operation as part of the procedure. This is for lengthening the soft palate and relaxation of these structures in order to aid in the restoration of normal speech.

The first operation accomplishes establishment of collateral circulation. The second, pushing back of the entire soft tissue of the palate and closure of the cleft. These authors use wiring between the dental arches to hold rubber sponges against the palate for pressure. Following the surgery, special training is always given which is considered a most important part of the procedure. Without this, the authors will not attempt surgery.

"After the palate is reconstructed, the capable surgeon produces a closed palate and a long flexible soft palate in which the muscles are able to function normally after which there is no organic reason why the cleft palate should persist. Surgery which leaves the palate scarred, tight, contracted and too short, does not relieve the mechanical difficulties with consonant formulations and therefore cannot be considered adequate. However, in such cases, speech training will improve the enunciation."

Conclusions: The authors have written an up-to-date opinion on cleft palate. The time of the operation is somewhat later than that practiced in this community.

It is gratifying to note that the authors are not content with a single surgical closure of the palate. It is now clearly understood that a successful outcome of cleft palate surgery includes the following factors. (1) Surgical closure with normal length, flexible tissue, and adequate palato-pharyngeal closure. (2) Adequate speech training. (3) Removal of mental handicap and tendency to development of inferiority complex.

ORTHOPAEDIC SURGERY
Edited by Earl D. McBride, M.D., F.A.C.S.
717 North Robinson Street, Oklahoma City

Cysts of the Semilunar Cartilage. George E. Bennett. American Journal of Surgery, XLIII, 512, February, 1939.

Cysts of the semilunar cartilage are comparatively rare. Authors agree on symptomatology, signs and treatment, but disagree on etiology. A limp or limitation of motion is seldom present, but easy fatigue of the involved leg is frequent. Cysts, themselves, are not responsible for relaxation of the ligaments of the knee. On examination, it is not common to find an increase in synovial fluid, atrophy of the thigh and calf, or flexion deformities. Diagnosis is not difficult as a rule. Differentiation from a bursa arising from the medial and lateral ligaments and true synovial outpouchings is the most common problem.

The author gives various theories concerning the etiology, including trauma, local changes in cell metabolism, and congenital causes. Treatment consists in complete removal of the cartilage with the cyst. Simple removal of the cyst is often followed by recurrence. The cysts are usually found to be multilocular. No signs of active inflammation are reported in the cysts. Dr. Bennett believes that the cyst arises in a traumatized area in the capsular border of the cartilage, which undergoes mucoid degeneration and cyst formation.

Acute Hematogenous Bursitis. Morris B. Cooperman. Annals of Surgery, CVIII, 1094, 1938.

Acute bursal infections of hematogenous origin are rare complications of acute infectious diseases or septicaemias, or are metastatic lesions secondary to infections in other parts of the body. They must be differentiated from acute infectious arthritis or acute osteomyelitis. Needling is an important diagnostic measure. One must have thorough knowledge of the anatomical location of the various bursae. Gluteal bursitis is most difficult to diagnose. The treatment is incision and drainage when fluctuation is present. The author reports six cases, four involving the subacromial bursa and two involving the prepatellar and gluteal bursae.

Chromicized Beef Tendon for Internal Fixation of Fractures. Frank P. Strickler. Annals of Surgery, CVIII, 1102, 1938.

The author describes the use of chromicized beef

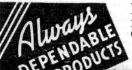

tendon prepared in plates, cuffs, and pegs for internal fixation in fractures. It is claimed to have the following advantages: it can be made absolutely sterile; it is easy to work with; it does not show on a roentgenogram; it will remain in position 60 to 90 days; if properly introduced, it has sufficient strength to maintain reduction of the fracture; and it is absorbed in about 90 days. Ten cases in which this material was used are reported.

Spatergebnisse Von Sehnennahten an Arm und Hand (Late Results of Tendon Suture in the Arm and Hand). Fritz Heck. Archiv Fur Orthopadische und UnfallChirurgie, XXXIX, 21, 1938.

On the basis of 75 cases of tendon suture in the arm and hand (59 primary and 16 delayed) and a review of the literature, the writer recommends primary suture where at all possible, except in cases of badly mangled flexor tendons. In the case of the extensor tendons, there was little difference between the results obtained by immediate suture and those following delayed suture. In the flexor tendons, the results were poorer with the delayed suture.

Die Bruche Des Korpernahen Oberarmendes (Fractures of the Proximal End of the Humerus). Franz Scheider. Archiv fur Orthopadishe und Unfall-Chirurgie, XXXIX, 29, 1938.

One hundred and twenty-five cases of fracture of the proximal end of the humerus are analyzed and tabulated, and the etiology and treatment are discussed at considerable length. These fractures are more frequent in older individuals, and two-thirds of them are extracapsular. They show typical displacements. Reduction is preferably accomplished under local anaesthesia with the patient in the sitting position. The subjects arms are clasped behind the back of the operator, who grasps them just below the shoulders. The fracture is held by an assistant, and the fracture is reduced by rotation of the operator's body. Fixation by an abduction plaster is preferred. In simple cases a splint is used. Open reduction is rarely indicated, and then only with nerve injuries or fracture dislocations which cannot be r e d u c e d by closed methods. Residual disability is rare and is usually caused by capsular changes rather than by malposition.

---o---

CARDIOLOGY
Edited by F. Redding Hood, M.D.
1200 N. Walker St., Oklahoma City

A Comprehensive Approach to the Diagnosis of Diseases of the Heart. Fredrick A. Willius. Medical Clinics of North America, July, 1939.

In this practical and common sense discussion, Dr. Willius warns against the dangers of over-mechanization of diagnosis and hopes that the time tested methods of physical diagnosis will remain a cardinal means of approach, yet weighing facts and contradictions, and arriving at a logical conclusion from the accumulation of unmistakable evidence from all possible sources.

The diagnostician must be equipped with a well founded knowledge of pathology and a practical understanding of the physiology of the cardiovascular system in order that he may be able to interpret and evaluate the varying expressions of disturbed functions.

He discusses the subject according to the time honored system and some of the points discussed are here outlined:

History: The age of the patient immediately narrows the scope of possibilities. The first ten years of life; rheumatic carditis and congenital heart disease predominate; 20 to 40 years, overwhelmingly rheumatic carditis; while cardio-vascular syphilis is encountered but the other forms of heart disease are infrequent; 40 to 60 years is the age group of coronary and hypertensive heart disease. It is in this age group that cardio-vascular syphilis most frequently manifests itself. Rheumatic heart disease is still encountered but congenital heart disease rarely. During the 60 to 80 age period, coronary and hypertensive heart disease hold sway.

Sex: Coronary and cardio-vascular diseases occur predominantly in the male, while rheumatic and hypertensive heart disease afflict the two sexes more nearly equal.

Family History: The degenerative cardia-vascular diseases are in a measure influenced by heredity. A family history of coronary disease or hypertension may arouse suspicion as to the condition of the patient.

Past Illnesses: Past rheumatic bouts or previous chancre are only two of the many examples which aid in the final conclusion.

Elicitation of Symptoms: No better example could be given than that of angina pectoris where the history of retrosternal pain or oppression of short duration, precipitated by accustomed effort and promptly relieved by rest, makes the diagnosis when all other sources of information fail.

Physical Examination: The sense of observation will reveal many valuable facts such as cyanosis, its intensity, and distribution. Cyanotic flushing of the malar eminences at once s u g g e s t s the presence of mitral stenosis. Central pallor of the face, intensified by cyanosis of adjacent areas and of the lips, suggests the possibility of aortic disease. Marked diffuse cyanosis, intensified by moderate exertion, would suggest the probability of congenital cardiac defect. Cyanosis of the digits with clubbing deformity suggests congenital cardiac defects or the possibility of subacute endocarditis.

The manner of respiration is of great value. The presence of dyspnea alone is important, and the distinction between expiratory and inspiratory effort aids in distinguishing between heart failure and bronchial asthma. Cheyne-Stokes type warns of serious disease. The sighing type of respiration identifies the functional dyspnea of the neurotic individual.

Inspection of the neck may reveal distended and tortuous jugular veins indicating retardation or obstruction of the venous return, and when associated with distention of the superficial veins of the upper extremities and some degree of cyanosis, indicate increased venous pressure. Irregular pulsation of the carotid arteries frequently permits recognition of premature contractions and auricular fibrillation. Extremely slow pulsations in the carotid arteries with rapid pulse waves in the jugular veins suggests the presence of heart block. Full pulsations of the peripheral arteries with a rapid drop of pulse stroke suggests the existence of aortic regurgitation.

A clearly visible apex beat displaced laterally in the sixth intercostal space is almost certain proof of enlargement of the left ventricle. Likewise, pulsations in the third or fourth inter-costal spaces, near the sternal border, are suggestive evidence of enlargement of the right ventricle. Broadbent's sign (the systolic retraction of the left thoracic wall) is occasionally observed in the presence of adherent pericarditis. Diastolic protrusion of the anterior portion of the thoracic wall frequently offers an early clue as to the presence of aneurysm.

The tactile sense verifies some of the observation already considered. Thrills invariably indicate passage of blood through a narrowed orifice or through a spurious channel, such as may occur in congenital cardiac defects. A presystolic or diastolic thrill at the apex immediately suggests mitral stenosis, while a rough systolic thrill at, or near, the second and third intercostal spaces, to the right of the sternum, is frequently a sign of stenosis of the aortic valve. A prolonged systolic thrill to the left of the lower or middle part of the sternum, would justify suspicion of the existence of a congenital cardiac defect. Palpation may confirm other observation regarding cardiac rhythm.

Although percussion may be considered inaccurate, there are many contingencies in which percussion is of paramount importance in arriving at an intelligent opinion as to heart size, when roentgenologic examination is not available. Determination of the heart size is many times a crucial point in distinguishing the diseased from the normal heart. An enlarged heart is a diseased heart.

An accentuated pulmonic second sound is normal in the infant or child but absolutely abnormal in the adult and the results from the forceful closure of the pulmonic valve due to increased pressure in the pulmonary circulation such as occurred in atherosclerosis of the pulmonary arterioles. In the mitral stenosis an absent aortic second sound always occurs in association with a systolic murmur. Results when the leaflets of the aortic valve do not move and with the exception of a rare congenital deformity this condition exists only in calcareous stenosis of the aortic valve. The accentuation of the aortic second sound at once suggests the presence of arterial hypertension.

Fluoroscopy is of extreme value in studying cardiac activity, abnormal dilatations and pulsations, would also permit recognition and localization of deposits of calcium.

Heart size may be determined. The normal heart being in its maximal transverse diameter less than 50 per cent of the transverse internal diameter of the thorax. Exceptions to this rule are that in the massively built, stocky, short-necked individual a relatively high diaphragm is the rule, reducing the vertical diameter of the thorax and displacing the heart upward giving an appearance of cardiac enlargement. In obese individuals the heart is actually larger than in a thin person or one of normal weight.

Although roentgenographic methods are of great importance and value they have their limitations and unless these restrictions are appreciated may lead to serious error.

Electrocardiography has advanced the accuracy of cardiac diagnosis. However, this method does not contain the answers to all questions. (This is merely another laboratory method as an aid to clinical diagnosis and should be interpreted as such). It is helpful in the diagnosis of myocardial infarction, in the identification of arrhythmia, and may produce a picture suggestive of disturbances of physiology as occur in hypertensive heart disease, mitral stenosis, congenital heart disease, etc., but caution should be used in interpreting results without clinical information. We must remember too that we may have serious heart disease such as angina pectoris without any positive findings by physical examination or from the laboratory. Dr. Willius concludes that the advantages of all methods must be utilized at all times in respective limitation under v a r y i n g conditions and their changing order of importance from case to case must be recognized. He emphasizes the necessity in stressing the value of the art and science of physical diagnosis in an era that is inclined to depend on mechanical devices.

INTERNAL MEDICINE
Edited by Hugh Jeter, M.D., 1200 North Walker, Oklahoma City

Advantages of Prozinsulin (Protamine Zinc Insulin) Therapy: Dietary Suggestions and Notes on the Management of Cases. By Herbert Pollack and Henry Dolger, New York, N. Y.

This appears to be a very practical report and is summarized in a very brief and clear manner by the authors as follows:

With proper dietary control, prozinsulin offers definite advantages for the routine case of diabetic patients. These advantages can be stated briefly as follows:

1. The single injection daily for patients.

2. Complete elimination of transient ketonuria.

3. Closer approximation to the normal carbohydrate metabolism.

4. Decrease in the incidence of hypoglycemic episodes.

5. Valuable as a supplementary agent in coma therapy.

6. Improvement in post-operative control of diabetic patients.

7. Obviates the absolute necessity of multifeeding schedules, yet permits optional midnight "snacks."

The essentials of the suggested dietary regimes are as follows:

1. The use of small breakfasts.

2. Division of carbohydrate into 1/5, 2/5, 2/5 for the respective morning, midday and evening meals.

3. Distribution of protein to allow for over one-half of the daily allowance at the evening meal.

4. Increased time interval between meals with particular reference to late suppers.

5. Elimination from the diet of rapidly available carbohydrate.

6. Specific use of fats in d e l a y i n g gastric-emptying time, such as cream with banana.

The majority of patients respond well, and are controlled with greater ease on such a regime. Frequent observation and meticulous attention to details of diet will be rewarded by better control of even the most unstable cases. The use of supplementary doses of old insulin can be almost completely avoided.

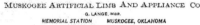

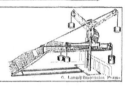

The Value of the Weltmann Serum Coagulation Reaction as a Laboratory Diagnostic Aid; Comparison with the Sedimentation Rate. By S. A. Levinson, M.D., F.A.C.P., and R. I. Klein, M.D., Chicago, Illinois.

The authors report a test which is apparently being used with the hopes of distinguishing between "exudative and fibrotic processes and to some extent parenchymal liver damage."

The test is simple and performed by addition of serum diluted 50 times with distilled water, added in graduated amounts to a solution of calcium chloride and boiled for 15 minutes. Coagulation of serum is thus determined.

In pathological conditions the coagulation band may be normal, shortened or lengthened. In inflammatory and exudative processes coagulation is shortened and the band is said to have shifted to the left, whereas in fibrotic processes and those conditions associated with parenchymal damage of the liver, a shift to the right or lengthening of the coagulation band is obtained. The authors have studied the reaction in 2,000 cases of various diseases and show interesting comparison of the reaction with that of the sedimentation rate as a diagnostic aid. The reports on the various types of diseases indicate that the test is a very helpful link in the chain of diagnosis.

Weltmann, who originated the disease, made his report in non-English foreign literature and consequently most of the publications which have followed have been foreign.

Comment: Our experience with the test is extremely limited, but it is a simple test and seems likely to prove just as satisfactory, if not more satisfactory and helpful, than the sedimentation rate.

UROLOGY

Edited by D. W. Branham, M.D.

514 Medical Arts Building, Oklahoma City

Gonorrhea in the Female: A Study of 3,838 Cases with Special Reference to Electrosurgical Treatment of Gonorrheal Endocervicitis. Samuel Goldblatt, M.D., M.S., Venereal Disease Consultant to the Cincinnati Health Department. Venereal Disease Information, Vol. 20, No. 6, June, 1939.

Summary: In this study 3,838 consecutive cases of gonorrheal endocervicitis were treated by various methods. This treatment was carried out from 1928 to 1937 in the Quarantine Hospital of the Cincinnati area, where observation was continuous and where such complicating factors as re-exposure, alcohol, and sexual activity were completely ruled out. An additional 149 cases from Shoemaker Clinic were ambulatory patients. The study may be summed up in the following manner:

1. The various types of diagnostic methods in accepted usage are found to be inadequate for dismissing a patient as not infected unless there is continuous repetition of these examinations.

2. The endocervix apparently is the primary site of infection.

3. Analyses of the occurrence of other venereal diseases complicating gonorrhea, and the frequency of genito-urinary lesions in gonorrhea, are presented.

4. Various antiseptic medications, such as topical applications and douches, do not give satisfactory results.

5. Simple bed rest, extending for as long as 15 weeks, is totally ineffective as a method of cure.

6. The hypodermic injection of autogenous vaccines into the submucosa of the cervix, tried in a comparatively small number of cases, has little value.

7. Neutral acriflavine, used intravenously, while producing some prompt results, has serious disadvantages.

8. The fertility rate of females with gonorrhea is included, because it seems to contradict the accepted idea of "one-child sterility." Abortions, though frequent, are practically always self-induced.

9. Electrosurgery is found to be the most successful method of obtaining prompt cures, without serious complications even when used in cases of gonorrhea where any stage of pregnancy is involved. The technic is performed as follows:

A ball electrode is fitted in the os rather snugly, the current from a high frequency endothermy apparatus turned on and with varying degree of pressure the ball is rotated and very slowly withdrawn. Care must be exercised to produce a wide base at the external os or atresia of the canal may result. Following the operation a slough separates after 10 days leaving a very vascular granulating area. In most cases the infected cervix is reduced in size with a marked lessening of the discharge within a very short length of time.

THE JOURNAL

OF THE

OKLAHOMA STATE MEDICAL ASSOCIATION

| VOLUME XXXII | McALESTER, OKLAHOMA, SEPTEMBER, 1939 | Number 9 |

Experiences with Internal Fixation in Fractures of the Hip*

C. R. ROUNTREE, M.D., F.A.C.S.
Assistant Professor of Orthopedic Surgery,
Oklahoma University School of Medicine
OKLAHOMA CITY, OKLAHOMA

Fractures about the hip may be divided into two groups: those which occur through the neck proper and situated within the joint, the so-called intracapsular type; and those which occur through the region of the trochanter, the so-called intertrochanteric fractures. The latter are prone to unite without difficulty regardless of the treatment used, but often result in shortening and deformity, due to loss of the normal angle between the neck and shaft.

Fractures of the neck of the f e m u r proper, present an entirely different problem. It is well known that they unite slowly, and frequently not at all. No other major fracture shows such a high percentage of non-union. The mortality rate is also quite high due to the advanced age and physical infirmities of this class of patients.

These cases have received more consideration in the past six years than at any time since Royal Whitman introduced his classical method of reduction plus abduction cast treatment. This was about 30 years ago. He was the first to prove that closed reduction could be accomplished and also that union could be obtained. Because his teachings were based upon sound anatomical and physiological principles, his method was widely accepted and for a time surpassed any other means used to solve this problem.

As carefully prepared statistics began to accumulate, it became increasingly more apparent that the percentage of union with this treatment is not nearly as high as we once believed. It is now generally recognized that with the best of treatment, including carefully planned and well executed follow-up management, that union is attained in only 60 to 65 per cent of cases where external fixation alone is depended upon.

Three basic requirements are necessary for the healing of any fracture:

1. Sufficient circulation to t h e fragments.

2. Adequate reduction.

3. Proper immobilization.

Much has been said about the inadequacy of the circulation to the head and neck of the femur.

Through the investigation of Wolcott[12], C h a n d l e r and Kreuscher[2], and many others, the circulation of the hip has been clearly worked out. In brief, it may be said that the chief blood supply comes from three sources.

First, branches of the nutrient artery which continue upward from the shaft into the neck, supplying the head and neck with fair-sized vessels.

Second, the capsular arteries which penetrate the capsule of the joint and enter the neck chiefly through the foramina situated

---

*Read at Annual Meeting Oklahoma State Medical Association, May 2, 1939.

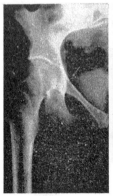

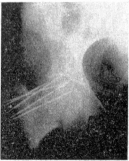

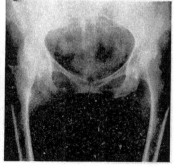

FIG. 1-B

After reduction and fixation
with Kirschner wires. One wire,
across joint into the pelvis, was
removed.

FIG. 1-A

Mrs. B. W., Age 58.
Fracture of right femur
before reduction.

FIG. 1-C

Solid union
19 months after operation.

on the posterior superior surface. The inspection of any dried specimen will clearly show their presence. They furnish an adequate supply and are constantly present.

Three, vessels contained in the ligamentum teres and entering the head through this medium. These are variable in size and are not constantly present, but undoubtedly provide more or less blood supply. The study of injected specimens by means of the roentgenograms show an anastamosis between these vessels and those entering from the capsule. Thus, under ordinary conditions, it is safe to assume that there is an abundant blood supply to the head and neck of the femur. It may be stated, therefore, that poor circulation is not a primary factor in failure to secure union.

In fractures of long bones generally, any degree of apposition, so long as the fragments touch, is sufficient for union. This is not true in fractures of the neck of the femur. The periosteum of the femoral neck is considered to be deficient or absent entirely. Callus formation is of the endosteal rather than periosteal variety. It is well known that this type of union occurs only where there is accurate reduction and replacement of the fragments. Thus, it follows that accurate reduction of the fracture is necessary before union can be reasonably expected to occur.

The question naturally arises—Is there any method whereby the fracture can be accurately reduced? The answer is in the affirmative. Surgeons who have opened the joint immediately following the reduction as practiced by Whitman, or who have carried out his technique following exposure of the fragments, have verified the fact that complete apposition of the fragments practically always takes place. Gaenslen[5], in an experimental study producing fractures of the neck, in dissecting room specimens found not infrequently a portion of the joint capsule interposed between the fragments, a condition which probably occurs more often than we realize and serves to inhibit union. Similar findings have been reported in the living subject by Cubbins[3] and his co-workers. Gaenslen stated that traction and extension (Whitman) failed to release the capsule, but release was invariably accomplished by traction, plus flexion of the hip to 90 degrees. This is the principle of the Leadbetter[6] technique. It is the author's conviction, based upon clinical observation, that too much emphasis cannot be placed on securing accurate and complete reduction. We routinely use the Leadbetter method because we feel that it embodies the Whitman principles and has the additional advantage of releasing the capsule in cases where interposition is present.

The third requirement, proper immobilization, is also one of paramount importance. Experience with the impacted type teaches us that u n i o n promptly occurs. This is due to the absence of displacement of the fragments, and, therefore, a minimum damage to the blood supply. Neither is there opportunity for inclusion of the capsule. The entanglement of the fragments provides complete fixation and this makes for uninterrupted healing. In the average case, displacement rather than impaction is the rule. Granting proper reduction, it is my belief that success or failure very often depends upon how efficiently the case is immobilized. It is almost impossible to attain this end by means of a plaster cast. No external dressing can be applied firmly enough to prevent some m o t i o n at the fracture. Most patients, especially those who tend to be obese, lose weight rapidly in a cast. In a short time it becomes so loose that the patient can turn and move about w i t h considerable freedom. Thus, the mechanical e f f e c - t i v e n e s s of the appliance is l o s t. Movements of t h e body, together with muscle p u l l about the hip, p r o d u c e m i n u t e displacements and stresses of a shearing character w h i c h unquestionably retard callus formation. Clinical observation and study of the cases contained in this report, convince me that too much consideration cannot be paid to this factor.

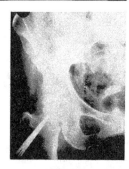

FIG. 2-B
After reduction. Fixation with Kirschner wires.

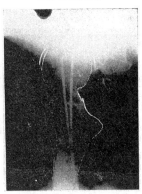

FIG. 2-A
Mrs. L. C. F., Age 76.
Before reduction.

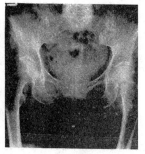

FIG. 2-C
Lateral view showing wires in neck of femur.

FIG. 2-D
Solid union. Excellent function.
Thirteen months post-operative.

Thus it is s e e n t h a t whereas suitable methods of reduction have b e e n devised, p e r h a p s failure to o b t a i n healing in a higher percentage of cases can be attributed to inadequate fixation of the fracture until union can occur.

In 1931, S m i t h- Peterson[9] of Boston r e v i v e d the procedure of internal fixation, a principle w h i c h has b e e n k n o w n for many years. Apparently, Von Langenbeck[11] in 1850 was the first to use transfixation of this fracture. The operation was not successful because the patient died. It is not within the scope of this paper to review the literature. A list of references is appended for those interested. Suffice it to say that the method was practiced with more or less indifferent results until recent years.

All sorts of wires, screws, nails, etc., were employed by the e a r l i e r investigators. Smith-Peterson suggested the use of an ingenious three flanged nail which he devised to hold the fragments securely together. At first, he advocated wide exposure of the joint, accurate reduction of the fracture under direct vision, followed by nailing. In r e c e n t years[10], he has changed his views and now believes that the operation can be successfully d o n e without opening the joint. His work was given an added impetus by the work of Leonard and George[7] who introduced a technique for obtaining lateral X-ray views of the hip. Although their original technique has been·replaced by that of Ferguson and Liebolt[4], due credit must be given Leonard and George for first c l e a r l y demonstrating that lateral views of the hip are possible. Without them, I do not b e l i e v e the operation could enjoy its present success. By m e a n s of anterior-

posterior and lateral roentgenograms, an absolute check is possible on the accuracy of reduction and serves as a guide to correct placement of internal fixation appliances.

Those who favor internal fixation belong to two schools: (1) Closed internal fixation, using screws, pins, bolts, three flanged nail, or Kirschner wires; (2) open internal fixation, using similar devices except that they are introduced after opening the joint and reducing the fracture.

The voluminous literature w h i c h has grown up in relation to this subject has been excellently reviewed by Callahan[1] in a recent article.

My experience is limited almost entirely to the first method. In only one case was open reduction resorted to. The case was a boy aged 13 years who sustained a severe fracture at the base of the femoral neck and, in addition, a complete avulsion of the greater trochanter. Attempts. at closed reduction by means of traction and manipulation failed. Open reduction was resorted to, using Kirschner wires to fix the fragments. An excellent result was obtained.

When this method was first adopted, we used Kirschner wires. Since then, I have tried Moore pins and the Smith-Peterson nail. The results in connection with each

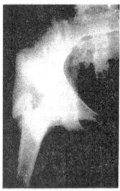
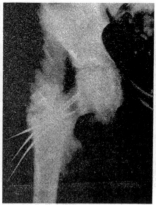
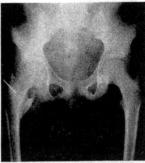

FIG. 3-A

L. B. Boy, age 13.
Before reduction.

FIG. 3-B
After reduction.

FIG. 3-C
Final result.
Solid union. Excellent function.

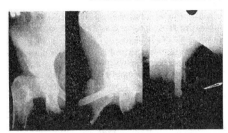

FIG. 4-A
Mrs. M. H. Age 60.
Fracture of neck of the right femur before reduction; and after reduction, showing fixation with Smith-Peterson nail.

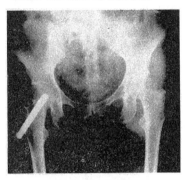

FIG. 4-B
Fracture eight months after operation. Excellent function. Apparently solid union. No pain or disability.

method are given in charts accompanying this paper. Which is the better type of fixation appliance has as yet not been definitely determined. In my opinion, it makes no difference whether one large nail or several smaller ones are used. The aggregate amount of metal is probably about the same in either case.

OPERATION

The technique we employ follows generally that described by Moore[8] and by Smith-Peterson[10]. Although the operation can be successfully performed under local anaesthetic, I prefer either gas (cyclopropane) or spinal anaesthesia. When properly administered, they are well tolerated and relatively safe. We have had no deaths which could be attributed to their use.

The patient is placed on an ordinary operating table, with the hips centered over a "cassette tunnel." This is a shallow box constructed of material not impervious to passage of X-rays. It is open at each end. By this means, the X-ray cassette can be placed under the affected hip from the opposite side of the table without disturbing the sterile draping.

The fracture is now reduced and roentgenograms of both the anterior-posterior and lateral views are taken to check the reduction. While the patient is being prepared and draped, the films are developed. Any adjustment of the fracture can be easily made without disturbing the patient or breaking the aseptic technique.

An incision is made from a point opposite the trochanter and extends down the lateral aspect of the thigh, parallel with the shaft of the femur, for about five or six inches. The attachment of the vastus externus muscle is identified. The femur is e x p o s e d subperiostally for about three inches below this point by separating the fibers of this muscle. An assistant holds the extremity in extension and about 25 degrees abduction, with 20 degrees of internal rotation. In this position, the neck of the femur is approximately parallel to the surface of the table. The central axis of the neck is l o c a t e d at a point about three-quarters of an inch below the superior attachment of the vastus externus muscle and at an angle of about 45 degrees with the lateral aspect of the shaft.

From here on, the technique varies with the type of fixation appliance used. If Kirschner w i r e s or pins are employed, they are drilled upward into the neck and head, using this point as the center of a small circle, care being taken to see that they are so placed as to be confined within the circumference of the neck and do not enter the acetabulum. Should this occur, they must be withdrawn so that the point of the pin, while engaging the compact bone of the head, does not enter the joint. Failure to observe this precaution results in post-operative pain and traumatic arthritis which may be a very serious complication. After one or two are placed, I always check with anterior-posterior and lateral roentgenograms to see that they are in proper position and do not enter the joint. It is desirable that they cross with-

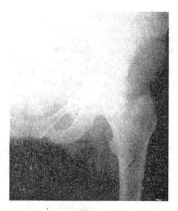

FIG. 5-A
Mrs. K. A. Age 61.
Fracture of neck of left femur before reduction.

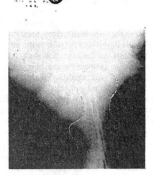

FIG. 5-B
Lateral view after reduction.
Moore nails maintaining position.

thus produced may assist in revascularizing the fracture.

Before the operation is completed, roentgenograms should be made in both planes to insure that proper reduction and nailing has been accomplished. The ends of the pins or wires are cut off close to the bone. The incision is closed in the usual manner and sterile dressing applied.

Many mechanical aids to d i r e c t the course and depth of the pin, wire, or nail, have been developed, but I have not found their use necessary. By a careful study of the X-ray, one can estimate fairly accurately the direction the appliance should take and its length. Although the impor-

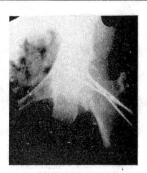

FIG. 5-C
AP view following nailing with Moore nails.

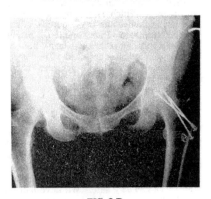

FIG. 5-D

One year after operation. Union of fracture with normal function of hip.

in the substance of the neck so as to fix the fragments more securely. As a rule, three or four are sufficient for fixation.

When the Smith-Peterson nail is used, a heavy guide wire is drilled in and its position verified. If satisfactory, the nail, which has a hole down the c e n t e r, is threaded over the wire and inserted. The purpose of the guide wire is to direct the nail in the proper course. Should the pins or wires go astray, no difficulty is experienced in reinserting them in the proper direction. The additional drill channels tance of impaction following nailing, has been stressed, I have not used it routinely.

In some of the earlier cases, we used external fixation in the form of traction or a Thomas splint, but at the present time we feel that no external fixation is necessary except a boot cast with a cross bar at the ankle which is built up on the outer side to prevent external rotation of the leg.

The post-operative management is directed toward keeping the patient comfortable and happy. We believe that in spite of the stability of the fracture following proper internal fixation, too much liberty should not be taken with it. Patient is kept in bed or a wheel chair for three months, after which crutches are permitted, but full weight-bearing is never encouraged or recommended under six months. We prefer not to remove the nails or pins under one year. As a matter of fact, they may remain in situ indefinitely if they cause no trouble.

In the early cases we used Kirschner wires, but soon found that these were unsuitable because of the tendency to loosen up and back out under the skin, causing pain and requiring early removal. Then, too, the heaviest Kirschner wire does not seem to be large enough to firmly fix the fragments.

Although a number of good results accrued from this method, it was soon discarded in favor of the Moore pins. Experience with this was, on the whole, satisfactory; but, for some reason, it seemed more difficult to properly introduce these pins than the Kirschner wires. They have the advantage, however, of not backing out, and I believe the mechanical principle to be sound. In no case where wire or pin was used, have we ever noted any tendency to migration into the pelvis, a complication which has been reported.

Recently, we have been using the Smith-Peterson nail. So far, the results have been satisfactory. It is my opinion that this is a much easier operation, especially when a guide wire is used to direct the course of the nail. Apparently, the fragments are thoroughly immobilized and there are no untoward effects from the presence of such a large piece of metal.

It has been stated that nailing of a fractured hip can be accomplished in a short space of time. In my experience, this is not true. The necessary steps are time consuming and must be controlled with frequent X-ray examinations during each step in order to insure success. While it may seem to be a simple procedure in the hands of experts, it is certainly difficult and complicated for the novice. The operation should not be undertaken except in a well equipped hospital where trained assistants are available and where portable X-ray equipment is at hand.

The advantages of internal fixation over cast treatment are many. The comfort of the patient is a factor of the greatest importance. They are not encumbered with an extensive cast which entails a prolonged stay in the hospital for weeks or months. The customary stiffness of the knee joint, seen following prolonged immobilization in plaster, is lacking. Complications which accompany the sudden withdrawal of activity in the aged, are reduced. The patient has the assurance of freedom of the bed and has the promise of a wheel chair in a short time. I have been impressed with the fact that these patients have practically no pain following operation and are able to move the extremity around with remarkable ease. Finally, this method is much less expensive. Not infrequently, the patient is able to leave the hospital within a week. He does not require the expert nursing care which is so essential to the cast treatment.

RESULTS

No case is reported as a result, in this paper, earlier than six months following operation.

An analysis of results shows that out of 21 cases, 16, or 76.16 per cent, obtained solid union. There were two deaths before union could occur, or 9.52 per cent. One patient died 12 days following operation, from uremia. The second death occurred in a 93-year-old woman who developed broncho-pneumonia three weeks following operation. There were three non-unions, or 14.28 per cent. In two of these cases, the fracture was not nailed until four and six weeks, respectively, following injury. In the third patient, failure to obtain accurate reduction probably accounted for the poor result.

There were three cases of impacted

CHART NO. 1 — KIRSCHNER WIRE

NAME	AGE	DATE INJURY	DATE TREATMENT	X-RAY	ANAES.	TREATMENT	EXTERNAL FIXATION	UNION	RESULT
Mrs. M. C.	75	2-22-35	2-23-35	Fracture neck (rt.), displaced	Ether	Reduction 4 Kirschner wires	Single spica cast 4 wks.	Yes	Solid union. No shortening. Normal motion in hip. Excellent functioning.
Mrs. M. M.	83	4-18-35	5-5-35	Trans. cerv. (lt.) displaced	Spinal	Reduction 4 Kirschner wires	Single spica 8 wks.	Yes	Solid union. No shortening. Normal motion. Excellent result.
Mr. J. N.	47	7-11-35	8-25-35	Trans. cerv. (lt.) displaced	Spinal	Reduction 2 Kirschner wires	Long leg casts with bar between	No	Painful hip. Fibrous union. Poor result.
L.B.	13	11-9-35	11-19-35	Fractured neck and greater trochanter, displaced, (rt.)	Ether	Closed traction & manip. Unsuccessful. Open reduc. 3 Kirschner wires	Plaster spica 9 wks.	Yes	Solid union. Excellent function. No shortening.
Mr. W. A. B.	76	12-26-35	12-30-35	Trans. cerv. (lt.) displaced	Gas	Reduction nailing— 4 Kirschner wires	None	Yes	Solid union. Perfect functional result. No shortening.
Mr. B. S.	46	2-7-36	2-9-36	Gunshot frac. (lt.) displaced	Ether	Reduc. & nailing. 4 Kirschner wires. Bullet not removed	Thomas splint 4 wks.	Yes	Sequestration of head. Painful hip. Union of fracture. Poor result.
Mrs. B. W.	58	11-14-36	11-16-36	Trans. cerv. (lt.) displaced	Gas	Reduction, 5 Kirschner wires	None	Yes	Solid union. Normal motion. No pain. Excellent result.
Mrs. Y.	58	3-3-37	3-5-37	Sub-capital displaced, (rt.)	Spinal	Reduction nailing 4 Kirschner wires	Buck's extension 4 wks.	Yes	Solid union. Limitation of motion due to healing with angulation of neck. Limp. No pain.

CHART NO. 2 — MOORE PINS

NAME	AGE	DATE INJURY	DATE TREATMENT	X-RAY	ANAES.	TREATMENT	EXTERNAL FIXATION	UNION	RESULT
Mrs. A. F.	90	4-18-37	4-19-37	Trans-cervical, displaced, (rt.)	Local 2% Nov.	Reduction 4 Moore pins	None	Yes	Hypertensive heart disease. Never walked. Union of frac. Lived 1 year after operation.
Mrs. F. R.	47	4-21-37	5-5-37	Frac. base of neck, (lt.)	Gas	Reduction, nailing 3 Moore pins	None	Yes	Developed infec. with painful hip and resultant ankylosis in spite of union of frac. Poor result.
Mrs. S.	72	8-7-37	9-4-37	Comminuted frac., displaced, (rt.)	Gas	Reduction, nailing 4 Moore pins	None	No	Non-union. Painful hip.
Miss J. O. L.	93	10-14-37	10-15-37	Trans-cervical, displaced, (lt.)	Local 2% Nov.	Reduction, nailing 4 Moore pins	None	Died before union	Death 3 wks. later. Broncho-pneumonia. Frac. holding. Pt. up in wheel chair
Mr. J. E. McK.	75	10-21-37	10-22-37	Oblique neck, (lt.)	Gas	Reduction, nailing 4 Moore pins	Buck's extension	Died before union	Death 12 days after operation. from uremia and pneumonia.
Mr. M. J. G.	84	5-8-38	5-8-38	Oblique neck (lt.) displaced	Spinal	Reduction 5 Moore pins	None	Yes	Union of fracture, but pt refuses to walk because of old age.
Mrs. E. McM.	74	4-8-38	4-9-38	Trans-cerv. comminuted displaced (rt.)	Gas	Reduction, impacted 3 Moore pins	Short leg cast	No	Non-union. Painful hip. Shortening.
Mrs. L. C. F.	76	2-21-37	2-21-37	Trans-cerv. displaced, (rt.)	Spinal	Reduction 4 Moore pins	None	Yes	Solid union. Perfect function 13 months after operation.

UNIMPACTED FRACTURES TREATED WITH SMITH-PETERSON NAILS

NAME	AGE	DATE INJURY	DATE TREATMENT	X-RAY	ANAES.	TREATMENT	EXTERNAL FIXATION	UNION	RESULT
Mrs. A. H.	67	10-4-38	10-4-38	Trans. cervical displaced	Gas	Reduction; Smith-Peterson nail	Short leg cast	Yes	Union and perfect function 8 months after operation.
Mrs. N. B.	72	11-5-38	11-8-38	Trans. cervical; extreme displacement	Gas	Reduction; Smith-Peterson nail	Short leg cast	Yes	Six months after operation, walking—no shortening or disability.

IMPACTED FRACTURES

NAME	AGE	DATE INJURY	DATE TREATMENT	X-RAY	ANAES.	TREATMENT	EXTERNAL FIXATION	UNION	RESULT
Mrs. L. A.	61	7-21-37	8-4-37	Impacted thru neck, (lk.)	Gas	Reduction; 3 Moore pins	None	Yes	Perfect function. No disability.
Mrs. A. McN.	56	5-27-38	5-30-38	Impacted thru neck, (lt.)	Gas	Reduction. Smith-Peterson nail	None	Yes	Perfect function. No disability.
Mrs. K. H.	69	8-29-38	8-31-38	Impacted thru neck, (rt.)	Gas	Reduction. Smith-Peterson nail	None	Yes	Perfect function. No disability.

fractures in this series, which united without any difficulty.

The mere fact that the fracture united, does not tell the whole story. A further analysis of the 16 cases which united reveals an excellent functional result in 13 cases. In three patients, union of the fracture occurred, but the functional result was poor. In one case, post-operative infection developed w h i c h resulted in a painful, arthritic hip. In one patient, a gunshot fracture of the neck of the femur, necrosis of the head occurred in spite of union, resulting in a painful hip. In one patient, a 90-year-old woman, union was obtained and she lived for one year following operation; but, due to her advanced age and poor physical condition, she was never able to walk.

BIBLIOGRAPHY

1. Callahan, James J.: Surg., Gyn. & Obstet., Vol. 68, No. 4, April, 1939, P. 411-18.
2. Chandler, S. B., and Kreuscher, P. H.: "Study of Blood Supply of Ligamentum Teres and Its Relation to Circulation of Head of Femur." Jrn. Bone & Joint Surg. 14:834-46, October, 1932.
3. Cubbins, W. K., and Callahan, J. J., and Scudin, Carlo S.: Surg., Gyn. & Ob., Vol. 68, January, 1939, No. 1, P. 87-94.
4. Ferguson, A. B., and Liebolt, F. L.: Radiology, Vol. 27, No. 6, P. 704-07, December, 1936.
5. Gaenslen, F. J.: "Fracture of the Neck of the Femur." Jrn. A.M.A., Vol. 107, July 11, 1936, p. 105-14.
6. Leadbetter, G. W.: "A Treatment for Fracture of the Neck of the Femur." Jrn. Bone & Joint Surg., Vol. 15, October, 1933.
7. Leonard, R. D., and George, A. W.: Jrn. Roentgenol., 1932.
8. Moore, A. T.: Surg., Gyn. & Obs., Vol. 64, p. 420-36, February, 1937.
9. Smith-Peterson, M. N., and Von Gorder, George W.: "Intra-capsular Fracture of the Neck of the Femur." Arch. Surg. 23:715-59, November, 1931.
10. Smith-Peterson, M. N.: "Treatment of Fracture of the Neck of the Femur by Internal Fixation." Surg., Gyn. & Ob., February 15, 1937, Vol. 64, p. 287-294.
11. Von Langenbeck: Verhandl. d. deutsch. Gesellsch. f. Chir., Seventh Congress 1:92, 1878.
12. Wolcott, W. E.: "Circulation of the Head and Neck of Femur; Its Relation to Non-Union in Fractures of the Femoral Neck." Jrn. A.M.A., 100:27-34, January 7, 1933.

ADDITIONAL REFERENCES

1. Brewster, W. R., and Martin, E. D.: Amer. Jrn. Surg., 1935, 30:420, 482.
2. Carrell, W. B.: South. Med. Jrn., 1935, 28:583.
3. Conwell, H. E., and Sherrill, J. D.: South. Surg., 1937, 6:194.
4. Dickson, F. D.: Jrn. Missouri State Med. Assoc., 1935, 32:481.
5. Gaenslen, F. J.: Jrn. Bone & Joint Surg., 1935, 17:739.
6. Harris, R. I.: Jrn. Bone & Joint Surg., 1938, 20:114.
7. Henderson, M. S.: Annals of Surg., 1931, 93:968.
8. Magnuson, P. B.: Jrn. Amer. Med. Assoc., 1936, 107:1439.
9. Moore, A. T.: Jrn. South Carolina Med. Assoc., October, 1934, Vol. XXX, No. 10.
10. Selig, Seth: Jrn. Bone & Joint Surg., Vol. XXI, No. 1, January, 1939, p. 182-186.
11. Telson, D. R., and Ransohoff, N. S.: Jrn. Bone & Joint Surgery, 1935, 17:727.
12. Thornton, L., and Sandison, C.: Southern Med. Jrn., 1936, 29:456. Amer. College of Surgeons' Meeting in Chicago, 1937.
13. Whitman, R. Blrt: M. J., 1936, 2:167.

The Removal of Non-Magnetic Foreign Bodies From the Vitreous With Report of a Case*

J. J. CAVINESS, M.D.

OKLAHOMA CITY, OKLAHOMA

Prior to the discovery of X-rays, attempts were made to remove foreign bodies from the vitreous by various methods. Most of the cases of which we have any record of r e m o v a l were those of magnetic substances.

In 1893 Norris and Oliver[1] reported 100 cases of Hirschbergs, giving a description of the methods of removal; these were all cases of magnetic substances.

In 1896 F. H. Williams[2] of Boston, made the first successful demonstration of intra ocular foreign body by means of the X-ray. Following this incident, there was a great stimulation of interest in the study of such injuries together with an increase in the literature on the subject of the diagnosis and treatment of intra ocular foreign bodies.

Localization of intra ocular f o r e i g n bodies, by means of X-ray, was made possible by Sweet[3] in 1909 and from that time dates the real beginning of our present knowledge of this subject.

Following this discovery many cases of intra vitreous foreign bodies were successfully removed by means of the magnet and extraction; these, however, were all magnetic substances and little was said during this same period, relative to the treatment of the v a r i o u s non-magnetic foreign bodies in the vitreous. The routine treatment in such injuries was the removal of the eye.

As late as 1927, E. C. Ellet[4], in an article in the Trans-American Ophthalmological Society, entitled "Wounds of The Eye By Projectiles of Small Caliber and Low Velocity," with special reference to bird shot, gave a very gloomy report of his opinion on the outcome of such injuries. He stated that such an eye is almost always lost;

that the injuries in which there were retained shot in the vitreous, give even a poorer prognosis than the c a s e s where through and through injuries occurred. He stated that such retained shot almost always caused loss of vision and ultimately loss of the eyeball, as a result of chronic infection.

In 1927 G. H. Cross[5] first made mention of the use of the biplane fluoroscope, as an aid in the removal of a lead shot from the vitreous. He was able by means of this procedure to locate the shot, which was removed by means of a specially designed cross action wire forceps inserted through an incision in the sclera.

He reported another such case[6] in 1929, in which a number eight lead shot was removed from the vitreous, with resulting vision of 20-20. He published other articles in 1930[7], 1930-31[8], and 1935[9], dealing with various phases of the subject, giving case reports and description of technique. He reported a total of 18 cases of non-magnetic foreign bodies of various nature, where removal was effected with the same general procedure, using the b i p l a n e fluoroscope and forceps to suit the particular case.

In 1934[10] and 1936[11] Harvey E. Thorpe reported an ocular endoscope and a new forceps for the removal of lead shot from the vitreous. He did not report any cases.

In 1937 Borley[12] and Leef of San Francisco, reported one case of a 50-year-old man in which a lead shot was removed from the vitreous of the right eye, by means of the biplane fluoroscope and a specially designed cross action wire forceps. The resulting vision was the same as before operation, namely, light perception.

In searching the literature we were unable to find any further case reports of similar cases up to the present time.

*Read before the Section on Eye, Ear, Nose and Throat, Annual Meeting, Oklahoma State Medical Association, Oklahoma City, May 2, 1939.

Foreign b o d i e s in the vitreous, non-magnetic in character, are by no means rare. They may consist of lead shot or other bits of lead, glass fragments, splinters of wood, bits of stone, gun caps and other substances.

Lead particles as well as copper and stone cast a definite shadow and are easily seen in X-ray films. Certain types of glass also cast very definite shadows while other types may not show in the least. The commonest injuries seen by the Ophthalmologist in intra vitreous non-magnetic foreign bodies are produced by lead shot, by particles of copper from gun caps, and by fragments of glass; u s u a l l y the last named is a result of automobile injuries.

While it would be absurd to state that all non-magnetic foreign b o d i e s in the vitreous, could or should be removed, one may state positively that we have made progress in the successful handling of such cases.

Where one finds severe destructive injuries in the globe with a retained foreign body in the vitreous, it would of course be a waste of time and poor judgment to even attempt removal of such foreign body. Where one finds a great loss of the vitreous body, such attempts are unsuccessful even from the standpoint of preservation of the globe. Where preservation of the globe is possible, removal of the foreign body is advisable, even though the vision may be lost.

Discovery of the X - r a y and Sweet's[3] method of localization of foreign bodies in the vitreous, has made the diagnosis and treatment of these injuries more rational. The handling of specific cases has become more nearly standardized. In c e r t a i n types of injuries the results have been gratifying, when one compares the results of present day treatment to t h o s e of a decade or more past.

The type of foreign bodies of non-magnetic nature in the vitreous that give the best chance for removal and preservation of vision and of the globe, are the various kinds of lead shot and other small bits of non-magnetic substances that cast enough shadow to be seen with the fluoroscope. In such cases the use of the biplane flouroscope together with the cross action wire forceps, molded to fit over the individual

foreign body, affords us an excellent chance for successful r e m o v a l of such foreign body. As I have stated before, removal of any foreign body should not be attempted if there has been too much damage to the eye structures.

It is the exception rather than the rule, where the eye does not react rather quickly to the presence of a f o r e i g n body, wherever the location may be. This is especially true of the vitreous, therefore prompt removal should be practiced whenever possible. Many cases are on record where foreign bodies may have remained in the vitreous over long periods without becoming active, but these should be discounted whenever the prognosis is considered.

There is less tendency to accept former opinions, regarding the probable sterility of an object such as a shot, at the time it enters the eye. There seems to be no real foundation for such opinion.

The infectiveness of the foreign body at the time of entrance into the vitreous, together with the chemical make up of such foreign body, influences the degree of irritation and inflammation in each particular injury.

The point of entrance of the foreign body may also influence the particular c a s e. The injuries that involve the so-called danger zone, around the limbus, give a less favorable prognostic outlook.

It is well known that copper fragments are poorly tolerated in the vitreous; this is proved by the many cases showing severe destructive inflammations following such injuries; the element of time in these injuries may have much bearing on the final outcome.

Before attempting the actual removal of these non-magnetic foreign bodies f r o m the vitreous, by m e a n s of the biplane fluoroscope and suitable forceps, there is always necessary a great amount of preliminary work on each case. The first step should be a careful study of the injured eye, the next step s h o u l d be a thorough physical examination, including necessary laboratory data.

One of the most important considerations preoperatively is that of p r a c t i c e with assistants and X-ray operators in order that one may develop the proper team work for the actual operation. This time spent is of vital importance and may mean the difference between success and failure.

By means of a cadaver or a special form for holding eyes, and with a reasonable amount of practice, one may develop some degree of precision in the location and removal of small objects from the vitreous cavity.

The procedure in any given case would necessarily vary and would depend on the type of injury, on the type of foreign body, and on the location of the foreign body in the vitreous. Where the foreign body has been retained over a period of weeks, such object may become enmeshed in adhesions, rendering the removal difficult. These adhesions may hinder one in the attempt to grasp the foreign body; they might offer resistance to the withdrawal after a grasp has been accomplished. Adhesions might actually pull the foreign body out of the grasp of the wire forceps. This happened in the case reported by Borley[12] and Leef and to a certain extent in my own case which will be reported later.

The incision in the conjunctiva should be sufficiently wide as to cause no interference. The scleral incision should be radial to the limbus, its length just sufficient to admit passage of the f o r c e p s with the foreign body enclosed in its grasp. This in the case of a number seven or eight shot, is approximately five millimeters.

The location of the scleral incision, as recommended by Cross[5], is s e v e n millimeters back of the limbus. The reason for this is that in this location there is least likelihood of injury to the lens and Ora Serrata.

Borley[12] and Leef in their case report, suggested and used a barrage of diathermy micro punctures around the proposed site of the scleral incision in order to lessen the danger of retinal detachment. This to the author seems to be a good point in technique and was carried out in my case, although the incision was made farther back from the limbus, because of possible injury to the lens and because of the fact that the foreign body was located far posterior on the nasal side; the incision in the location as used by Cross[5] would have made it extremely difficult to reach the foreign body, and would have interfered with free movements while manipulating the cross action forceps in the act of grasping the foreign body.

This case had in addition, an already existing detachment of the retina, so that the admonition of Cross[5] regarding the d a n g e r of causing detachment did not enter into the picture of this case.

* * * *

CASE REPORT

E. P., white, male, age 14; was admitted to St. Anthony Hospital at 8:30 p.m., September 25, 1938, with a history of having been struck in the face with scattered bird shot from a companion's gun, from a distance approximated at 60 yards. The time of accident was two hours previous to admission to the hospital.

FINDINGS ON ADMISSION

Right Eye. There was a small cut on the center of the lower lid about six millimeters below the lid edge. Beneath this some four millimeters a small hard mass could be felt. There was no evidence of injury to the eyeball.

Left Eye. The lids were kept closed. There was slight blepharospasm, photophobia, and lacrymation. There was no external evidence of injury. The cornea appeared normal except at a point at the limbus at four o'clock. At this location there was a very small wound through the corneo scleral j u n c t i o n and it was thought that a small opening could be seen through the iris b e n e a t h the external wound. There was slight hyphemia. The pupil was contracted and showed a slight irregularity at four o'clock.

X-RAY FINDINGS

There was a small foreign body lodged in the right lower lid. The left eye showed the same type foreign body, located in the posterior part of the vitreous cavity, 18 millimeters behind, 6 millimeters to the nasal side, and 6 millimeters below the center of the cornea.

The patient was hospitalized and was given the usual treatment for such injuries. He was given anti-tetanus vaccine at once, the eye was atropinized, cold compresses were used and he was kept at complete rest in bed.

On the third day in the hospital, the hyphemia had cleared sufficiently to allow

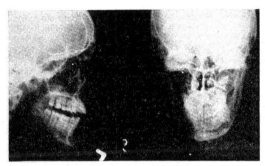

FIG. 1.—Reontgenogram showing anterior and lateral view of the shot in vitreous.

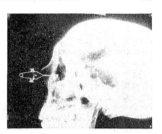

FIG. 3.—Showing shot in grasp of cross action forceps, ready for removal.

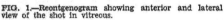

FIG. 2.—Showing localization of the shot in vitreous of left eye.

an examination of the fundus. The pupil still showed a slight irregularity at four o'clock. The fundus could be seen clearly in the upper part, less clearly in the lower and inner quadrant. There was a slight cloudy appearance of the media in this location and there were several s m a l l hemorrhagic areas seen. In the posterior inferior nasal part of the eye and at the location mentioned in the X-ray report, a small glistening object could be seen. This was thought to be the foreign body.

The patient continued to improve. In a few days, the external wound was barely visible and the media had cleared to a great extent. There was no evidence of infection. No attempt was made to determine the exact amount of vision but he was able to recognize small objects, colors, etc. He was discharged from the hospital 10 days after admission and was advised to remain in bed at home.

Two weeks after the injury, a detachment of the retina was noted in the lower half followed in a few days by detachment almost complete.

In the following weeks the media became less clear and vision diminished.

At this time it was decided that removal of the shot, if successful, might prevent removal of the eye. He reentered the hospital on December 12. On December 16, he was given a general anesthetic and the shot was successfully removed. An operating room was set up in the fluoroscopic room, using regular operating room technique.

A large conjunctival incision was made eight millimeters back from the limbus on the nasal side. The medial rectus muscle was s e v e r e d, leaving a good stump; a heavy black silk suture was passed from below and brought out through the upper and lower third of the muscle. The eye was then rotated out, the suture acting as an anchor. The sclera was carefully exposed and dried. At a point 10 millimeters from the limbus and midway vertically, a barrage of diathermy micro punctures was made through the sclera around the proposed site of scleral incision. With a cataract knife, a five millimeter incision was made radial to the limbus; a Cross[5], cross action wire forceps was introduced into the vitreous cavity; the biplane fluoroscope was put into place and the l i g h t s extinguished.

The vertical plane was manipulated by

Dr. J. E. Heatley, while the author used the horizontal plane. The shot could be easily seen; however, attempts to grasp it were difficult; the shot could be seen to move in front of the forceps at each attempt to grasp. It was grasped and slowly brought out to the scleral wound; at this point slight traction could be felt which interfered with easy delivery. No attempt was made to forcibly pull the foreign body through the wound. At this point an iris scissors was used to snip away the tissue between the scleral wound and the end of the wire forceps, thus delivering the shot.

No attempt was made to s u t u r e the scleral wound; the ends of the medial rectus muscle were sutured with the already placed silk suture and this brought out through the conjunctival flaps.

The post operative course was smooth and uneventful; the patient was sent home two weeks after the operation. He was kept in bed for three more weeks.

Examination postoperative, s h o w s a coloboma of the retina at the point of incision; around this point the retina shows points of attachment but elsewhere the retina is detached. The tension is good. There has not been any pain or irritation since soon after the operation. He has good light perception and fair light projection. Examination May 1, 1939. Patient counts fingers at six feet.

REFERENCES

1. Norris, W. F., and Oliver, C. A.: A Textbook of Ophthalmology. Lea Bros. Co., 1893, pp. 296-299.
2. The American Encyclopedia of Ophthalmology. 1917, v. 10, p. 7503.
3. The American Encyclopedia of Ophthalmology. 1917, v. 10, p. 7512.
4. Ellett, E. C. Wounds of the Eye by Projectiles of Small Caliber and Low Velocity. Trans Amer. Opthal. Soc. 1927, v. 25, p. 64.
5. Cross, G. H. Removal of No. 6 Lead Shot from Within the Eyeball by Specially Designed Forceps with the Aid of the Double Plane Fluoroscope. Trans. Amer. Opthal. Soc., 1927, v. 25, p. 80.
6. Cross, G. H. Removal of a No. 8 Lead Shot from the Vitreous with 20-20 Vision in One Case. Trans. Amer. Acad. Opthal. and Otolaryng., 1929, p. 173.
7. Cross, G. H. Removal of Lead Shot from the Vitreous. Amer. Jour. Opthal., 1930, v. 13, p. 41.
8. Cross, G. H. Removal of Non-Magnetic Foreign Bodies from the Vitreous. The Penn. Med. Jour., 1930-31, v. 34, p. 480.
9. Cross, G. H. Intraocular Non-Magnetic Foreign Bodies with Special Reference to Their Removal. Journal Med. Soc. of New Jersey, 1935, v. 32, p. 697.
10. Thorpe, H. E. Ocular Endoscope. Trans. Sec. Opthal. Amer. Med. Assoc., 1934, p. 290.
11. Thorpe, H. E. A New Forceps for the Removal of Lead Shot from the Vitreous. Arch. Opthal., 1936, v. 15, p. 308.
12. Borley, W. E., and Leef, Edward. Removal of Lead Shot from the Vitreous by Use of the Biplane Fluoroscope. Amer. Jour. Opthal., vol. 20, p. 1232.

—————o—————

Practical Management in Peripheral Vascular Disease*

B. E. MULVEY, M.D.
OKLAHOMA CITY, OKLAHOMA

Peripheral vascular disease is a widespread affliction. Interest and study in diseases affecting the peripheral vascular system have disclosed a prevalence which is truly astounding. For one outstanding case with marked morbidity there are perhaps 10 or 15 cases of minor or moderate severity which are missed unless care is taken in following up leading symptoms.

During the last four years at the University Hospital we have followed many

*Read before the Section on General Medicine, Annual Meeting, Oklahoma State Medical Association, Oklahoma City, May, 1939. From the University of Oklahoma Medical School Research No. 1.

of these cases. For the first two years most of the patients seen were those with advanced lesions, usually gangrene, or those with severe crippling pain; these were hospital patients. During the last two years we have been seeing and recognizing patients at an earlier stage, in the dispensary, and many of these remain dispensary patients. We attribute this to a greater current interest and therefore a g r e a t e r knowledge concerning these diseases.

There has been hitherto too great a tendency to classify diseases of the peripheral vascular system under men's names. One advancement has resulted from the desire to arrive at a diagnosis through an understanding of the actual pathology or pathological physiology underlying the subjective and objective symptoms, in this way a more rational therapy can be devised.

Interference in blood supply to a part may result from spasm of blood vessels, occlusion of these canals or a combination of spasm and occlusion. Spasm may exist alone but o c c l u s i o n rarely ever exists alone. Occlusive vascular disorders are more common than those with pure spasm. Most of the patients we see exhibit degenerative blood vessel disease, namely arteriosclerosis, with or without diabetes; therefore from sheer numbers we feel that this group is most important.

When one loses a patient with gangrene of an extremity after amputation he is not greatly impressed, because after all, he reasons, the patient was rather far advanced in years and subject to complications. Another physician has the same experience and perhaps the same feeling. But when these individual experiences are added together as we have done on a series of patients, we find that the mortality is about 60 per cent, a rather shocking percentage. The morbidity in the remaining 40 per cent consists of course, on an average, of loss of at least one-half of an extremity.

This situation at the end stage will probably not be improved upon. Our hope for better results must be in earlier diagnosis; this is quite possible in most instances. In our series of patients we have noted from the histories an average duration of symptoms of four years from onset to gangrene, with a range of a few months to 12 years. In nearly every case there has been ample time for diagnosis.

In talking to a great number of these patients one is impressed with the information that no examination had been made of the extremity until the actual discoloration of early gangrene had occurred. In m a n y instances, enough complaint had been registered to call for treatment of fallen arches, sciatica, n e u r i t i s, etc.; whereas an examination would have disclosed impairment of blood supply as actual cause of symptoms.

In patients with recurring paronychia, leg fatigue, pains and cramps, and above all in those of the older age group who complain of parasthesias of the extremity, a vascular evaluation s h o u l d be undertaken. We have found that parasthesias are more important early; in degenerative blood vessel changes pain is frequently only a late manifestation.

In making this last statement I wish to reemphasize that most of the patients we see are those with arteriosclerotic vascular disease. Pain, cramping and intermittent claudication as early symptoms are more prominent in the younger individual in whom actual inflammation is causing the spasm and occlusion, rather than degeneration.

In general one might say the disease process in the older groups is more arteriolar, whereas the inflammatory lesions of the younger group is not only arteriolar but also involves the larger vessels. It is not at all uncommon to find an arteriosclerotic individual with gangrene of the toes and at the same time nicely pulsating dorsalis pedis and posterior tibial arteries, but not so the young i n d i v i d u a l with thrombo-angiitis obliterans who has gangrene of the toes; no dorsalis pedis or posterior tibial can be found in him; he usually has in addition, a phlebitis.

The parasthesias are in both instances due to ischemia of the peripheral vessels from arteriolar occlusion; the younger man has claudication early because the large vessels are also occluded. Pain overshadows parethesia.

The elderly patient who complains of burning of the feet when these members are actually cold is misinterpreting sensation because of nerve ischemia. He may complain of extreme coldness or tingling for the same reason.

The patient who complains of pain or parasthesias accompanied by color changes, pallor, cyanosis or redness, in one or more extremities, on exposure to a moderate coldness, comfortable to a normal individual, is over reacting; he has spasm of his blood vessels. His diagnosis rests on his story and his contention can be proven by exposing him to cold.

The patient with occlusive vascular disease usually exhibits some very characteristic phenomena. The distal parts of the extremities are usually colder than the proximal p a r t s, the examiner can very easily detect differences of one degree in temperature by palpation, therefore he palpates at various levels and at symmetrical areas on the two limbs. A difference in temperature of similar areas on both limbs is more important than a difference between proximal and distal portions of the same limb. The temperature of an area is directly proportional to the a m o u n t of blood and its speed of circulation in that particular area.

The examiner palpates for the brachial, the radial, the ulnar, femoral, popliteal, dorsalis pedis and posterior tibial, taking note of difference between or absence of pulsation in these vessels. He should not be misled by the presence of pulsation, particularly in the elderly.

The extremity on c a s u a l observation may appear perfectly normal, especially with the patient in a supine position. Careful examination for parasitic infection between the toes, on the soles of the feet and around the nails, should be undertaken. Any unhealthy appearance of the nails should be noted.

After this examination the legs should be elevated at an angle of about 30 degrees and the patient instructed to flex and dorsi flex his feet. If marked pallor, at times a marble appearance, becomes quickly present in one or both feet, we are rather certain that occlusive disease exists, especially if the environmental temperature is warm.

If the feet are then placed in a dependent position in relation to the body and redness or cyanosis accompanied by coldness to palpation is noted we are certain of occlusive vascular disease.

Conservative treatment in most cases, if undertaken early enough, is usually all that is needed. The little things count the most. Warm clothing, and particularly warm covering of the hands and feet, will take care of most cases of pure spasm of moderate severity. A small percentage will, however, be so miserable and over react so greatly that some interruption of the nerve tracts will be necessary. The most successful operations are those done on the sympathetic nervous system, by a neuro-surgeon. These procedures should only be attempted after a careful evaluation of the degree of spasm, and this can only be done in laboratories equipped with instruments designed for this p u r p o s e.

Such examinations should consist of temperature studies by thermocouple devices, in a constant temperature room. A good rise in temperature in an extremity after t e m p o r a r y nerve block or intravenous typhoid injection indicates that operation may be successful.

A patient with pure spasm has potentially a good circulation; if he injures his foot, heat will relax the spasm and a good blood supply results. This is not true of those with degenerative vascular diseases. If a toe is injured or an infection occurs, blood supply is not always ample for healing. The time honored but ill founded treatment for all diseases of the extremity, namely heat plus elevation, adds insult to injury. The former increases metabolism to a greater extent than can be taken care of by the nutrient material at hand, and the elevation adds its burden due to gravity. One can see gangrene speed up under this treatment. The habit many old people have of taking hot irons and electric pads to bed is a dangerous thing. Heavy bed socks are safer and serve the purpose. Rest in the presence of infection accomplishes a great deal.

Simple contrast baths where the limbs are alternately placed in vessels containing hot and cold water respectively, for periods, twice daily, followed by gentle massage and application of cocoa butter improves the circulation and gives a surprising amount of comfort.

Some set of exercises similar to those suggested by Buerger[1] help a great deal. In short these have to do with elevation of the extremities above the plane of the body on pillows or a board for two or three minutes and then placing them in a dependent position for the same length of time. Exercises such as this should be undertaken one or more times daily for 30 minutes at a time.

One of the most satisfactory office treatments is that of giving hypertonic saline intravenously[2], this seems helpful in all cases except those due to pure spasm. It may be given at all ages except where nephritis or heart disease contraindicates the use of sodium chloride. The strength varies from two to five per cent in 200-500 c.c. lots. The younger the p a t i e n t the stronger the solution. It may be given two or three times a week or at longer intervals, depending on the severity of the condition. These solutions are r e a d i l y available from many drug houses as are also the intra venous outfits.

Many vascular accidents are going to occur in spite of treatment, an already narrowed vessel may easily close with a small thrombus and gangrene will result. When such a condition occurs we have two choices, one is to wait weeks and even months for the gangrenous m e m b e r to undergo self amputation or to remove the offending part surgically well above the area of involvement w h e r e circulation seems ample. This usually means at the level of the knee or in the thigh. If only one or two toes are involved it is probably better to permit self amputation, surgical amputation of one or two toes in arterio-sclerotic pheripheral vascular disease, at the area of demarcation, is a mistake. If more than a third of a foot is involved amputation high is the best procedure.

It has been found that histamine inject-ed intradermally in very small amounts will c a u s e dilatation of capillaries and small arterioles in the immediate vicinity of the injection. This dilatation is made manifest by an area of erythema surround-ing the site of injection. If blood supply to this site is impaired due to occlusion the flare will be reduced. We routinely make this test in finding the level for amputa-tion; it is preferable for surgery to be done at the level of a good flare.

CONCLUSIONS

1. The mortality in arteriosclerotic gan-grene of the extremity is quite high in our series.

2. We feel that this mortality cannot be greatly decreased at this time.

3. Earlier diagnosis and simple thera-peutic procedures will benefit many of these individuals and decrease the preva-lence of gangrene.

4. Under the best of available treat-ment these patients are very susceptible to thrombosis and resultant gangrene.

REFERENCES

1. Buerger, L.: The Circulatory Disturbances of the Extremities. W. B. Sanders Co., Philadelphia, 1924.

2. Silbert, S.: The Treatment of Thrombo-angiitis Oblit-erans by Intravenous Injection of Hypertonic Salt Solu-tion. J.A.M.A., 1926-86-1759.

DISCUSSION

Dr. Lea A. Riely: You can see from Dr. Mulvey's paper that medical nosography and practice has a new specialty which may be called angiology. This has to do with the dealing with arteries and veins and capillaries, in their vagaries of anato-mic, physiologic and pathologic evaluation. It has come into notice so rapidly that its literature is voluminous; it runs a con-current and interlocking interest in heart diseases. Peripheral vascular disease also insinuates itself into all the specialties and all the organs and brings within its aegis many diseases that previously did not have any obvious connection with it.

The vasomotor nervous system which has its centers in the medulla and in the spinal cord is distributed chiefly in the arterioles and capillaries, but also the veins and larger arteries. The nervous appa-ratus in the vessel walls regulates the tonus of the vessels. This tonus, together with the force of the heart, maintains the blood pressure. This vasomotor system, including its intrinsic and extrinsic mech-anism, is very sensitive and readily in-fluenced by many factors as hormones, temperature, emotions and sensations, also the activity of the muscles of the internal organs; hence the proper evaluation of these troubles may lead us far afield. It shows that by immersing any one of the extremities, either partially or wholly, in cold water would cause the temperature to fall rapidly in the unimmersed portion. George Brown thought a trigger like re-sponse to cold presaged an essential or malignant hypertension in later years.

With the instruments of precision that we have for the study of these vessels we have found that the classifications are not clean-cut. The arterioscleratic, senile and diabetic group may show an absence of vasospasm and no vasoconstrictor gradient after tests. But the presence of arterio-sclerosis and diabetes does not mean that there is no element of spasm or that that is unimportant.

Again the vasoconstrictor group after anesthesia, general, spinal, or nerve block may show a very definite change of tem-perature. Alcohol is one of the best medi-cinal dialators while cigarets or nicotine is a splendid constrictor. Physiologically this group responds to pure spasm.

Raynaud's d i s e a s e clinically mild is classified in this group, but the arterial spasm in Raynaud's disease is a very complicated type of reaction not caused entirely by sympathetic activity.

The mixed group includes a majority of presenile types of arterial d i s e a s e as thrombo-angiitis obliterans in the stage most often seen. Let me emphasize the fact that not only the arteries but also the veins and capillaries are complicated in the pathological process.

We find that most all of these cases give ample warning of their ultimate devastation so that if they were properly interpreted and treated they may save many a more serious complication later.

We find these complications are precipitated by ill fitting shoes, lack of cleanliness, infection, tobacco, untreated diabetics, trauma, and trimming corns and callouses.

I want to emphasize the harm done to these gangrenous feet with obstructed arteries by applying heat and increasing the

metabolism in a condition when the circulation is much impaired and the gangrene rapidly spreads due to the increased work.

Our equipment for the study of these problems is quite complete, and we see many of these cases in the University Hospital. We are not as enthusiastic as others on the suction and compression machine (Pavex type). We see vast benefit from repeated NaCl2 five per cent s o l u t i o n ranging in amount from 150 c.c. to 300 c.c. even in the aged and the advanced sclerotic types.

Berger's exercises are used in most cases at times, but after any acute complication the rest is imperative. We have a high mortality with amputation so we usually let those with dry gangrene go until a line of demarcation. Histamine flures and the oscillometer guide us in determining the height of amputation, and that is generally at or above the knee.

These cases are always of long duration and a big economic problem in those so afflicted.

———————o———————

Interstitial Radium Treatment of Cancer of the Lower Lip*

L. K. CHONT, M.D.
OKLAHOMA CITY, OKLAHOMA

The clinical material of this study consists of 69 cases treated by radiation alone by the Department of Radiology of the Oklahoma State University Hospital, during the period 1932-1937 inclusive.

The lip cancer is a squamous cell epithelioma at least in 95 per cent but, certain authors believe it is 100 per cent[1-2]. Only a few cases of lip sarcoma are reported. Clinically they so closely resemble the epithelioma that it is impossible to differentiate them w i t h o u t a microscopic examination[3].

All squamous cell epithelioma metasta-

size sooner or later through the regional lymphatics, sometimes in a very e a r l y stage of the primary lesion. Lip cancers metastasize comparatively l a t e but, the exceptions are not rare. Metastasis occur to the submaxillary, sublingual and cervical glands. Remote metastasis are uncommon.

It is generally known that almost 100 per cent of the epitheliomas c o u l d be cured if treated early but, a favorable result requires an-early diagnosis and adequate treatment.

The diagnosis, even in the earliest stage, is usually easy since only a few diseases such as syphilis, tuberculosis, keratosis,

*From the Department of Radiology, University of Oklahoma State Hospital. Chief of Service—William E. Eastland, M.D.

and leukoplakia s h o u l d be eliminated. Every lesion of the lip, lasting more than three weeks, should be suspected of malignancy.

(1). Primary lesions of lues may imitate a cancer strikingly but the rapid development of the ulcer, with early enlargement of the regional lymph nodes and a careful history, shall prevent a diagnostic error. In doubtful cases, a microscopic and dark field examination is indicated.

(2). Gumma has soft, undermined edges and is more common on the upper lip. A Wassermann test of the blood is a routine examination in our tumor clinic.

(3). Tuberculosis of the lip is rare, occurs in childhood and, often accompanied by pulmonary phthisis. The base of the t u b e r c u l o u s ulcer shows soft brown nodules[1].

Keratoses, very often the forerunner of eiptheliomas, r e q u i r e special attention. They are superficial, coarse, scaly lesions which easily undergo malignant degeneration, indicated by intradermal induration and often a thin z o n e of inflammation. Pure keratoses respond readily to moderate doses of X-ray or radium but if they have already undergone malignant changes and become squamous cell epitheliomas, yet are treated with minimal or inadequate dosages of irridiation as if a benign lesion, they become radio-resistant and require surgical removal. Similar unfavorable processes occur in any stage of an epithelioma if radiated with under dosage for fear of roentgen or radium ulcers and other permanent disfiguring sequelae of radio-dermitis. Since a lethal dose of a squamous cell eipthelioma is about five times more than that of a keratosis, an accurate diagnosis is invaluable in the prognosis.

Leukoplakia occurs as an elevated, flat, smooth lesion on the lip and often undergoes malignant degeneration. It may be c u r e d by mild doses of radiation when small in size but tends to recur. No extensive leukoplakia has been cured by radiation, according to reports in medical literature. We p r e f e r electro-coagulation of these lesions.

The epitheliomas of the lip produce two different clinical pictures, (1) the hypertrophic or proliferative and (2) the deeply infiltrating types. The hypertrophic is more frequent and less malignant. It occurs as an elevated, papillary growth projecting out from the vermilion surface of the lip and is, sometimes, very large. We have seen such tumors protruding from the lower lip with a broad base extending five centimeters high.

The deeply infiltrating type as indicated by its name extends downward into the lip producing a deep infiltrating destruction. This type is more malignant and metastasizes early.

The choice of treatment of lip cancers has been discussed many times without definite conclusion and unison of opinion as to treatment. Our purpose is to add our experience, m e t h o d, technique of treatment and statistics to previous reports.

The older and technically more crystallized method of treatment is surgical. It consists of wide excision of the growth and a bilateral block excision of the neck which has an operative mortality of 11 per cent[4] and, often unsatisfacfory cosmetic results.

Radiation therapy is much younger. The first roentgen treatment was applied to an epithelioma in 1899 by Stenbeck,[5] of Stockholm. Danlos, of Paris, used radium on skin cancers in 1901, having been inspired by the famous radio-dermatitis of Becquerel. The type and technique of radiation is not as uniform as that of surgery. X-ray, gamma rays of radium and a combination of them are used in about equal proportions. The application of rays varies greatly. Low and high voltage X-rays, surface applicators, radium needles containing 0.6 to 8 milligrams of radium for each centimeter of length, and radon seeds are in use at various institutions.

Both surgical and radiation therapy give satisfactory results if applied early and adequately but, a thorough search in the literature reveals that radium treatment gives a higher per cent of cure than other treatment. J. Lane-Clayson's[7] statistical study is especially interesting and thorough in the "Reports on Public Health and Medical Subjects," Great Britain Ministry of Health, 1930, who reports 71.1 per cent of five year survival of lip cancers treated with radiation against 62 per cent treated by surgery. Higher percentage of cures are reported with radium treatment, up to 97.7 per cent by various dependable authors. Probably the statistics would be better if the radiologist could deal with selected cases like surgeons do as the cases declared inoperable by surgeons do not affect their statistics. It is interesting to note that Schreiner[8] reports 11.1 per cent of five year cure in inoperable cases with advanced metastasis.

The result of radiation therapy depends primarily upon the radio-sensitivity of the tumor, more correctly of every individual malignant cell. The radio-sensitivity of a malignant cell varies greatly from time to time, being more resistant during rest and less resistant just after and during mitosis. The most favorable results, that is complete destruction of all malignant cells with less damage to normal tissue, is obtained when the irradiation is continuous and uninterrupted for several days.

The physiological action of radiation on the cell has been thoroughly studied. Histological examination r e v e a l s that the plasma does not show gross changes first but, the n u c l e a r chromatin undergoes granular changes and fragmentation. The vital functions of the cell as nutrition and mitosis are not affected. Erhlich, trying to apply his side chain theory to these phenomena believe that the "nutriceptors" of the cell are radio-resistant while the "genoceptors" are radio-sensitive. Regaud and Lacassagne[8] divided the action of radiation into four groups as follows:

1. Cyto-caustic action, a similar coagulation necrosis of the cell as caused by heat and strong chemical agents.

2. Granular cytolysis, starting fragmentation of the nuclear chromatin followed by liquifaction of the cytoplasm and absorption of granulated, fragmented nucleus.

3. Abnormal mitosis and suspension of mitosis for a varying time.

4. Latent disability, indicated lessened reproductive ability s e v e r a l months or years later.

Our p r e s e n t technique of treatment consists of two external irradiations of the tumor and surrounding uninvolved tissue in a zone one centimeter around the lesion on two consecutive days, giving about one-half erythema dose of heavily filtered X-ray, generated at high v o l t a g e. Then,

radium needles containing 0.6 milligrams of radium screened by one-half millimeter of platinum are applied interstitially giving between 90-100 milligram hours per cubic centimeter.

Secondary infection has a definite detrimental effect on the radio-sensitivity of the lip cancer, and should be treated by wet dressings before radium application. External irradiation shortens the duration of this infection markedly.

A common cause of failure in the radiation treatment of these epitheliomas is the incomplete destruction of the peripheral cells. This failure is easily avoided if the marginal needles are i n s e r t e d in the healthy tissue at the border of the lesion. It is very important to notice that a sheer inspection is not sufficient and, very often misleading in the estimation of the extent of the tumor of the lip. Palpation gives a far more a c c u r a t e determination and should always be done.

Opinions are divergent concerning preventive radiation of regional glands. Some of the competent radiologists prefer a moderate dose of deep X-ray to both sides of the neck and sublingual regions, others oppose it. We do not usually irradiate the r e g i o n a l lymphatics preventively, believing that it is impossible to give a sufficient dose to such a large area and, better to save the condition of the skin for the time when metastasis may develop. Dependable statistics from various c l i n i c s state the metastasis of early and adequately treated epitheliomas of the lip is about five per cent.

When suspicious or definite glandular metastasis is a l r e a d y present, the involved glands should be treated by radium application or external radiation. We prefer large doses of deep X-ray, administered by Coutard method in a period of three to four weeks, depending upon the size of the field to be radiated.

In brief, our statistical data is as follows. It is, however, not complete since all of the patients have not passed the five year period after treatment.

Two of our 69 patients, less than two per cent, were women and both denied they had ever smoked.

The age scale showed a wider distribution than in other kinds of carcinomas.

Sixty-one per cent of our cases occurred between the ages of 40 and 70. The fifth decade was the most frequented and represented 36 per cent of all the cases. Eight per cent were under 30 years of age, the youngest 21 and the oldest 88 years of age.

Twenty-eight patients (41 per cent) had palpable glands when admitted. Eight out of all the patients never returned after treatment, as they moved from the county and it was impossible to locate them. They are discarded from the further statistical data.

For comparison, we have divided the cases into two groups. Group one represents those not h a v i n g metastasis and group two represents those having metastasis at admission.

We have failed to control the primary lesion in four cases, all of them having advanced metastasis at admission. These belong to group two.

Thirty-six out of 38 patients in the first group (97.6 per cent) showed apparent cure and only two of this group developed uncontrollable metastases. Three of them died with intercurrent disease, without any sign of metastasis or recurrence.

Sixteen out of 23 cases (69 per cent) of the second group showed apparent cure. Three of them died with intercurrent disease without any sign of metastasis or recurrence. Probably, some of these patients

should belong to group one as some of the palpable glands were undoubtedly inflammatory.

Our final statistics showed 86.8 per cent cure up to recent date including six deaths caused by intercurrent disease and, 75.4 per cent cured, discarding six deaths.

SUMMARY

A series of 69 cases has been presented on carcinoma of the lower lip, treated by interstitial radium implant.

Our statistical results compare favorably with those reported from other clinics, based on unselected cases.

We hope that our percentage of cures will be increased by the use of external X-ray radiation in addition to radium implant. A few of the above mentioned series have received both forms of radiation.

The answer to the entire problem will be, of course, the treatment of early cases.

REFERENCES

1. Sutton, R. L., and Sutton, R. L., Jr.: An Introduction to Dermatology. Third Edition, C. V. Mosby, 1937.
2. Eastland, Wm. E.: Personal communication.
3. Richards, G. E.: Carcinoma of the Lips, Canadian M. A. Journal, 35:593, December, 1936.
4. Kennedy, R. H.: Epithelioma of the Lip, Ann. Surgery, 99:81, 1934.
5. MacKee, G. M.: X-rays and Radium in Treatment of Diseases of the Skin, Lea and Febiger, Third Edition, 1938.
6. Ward, W. R., and Smith, A. J. D.: Recent Advances in Radium, pp. 174, P. Blakistons' Son and Co., 1934.
7. Lane, Clayson J.: cited by MacKee.
8. Schreiner, cited by MacKee.
9. Regaud and Lacassagne, cited by Ward and Smith on pp. 28.

―――――――――0―――――――――

The Use of Autohemotherapy Reinforced With Artificial Fever in the Treatment of Rheumatic Disease*

WILLIAM K. ISHMAEL, M.D.
OKLAHOMA CITY, OKLAHOMA

It is a well known principle of nature that any organism has the intrinsic ability to offer protection to itself against the changing effects of its environment.

*Read before the Section on Internal Medicine, Annual Meeting, Oklahoma State Medical Association, Oklahoma City, May, 1939.

The mechanism by which i n f e c t i o n brings about inflamed j o i n t s has never been satisfactorily explained, nor do we understand how exacerbations and remissions in the course of the d i s e a s e are brought about. We have all observed that the removal of the infection results in an unpredictable reaction — remission, flare up, or no effect w h a t e v e r; and that a permanent relief from the disease is rarely seen.

Realizing, therefore, that extinction of the disease must depend upon this intrinsic ability of the organism to develop its own protective powers, great effort has been put forth to provoke some reaction which would alter this abnormally disrupted immunity response of the b o d y toward an infection.

Chemo - therapy, immunological measures, physical applications and many others have failed to alter completely, with any consistency, the irreversible progress of this disease, yet nature alone, as repeatedly pointed out by Hench, by the effect of jaundice and pregnancy[26-28-30] on arthritis, has taught us that the progress of a rheumatic process can be retractable and is not necessarily an irreversible one. As yet, efforts to reproduce these two states have failed[29-30].

Remissions are also n o t e d frequently following any type of surgical procedure, this being explained by such theories as the effect of the infection removal, lowered blood sugar, rest in bed, the anesthetic and others. In consideration of the possibility that the e f f e c t of the extravasation of blood into the tissues may be responsible for this reaction, it was quite easy to simulate this phenomena by simply withdrawing the patient's blood and injecting it back in his own t i s s u e s. This procedure is termed autohemotherapy.

The process of autohemotherapy is an established measure of desensitization[1-2-3-4-5-6] and has been tried in the treatment of v a r i o u s rheumatic phenomena[7] Used alone, it has fallen short of expectations and various substances have been added to the blood[7] but without satisfactory results.

Being mindful of the fact that an increase in the body temperature is a natural defense mechanism and very frequently follows any surgical procedure, it occurred to us that the artificial stimulation of fever

to reinforce the reaction of the injected blood would bring about a change which would interrupt this deranged immunity response[23-24-25] seen in certain t y p e s of rheumatic disease.

Based upon this idea, these measures were applied to a series of 168 rheumatic patients.

METHOD OF TREATMENT

Autohemotherapy is a very simple procedure and can be employed safely without fear of untoward reaction. The technique employed is as follows: 10 to 20 c.c. of blood is withdrawn from the patient's vein and immediately injected into the muscles of the same patient's hip. This is done before clotting takes place and nothing need be added to the blood. The artificial fever is given immediately following the autohemotherapy and it was f o u n d that a relatively low level for one hour was adequate. Various degrees of fever and methods of administration were used, but 101.5 degrees for one hour, using the inductotherm in adults and intravenous typhoid vaccine in children to produce the fever, proved to be most satisfactory in all cases, except those with rheumatic fever where 104 degrees for four hours was used. W i t h inductothermy approximately one hour was used to reach 101.5 degrees, the temperature maintained for one hour and around two hours allowed for the temperature to return to normal, making a total of four hours involved. In using the inductotherm, each patient was allowed to eat a normal meal before the fever was started and occasionally 10 to 25 grains of sodium chloride was supplied along with ample fluids. No untoward reactions have been experienced to date and the patient is able to resume his normal activities as soon as his temperature has returned to normal. Optimum results were obtained when the procedure was repeated every four days. In the average case, six to ten treatments were given.

The results obtained in these cases are tabulated in chart number one immediately following.

CHART NO. 1 DIAGNOSIS	Total No.	Combined Therapy, Autohemo Plus Fever			Autohemother Only			Fever Only			Total		
	Total	Comp. Remission	Improved	No Response	Comp. Remission	Improved	Not Improved	Comp. Remission	Improved	Not Improved	Comp. Remission	Improved	Not Improved
Acute Gonorrheal Arthritis	7	5	0	0	1	1	0	0	0	0	6	1	0
Acute Infectious Arthritis	15	10	0	0	3	2	0	0	0	0	13	2	0
Acute Fibrositis	22	18	0	0	1	1	0	1*	1	0	20	2	0
Acute Gouty Arthritis	2	2	0	0	0	0	0	0	0	0	2	0	0
Rheumatic Fever	24	0	0	0	2	0	2	15*	5	0	17	5	2
Infectious Arthritis In Children (Still's Disease)	9	7	0	0	0	1	0	0	1	0	7	2	0
Premenstrual Rheumatic Exacerbation Syndrome	39	8	1	0	26	3	1	0	0	0	34	4	1
Menopausal Arthralgia	4	2	0	1	0	1	0	0	0	0	2	1	1
Chronic Fibrositis	30	12	1	0	0	2	0	14	0	1	26	3	1
Chronic Infectious Arthritis	16	1	4	5	0	2	1	0	1	2	1	7	8
TOTAL	168	65	6	6	33	13	4	30	3	3	128	27	13

The most striking results are seen in the cases with the acutely inflamed joints. Forty-four cases in all were treated by this combined r a p i d desensitization method and all responded completely in an average of 76 hours. In none have there been any recurrences. To date the types of joints treated in the acute phase included seven of acute G. C. arthritis, two acute gouty arthritis, 15 of acute infectious (atrophic) arthritis and 20 diagnosed as acute fibrositis. All these cases were in the acute p h a s e and not exacerbations in chronic cases.

DISCUSSION

1. In the acute gonorrheal cases, it will be noted that three had had sulfanilamide prior to the autohemotherapy fever treatment with no results and four had had no previous treatment at all. In all t h e s e cases, no treatment, in addition to the combined desensitization, was given during the management. The urethritis was not affected by the treatment and had to be treated by other measures after the joint and sedimentation time had returned to normal.

Case History: A 30-year-old colored male was seen complaining of severe pain and swelling in right knee. He stated that he had had a profuse urethral discharge for the past ten days and that for four days prior to admission the knee had become acutely swollen and painful. Examination revealed the right knee to be acutely painful with a great amount of effusion. Examination otherwise negative, except for the profuse urethral discharge which contained innumerable intra and e x t r a cellular gram negative diplococci which were diagnosed as gonococci by the laboratory. Wassermann, blood and u r i n e negative. He was given 10 c.c. autohemotherapy and told to take a hot tub bath at home with the water 103 degrees lasting for one hour. He returned in 48 hours and examination at that time revealed all the e f f u s i o n and tenderness gone from the knee. He stated that the pain and swelling disappeared within 12 hours following the autohemotherapy and heat. The urethritis was not affected and continued to drain throughout the 14 day observation period. No pain or swelling returned to the joint. Fourteen days following the remission he was referred to the G.U. department for treatment of his gonorrheal urethritis.

2. The remission of the acute g o u t y cases was singular in that any surgical procedure or foreign protein reaction may precipitate an attack of arthritis. As a matter of fact, the blood uric acid level in both cases became elevated 24 hours following the autohemotherapy and f e v e r. No conclusions should be drawn on a series as small as this one, but the reactions seen in these cases w a r r a n t further study. Slocumb[27] has pointed out that in these cases the systemic gout was not controlled although the arthritis was.

Case Report: White female 45 years of age complaining of intense pain in her left wrist which had not been relieved by morphine. History of sudden onset two days prior to admission. Past history negative except for three previous similar attacks, less severe than the present one. Examination revealed the left wrist to be of a dusky red color, markedly swollen and motion in the wrist and hand to be limited by the acute pain. Temperature 100.8 degrees. Examination otherwise negative. Laboratory: Urine negative, blood count negative, blood uric acid 4.6 mg per cent and the sedimentation rate fall of 52 mm in one hour. X-ray of the left wrist revealed an irregularity or roughening of the articular surface of the dorsal margin of the radius and the distal margin of the ulna. She was given 10 c.c. autohemotherapy followed by one hour of 101 degrees artificial fever. Six hours following this treatment all the swelling had subsided and about 10 to 20

per cent of the pain remained. Within 24 hours all the pain had subsided and the temperature was 98 degrees. The blood uric acid was repeated 24 hours following the autohemotherapy at which time she was in complete remission and was found to be 5.0 mg per cent.

' 3. In those cases diagnosed as acute nonspecific (atrophic) arthritis, the r e s u l t s were equally good. The average time for complete remission was two weeks, however, but the end result was comparable with the other types of acute joints. Those in this group were the early acute joints and not exacerbations of l o n g standing chronic ones.

4. The group diagnosed as acute fibrositis responded more quickly than any of the others to the combined rapid desensitization treatment. The average length of time before the remission was from four to 12 hours. All were complete within 48 hours. This group included five cases of "sciatica," 12 of acute "lumbago" and three of acute torticollis. All were within the age group between 24 and 35 years. In all the remissions were complete and have continued to the present period of observation.

Case Report: White male, 26 years of age, complaining of intense pain in the left side of his neck and left scapular region. It had appeared suddenly following a mild strain three days prior to admission and had become progressively worse. General examination negative except for torticollis and m u s c l e spasm of the left scapular group of muscles. He was given 10 c.c. autohemotherapy and this was followed by one hour of inductothermy. Five hours following this, all pain had subsided and he had free motion in his neck. There has been no return of symptoms to date.

The results seen in the chronic types were not so striking, except in the group diagnosed as chronic infectious arthritis in c h i l d r e n ("Still's disease") where probably the most interesting phenomena encountered was seen. Of the seven cases of "Still's disease" treated by the combined autohemotherapy—fever treatments, all seven had a complete remission in an average of 22 days. All cases were confined

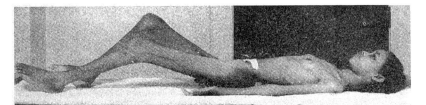

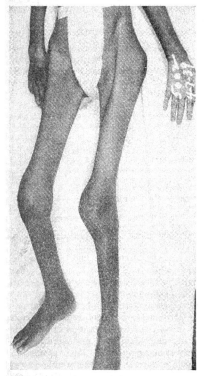

Figures 1 and 2

Photograph of patient with chronic juvenile infectious arthritis before treatment begun, April 7, 1939.

to bed by their disability when treatment was begun and in the seven remissions, the pain and swelling subsided and the deformities disappeared, leaving the joints with normal function and appearance.

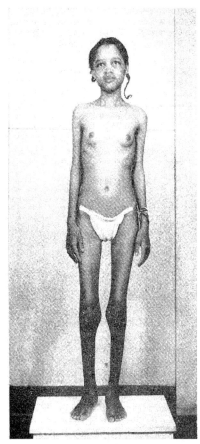

Figure 3

Photograph of same patient as in figure one, taken on May 24, 1939, following treatment consisting of autohemotherapy followed by artificial fever.

All cases were under seven years of age. This work on Still's disease is under intense study at the present time with a more a d e q u a t e control group. In the above series, only two controls were used, one receiving the fever only and one the autohemotherapy only. Neither of these controls had a remission in a period of 12 weeks, although both were "improved" in that pain and swelling had decreased but the deformities had not. It is impossible to draw any conclusions from this short series and it will require several years to arrive at any definite impression.

6. In rheumatic fever the results were hard to evaluate in that artificial fever is already of reported value[31-32-33-34]. Twenty cases received artificial fever of 104 degrees for the average total of eight hours. Fifteen had complete remission, five were "improved" and none had no change. Those receiving autohemotherapy only or fever of 101.5 degrees or less failed to improve.

7. In the cases of c h r o n i c infectious arthritis, the results are extremely difficult to judge due to the remissions and exacerbations seen normally in the course of the disease. Only 10 cases of this type were treated, using the combined autohemotherapy with fever. In addition to these, three received only the autohemotherapy and three only the fever.

Ten receiving the combined therapy:

One had a remission in four weeks and four were improved.

Five had no effect and none suffered exacerbation.

Three receiving fever only (101 degrees for one hour): No remissions, one improved, two no effect and none flared up.

Three receiving autohemotherapy only: No remissions, two "improved," one unchanged and none flared up.

Special attention will be called to a certain group of chronic infectious arthritis cases which had exacerbation three to five days prior to each menstrual period. These will be discussed in a separate group.

8. In the group diagnosed as chronic fibrositis, the r e s u l t s were favorable. Thirteen cases r e c e i v e d the combined therapy, 15 the fever only and two the autohemotherapy only. Twelve of the 13 receiving the combined therapy had a remission and one was improved. Of the 15 receiving the fever only, 14 had a remission and one was improved. Of the two receiving the autohemotherapy only, none had a remission and two were "improved." A group of cases diagnosed as fibrositis is now under o b s e r v a t i o n in which fever alone is being used and will be reported at a later date.

9. In the group diagnosed as hypertrophic arthritis, only that type known as "menopause arthralgias" was included in this series. Abrami[6] et al in 1937, reported the use of autohemotherapy to relieve the "reactions" of the menopause. Hall[20-21] and others[8-9-10-11-12-13-14-15-16-17-18-19-20] h a v e reported the use of the estrin complex to relieve the symptoms of m e n o p a u s e arthralgia with good results. Our results with estrin compare favorably with those reported by Hall[20-21]. The main effects of the autohemotherapy seems to be in the delayed absorption afforded by the presence of the blood about the e s t r i n and the "relief" reported by Abrami[6].

10. The tenth group studied, termed as the "premenstrual rheumatic syndrome" was of extreme interest and bears further study. John F. Kuhn, Jr.,[35] observing that urticaria occasionally precedes and accompanies catamenia, has e m p l o y e d autohemotherapy in the relief of this syndrome. He reports 100 per cent remissions from this management and s u g g e s t e d to the author the likelihood of a similar phenomena being present in the premenstrual rheumatic syndrome. Thirty-nine c a s e s exhibiting rheumatic exacerbations in the period three to five days prior to and during each menstrual period were selected by Dr. Kuhn and the author for study. In this group, where autohemotherapy alone was used, complete remissions were seen in 26 of the 30 cases treated. Three were "improved" and one was u n i m p r o v e d. Nine of these cases received the combined therapy with eight having complete remission and one was "improved."

CONCLUSIONS

1. A new technique of rapid desensitization is described which embodies the effects of autohemotherapy reinforced with a low degree of artificial fever.

2. Beneficial effects from this management are seen in the following conditions:

(a). Acutely inflamed joints.

(b). Still's disease.

(c). The "premenstrual r h e u m a t i c" exacerbation.

(d). Rheumatic fever if the temperature is elevated to 104 degrees.

3. No consistent beneficial effects were seen in:

(a). Chronic joints (except Still's disease).

(b). Rheumatic fever, when the temperature does not go above 101.5 degrees.

BIBLIOGRAPHY

1. Revent, P.: Autohemotherapy in Some Dermatoses, ann. de dermat et syph., 4:292, 1913.

2. Sicard, J. A.: Subcutaneous Homohemotherapy, La-Prasse Medicale, 26:304, June 13, 1918.

3. Levy-Solal, E.: Autohemotherapy in the dermatitis of Pregnancy, Gynec at Obst., 6:330 (Nov.) 1922.

4. Lyon, G.: Auto and Hetero-serotherapy, auto and heterohemotherapy, Bull. Med., Paris, 37:423, 1923.

5. Sternheim, L.: Harmonal Improvement Due to Ovarian Extracts and Autoblood Injections, Med. Welt, 6:164, January 30, 1932.

6. Abrami, P., Delacce, Jean, and Wallich, Robert: New Indications of Autohemotherapy in the Female, La Presse Medicale, 45:713 (May 12), 1937.

7. Le Calve, J.: The Rheumatism and Their Treatment, La Presse Medicale, 45:1409 (October 6), 1937.

8. Fox, R. F.: Arthritis in Women. J. State Med., 44:275-301, 1936.

9. Weil, M. P.: Le rhumatisme de la menopause. Bruxelles med. 8:1629-1640, 1697, 1928.

10. Charcot, J. M.: Etudes pour servir a Phistoire de l'affection decrite sous les noms de goutte asthenique primitive, nodosities des jointures, rheumastisme articulaire chronique (forms primitive). 59 pp. These de Paris, 1853.

11. Dalche, P.: Accidents osseux et articulaires d'origine genitale chez la femme. Gynecologie 8:487-506, 1903. Dysmenorrhee, rhumatisme noueux et retroflexion uterine. Rev. intrnat. de med. et de chir. 14:236, 1903.

12. Thomson, F. G.: Rheumatoid and Climacteric Arthritis. Brit. M. J. 1:1171, 1936.

13. Mouriquand, G.: Le Menopause dans ses rapports avec le rhumatisme chronique. Lyon med. 154:257-260, 1934.

14. Leriche, R.: Traitement de certaines doulcurs osseuses et musculaires consecutives a la castration (faux rhumatismes par carence). J. de med., de Lyon, 120:17, 1925.

15. Mazer, C., and Israel, S. L.: Symptoms and Treatment of Menopause. M. Clin. North American, 19:205, 1935.

16. Temperaar, H. C.G., and van Breemen, J.: On the Influence of Ovarnon on Climacteric Arthritis. Acta rheumatol., 3:13-18, 1931.

17. Lauber, H. J., and Ramm, C.: Prognose and Therapie der Arthropathia ovaripriva. Muchen. med. Wchnschr., 77:89, 1930.

18. Fliegel, O., and Strauss, R.: Zur "Arthropathia ovaripriva" Menge's. Zentralbl. f. Gynsk, 49:633, 1925.

19. Gillet, P.: Le rhumatisme chronique ovarien. Bull. med. 40:873-877, 1926.

20. Hall, F. C., and Monroe, R. T.: Thyroid Gland Deficiency in Chronic Arthritis. J. Lab. & Clin. Med., 18:439-457, 1933.

21. Hall, F. C.: The Value of Estrogenic Substance in "Menopausal Arthritis." Christian Birthday Volume, Baltimore: Waverly Press, Inc., 1936. Pp. 928-935. Oestrogena Substansers Varde vid "Menopaus-arthrit." Nord. med. tidskr. 12:1430, 1936.

23. Ishmael, Wm. K.: Discussion, J.A.M.A., 109-15, October 9, 1937, page 1029.

24. Ishmael, Wm. K., and McBride, Earl D.: The Regimented Rationale in the Treatment of Rheumatic Disease. Jour. Okla. State Med. Assn., October, 1937.

25. Small, J. C.: The Desensitization Treatment of Chronic Arthritis. Proc. Conf. Rheum. Dis. Acta. Rheumat., 5:26, 1932.

26. Hench, P. S.: Ann. Int. Med., April, 1934, 1278: Analgesic Effect of Hepatitis and Jaundice in Chronic Arthritis, Fibrositis and Sciatic Pain.

27. Slocumb, Charles H.: Correspondence from Mayo Clinic, Rochester, 1939.

28. Hench, P. S.: Med. Clin. N. Amer., 1935, 19, 551-583.

29. Thompson, H. E., and Wyatt, B. L.: Jour. Am. Med. Assn., 109:1482-4 (October 30), 1937; Arch. Int. Med., 61:481-500 (March), 1938.

30. Hench, P. S.: Arch. Int. Med. 61:451-480 and 495-500 (March), 1938.

31. Sutton, L. P., and Dodge, K. G.: Jour. Pedlat., 935, 6,494.

32. Sutton, L. P.: Med. Clinic N. A., 1935, 19,771-784.

33. Bland, E. F., and Jones, T. D.: Jour. Clin. Investigation, 1935, 14,683-648.

34. Report of Fifth Annual Fever Conf., May, 1935, pp. 1-117.

35. Kuhn, J. F., Jr.: Oklahoma City, Oklahoma. Communication, work now under investigation: "Treatment of Primary Dysmenorrhea."

———o———

DECREASE IN MATERNAL DEATHS SHOWS INFLUENCE OF CAMPAIGN

Intensive Efforts of Governmental, Lay and Medical Groups Are Beginning to Reveal Their Effects

Recent maternal mortality statistics indicate that the intensive efforts by physicians, various government health agencies and numerous lay groups to reduce such deaths in the United States are beginning to show their effects, Edwin F. Daily, M.D., Washington, D.C., states in The Journal of the American Medical Association for June 10.

"Official statistics of the Bureau of the Census for the year 1937," he continues, "give a maternal mortality rate of 49 per 10,000 live births. This rate is 14 per cent lower than the rate for 1936 (57), which was the previous low rate for the United States. If the maternal mortality rate for 1937 had remained the same as in 1936 there would have been 1,746 more maternal deaths in 1937 than actually occurred.

"This decrease in maternal mortality in 1937 is especially significant, since the death rate among women of child-bearing ages (from 15 to 49 years of age) from all other causes decreased by only 4 per cent. The birth rate in 1937 (17.0) was higher than the birth rate for 1936 (16.7)."

The only recent scientific discovery which aids the obstetrician is sulfanilamide. This drug in the future will be likely to save many lives from certain types of child-bed fever, but its use in 1937 for the treatment of this fever was not widespread in the United States.

Of the 14,296 deaths in 1935 certified as being associated with pregnancy and childbirth, 87.7 per cent were classified as directly due to child-bed fever. The remainder included deaths due to criminal abortion and tuberculosis, diabetes, chronic infection of the kidneys and syphilis. These latter diseases might or might not have proved fatal if the women had not become pregnant.

THE JOURNAL
OF THE
Oklahoma State Medical Association

Issued Monthly at McAlester, Oklahoma, under direction of the Council.

Copyright, 1939, by Oklahoma State Medical Association, McAlester, Oklahoma.

| Vol. XXXII | SEPTEMBER | Number 9 |

EDITORIAL BOARD
Dr. Ned Smith...Tulsa
Dr. L. J. Moorman..Oklahoma City
Dr. L. S. Willour, Chairman and Editor-in-Chief....McAlester

Entered at the Post Office at McAlester, Oklahoma, as second-class matter under the act of March 3rd, 1879.

This is the official Journal of the Oklahoma State Medical Association. All communications should be addressed to The Journal of the Oklahoma State Medical Association, McAlester Clinic, McAlester, Oklahoma. $4.00 per year; 40c per copy.

The editorial department is not responsible for the opinions expressed in the original articles of contributors.

Reprints of original articles will be supplied at actual cost provided request for them is attached to manuscripts or made in sufficient time before publication.

Articles sent this Journal for publication and all those read at the annual meetings of the State Association are the sole property of this Journal. The Journal relies on each individual contributor's strict adherence to this well-known rule of medical journalism. In the event an article sent this Journal for publication is published before appearance in The Journal the manuscript will be returned to the writer.

Failure to receive The Journal should call for immediate notification of the Editor, McAlester Clinic, McAlester, Oklahoma.

Local news of possible interest to the medical profession, notes on removals, changes of addresses, births, deaths and weddings will be gratefully received.

Advertising of articles, drugs or compounds unapproved by the Council on Pharmacy of the A. M. A., will not be accepted.

Advertising rates will be supplied on application.

It is suggested that wherever possible members of the State Association should patronize our advertisers in preference to others as a matter of fair reciprocity.

Printed by News-Capital Company, McAlester.

EDITORIAL

BREAD AND BOOKS
LEWIS J. MOORMAN, M.D.

John Muir, while spending his summers in the High Sierras studying glacial formations, always looked forward to the coming of winter, because he could then be warmly snow-bound in his Yosemite cabin with "plenty of bread and books." Obviously a busy doctor cannot hibernate, but while engaged in the pursuit of bread, he can always find time for books.

William Osler insisted upon the habit of daily reading, and it was he who said: "To study the phenomena of disease without books is to sail an uncharted sea, while to study books without patients is not to go to sea at all." To be reasonably well informed in the medical field of his endeavor, is every physician's duty. He should also seek a general knowledge of medicine with historical continuity. Our response to the new should be conditioned by what has gone before.

The art of medicine must not be neglected. Pondering over the phenomena of health and disease, and the intimate relationshp of patient and physician, Hippocrates said, "A doctor who is also a philosopher becomes god-like." There are few good philosophers who do not live with books. One's own sagacity must be checked with the recorded wisdom of the world, and chastened by "the touch divine of noble natures gone." Bacon has said: "Books will speak plain when councilors blanch." According to Timotheus, "They who dine with Plato never complain the next morning." Zeus consulted the oracle for a manner of living, "The answer was, that he should inquire of the dead." The latter is from the renowned Plutarch. The number of authors he quoted, in a period when printing was unknown, and manuscripts were rare and difficult to obtain, seems incredible, and should put to shame all who make excuses in this day of plenty.

In spite of modern self-sufficiency, founded on reason and science, serious illness may still result in psychological conflicts which should be resolved through the art of medicine. While medicine may successfully meet the needs of the body, only sound sagacity can succor the sick soul.

It is said that William Osler seldom went to sleep without a literary nightcap and in the morning there was always a book on his dressing table. Francis Adams, a busy country doctor, spent nine hours a day on his English translation of Hippocrates. The following quotation is from a recent letter written by the medical historian, Dr. Charles Singer of London: "Dr. Adams always took a few classical books with him and read while on horseback. This seems incredible, but I have been assured that it is true. He appeared to be a very poor rider, but never fell off his horse. The old doctor, reading his books on horseback, was a well-known sight to the village boys, and a source of endless amusement to them. Sir Donald McAlister, who died at a very advanced age, only a few years ago, could remember it." Dr. Singer also reports that after his days work was done, "He would then gather all his n e e d e d books together and take them to bed with him. He would often be asleep by eight p.m. and sleep perhaps 'till 11 or 12. He would then work right through the night, falling asleep at six or seven in the morning, to rise at nine. He continued in this course for years."

On his first trip across the American continent, Robert Louis Stevenson went hungry and traveled on an emigrant train in order that he might have money for the purchase of a six volume "Bancrofts History of the United States," before leaving New York City. Shelley's body was washed up from the sea with a small volume of Sophocles in one pocket and Keats in the other. Francis Thompson, English poet, while still enslaved by poverty, opium and tuberculosis, made the r o u n d s between cold park benches and London dump heaps with frayed copies of Aeschylus and Blake in his pocket.

Many more examples could be cited, but these are sufficient to show that "where there is a will, there is a way." One hour a day for 24 years would supply three full years of reading, counting eight hours a day.

In contemplation, we exclaim with Plutarch:

"Ye Gods! What greater pleasure?
What happier road to virtue."

William Osler, in his "Bed-side Library for M e d i c a l Students" recommends, in addition to professional training, at least half an hours reading before going to sleep at night, in order that the student may "get the education, if not of a scholar, at least of a gentleman." He then offers the following list of books.

"1. Old and New Testament.
2. Shakespeare.
3. Montaigne.
4. Plutarch's Lives.
5. Marcus Aurelius.
6. Epictetus.
7. *Religio Medici.*
8. *Don Quixote.*
9. Emerson.
10. Oliver Wendell Holmes—"Breakfast Table Series."

Many could be added. In memory of this great humanist, certainly his delightful "Aequanimitas, With Other Addresses," should head the list.

---o---

Ninth Annual Fall Clinical Conference

The Ninth Annual Fall Clinical Conference of the Oklahoma City Clinical Society will be held October 30, 31, November 1, 2, at the Biltmore Hotel in Oklahoma City. This post-graduate medical assembly again offers the profession of the Southwest another series of intensive clinics and lectures covering the most important fields of medicine, surgery, and the specialties. The 16 guest lecturers this year are among the recognized leaders in their respective fields and have chosen very practical subjects. In addition to the distinguished guests, the program includes 72 lecturers selected from local members of the Society, all of whom have teaching ability and practical experience in their particular subjects.

The officers and members of the Oklahoma City Clinical Society, being cognizant that the rapid development of new facts and theories in the field of medicine necessitates frequent post-graduate instruction for those who would progress, have arranged in this course a four-day period of very intensive instruction at a most nominal expenditure of time and money for those who attend. Those of us who have attended this conference in the past have been impressed with the precision in which the program is carried on, the diversity of it, the practical experience gained from the lecturers and our direct association with them, and the whole-hearted hospitality accorded all visitors. We feel that the stimulation received from attending these meetings always tends to bring the profession into a closer understanding of its problems and into a closer fellowship as members of our great profession.

The announcement of the coming meeting will be found on the front cover of this issue of the Journal, and we are sure you will be impressed with the prominence of the guest speakers and the program in general. We believe you should attend this meeting and that you will be well repaid for the time spent there.

---o---

Trade or Profession?

Every layman will feel that the federal judge of Washington who holds the practice of medicine is a profession and not a trade or commercial venture interpreted our country's anti-trust laws correctly.

And if the practice of medicine is a trade, it is difficult to see how the practice of law and theology and pedagogy are not trades also. If physicians can be prosecuted for violating a law forbidding the illegal restraint of trade, why will not a similar prosecution lie against lawyers and ministers and teachers? And why would it not be in order to prosecute carpenters who agree upon a uniform price and miners who set a definite rate for mining coal?

Moreover, the physician who follows a rate card in treating typhoid in Massachusetts or combatting a case of mumps in Oklahoma is no more engaged in interstate commerce than the lawyer who defends a negro for shooting craps in Little Rock or the well digger who seeks for living water in the valley of the Sangamon.

In their zeal for obliterating state lines in order to promote the more abundant life our lawmakers have assaulted more than the constitution of the United States: They have delivered a furious assault on the unabridged dictionary and the art of accurate definition—The Oklahoman.

Due to the necessary extra work and time entailed in moving and establishing the office of the Executive Secretary to Oklahoma City, the reports of the Meetings of the House of Delegates have been deferred until this issue of the Journal.

* * * *

MINUTES OF THE MEETING OF THE HOUSE OF DELEGATES

Oklahoma State Medical Association

Skirvin Tower Hotel

8:00 P.M.

May 1, 1939

The first meeting of the House of Delegates of the Oklahoma State Medical Association was held at the Skirvin Tower Hotel, Oklahoma City, May 1, 1939.

The meeting was called to order by Dr. J. D. Osborn, Jr., Speaker of the House of Delegates. Before the regular order of business was brought before the House, Dr. Osborn made several announcements relative to the procedure to be followed during the coming meetings of the House. The Speaker then announced his appointment of assistants and committees for the conducting of the business of the Association. These appointments were: Doctors H. F. Vandever and Ned Smith, Sergeant at Arms; Doctors E. Albert Aisenstadt, G. H. Garrison, Geo. K. Hemphill, and S. C. Sheppard, Reference Committee; Doctors C. P. Bondurant and McLain Rogers, Credentials Committee. The Speaker further stated that the meetings of the House of Delegates would be conducted according to Roberts Rules of Order.

Following these preliminary remarks the Credentials called the roll and advised the Chair there were eighty (80) delegates present and qualified, and moved that this number constituted a quorum. On motion of Dr. Walker, seconded by Dr. Tisdal, this report was accepted.

The next order of business was the reading of the minutes of the previous Annual Meeting which was done by the Secretary and on motion, duly seconded, were accepted.

The Chair next called for a report of the Standing Committees but before such reports were made Dr. Vandever addressed a motion to the Chair that the Report of the Committee on Revision of the Constitution and By-Laws be made special order of business and remain special order until disposed of. This motion was seconded by Dr. Watson, and carried.

Dr. Osborn then called for the report of the Committee on the Revision of the Constitution and By-Laws. Dr. Ritzhaupt, as Chairman of this Committee, after some introductory remarks, submitted the written report of the Committee together with the completed revision. This revision was read by Dr. Ritzhaupt and on concluding, the question of whether or not the articles could be acted upon as read was asked by Dr. White of Muskogee. The Chair in answer to this question stated that unless overruled by the House—the proper procedure would be to complete the first reading whereupon the House of Delegates would then accept or adopt the report—that it would then be read again and the House would have the right to amend each section as read, but not vote on the amendments for adoption.

Dr. McCarley, moved, that in order to save time, the By-Laws be read by title, the purpose being to accept the report of the Committee and proceed to pass on each Article and Section. Seconded by Dr. Ritzhaupt.

Dr. Fulton, spoke on the subject of making the revision but made no motion.

Dr. Ned Smith, pointed out that the present Constitution was very definite on the procedure to follow and requested Dr. McCarley to yield his motion for a substitute motion that would embody the same action. Dr. McCarley yielded and Dr. Smith

moved that the Constitution as read lay on the table for one year, or until the first meeting of the House of Delegates next year. This motion was seconded by Dr. Walker.

Dr. Speed asked if the Constitution lay over without being amended, would it not be necessary for it to lay over another year in the event any amendments were made next year. Dr. Smith and Dr. McNeill, discussed this question at some length. Dr. Ritzhaupt on a point of order, pointed out that Dr. McCarley's motion pertained to the By-Laws and not to the Constitution and that the By-Laws could be amended and lay on the table over night and be acted upon the following morning. Dr. Ritzhaupt stated that the entire report of the Committee would not be adopted until Dr. McCarley's motion had been accepted. Dr. McCarley's motion was then put before the House and passed.

Dr. Ritzhaupt then moved that the report of the Committee be adopted as stated in its written report. The motion was seconded by Dr. Aisenstadt and passed.

Dr. Ritzhaupt next moved that the Constitution be read Article by Article and any amendments desired by the Delegates be submitted in writing. Dr. Ritzhaupt made a few remarks in support of his motion, stating that if this procedure were adopted the amendments could be adopted next year. Carried unanimously.

Speaker of the House note: (Copies of the Constitution and By-Laws, with the changes in the By-Laws and amendments to the Constitution to be acted upon next year, will be sent to the officers of the Association, Councilors, Presidents and Secretaries of all County Medical Societies and Delegates. Anyone else desiring a copy may receive same by writing the Executive Secretary, 210 Plaza Court, Oklahoma City. The Speaker of the House requests that they be read at the next session of the different county society meetings.)

Dr. Willour, next read the Constitution and amendments were made by a number of the delegates. (A full copy of the amendments can be obtained from your County Secretary.) Upon completion of the reading of the Constitution and amendments, made from the floor, Dr. Cook, moved the adoption of the Committee report as amended and that same be tabled for one year. The motion was seconded by Dr. Walker, and passed.

Dr. McKeel, was then recognized by the Chair and stated that inasmuch as action on the By-Laws could not be made until the new Constitution was adopted the following year, that the reading of the By-Laws be dispensed with and the next order of business considered. Dr. Stevenson and Dr. Ritzhaupt pointed out that these proposed By-Laws were not "new" By-Laws but amendments to the old By-Laws and could be acted upon at this time. Dr. McKeel's motion was lost for want of a second.

Dr. Walker, moved that the By-Laws be read by title and laid on the table until the next morning. Dr. Fulton spoke on the advisability of delaying action until a later date as it was growing late. Dr. Ritzhaupt pointed out that the motion by Dr. Vandever, and carried, had made this matter special business until completed. The Secretary then read the proposed amendments to the present By-Laws and additional amendments were offered by delegates from the floor. (NOTE: These amendments are available from the Secretary of your County Society or from the Executive Secretary of the State Association.)

After a short discussion Dr. Ned Smith, moved that the consideration of the By-Laws be made special order of business for the next day and made so until disposed of. The motion was seconded by Dr. Aisenstadt and carried.

The House adjourned until the next morning, May 2nd.

MINUTES OF THE MEETING OF THE HOUSE OF DELEGATES

May 2, 1939

The second meeting of the House of Delegates was called to order by the Speaker of the House of Delegates, Dr. J. D. Osborn, Jr.

A roll call of the Delegates was made and the tellers reported seventy-four (74) present and voting.

The first order of business was the consideration of the amendments to the By-Laws which were submitted at the previous meeting, May 1st, and were now ready for action.

Dr. Ned Smith moved that consideration and action of the House be limited to Chapter 6, Section 6 and 7; Chapter 7, Section 7; and Chapter 8 as a whole; and that the remainder of the By-Laws, together with the proposed amendments lay over until the next House of Delegates meeting in 1940.

Dr. Ritzhaupt amended this motion to have the House recess at 10 o'clock to attend the scientific meetings and to reconvene. This amendment lost on vote and the original motion prevailed.

Dr. Ritzhaupt as Chairman of the Committee, then read to the House the proposed amendments to the By-Laws as per Dr. Smith's motion. (Those acted upon favorably now comprise the changes in the previous By-Laws of the Oklahoma State Medical Association. A copy of the new changes in the By-Laws can be had by getting in touch with the Ssecretary of your County Society or the Executive Secretary's office.)

Upon completion of this business on special order, Dr. Vandever was recognized by the Chair and offered a motion relating to the employment of two paid secretaries, pointing out the necessity of economy and the desirability for the establishment of a business office and that the necessary time could not be given by a practicing physician. That this motion was in no way to be considered disapproval of the past valuable services of the present Secretary, Dr. Willour, but that its sole purpose was in the interests of economy and for the good of the Association.

Dr. Fulton spoke against the motion, pointing out that the Journal should be edited by a doctor and that the decision was up to the Council.

Dr. Ned Smith spoke in behalf of the motion commending Dr. Willour for his work and pointed out the By-Laws provided for the handling of the scientific part of the Journal by the creation of an Editorial Board composed of doctors. Dr. Smith then offered an amendment to Dr. Vandever's motion, that Dr. Willour continue in his elected position as Secretary-Treasurer until his term expired or the Constitution changed and that he act as Editor-in-Chief of the Editorial Board, his salary to be determined by the Council.

Dr. Stevenson spoke in behalf of the amended motion and Dr. Willour requested that he did not desire any personal consideration and for the Delegates to act for the good of the Association.

Dr. Vandever accepted the amendment to his motion and the motion as amended carried.

The next order of business was the election of officers. Dr. C. R. Rountree, nominated Dr. Henry H. Turner, for President-Elect. The nomination was seconded by Dr. Watson of Enid. Dr. Ritzhaupt moved the nominations be closed and the Secretary instructed to announce the election unanimous by acclamation.

Dr. Turner upon being advised of his election was brought before the House and thanked the Delegates for this high honor.

Dr. Osborn next ruled the House would recess for the election of Councilors. Caucuses by Councilor Districts were held and upon reconvening the elected Councilors from their respective districts were announced to be: District No. 2, V. C. Tisdal,

Elk City; District No. 7, J. A. Walker, Shawnee; District No. 8, F. W. Ewing, Muskogee; District No. 9, L. C. Kuyrkendall, McAlester; District No. 10, J. S. Fulton, Atoka.

Following the election of the Councilors the election of Delegates to the American Medical Association was next in order and Dr. J. A. Walker, nominated Dr. Horace Reed, Oklahoma City. Dr. Haralson, moved that the term of Dr. W. Albert Cook, be extended one year in order that a delegate may be elected each year to serve for a term of two years. The chair ruled this motion out of order. Dr. Ritzhaupt nominated Dr. McLain Rogers, Clinton. The nominations were then declared closed, the ballot taken and Dr. Rogers declared elected.

The Speaker next asked for resolutions of thanks be drawn for those persons and agencies which were of help to the Association during the past year. A motion to this effect was made by Dr. Sugg, amended by Dr. Ritzhaupt and passed.

Dr. McNeill, as Councilor, asked for instruction from the House concerning an alternate from Okmulgee living in Oklahoma County. The delegate from Okmulgee explained the history of the case in question and Dr. Ritzhaupt moved the matter be referred to the Council. The motion of Dr. Ritzhaupt prevailed and the House adjourned until the next morning, May 3, 1939.

MINUTES OF THE MEETING OF THE HOUSE OF DELEGATES

May 3, 1939

The third meeting of the House of Delegates was called to order by the Speaker of the House, Dr. J. D. Osborn, Jr.

A quorum was declared present by the tellers and the meeting proceeded with the regular order of business.

Reports were received by the House from Drs. Speed and Willour, Dr. Speed giving a report on the matters of the Association, conducted during his administration by the Council and Dr. Willour presented resolutions passed by members of the Council. Their reports and resolutions were accepted by vote of the House.

The Chair next asked the pleasure of the House on the disposition of the minutes of the last meeting. Dr. Fulton moved the reading of the minutes be dispensed with, and on seconding said motion was adopted.

The next order of business was the report of the Standing Committees. Dr. McNeill moved said reports be accepted as reported in the Journal. The motion was seconded and carried.

Dr. Speed was recognized by the Chair and requested the report of the Necrology Committee. Dr. Willour read the report and Dr. Fulton spoke in eulogy of the deceased members. Dr. Fulton also moved the report be accepted and any additional names of deceased members that might not have been included added to the list. The motion carried and a moment of silence was observed in memory of the deceased members.

The next order of business was the report of the Special Committees. Dr. Turner gave the report of the Post Graduate Committee and made additional remarks, relative to the work accomplished by this Committee. Dr. Risser praised the Committee's work and made a few remarks on the advantages of this course to the rural doctors, and moved that the House instruct the Council to continue the work of the Committee and make an appropriation of $2,000.00 per year for the next two years for its work. The motion was seconded and carried.

Dr. Willour then presented the report of the Committee on Control of Cancer and Dr. Carl Puckett stated the report of the Committee on

Control of Tuberculosis would appear in the next issue of the Journal.

Dr. L. J. Moorman was next accorded the floor and presented the name of Dr. A. J. Coley, Oklahoma City, for honorary membership in the Association. The presentation was then filed in the form of a motion, seconded and carried. Dr. C. M. Pounders, presented the names of Drs. Virgil F. Dougherty and R. J. Fitz, who are in missionary work, as honorary members. Dr. Willour moved they be made honorary members for the term of their foreign duty. This was seconded and carried. Dr. Moorman was again recognized and moved the delegates to the American Medical Association present the name of Dr. D. D. McHenry, Oklahoma City, for election to Fellowship in the American Medical Association; this was seconded and carried. Dr. Willour presented the name of Dr. J. E. Cullum, Earlsboro, for honorary membership in the Association; this was seconded and carried.

The next order of business was the consideration of the amendment to the Constitution that had been introduced at the last annual meeting of the Association. This was voted upon and failed of passage.

Dr. A. Ray Wiley, President of the Tulsa County Medical Society, was next recognized and extended an invitation to the Association to meet in Tulsa in 1940. The motion was seconded and carried.

Action on the motion offered by Dr. Haralson on the preceding day, extending Dr. Rogers' appointed term to three years and Dr. Cook's one, so that thereafter a delegate could be elected every year to serve two years, was sconded by Dr. Willour and carried.

Dr. Aisenstadt moved that the dues for 1940 be set and Dr. Ned Smith, moved they be ten ($10.00) dollars. The motion was seconded and carried.

Dr. Risser was next recognized and spoke on County organization work. The necessity for all doctors to become members of their Association and be united in their many efforts. Drs. Ritzhaupt, Ewing, and McKeel, likewise spoke on the interests the doctors should take in the affairs of their respective localities.

Dr. Willour next presented the budget for the coming year which was accepted. Dr. Wiley nominated Drs. Willour and Horace Reed as Alternates to the American Medical Association; these were seconded and carried.

A letter was read from Dr. LeRoy Long, expressing his appreciation for the kindnesses extended him during his illness.

A letter was read from the American Medical Association seeking the support of the Association in urging Congress to make an appropriation for housing a Medical Library of Congress. Such recommendation was made, seconded and carried.

After a short presentation of the Tulsa County's malpractice insurance plan by Mr. Lloyd Stone, Executive Secretary of the Tulsa County Medical Society, the meeting adjourned.

* * * *

This is to certify that I have carefully reviewed the abstracted minutes of the meetings of the House of Delegates of the last Annual Meeting of the Oklahoma State Medical Association, together with the original transcription, and they are correctly recorded to the best of my knowledge and belief.

JAS. D. OSBORN, JR., Speaker, House of Delegates.

———————o———————

Council Convenes

The Council of the Oklahoma State Medical Association convened on August 10, 1939, in the offices of the Association, 210 Plaza Court, Oklahoma City, on the call of the President, W. A. Howard.

Councilors present were W. A. Howard, Henry H. Turner, L. S. Willour, James Stevenson, Walter

Hardy, E. Albert Aisenstadt, L. C. Kuyrkendall, A. S. Risser and V. C. Tisdall.

The Council convened to receive the report of the Committee on Group Hospitalization Insurance. This report was read by V. K. Allen, Tulsa, following this each Councilor was given a chance to ask questions of the Committee. All Committee members were present in the persons of V. K. Allen, Tulsa, John E. Heatley, Oklahoma City, and John Carson, Shawnee. After a general discussion of the topic a letter from Councilor Philip M. McNeill was read and the following motion was made by A. S. Risser:

"In view of circumstances throughout the State, that it be the action of the Council to endorse the general plan of the Committee on Hospitalization Insurance; and instruct the President to appoint a Committee to work out a plan of organization and report back to the Council; and, that they be allowed to draw on the Treasury of the State Medical Association in an amount not to exceed $500, this to be paid back if and when the organization is completed and in running order."

Dr. Aisenstadt spoke against the motion and Dr. Stevenson for it.

All Councilors voted "aye" on the motion and Dr. Aisenstadt requested that his vote be explained. He desired to state for the record that he was opposed to the voting of the sum of $500 for the use of the Committee.

In compliance with the above motion the following Committee was appointed by the president: A. S. Risser, Chairman, Blackwell; P. M. McNeill, Oklahoma City; J. A. Walker, Shawnee; James Stevenson, Tulsa; V. C. Tisdal, Elk City.

A transcript of the discussion by Councilors Stevenson and Aisenstadt is on file in the office of the Association.

On motion the Council adjourned.

L. S. WILLOUR, Secretary.

———————o———————

Editorial Notes—Personal and General

Word has just been received from Dr. Geo. J. Seibold that he is now located in Wichita Falls, Texas, with the Medical and Surgical Clinic. Dr. Seibold will specialize in the practice of allergy at his new location.

———————

DR. J. A. MORROW, Sallisaw, appointed by Governor Leon C. Phillips as a member of the Oklahoma Public Welfare Commission, has resigned to accept the position of Deputy Health Commissioner of the Oklahoma State Department of Health. Dr. and Mrs. Morrow will make their home in Oklahoma City during his tenure of office.

———————

The Southwestern Clinic Hospital of Lawton has recently been enlarged and modernized and a formal opening for inspection by the public was recently held. The physician personnel consists of Drs. E. B. Dunlap, O. L. Parsons, Fred T. Fox, George Barber, L. W. Ferguson and G. G. Downing. Opening of this newly renovated hospital with the finest of new modern equipment increases the medical services available to the people of the southwest. Lawton's two hospitals, the Angus and the Southwest, now present facilities on a par with any hospital anywhere.

———————

John Steinbeck's novel, "The Grapes of Wrath" has not only caused great furor in the literary world but has also greatly affected the practice of medicine in at least one state. The conditions existing among roving families as presented by this novel has caused the state of California to purchase and equip four auto-clinics for the purpose of immunization among this group. Each unit is staffed by a physician, a nurse and a sanitation expert. Since 1937 the state department of health has vaccinated 23,701 against small-pox and innoculated 74,257 against typhoid fever, thus bringing the state's death rate in these two fields to the lowest point in history.

DR. W. W. COTTON, Walters, and DR. R. M. VAN MATRE, formerly of Lawton, have established practice in Temple. Dr. Cotton is a graduate of the University of Oklahoma School of Medicine and Dr. Van Matre received his medical education at Washington University, St. Louis, Mo.

DR. JOHN F. PARK of the McAlester Clinic has just returned from a visit to London, England, where he attended the surgical clinics.

City Commissioners of Stillwater recently purchased an X-ray machine and are in hopes of having the new hospital constructed in that city open by the first part of September. The hospital will be under the management of the Sisters of the Most Most Sacred Blood.

Dr. Ralph Bowen, connected since 1932 with the Balyeat-Bowen Clinic in Oklahoma City, has recently established his own office in Houston, Texas. Dr. Bowen's work in his new location will be limited exclusively to asthma, hay-fever, and other diseases of allergy.

Dr. Grady Mathews announces the appointment of Dr. J. Dorrough of McAlester as county health superintendent of Pittsburg County and Dr. W. K. Haynie of Durant as county health officer of Bryan County.

DR. and MRS. W. ALBERT COOK of Tulsa have been spending July and August in the mountains near Chattanooga, Tennessee, and the Smoky Mountains of North Carolina. They expect to return home about September 1st.

OBITUARIES

Dr. James L. Shuler

Dr. James L. Shuler of Durant, Oklahoma, died at the home of his son in Hobbs, New Mexico, August 24, 1939, about 6 p.m. Dr. Shuler had been in rather poor health for some months following an acute septicemia from an infected wound of the finger.

Dr. Shuler was born in Cartersville, Georgia, in 1860, and had resided in Durant since 1900. He was a graduate of the University of Arkansas Medical School. He was married to Miss Lucy Hickman, at Poscola, Indian Territory, January 11, 1896. To this union was born one son, Dr. A. C. Shuler of Hobbs, New Mexico.

Dr. Shuler has been an active member of organized medicine in Oklahoma since his location in Durant nearly 40 years ago. He has served as President for several terms and at the time of his death was secretary of his County Society. For many years he was a Councilor of the Oklahoma State Medical Association and he served as President in 1912. It is consequently evident that he has given liberally of his time and talent in the support of his profession. Dr. Shuler was also a member of the Masonic Order, holding membership in the Blue Lodge, Knight's Templar, Scottish Rite and Shrine and he has always been a very active and consistent member of the Methodist Church.

The funeral services were held Saturday, August 26, from the Methodist Church of Durant. Rev. W. L. Broome and Rev. W. L. Blackburn officiated and interment was in the Durant Highland cemetery.

Dr. Shuler is survived by his widow, Mrs. Lucy Shuler of Durant, and one son, Dr. A. C. Shuler, of New Mexico.

Organized medicine in Oklahoma has lost one of its original members and his presence and council will be decidedly missed.

New Books

THE ART OF ANAESTHESIA: By Paluel J. Flagg, M.D., Visiting Anaesthetist to Manhattan Eye and Ear Hospital; Consulting Anaesthetist to St. Vincent's Hospital, New York, N. Y.; Consulting Anaesthetist to the Woman's Hospital, Sea View Hospital, Jamaica Hospital, Mount Vernon Hospital, Flushing Hospital, Mary Immaculate Hospital, St. Mary's Hospital, Far Rockaway, N. Y.; Nassau Hospital, L. I.; Director of Pneumatology, World's Fair, New York City, and Chairman of Committee on Asphyxia of the American Medical Association. Sixth Edition, Revised. 491 pages with 161 illustrations. Philadelphia, London and Montreal. J. B. Lippincott Company, 1939.

In the sixth edition of The Art of Anaesthesia, Dr. Flagg gives us the basic principles of anesthesia in a most comprehensive manner which should be appreciated by both the trained and untrained anesthetist. The introduction gives the history of the pre-anesthetic period then takes up the anesthetic period from 1842 to the present date.

Dr. Flagg neatly classifies anesthesia; gives the characteristic signs and various methods of administration, taking ether as the more commonly used anesthetic agent.

The chapter on chloroform is especially interesting, particularly so for the average small town and country doctor. Quote, "Chloroform, while ideal in efficiency, is a dangerous poison. In the light of present day pathology, chloroform should cease to be used as an anesthetic in obstetrics."

The second part of this edition contains material bearing upon factors incidental to the actual administration of the anesthetic; as, preliminary medication (which is too often treated very lightly); post-operative treatment and duties of the nurse; Co2 and rebreathing; pre-anesthetic examination (which should be a routine for every one). The improved method of intratracheal anesthesia is very helpful for the anesthetist who does not have occasion to use this method every day.

The patient's point of view is brought out in an elaborate but not too lengthy manner. Dr. Flagg says, "One need not follow the isms of the faddist to be up to date. Truth is not a matter of time or place, it is unchangeable. The acknowledgement of the existence of the supernatural in the soul of man is not an evidence of revision of type. It is but the result of the acceptance and of the intelligent correlation of a host of facts which we see about us."

The author treats the basal anesthetics and cyclopropane with great interest, then touches on dental anesthesias; intubation and causes of death in anesthesia.

The last chapter dealing with pneumotology is extremely interesting and certainly worthy of much consideration by hospital superintendents, municipal heads and boards of health.

In all "The Art of Anaesthesia," is a splendid and well written book, and should be a prized possession of any one practicing anesthesia.

ABSTRACTS : REVIEWS : COMMENTS
and CORRESPONDENCE

SURGERY AND GYNECOLOGY
Abstracts, Reviews and Comments from
LeRoy Long Clinic
714 Medical Arts Building, Oklahoma City

Calcification of the Supraspinatus Tendon: W. A. Bishop, Jr., M.D., Oklahoma City, Archives of Surgery, August, 1939, Vol. 39, No. 2, page 231.

The author has made an attempt to correlate the pathologic lesion with the symptoms produced and to rationalize the treatment.

This article is based on a series of 27 patients, nine of whom had bilateral deposits, while the author was working under the supervision of Dr. J. A. Freiberg in the Department of Orthopedic Surgery at the University of Cincinnati.

The author's summary and conclusions follow:

"No attempt has been made to discuss a differential diagnosis of lesions of the shoulder except in connection with cases in which calcareous deposits are present. As was shown by Codman, such deposits are most often located in the tendon of the supraspinatus muscle at the usual site of rupture, near its attachment into the greater tuberosity of the humerus. Occasionally the tendon of the infraspinatus or the subscapularis muscle is involved. The calcium salts are thought to be laid down slowly over a period of months or even years in the hyaline connective tissue subsequent to repair of repeated minor traumas. The masses are asymptomatic until they are large enough to produce mechanical disturbances or until a minor trauma tears a few of the adjacent tendon fibers and produces mechanical irritation with the accumulation of serum and inflammatory cells to activate the process.

"A case is presented to illustrate the types of pain encountered. Pain in the region of the insertion of the deltoid muscle is thought to be referred from the subacromial bursa. The increased pressure within the t e n d o n and the stretching of the overlying synovial membrane which lines the base of the bursa seem to account for the occurrence of constant dull, boring or aching pain localized to the point of the shoulder. The third type of pain encountered in this condition is really the result of a complication. It consists of pain throughout the distribution of the brachial plexus. The most severe symptom is a burning, shooting or tingling sensation down the arm, most often in the distribution of the ulnar nerve but also encountered in the areas innervated by the median and radial nerves. It is often associated with swelling of the involved hand. Oscillometric tracings may show some decrease in the vascular pulsations on the affected side. Sensory and other subjective neurologic changes are not uncommon. The entire picture is that presented by the scalenus anticus syndrome and is thought to result from reflex spasm of the scalenus anticus muscle of the affected side.

"The diagnosis depends on a carefully taken history and on the physical findings, which, however, differ little from those associated with other painful conditions of the s h o u l d e r. Roentgen examination should consist of the taking of anteroposterior views of the shoulder with the humerus in the neutral position and in lateral rotation, a "semisoft' technic being advisable.

"Routine treatment is considered radical. The acute condition should be treated immediately by lavage. In the subacute or chronic stages, a decision must be made to give diathermy a trial or to resort to lavage if it has not been used previously. In a small percentage of cases the condition cannot be satisfactorily treated except by surgical removal of the deposit."

LeRoy D. Long.

Penetrating Stab Wounds of the Abdomen and Stab Wounds of the Abdominal Wall, A Review of 184 Consecutive Cases: Louis T. Wright, M.D., Robert S. Wilkinson, M.D., and Joseph L. Gaster, M.D., New York, N. Y.; Surgery, August, 1939, Vol. 6, No. 2, page 241.

Stab wounds that penetrate the peritoneal cavity demand immediate laparotomy because of the possibility of injury to some abdominal viscus or blood vessel.

Whereas the majority of cases at the time of admission to hospital shows adequate clinical proof of intra-abdominal injury, the borderline group of cases, where uncertainty exists as to the presence of intra-abdominal injury, causes great anxiety and in the past (because of watchful-waiting policy) added to mortality.

At the Harlem Hospital these men in previous years customarily waited and attempted clinically to tell whether penetration of the abdomen was present or not. This was felt to be wrong, and it was, therefore, decided to operate upon every case of stab wound in the following fashion: to open the abdominal wall down to the peritoneum without opening the peritoneal cavity, and, if there was no sign of penetration of the parietal peritoneum, the operator would gently peel the peritoneum away from the abdominal parietes and look for (a) intraperitoneal hemorrhage and (b) if there was evidence of penetration of the peritoneum. Of course, if the peritoneum had been entered, the patient received thorough surgical exploration. The skin incision was made closely adjacent to the stab wound itself and in some instances the stab wound was made part of the incision. It was assumed that in all of these cases, if the knife entered the peritoneal cavity, the abdominal cavity was infected and, therefore, it was safe for the surgeon to investigate. In the event it was found that the abdominal cavity had not been opened, the muscles of the abdominal wall were closed in the usual fashion and one or two Penrose drains were inserted down to the peritoneum. Following this procedure, their total mortality was reduced for all types of cases.

In this way the total mortality of penetrating stab wounds of the abdomen was lowered because in no instance was penetration missed or operation delayed while waiting for symptoms to develop.

The only site where this procedure caused technical difficulties was along the anterior costal margins and in the back.

The authors urge the routine X-ray of abdomen and chest, blood banks, intravenous glucose and saline by slow drip method and avoidance of spinal anesthesia while taking care of this type of case.

LeRoy D. Long.

Sulfapyridine in Treatment of Pneumonia, With Special Reference to Postoperative Pneumonia: By H. Corwin Hinshaw, M.D., Ph.D., and Herman J. Moersch, M.D., Rochester, Minnesota; Archives of Surgery, August, 1939, Vol. 39, No. 2, page 275.

This is a very important and practical contribution, based upon the experience of the authors in the treatment of 21 cases of postoperative pneumonia and six cases of primary pneumonia in the Mayo Clinic.

The average patient was given 15 grains of sulfapyridine by mouth every four hours, day and night. "The first dose, and sometimes the second dose also, was doubled, making a total of either 105 or 120 grains during the first 24 hours."

In connection with unfavorable e f f e c t s, the authors report that in this group there was no significant leukopenia, cyanosis, hemolytic anemia, drug rash, drug fever, or other annoying complications.

About half of the patients complained of nausea. The treatment was shortened in about half the cases complaining of nausea, but it appears that the authors believe that nausea does not usually make it necessary to discontinue the drug. They expressed themselves as believing that nausea "is merely an uncomfortable reaction."

In about half of the patients the temperature returned to around normal within 24 hours after the beginning of the treatment, and "the condition of most of the remainder was significantly improved in 48 to 72 hours."

There was one death in the group. "This was in a case of early fulminating postoperative pneumonia which developed on the second day after extraperitoneal resection of a carcinoma of the colon." In the case of this patient sulfanilamide, together with rabbit serum were given before the employment of the sulfapyridine, the patient having had 100 grains of sulfanilamide, and 100,000 units, type 13, of rabbit serum on the second day of the pneumonia. The administration of sulfapyridine was started 30 hours before death. The patient was comatose, and for that reason the drug was given per duodenal tube. Autopsy revealed extensive bilateral pneumonia.

In all the patients treated, there was striking reduction of the abnormally high temperature following the administration of sulfapyridine.

The authors say, "It must be emphasized that other patients, whose cases were not reported here, responded satisfactorily to serum, sulfanilamide or neoprontosil and, therefore, did not receive sulfapyridine." At the same time, attention is called to the important fact that some patients who did not respond to other treatment did subsequently respond to sulfapyridine.

Notwithstanding the very satisfactory results, it is clear that the authors do not believe that sulfapyridine is a panacea, and there is a swift and significant reference to preventive measures in the following statement: "Efforts to avoid atelectasis and aspiration may prevent, or even abort, very early postoperative pneumonia." If these efforts are not effectual, then sulfapyridine occupies an important place in the treatment of postoperative pneumonia in the case of all patients where the drug may be given per orum. "Sulfapyridine cannot be administered parenterally because of its insolubility."

The following is a summary of the article: "Sulfapyridine may promptly arrest the progress of postoperative as well as primary pneumonia. It may be successful when other chemotherapeutic agents apparently have failed. It is effective in the treatment of elderly as well as the young patients. Pneumococci are frequently the predominant organisms in the sputum of patients with postoperative pneumonia. The drug appears to be equally effective when pneumococci are not identified in the sputum."

Notes:—Our experience convinces us that sulfapyridine is an agent of remarkable and striking value in the treatment of postoperative pneumonia.

Leroy Long.

The Treatment of Dysmenorrhea With Testosterone Propionate: Udall J. Salmon, M.D., Samuel H. Geist, M.D., and Robert I. Walter, M.D., New York, N. Y.; American Journal of Obstetrics and Gynecology, August, 1939, Vol. 38, No. 2, page 264.

These authors begin their discussion by stating that the subject of dysmenorrhea has engaged the attention of numerous investigators and an extensive literature has accumulated on the subject. There are three current theories as regards the etiology of dysmenorrhea: (a) deficiency of progesterone, permitting the unopposed action of estrogenic hormone upon the uterine muscles; (b) excessive estrogen production resulting in hypermotility of uterine musculature; and (c) excessive progesterone activity. None of these are, however, adequately supported by controlled experimental studies. The authors advance still another theory: that dysmenorrhea may be due to an androgen deficiency (male hormone) resulting in the unopposed action of ovarian hormones.

The rationale for the androgen theory is based on the observation that testosterone counteracts certain of the physiologic effects of the estrogens in animals and human beings. Also favoring this theory are studies reported by Koch recently in which it was found that normal young women excrete daily an average of 26 international units of androgenic substance as compared with an average of 40 international units per day by men of the same age. Only traces are excreted by girls before puberty.

The present study was conducted on a series of 30 patients from 15 to 45 years of age. Seventeen were under 30, 10 between 30 and 40, and three over 40. In all but five the dysmenorrhea had been present since puberty. Twenty-seven had no palpable evidence of pelvic disease; two had suggestive signs of chronic adnexitis; and one had several small myomas. Nineteen had normal, regular menstrual cycles; 11 had various degrees of menorrhagia.

Satisfactory clinical results occurred during the course of treatment in 26 of the 30 cases. Twenty-two had complete relief; four were considerably improved; and in four cases there was no improvement. Following the discontinuation of treatment 17 patients remained symptom-free during the period of observation which varied from three to 24 months. In eight cases there was slight recurrence of pain within two months after discontinuation of testosterone. In one there was complete recurrence of pain one month after the last injection.

Of the four patients who failed to respond, one had uterine myomas; one had chronic adnexitis; and the remaining two exhibited no palpable sign of pelvic disease.

The authors feel that the optimal dosage for relief of dysmenorrhea is in the neighborhood of 250 to 350 mg. of testosterone proprionate given in divided doses during one cycle. If the pain is relieved completely or partially with this dosage, it is advisable to give an additional course of therapy decreasing the amount by half. If only slight or no improvement is obtained, a second course should be given.

In conclusion, dysmenorrhea is attributed to an androgen deficiency resulting in the unopposed or unmodified action of the ovarian hormones. The following evidence is offered in support of this theory: (a) androgens play an important part in normal hormonal economy of the sexually mature female; (b) there is experimental evidence indicating a definite antagonism in the human female between estrogens and androgens; (c) 86 per cent of the cases of functional dysmenorrhea in this series were relieved when treated with a potent androgen (testosterone proprionate).

Although their results in this series have been gratifying, the authors do not believe that testosterone is the complete answer to the problem of dysmenorrhea. They do feel, however, that testosterone is a valuable addition to our therapeutic armamentarium.

Warren Poole.

Recent Developments In Diagnosis and Treatment of Hydatidiform Mole and Chorioepithelioma: By Albert Mathieu, M.D., F.A.C.S., Portland, Oregon; American Journal of Obstetrics and Gynecology, April, 1939, Vol. 37, No. 4, page 654.

An extensive analysis of the literature prior to 1930 including about 1,500 cases of chorioepithelioma and probably 10 times as many moles showed a mortality rate for hydatidiform mole of approximately 12 per cent and that of chorioepithelioma 60 per cent.

Since 1929 when Zondek discovered that gonadotropic hormone was present in the urine of patients with hydatidiform mole, and was greatly increased in amount over that of normal pregnancy, and since 1930, when this same discovery was made in relation to chorioepithelioma, diagnosis, treatment, and prognosis of these diseases changed remarkably.

The author's review of the world's literature for the three years, 1935, 1936 and 1937, involving 576 cases of mole and 266 of chorioepithelioma shows the mortality to be approximately two per cent and 10 per cent respectively.

His analysis of the literature indicates the fact that the decreased mortality is the result of early diagnosis by means of the various biological pregnancy tests and early treatment by hysterectomy.

The author gives a long list of the precautions that should be taken in using these biological tests from a qualitative standpoint. Because of the importance of these precautions, they are quoted: "(1) the test is positive in the presence of living chorionic tissue, which includes normal pregnancy; (2) the test is also positive in hydatidiform mole, chorioepithelioma, or metastases of either disease; (3) the test may be negative in missed molar abortion; (4) the test may be positive for six weeks following the passage of a mole because of stored hormone in the body; (5) if a test is positive two months after the passage of the mole, and normal pregnancy has been excluded, it is likely that living molar tissue is still present or chorioepithelioma has developed; (6) in the presence of lutein cysts after all living chorionic tissue has been removed, the test will be positive until these cysts regress because the hormone is stored in them; (7) a positive test one month after the removal of a chorioepithelioma is strong evidence of metastasis; (8) the spinal fluid gives a negative test in normal pregnancy and a positive test in mole or chorioepithelioma; (9) absolute reliance should not be placed on one test, and in questionable cases the test should be checked and rechecked; (10) the test should be used in all questionable conditions where the element of chorioepithelioma might exist; and (11) the biologic test should overrule contrary clinical and pathologic findings. During a period of a week or so following mole, there might exist a nidus of chorioepithelioma which is too small to produce a sufficient quantity of hormone to be detectable by methods now extant. Al-

though such a nidus is a rarity, it probably explains those few cases reported in which there was a negative test at some period during the transition of mole into chorioepithelioma. If such a nidus exists, it will not be long before it grows sufficiently to give a positive test, or, the test will be positive before the disease gets beyond easy clinical control."

The diagnosis and treatment of hydatidiform mole is concisely given in the following quotation: "When the diagnosis of mole is uncertain the patient should be treated conservatively, but once the diagnosis is certain, it is probably best to empty the uterus at once through the vagina. An important part of the treatment of mole is watchfulness for the advent or presence of chorioepithelioma. Evidence indicates that there are many cases of simultaneous occurrence of these two diseases. In the follow-up treatment there should be repeated biologic pregnancy tests which, when correlated with the clinical findings, will show the presence or absence of chorioepithelioma. The greatest pitfalls in the follow-up treatment of mole are lack of knowledge that chorioepithelioma may ensue and the misconception of the biologic pregnancy test."

Early diagnosis and immediate hysterectomy is the preferable treatment for chorioepithelioma.

The author believes that there is sufficient evidence in the literature to show it is safe to leave the ovaries when hysterectomy is performed, except when there is primary chorioepithelioma of the ovary. In the discussion of this paper, practically all those who discussed it disagreed with him upon this point and felt that bilateral oophorectomy should be performed in the presence of a chorioepithelioma.

The author is quite optimistic in looking forward to a time when the cure of chorioepithelioma will range in the neighborhood of 95 per cent, made possible by early diagnosis and treatment. He not only feels that this may be true, but that the ovaries may also be preserved.

Comment: This author has made a most extensive study of this disease and for a collective review of the literature for the years 1935, 1936, and 1937, on these subjects you are referred to his articles in the International Abstract of Surgery, January, 1939, Vol. 68, pages 52-70, and February 1, 1939, Vol. 68, pages 181-198.

The evidence as shown from this review of literature reveals most amazing improvement in the results in the treatment of these diseases and even these figures do not give full credit as hydatid mole is now being treated conservatively with evacuation of the uterus only and observation by biologic tests, whereas many of these patients were formerly subjected to radical surgery.

However, it is in this very field of conservatism that the greatest precaution should be taken. Full knowledge of the biologic tests employed and their clinical significance, as well as clinical observation of the patient, is fundamental to proper treatment. For example, a patient has come to my attention who had the uterus evacuated, and shortly thereafter a negative Friedmann test. Though she persisted in having vaginal discharge of bloody character, no additional Friedmann tests were done, and the patient succumbed to chorioepithelioma.

In spite of the great improvement that has been made and also the satisfactory conservative management of hydatid mole when precautions are taken, I cannot quite agree with this author in leaving the uterine adnexa behind as they are frequently the site of invasion.

Wendell Long.

EYE, EAR, NOSE AND THROAT
Edited by Marvin D. Henley, M.D.
911 Medical Arts Building, Tulsa

Ocular Manifestations of Brucellosis (Malta Fever; Undulant Fever). Original paper by John Green, M.D., St. Louis, Mo. Published in Digest of Ophthalmology and Otolaryngology, August, 1939. Digested from Trans. of the American Ophthalmological Society, 1938, Pp. 104-126.

An epidemic form of fever in man had long existed in the Mediterranean area and was especially noticed in the island of Malta. Organisms belonging to this group have been given the generic name of Brucella in honor of Sir David Bruce who in 1886 proved the etiologic factor which he called Micrococcus melitensis. In the human being the disease was variously termed Mediterranean, Gibraltar, Malta, undulating, undulant and goat fever.

Human beings may become infected by consuming unpasteurized milk or other dairy products containing Brucella abortus or by infection through skin abrasions and other wounds. The incubation period lasts from five to 15 days. The onset is gradual, with weakness, general malaise, headache, backache, anorexia, and constipation, followed by fever, chills, sweats, aching of the muscles, bones, and joints, and loss of weight. One characteristic is that the appearance and general condition of the patient may be good despite a rapid pulse and high temperature. Physical signs consist of an enlarged spleen, enlarged lymph glands (less frequent), swelling of the joints without redness or pain, and abdominal distress suggestive of appendicitis or cholecystitis.

Positive diagnosis cannot be made on clinical signs alone but, by means of the Opsonocytophagic test, the blood-agglutination test or the skin test it can definitely be determined that a patient has or has had the disease.

Fever therapy, by means of the Kettering hypertherm, has been effective in treatment of some acute cases and probably acts by raising the phagocytic power of the blood. Recently Dr. Lee Foshay of Cincinnati General Hospital has developed an effective serum for acute cases and a vaccine for chronic cases.

Comparatively few ophthalmologists are taking advantage of the opportunity to determine by laboratory methods the presence or absence of past or present Brucella infection although the occurrence of ocular manifestations in the course of brucellosis is now well established. Those who have studied the disease become enthusiastic about the possibilities and implications of the disease. Evidence is accumulating that some ocular maladies hitherto ascribed to other origins may be caused by brucellosis.

It is noted that most ocular lesions occurring in the course of brucellosis do not destroy the integrity of the globe—hence enucleation is not demanded. Clinically and pathologically the eye with melitensis bears great similarity to ocular tuberculosis.

The external ocular muscles, the cornea, the retina, and the optic nerve have all proved to be vulnerable to infection by Brucella. Should not the ophthalmologist include in his list of possible etiologic factors a disease that is so widespread and one that has been proved to be capable of affecting almost every tissue of the body?

The Intra-Capsular Extraction of Cataract with Forceps: Is Its Use Justifiable? Robert Buxton, Weston-Super-Mare. The British Journal of Ophthalmology, August, 1939.

This controversial question is discussed under the following headings:

(1). Historical and general considerations.

(2). Certain complications: their i n c i d e n c e, causes and avoidance.

(3). Choice of cases.

(4). Important details of technique.

This article is about 35 pages in length and is discussed in much detail. There are accompanying illustrations and a long bibliography appended. The author's own summary is as follows:

(1). The advantages and disadvantages of the intra-capsular extraction of cataract with forceps are discussed.

(2). The incidence of certain complications of the operation is investigated.

(3). The importance of a careful selection of cases and attention to minute details of technique is emphasized.

(4). Not until further statistics are published, showing the end-results of selected cases compared with the end-results of the classical operation, can any conclusions be arrived at as to whether the use of the intracapsular operation is justified.

(5). While posessing certain advantages, the intra-capsular operation carries with it an increased risk of certain complications.

(6). The results of the classical operation are so satisfactory that it is doubtful whether it will be superceded by the intracapsular operation even in selected cases.

(7). It is probable that under poor conditions where increased risks have to be taken, e.g., in India, the intra-capsular operation in selected cases is preferable.

Double Injury To The Ear. By Th. De Szentlorinczi-Liebermann and G. Kelemen, Budapest. The Journal of Laryngology and Otology, July, 1939.

This interesting article is most suitably summarized by the authors as follows:

Owing to a fall on the head from a height and the simultaneous penetration of a hairpin into the ear, a double injury occurred, the fall having caused a fracture of the middle and inner ear, whereas the pin penetrating into the ear had brought about a luxation of the stapes. Death occurred after three weeks. Dissection, completed by microscopic investigation of the p e t r o u s bone, showed that the opening of the oval window, caused by the luxation of the stapes, was blocked by granulations. No symptoms of meningitis were found either clinically or as a result of dissection. Death occurred owing to increasing intracranial pressure, caused by a haematoma in the scala posterior. This haematoma followed a rupture in the sinus wall and constantly increased in volume owing to the fact that the irrepressible vomiting pressed fresh quantities of blood through the sinus rupture. The most remarkable phenomenon was that the double nature of the injury was clearly traceable on microscopic examination. Luxation of the stapes without any fracture of the latter must be regarded as a rare condition in the case of non-operative traumata.

PLASTIC SURGERY
Edited by
GEO. H. KIMBALL, M.D., F.A.C.S.
404 Medical Arts Building, Oklahoma City

Lesions of the Tongue: A Collective Review. J. B. Brown, M.D., F.A.C.S., and H. Haffner, M.D., St. Louis, Mo. S. G. & O., August, 1939, Vol. 69, No. 2.

Radical operative removal of the tongue for carcinoma is a rapidly decreasing type of operation but it is interesting to note that most authors recommend a radical dissection of the cervical lymphatics if there is any local cure with radium or local operation possible. Such uniformity of opinion points to the conclusion, at least for the present, that dissection should always be done on the side of involvement and the opposite side closely observed for any evidence of growth in the lymphatic system. Unanimous opinion seems to be that in the early forms of this disease, local treatment with radiation should be carried out and followed by operative dissection of the entire cervical lymphatics.

It would seem from this review that carcinoma of the oral cavity can be divided into three groups according to their amount of extension. (1) Group with a definitely proved local lesion and without palpable glands. (2) Proven local lesions with palpable glands which are small and mobile lending themselves to operative removal. (3) Advanced local lesion with extensive metastisis.

Sanford Cade quotes Wallace's s u m m a r y on glands. Of the first group mentioned in the classification above after the local lesion has been treated the lympahatic area of the neck is given surface radiation. In the second group the glands are radically removed if the condition of the patient permits; if not, interstitial radiation is used. Of the third group those with extensive and gross metastisis treatment of the lymphatic region is by deep X-ray.

If one in considering the reports contained in this article were to attempt to establish some fairly routine procedure in treatment of a carcinoma of the tongue it would most probably be a local treatment of the lesion by operative removal or interstitial radiation followed by a rest period of from four to six weeks and a radical dissection of the cervical lymphatics.

Statistical reports included in the article indicate an improvement of 10 to 15 per cent mortality where early dissection is carried out. One author states that approximately 30 per cent five-year cures should be obtained without nodal involvement whereas those with nodal involvement would probably be less than 10 per cent. This author maintains that successful treatment depends on keeping ahead of the disease and this should best be done by routine neck dissection whether the glands are palpable or not.

Muscle tumors of the tongue fall into two groups:

Rhabdo myoma and myoblastoma. Cappell and Montgomery believe the tongue to be the most common site of tumors arising from muscle cells and emphasize the importance prognostically of differentiation of rhabdomyomas f r o m myoblastomas. The f o r m e r grow as pedunculated small tabloid masses on the tongue and frequently recur and metastisize through the lymphatics in spite of early radical removal. The latter are generally rounded nodules within the substance of the tongue and are frequently cured by local removal.

Congenital lesions of the tongue may be of almost any character, one complete cleft of the tongue has been reported associated with a cleft palate. Congenital cavernous hemangioma is a rather infrequent occurrence usually small at birth but takes on periods of rapid growth. Early treatment is urgent whether in the form of surgery, chemical, physical extirpation.

Macroglossia producing anomalies of occlusion and respiration may occur and should be treated by partial excision sufficient to reduce the tongue to somewhat near normal size as early as the condition of the patient permits.

Chondromas of the tongue are rare, eight cases having reported at the present time; excision is the treatment. Lipomas are a rare occurrence but have been reported.

Tuberculosis of the tongue usually appears in association with advanced pulmonary tuberculosis but occasionally the large ulcerated lesion of the tongue should have a biopsy performed. Tuberculosis may be cured by radical excision of the ulcer site. One case is reported which is presumed to be primary tuberculosis.

Syphilitic ulcers occur on the tongue in association with generalized syphilitic infection and Thuzuki found that 70 per cent of ranula cases are syphilitic. These cases respond to general antiluetic treatment.

Infections of the tongue occur as acute glossitis and primary and secondary abscesses. These conditions are treated in accordance with infections elsewhere in the body.

Comment: This is an exhaustive collective review of lesions of the tongue which represents a very intensive study of the literature and gives some uniformity in the treatment of the various lesions. Carcinoma occupies most of the article and for the most part the authorities agree to treatment of the local lesion followed by a radical removal of the cervical lymphatics. Other lesions of the tongue are given representative consideration with some suggestions as to their management.

───────o───────

ORTHOPAEDIC SURGERY
Edited by Earl D. McBride, M.D., F.A.C.S.
717 North Robinson Street, Oklahoma City

"Calcification of the Supraspinatus Tendon: Cause, Pathologic Picture and Relation to the Scalenus Anticus Syndrome," W. A. Bishop, Jr., Oklahoma City, Oklahoma. Archives of Surgery, Vol. 39, No. 2, August, 1939.

The author discusses the incidence of calcareous deposits of the shoulder, giving a new routine of examination of the shoulder, through which during the past year 27 patients were found to have calcareous deposits. This occurs most commonly between the ages of 30 and 50 years. Men are found to have the condition twice as often as women.

Anatomy of the shoulder region is discussed, primarily with relation to the tendon of the supraspinatus muscle which reenforces the central upper portion of the capsule and is inserted into the anterior and uppermost part of the greater tuberosity.

Discussion of the etiology of this reviewed the controversy of opinions as to the cause. Some feel that calcium is laid down in the unabsorbed hemorrhage which fills the defect in an abortive attempt at repair of minor injuries to the tendon tissue. Others state due to a tendinitis, local necrosis of the tendon and calcification produced by often repeated occupational traumas which squeeze the supraspinatus tendon between the tuberosity of the humerus and the roof of the subacromial bursa. Still others advance the hypothesis of a metabolic factor.

The author feels that deposits are laid down

slowly in the areas of hyaline degeneration subsequent to repair of repeated minor injuries.

Details of pathology follow, after which the symptoms are discussed.

In general the onset is abrupt and very painful, but the history in a very large number of cases elicits an insidious beginning. Abduction and medial rotation are the first motions which are limited and cause pain. Three types of pain are described. They vary in degree from mild to agonizing. 1. Pain at the insertion of the deltoid muscle. It is sharp, cutting or stabbing and is compared to the pain which accompanies motion in an arthritic joint. 2. The greater percentage of patients complain of a constant dull, boring or aching pain localized at the tip of the shoulder at the point of greatest tenderness. 3. This type is associated with this and other lesions about the shoulder consists of pain in the muscles of the neck, in the scapular region and occasionally down the arm as far as the finger tips. This often follows the distribution of the ulnar nerve, with occasionally a numbness which suggest the extremity has "gone to sleep." There may be swelling of the involved hand. These findings are identical with those encountered in the "scalenus anticus syndrome," believed to be due to reflex spasm of the scalenus anticus muscle on the affected side.

Diagnosis of this condition is made on the history and physical findings which consist of tenderness below the tip of the acromion, painful "hitch" on abduction and again on descent of the arm, and the X-ray findings. "Soft" or "semisoft" technique should be used in roentgen examination of the shoulder.

In treatment with the acute onset, the Smith-Petersen type lavage is recommended. In the less severe attacks, sedative and ice bags relieve pain. In the chronic stage diathermy or roentgen therapy is used or the lavage may be used.

A case is reported with the particular symptoms resembling the anterior scalenus syndrome.

If lavage or diathermy does not relieve the condition, surgical removal of the deposit is necessary.

"The Colonna Reconstruction Operation for Ununited Fractures of the Neck of the Femur," Paul C. Colonna, Oklahoma City, Oklahoma. The Jr. Bone & Joint Surg., Vol. XXI, No. 3, July, 1939.

The type of operation as advised by Dr. Colonna has been reviewed in a previous abstract in this Journal. Consequently will not be dealt with in detail, other than the results he has obtained in the past year or so, particularly that done by other men. He sent questionnaires to several orthopedic surgeons and has classified the end-results with reference to: (1) those with surgery performed previous to the reconstruction operation and those without; (2) those with preoperative evidence of arthritis, and those without; (3) those with absorption of the neck and those without.

The best results were obtained in the case where there was no preoperative evidence of arthritis about the joint and without previous hip joint surgery. However, excellent results were obtained in other cases and the author presents definite evidence that this type of reconstruction operation has proved suitable for those cases of old ununited fractures of the neck of the femur which have complete absorption of the neck and necrosis of the head.

Briefly, the operation consists of removal of the head of the femur and insertion of the trochanter immediately into the acetabulum, without removal of the muscles immediately from the trochanter.

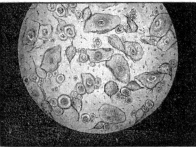
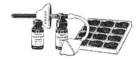

CARDIOLOGY

Edited by F. Redding Hood, M.D.
1200 N. Walker St., Oklahoma City

The Treatment of Hypertension. Nelson W. Barker and Robert W. Graham. Medical Clinics of North America. July, 1939. Mayo Clinic Number.

It has been estimated that approximately 15 per cent of all adults have hypertension and that 23 per cent of those above 53 years of age die as a result of this condition. Knowledge concerning the cause is still imperfect and the large number of drugs, diets and regimens which have been used in the treatment of hypertension, is in itself an indictment.

There have been four theories regarding the cause of essential hypertension. These are: (1) Hyperirritability of the sympathetic vasomotor system. (2) Excessive secretion of the endocrine glands. (Pituitary body, suprarenal gland, thyroid gland.) (3) Exogenous toxins or infections. (4) Obstruction of renal circulation as a result of ischemia, a vasopressor substance, acting directly on the arterioles is liberated into the blood stream. It is possible that essential hypertension may be produced by any one of these four ways.

Essential hypertension first passes through the so-called functional stage in which there is no evidence of organic disease of the arterioles, and in which the blood pressure fluctuates greatly and even returns to normal for short periods. As the disease progresses, organic changes appear in the arterioles and finally there may arise three types of dangerous complications, namely, myocardial insufficiency with congestive heart failure, chronic renal ischemia with renal insufficiency, and cerebral or coronary arterial accidents. In the functional and even in the early organic stages there may be no symptoms; hence the patient usually consults the doctor when the disease is well advanced. Obviously if any treatment is to be successful, it should be instituted as early as possible, and before cardiovascular changes have taken place.

Keith and Wagener have divided cases with essential hypertension into four groups: (1) those with little or no sclerosis of the retinal arteries and without retinitis; (2) those with definite sclerosis of the retinal arteries but without retinitis; (3) those with definite sclerosis of the retinal arteries with retinitis (hemorrhages and exudates) but without edema of the optic disks, and (4) those with definite sclerosis of the retinal arteries with retinitis and edema of the disks. It has been found that in cases in group four, the prognosis is very poor and the disease is extremely refractory to all types of treatment.

In evaluating the results of treatment in hypertension it is necessary to emphasize the fact that the blood pressure in these cases may undergo spontaneous fluctuations. The cold pressor test (Hines) has been valuable in estimating maximal blood pressure and the administrations of barbiturates together with rest in bed, has been valuable in estimating minimal blood pressures in cases of hypertension. The treatment of hypertension may be divided into four parts: (1) general and dietary measures, (2) the use of drugs and biological preparations, (3) surgical procedures and (4) treatment of complications.

General and Dietary Measures:

It has long been recognized that rest and the reduction of nervous stresses and strains are important in the treatment of hypertensive patients. Such a program has to be adapted to the individual case. In general, patients with hypertension should be advised to get adequate sleep at night, to take a short rest following their noon meal, to avoid excitement, and if possible, to limit their business responsibilities. When the patients are young, it may be possible for them to select occupations which entail a minimal degree of nervous strain. In cases of severe or advanced hypertension further nervous relaxation may be obtained by prolonged quiet vacations, sojourns to warm climates during the winter, the use of hot baths, and occasional days spent in bed. There is no justification for stating a gloomy prognosis to the patient or for discussing the possibility of a cerebral vascular accident, as anxiety may be a definite factor in exaggerating the hypertension.

Evidence that anything may be definitely gained from reduction of protein intake in uncomplicated cases is lacking. The question of intake of sodium chloride is debatable, but a low sodium chloride is probably advisable. Hypertension with obesity constitutes a definite dietary management with the aim of reduction of weight. Patients with hypertension should not take coffee or alcohol in amounts to produce insomnia or nervous excitement. There is increasing evidence to show that the use of tobacco is harmful and may be the main factor in augmenting the blood pressure.

The Use of Drugs and Biologic Preparations:

In a general way, results as indicated by careful studies over a period of time have been disappointing.

Sedatives: Barbiturates and bromides have been used extensively because of their depressant action on the sympathetic nervous system, avoiding as much depression of the higher cortical centers as possible. Barbiturates have less danger of toxic effects.

Sulfocyanates: The exact method of action has not been determined and should only be used when patients can be kept under close observation, and where tests for concentration in the blood can be made periodically. There is a definite tendency toward accumulation and serious toxic effects may occur when a concentration reaches 18 mg. per 100 cc's. Concentration should be maintained between six and 12 mg. per 100 cc.

Nitrites and Nitrates: They produce a definite fall in the blood pressure due to peripheral vasodilitation, but their effects are too transient to produce any definite therapeutic effect.

The Methyl Purines: Caffeine, theobromine and theophylline have been used for their vasodilitation effect, and are usually combined with some barbiturate.

Iodides: Have been used empirically but their physiological action is questionable.

Tissue Extracts: Pancreatic tissue extract, liver

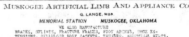
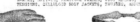

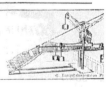

extract, various muscle extracts and others have been known to give a definite fall in blood pressure when given intravenously to animals. However, they are not safe to use on human beings, but when given intramuscularly or subcutaneously may have little or no effect.

Ovarian Hormones: The administration of estrogenic hormone has relieved symptoms in many instances where hypertension has come on with the menopause but has been very disappointing in its effect on blood pressure.

Surgical Treatment of Hypertension:

At present the operation of choice is sympathectomy, however, it will be necessary to wait several years longer before making a critical evaluation of this treatment for hypertension. In those cases in which definite unilateral renal disease associated with hypertension, if the blood pressure has returned to normal following nephrectomy and in rare instances where hypertension is associated with renal tumors, operation of such tumors is justified.

Treatment of Complications:

In most cases where hypertension has progressed to the stage where cardiac, renal or vascular complications have occurred, it is necessary to direct treatment chiefly toward these complications and therapy is largely a matter of conservation. The treatment of coronary and vascular accidents is essentially the same as when hypertension does exist. The outlook in cases of hypertensive heart disease and congestive heart failure is poor. It is often possible, by prolonged periods of long rest in bed and by the use of dieuretics and occasionally digitalis, to restore compensation but it usually only a matter of months before the condition recurs. When renal insufficiency is present without edema, the intake of fluids should be high (3,000 cc) and the intake of protein should be restricted to approximately 50 mg. daily. The occurrence of renal insufficiency is an extremely bad prognostic sign as it is usually evidence of advanced chronic renal ischemia of a progressive type.

---o---

INTERNAL MEDICINE
Edited by Hugh Jeter, M.D., 1200 North Walker, Oklahoma City

The Incidence of Intestinal Parasites—An Analysis of 2,265 Routine, Consecutive Stool Examinations In the Outpatient Dispensaries of Charity Hospital of Louisiana at New Orleans. Emma S. Moss. (American Journal of Clinical Pathology, July, 1939, Volume 9, Number 4.)

In this the authors have made an extremely interesting and valuable analysis of 2,265 routine stool examinations for parasites. Many very valuable tables have been prepared showing the incidence of parasites as to race, age and sex.

Nine hundred and nineteen of the 2,265 stool specimens, or 40.5 per cent, were positive for at least one parasite.

It is interesting to note that of the 146 cases of ascaris, 138 of them were in patients over 16 years of age. Twenty-eight of the patients were white males and 47 white females. Thirty-seven were colored males and 34 colored females. The sex and race incidence is practically parallel.

Trichocephalus trichiurus is the most frequent helminth encountered.

Endamoeba coli is the most frequent protozoa.

Giardia lamblia was present in 182 cases.

Ascaris lumbricoides appeared alone 63 times and in association with other parasites 80 times.

Endamoeba histolytica showed an absolute incidence of 3.4 per cent. This is based on the finding of typical cysts and is therefore somewhat lower than the figures usually achieved, which take into consideration precystic forms.

Strongyloides stercoralis appeared more frequently alone than in association with other parasites and more common in males and in patients over 20 years of age and only three times in negro subjects.

Enterobius vermicularis. This parasite appeared 27 times alone and 18 times in association with other parasites. Eighteen were males and 27 females. Thirty-nine were under 20 years and six over 20 years of age.

Necator americanus. A casual check of the data reveals that the majority of subjects studied belonged to the urban population from rural districts.

Endolimax nana. This parasite appeared 53 times and its chief importance seems to lie in the fact that it may be confused with amoeba histolytica.

Taenia saginata. Of the 10 infections with this parasite, only one was in association with other parasites. Only two of the 10 subjects were over 20 years of age.

Progress in Internal Medicine. Blood—A Review of the Literature. Cyrus C. Sturgis, M.D., Raphael Isaacs, M.D., S. Milton Goldhamer, M.D., and Frank H. Bethell, M.D., Ann Arbor, Mich. (Archives of Internal Medicine, July, 1939, Volume 64, Number 1.)

This is a continuation of this report, the first part being in the preceding journal.

As is the yearly custom the authors have reviewed many articles, 512 in all, which have been published recently on the subject of blood and allied diseases. Much recent data has been collected, such as the effects of certain recent drugs.

Kracke's work is outstanding in connection with the study of granulocytopenia. Two important diagnostic points are emphasized by Kracke, the first being that the patient with granulocytopenia shows no disturbance of the hemoglobin, erythrocytes or platelets, unless the process is prolonged. The second point is that there seems to be general agreement that these patients exhibit a marked degree of prostration entirely out of proportion to physical signs. Kracke also considers the present method of treating granulocytopenia as highly unsatisfactory and states, "No one man probably has treated a sufficient number of cases to form a proper evaluation of therapeutic agents." He points out that the granulocytopenic patient is suffering from two distinct diseases. One is depletion of white cells and the other, an invasion of organisms resulting from the lowered resistance.

He gives ten times the usual doses of liver extract in connection with the treatment.

Considerable emphasis has been placed and is herein reported in connection with the relation between sulfanilamide and granulocytopenia. Reznikoff considers that there are four important factors in connection with the causation of granulocytopenia: (1) fatigue, (2) drugs, (3) menstruation and (4) infection.

Reviews of work on anemia, pregnancy, Hodgkin's disease, lymphosarcoma, leukemia, leukemoid conditions, bone marrow and hematological methods are also abstracted.

---o---

UROLOGY
Edited by D. W. Branham, M.D.
514 Medical Arts Building, Oklahoma City

Urologic and Cutaneous Review. Lithiasis number. August, 1939.

This issue is devoted entirely to the consideration of urinary lithiasis and the majority of the articles consider various clinical and pathological aspects of renal and ureteral calculi.

Kahle and Maltry analyze 66 cases of large ureteral calculi from a clinical standpoint. The statistical data obtained is interesting.

Bowers discusses urinary calculi and concludes that urinary calculi are not a product of modern civilization and that no single simple explanation for calculous formation can be advanced. He is convinced that many ureteral and vesical calculi can be removed by conservative surgical methods. So called "silent" renal stones should not be treated expectantly but should be removed before they produce additional damage to the kidney. Incisions made in the kidney and ureter in order to remove stones should be allowed to close without suture.

Turner presents a very comprehensive article on the management of stone in the ureter. The multiple catheter has in his hands been the most successful method for the removal of such calculi. As far as the prevention of recurrent calculi he shares the same belief as many others that ones efforts in this direction are limited, but particular attention should be paid to the eradication of infection of the urinary tract, the correction of metabolic dysfunction and the promotion of better drainage to correct stasis.

Deakin presents a case which demonstrates the value of a permanent nephrostomy in an individual afflicted with recurrent stone of the kidney. The same procedure was shown to be of benefit in four cases of solitary kidney in an article by Wright.

Lazarus discusses the etiological factor of trauma in the formation of renal stone. He cites one case in detail which definitely proved that trauma was the predominant factor for the formation of a large stone in the kidney.

An important article was one by Abeshouse and Zinberg in which was discussed the similarity of the distribution of pain in herpes zoster and renal lithiasis. Case reports are presented which demonstrate the close similarity of the neurologic attack of herpes zoster to that of renal colic.

Prostatic calculi are considered in the article by Lynch and Thompson. They discuss the etiology, symptoms, diagnosis and treatment and cite typical case histories.

Comment: Recent literature on urinary calculi has placed much emphasis on the etiological factors of diet and vitamin deficiency towards the formation of stones. Reading this particular issue gives one the impression that the contributors of these articles hold little confidence that diet or vitamins have very much to do with calculous formations. Undoubtedly this phase of study has been overly exaggerated by enthusiastic investigators. Most of the essayists are of the opinion that in instances of recurrent calculi chief dependence for prophylaxis can hardly be placed on diet or vitamins in order to prevent recurrence. Eradicating infection and the correction of urinary stasis is fundamentally important for the prophylaxis of stone.

As far as the actual removal of ureteral stones is concerned the majority of urologists are of the opinion that the simple catheter or multiple catheter method is the safest. With this procedure a goodly percentage can be removed or encouraged to pass spontaneously. Failure in this method of removal warrants recourse to open surgery.

---o---

Index to Advertisers

THE JOURNAL
OF THE
OKLAHOMA STATE MEDICAL ASSOCIATION

| VOLUME XXXII | McALESTER, OKLAHOMA, OCTOBER, 1939 | Number 10 |

Pseudomycotic Leg Ulcers*

J. F. HAMILTON, M.D.†
Instructor In Medicine, University of Tennessee
MEMPHIS, TENNESSEE

A peculiar variety of indolent leg ulcer has held the writer's attention and has been of much interest to him for the past 12 years. In December, 1927[1], a study was made of the ulcers of two patients, the like of which had never been seen before. It later developed that the name of neither the disease nor its etiological agent had ever been put in print. To Castellani goes the credit of naming the disease and its causative micro-organism which was recorded in his case report published in December, 1928[2].

Pseudomycosis is characterized by the formation of more or less superficial ulcers with the constant tendency for the ulcers to become chronic and from which may be isolated micro-organisms resembling the hemolytic streptococcus. Furthermore, the pre-ulcer stage in some patients is accompanied by a systemic reaction with fever and rigors. These systemic reactions are usually associated with the infection when it manifests itself in the form of a diffuse cellulitis. As a rule, however, the disease is manifested by the formation of an ulcer with local pain, swelling, redness, and with very little or no general systemic reaction.

The name "pseudomycosis" given the disease by Castellani[2], implies the presence of a mycotic-like ulcer but never having recovered a yeast or fungus from the ulcers, it can not be classified as a true mycosis. This fact, no doubt, prompted Castellani, whose experience with the disease dated back to 1910 when in Ceylon[3], to give it the name pseudomycosis. Castellani also named the micro-organism so constantly associated with the ulcer, the "micrococcus (streptococcus) myceticus" which is considered to be the causative agent. Lancefield[4], of the Rockefeller Institute, New York, after studying a culture we sent her, classified the micrococcus as a hemolytic streptococcus belonging to group A, but was unable to classify it as to type in this group.

There is strong reason to believe that the same entity about which we have written under the caption "pseudomycosis" has been considered under other titles, such as , "lacunar ulcer" by Kilbourne[5], "chronic undermining ulcer" by Meleney[6-7], and Goodman[8] on "chronic streptococcus ulcer of the skin." It is felt that the name pseudomycosis as applied to the indolent leg ulcer previously described[1-2] needs no defense.

A large number of our patients present multiple ulcers with a definite mycotic-like appearance with the bases covered with pale to pink granulations, or greyish-white necrotic material, and thick undermined skin edges with intercommunicating daughter ulcers near the main ulcer and from which, in every case, micrococcus (streptococcus) myceticus is isolated —obtaining many times a pure growth on direct culture[9-10]. There are other ulcers, however, less mycotic in appearance from which the same micro-organism morpho-

*Presented before the General Session, Annual Meeting, Oklahoma State Medical Association, Oklahoma City, Oklahoma, May 3, 1939.
†Dr. Willis C. Campbell Clinic.

logically and biochemically to that found in the undermined ulcers, have been isolated. It is in the discrete smooth edged ulcer which has had various medicaments applied before coming to the clinic that we may fail to find the micrococcus myceticus. But in the actively undermining form, r e c o v e r y of the micro-organism never has failed if the material for cul-

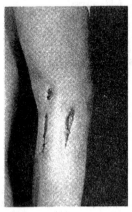

FIG. I

Mr. B. B. H., No. 29297, age 23, photograph 3-21-32 showing three ulcers which intercommunicate through subcutaneous sinuses. Duration of disease four months.

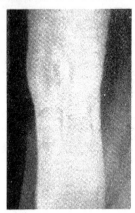

FIG. II

Mr. B. B. H., No. 29297, age 23, photograph 7-6-32 showing scars five weeks following incision of skin overlying sinuses. Duration of treatment four months. Duration of disease eight months.

ture is taken from the undermined area. Many cultures, if made from open ulcers, show a mixed bacterial flora. This fact is probably responsible for the term "symbiotic ulcer" as used by some authors.

There has been no history obtained in any patient of the occurrence of spontaneous multiple ulcers at the onset. The onset is usually quite insidious with local itching or stinging to which the patient pays little attention. But in the following 24 to 48 hours, a small pustule accompanied by local increased skin temperature, swelling, redness or tenderness may be seen. If the pustule is visible, it usually opens itself spontaneously in a short time resulting in a small ulcer and instead of beginning to resolve and heal, after liberating itself of the visible pus, the opposite takes place — namely; the ulcer spreads equally or irregularly in all directions frequently undermining the skin for a variable distance. Once an ulcer is formed and r e m a i n s open, the discharge is no longer purulent but assumes a serosanguinous character. The s k i n overlying the subcutaneous sinus is frequently thickened with a rolled edge. At the blind end of the sinus, perhaps an inch or more removed from the main ulcer may appear a daughter ulcer, the first indication of which will be a small tender red spot.

This daughter ulcer reminds o n e o f a perforation made by a shot, as it is so smooth and round. If the ulcer enlarges by an undermining of the skin, its outline will naturally be irregular as the tendency is for the main ulcer and the daughter ulcers to merge together forming one large ulcer. If the main ulcer does not enlarge by the undermining of the skin, its outline is more even, it increases in size much slower, its skin edge less thick, and it presents more of a scooped out appearance. With either of the above forms of the ulcer, they may be multiple on a single limb on admission. They may be several inches apart, suggesting either auto-inoculation, or a lymphatic mode of distribution.

Personal observation is convincing that auto-inoculation can occur from one leg to another by even the apposition of the ulcer against the healthy skin of the uninvolved leg[10]. Auto-inoculation by means of contaminated fingers is highly probable also. One wonders why more auto-inoculation especially to distant parts of the body does not take place.

The powerful necrotising effect of the infection upon the skin in some patients has been appalling. This has been seen to occur in spite of the application of all forms of treatment. Indeed, it is our opinion that this property of the c a u s a t i v e micro-organism together with the sinus produc-ing effect are reasons why treatment is so

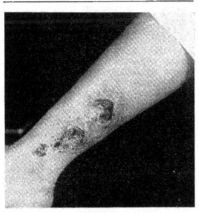

FIG. III

Miss P. B., No. 05753, age 11, photograph 12-13-34. Multiple ulcers with excoriation of surrounding skin. Duration, 24 months.

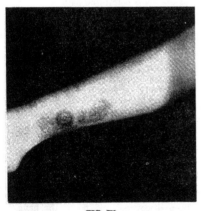

FIG. IV

Miss P. B., No. 05753, age 11, photograph 2-5-35, showing ulcer healed. Duration of treatment seven weeks. Duration of disease about 26 months.

ineffective and the morbidity rate is so high.

The ulcerations are strikingly unilateral. In an analysis of 44 patients previously re-ported[9-10], there were only two who had bilateral limb involvement. In only one patient, has an ulcer been seen on the body above the level of the knee. In our series of about 75 patients, only two have had re-currences. In both of these, there were ulcers of both legs at the time of their re-currences, and in one there was an ulcer at the level of the knee of the nearby in-volved limb and several in the upper third of the thigh. Fifteen to 24 months inter-vened between these recurrences.

The mode of entrance of the micrococcus myceticus into the body is not known. The history in certain patients would lead one to believe the bacterium is capable of en-tering through the unbroken skin. How-ever, there is no proof of this a c t u a l l y taking place. The cause of the disease has been attributed to many different and ab-surd agents such as shoe dye[1], nail punc-ture[11], and insect bites (mosquito, spi-der)[9].

Gram's stain of a direct smear of the mi-crococcus (streptococcus) m y c e t i c u s is usually gram negative appearing as diplo-cocci and in short chains. Some smears may contain both gram negative and gram positive diplococci. The large number of intracellular gram negative diplococci and their arrangement within the pus cells are striking observations and moreover may be quite confusing to the inexperienced ob-server; so much so, that one may suspect their being gonococci. Diligent search will be rewarded by the finding of short chains of gram negative cocci and, perhaps, gram positive diplococci in the same smear. This should aid in preventing one from making a diagnosis of gonococci from the smear alone. We have a record of a patient who was told he had gonococcic arthritis of the knee because of swelling and tenderness of the soft tissues and who upon admis-sion had no evidence of having had an arthritis, but who did have a d r a i n i n g sinus of several months' duration follow- · ing surgical i n c i s i o n of what was most likely a micrococcus myceticus cellulitis. Further suggestive evidence of this being the case, was the fact that the patient was told only bloody fluid was obtained at the time the surgical incision was made. We recovered the micrococcus myceticus in smear and culture from the sinus at the time this p a t i e n t was admitted to the Clinic. The o n s e t of his disability was nine months before admission. It took us three months to cure him.

We have had very little difficulty in growing the micrococcus myceticus. Special media such as dextrose brain broth, Loeffler's blood s e r u m and blood agar plates serve satisfactorily to grow it as well as to perpetuate the culture. Caution must be exercised in that transplants must be made every few days in order to consistently preserve the stock c u l t u r e. Cultures of the coccus may be trained to grow, eventually, on ordinary media such as plain agar, but one will not o b t a i n growth on this medium upon direct inoculation from the ulcer.

In dextrose brain broth, growth is fluent and in the form of long chains which tend to become entangled to form visible flocculi which eventually settle to the bottom of the tube, leaving a clear supernatant medium above.

Growth on blood agar plate appears in from 18 to 48 hours and invariably hemolyzes the blood. The colonies at first are pinpoint greyish-white, moist, smooth, and becoming granular at the b o r d e r later, with the tendency to become c o n f l u e n t later.

The cocci isolated from the pseudomycotic ulcers grow better under anaerobic conditions. This has been demonstrated by inoculating two p o u r e d blood agar plates at the same time and incubating one in a Novy jar and the other under aerobic conditions.

One needs all available information in diagnosing pseudomycosis. The diagnosis must rely upon the history, clinical findings and laboratory data. A history of long standing ulceration of the leg is pertinent. Especially is this true if the consistent conventional forms of treatment have been applied. There may be a history of one or more of the ulcers having healed while at the same time new ones made their appearance. To one familiar with the disease the very appearance of these ulcers is peculiar and different to the usual run of ulcers. They are often multiple and frequently seen in the 'teen age and in

young adults. Thirty-one of 44 patients analysed and reported elsewhere[9-10] were less than 31 years old. The period of morbidity will be greatly extended if one relies upon the laboratory diagnosis alone to guide him in his therapy. This is due to the likelihood of the laboratory reporting the culture as being an ordinary hemolytic streptococcus and the unsuspecting physician being disregardful of its presence and importance in such a lesion, applies the usual ointments or salves to the ulcer and allows the patient to go on about his affairs. This is especially true if the ulcer is of the more uniform rounded nonundermined form. On the other hand, let it be e m p h a s i z e d that one should suspect pseudomycosis in any patient with an ulcer of the leg from which an hemolytic streptococcus is reported as having been recovered by the laboratory.

A few patients with chronic skin syphilis have been encountered in the Clinic which were somewhat c o n f u s i n g with pseudomycosis, clinically, but were ruled out by obtaining a p o s i t i v e complement fixation test and by not finding the micrococcus myceticus on culture. The true mycoses and streptothricoses are ruled out by careful clinical and laboratory studies.

Varicose ulcers should give little or no trouble in differential diagnosis, especially if no special treatment has been applied to the veins before the patient is seen. It is conceded that pseudomycosis may coexist with varicose ulcers in which case, if the micrococcus (streptococcus) myceticus is found in the ulcer, it may be exceedingly difficult or impossible to determine which condition was primary. In such a case, treatment directed at the eradication of the infection should take precedence over all other therapy.

Tuberculosis of the skin is very rare and may be ruled out by biopsy and animal inoculation.

Out of the 44 patients, analysed as referred to above, 39 of them had no complicating factors whatever.

The prognosis in pseudomycosis is favorable in all patients. No bacteremia has been discovered and no deaths have occurred in our series.

The degree of resistance of the micrococcus myceticus infections to all kinds of therapy so far tried is amazing. Moreover, the slowness with which healing occurs is disappointing. A high morbidity rate is a natural consequence. It was not at all uncommon in our series of patients[9-10] for the disease to have run a course of from a few months to several years. The s h o r t e s t duration of the disease in the 44 patients previously reported was four weeks; the longest, 10 years, giving an average of 13.2 months. The shortest period of treatment before healing was established in our series was two weeks; the longest, 14.5 months, with the average being 2.7 months. We have used practically all of the different chemotherapeutic agents, as well as vaccines, X-rays and heliotherapy in an attempt to find the most effective method of treatment. Under p r e s e n t methods of treatment, the morbidity is still too high.

Although we have been unable to associate an i m p a i r e d circulation with the chronic ulceration, it is imperative that the patient be put to bed. This can not be over emphasized. Failing to demand absolute bed rest, but attempting to treat the patient while ambulant, will bring disappointment to the patient and reflection upon the physician's success. One wonders if some of these ulcers would ever heal if bed rest were not demanded of the patient.

If upon examination, the ulcer is found to be dirty and covered with a crust, it is necessary to r e m o v e this immediately. This may be done manually or by means of a wet dressing of 10 to 25 per cent urea solution. This solution is very effective in removing all exudative material and may also aid in the production of granulation tissue. The wet dressing should be applied for one or two hours, three times a day, until it has accomplished its purpose. If the ulcer on admission is fairly clean, urea may not be necessary, but a continuous wet dressing of potassium permanganate solution of 1 to 1,500 dilution may be applied for the first 48 to 72 hours, changing the dressing once daily. After this initial period is passed, it may be used at night and at intervals during the day. We have found this highly effective in the open ulcers.

For the past four years we have been using Cysteine hydrochloride[12] in one-half of one per cent solution as a wet dressing for one hour three times a day. This is probably the most effective single therapeutic agent that we have used. The solution must be used while fresh and it is recommended that the part of the dressing next to the ulcer be discarded every 15 to 30 minutes during the treatment.

During the intervals between the wet dressings, cradle heat should be applied. In fact, it may be left over the affected limb continuously night and day.

In order to effectively treat the undermining dissecting type of ulcer, the above measures may be used but with little or no effect unless and until the actively infected undermined tissue is made accessible to the therapeutic agent by laying open the sinus. Even though surgical incision may be necessary, it must be said that the least surgery done is by far the safer. It is in this type of patient and those with diffuse cellulitis following surgical procedures, that we have seen the most extensive ulceration, and the severest systemic reactions. The electric cautery probably is the best choice of instrument to use in opening the sinus. If this is not accessible, immediate chemical cauterization of the freshly incised tissue is advised.

If skin grafting is contemplated it should be done with safety only after a number of bacterial c o u n t s have been made in which no gram-negative or gram-positive intracellular or extracellular diplococci are found in the ulcer. If these c o c c i are present in the ulcer when the grafts are applied many, if not all, of the grafts will probably be destroyed. This has happened repeatedly[9].

Zinc peroxide has not given any marked results in our experience although we have not used it in a large number of patients. The same thing is true in regard to sulfanilamide. Further use shall be made of it as opportunity p e r m i t s. Goodman's[8] work with sulfanilamide in his ulcer patients, granting the etiology is the same in both, in so far as its s h o r t e n i n g the period of morbidity, did not seem to be any more effective than our therapeutic regime. However, a larger series of patients treated with it may prove the supposition erroneous.

If interest is not aroused in this disease among physicians, especially general practitioners, surgeons, internes, and dermatologists, the condition will continue to exist unrecognized and the patient may thus nurse his ulcers for years. For it is the doctor who is treating the patient who must first suspect the type of ulcer he sees and in turn make the laboratory personnel wise as to his suspicion. If haemolytic streptococci are cultured from an ulcer one should immediately become suspicious that the condition may be pseudomycosis.

CONCLUSIONS

1. Pseudomycosis is a d e f i n i t e entity with a definite known etiology.

2. It is characterized locally either by the formation of a single pustule followed by an ulcer with no systemic reaction, or by a marked tissue reaction simulating a cellulitis accompanied by rigors, fever and leucocytosis. An undermining necrotizing effect to the skin is almost pathognomonic of pseudomycosis.

3. Micrococcus (streptococcus) myceticus has been recovered consistently from open as well as closed lesions.

4. The infection is believed to gain entrance into the body through the skin and not by way of the blood stream.

5. Locally the infection is thought to spread through the tissue spaces by direct continuity and by way of the lymphatics. Furthermore, there is strong evidence that auto-inoculation can and does occur.

6. The marked resistance to all forms of therapy is striking.

7. The disease has recurred as long as two years following the first infection.

8. Data concerning diagnosis and treatment are recorded.

BIBLIOGRAPHY

1. Hamilton, J. F. Pseudomycosis Due to Micrococcus Myceticus: Preliminary Report. Journ. of So. Med. Association, Birmingham, Ala., March, 1931, 195-200.

2. Castellani, Aldo: Pseudomycosis Due to Coccus: Micrococcus Myceticus. Arch. Dermat. & Syph., 18:857, Dec., 1928. Abstract in the International Med. Digest, Tice, 14:140, March, 1929.

3. Castellani, Aldo: Personal Communication.

4. Lancefield, Rebecca C.: Correspondence.

5. Kilbourne, N. J.: Leg Ulcers of Unrecognized Etiology. J.A.M.A., 98:1955, June 4, 1932.

6. Meleney, Frank L.: Zinc Peroxide in the Treatment of Microaerophilic and Anaerobic Infections, with Special Reference to a Group of Chronic, Ulcerative, Burrowing, Non-Gangrenous Lesions of the Abdominal Wall Apparently Due to a Microaerophilic Hemolytic Streptococcus. Ann. Surg., 101:997, April, 1935.

7. Meleney, Frank L., and Johnson, B. A.: Further Laboratory and Clinical Experiences in the Treatment of Chronic, Undermining, Burrowing Ulcers with Zinc Peroxide. Surgery 1:169, Feb., 1937.

8. Goodman, M. H.: Correspondence. Chronic Streptococcic Ulcer of the Skin, Unresponsive to Local Therapy, But Cured by Sulfanilamide, Report of Two Cases. J.A.M.A., 111:1427-1431, October 15, 1938.

9. Hamilton, J. F.: Further Report on Pseudomycosis: Indolent Leg Ulcer Based on a Study of 54 Patients. Journ. of Tropical Med. and Hygiene, January 1, 1938.

10. Hamilton, J. F.: Pseudomycosis: Indolent Leg Ulcer. A Study of 54 Patients. South. Med. Journal, June, 1938, 579-590.

11. Hamilton, J. F.: Pseudomycosis: Case Report. Memphis Med. Journal, August, 1931.

12. Brunsting, L. A., and Simonsen, D. G.: Cutaneous Ulcers Treated by the Sulphydryl Containing Amino Acid Cysteine. Proc. Staff Meet. of the Mayo Clinic, 8:508, August 23, 1933.

Hospital Care and Schizophrenia

The importance of early hospitalization in bringing about recovery from schizophrenia (cleavage of mental functions) is emphasized in The Journal of the American Medical Association for June 10 by Jules Gelperin, M.D., Cincinnati, who made a study of 235 patients in the Cincinnati General Hospital.

The greater tendency for recovery among patients hospitalized soon after the onset of symptoms, he points out, is apparently not related to any specific treatment but rather to general care.

Of 103 patients whose symptoms were of less than six months' duration prior to hospital admission, 53 were discharged from the hospital improved. Of 30 patients whose symptoms were present for from six to 24 months prior to hospital admission, nine were discharged as improved. Twenty-seven patients showed improvement among the 90 whose symptoms were present for more than 24 months prior to hospitalization. Five of 12 patients whose symptoms were of undetermined duration were improved at the time of discharge from the hospital.

Dr. Gelperin later tried to interview all of the 94 improved patients, but only 21 could be located in the comumnity. Three had reentered the hospital because of recurrence of the condition, 12 months, 22 months and four years after the first discharge.

The 18 patients (14 men and four women) who remained in the community with no return of their symptoms were interviewed. Eleven of the men were working full time and three part time. One woman was working full time outside her home and three were carrying on their household duties.

These improved patients had remained out of the hospital from one to 55 months, the average being 25.9 months.

Sulfapyridine Brings About Recovery of Girl With Influenzal Meningitis

Treatment with sulfapyridine resulted in the recovery of a girl of 2 from influenzal meningitis with bacteria in the blood stream, Tom R. Hamilton, M.D., and Frank C. Neff, M.D., Kansas City, report in The Journal of the American Medical Association for Sept. 16.

The authors knew of no published report of this type of meningitis in which treatment with sulfapyridine had been successful but said it seemed advisable to try it, especially since serum treatment offered little benefit.

Their patient's temperature became normal on the sixteenth day of illness, up to which time sulfapyridine was used in large doses and then reduced. Recovery has been complete without any remaining detrimental signs.

Pregnant Woman May Eat Cucumbers

There is no basis for the idea that cucumbers and melons should be avoided during pregnancy, according to The Journal of the American Medical Association.

Conditions Involving the External Ear*

HUGH EVANS, M.D.
TULSA, OKLAHOMA
Discussed By A. H. DAVIS, M.D.
TULSA, OKLAHOMA

By far the most common o r g a n i s m s which invade the ear canal are the well known pyogens, streptococcus and staphylococcus. Of the former, streptococcus hemolyticus has been cited as the offender in the greatest number of cases, while of the latter, staphylococcus aureus is most often encountered.

Corneybasterium diptheria, corneybacterium a c n e s, plaut-vincent's organism, bacillus funduliformis, pneumococci and in rare instances the tubercle bacillus are among the bacteriological factors involved. While some reports give the influenza bacillus as a causative organism, the consensus of opinion is to the effect that an influenzal filterable virus alone without the interference of the influenzal bacillus is the etiological factor, and that when the latter occurs it is only incidental. Some authors, however, maintain that both the virus and the bacterium must be present, and the matter resolves itself into a moot question.

Pathogenic fungi and yeasts, as well as many which seemingly play the roles of harmless saprophytes in nature, but which are capable of producing lesions in the animal body, have been cited more and more frequently in the literature, and are classified under the general heading as otomycosis. It o c c u r s more frequently than is ordinarily suspected and is often unrecognized, but may cause considerable discomfort. A s p e r g i l l i, penicillia, the pathogenic yeasts and mucoracea, and certain of the tinea group of organisms, are most commonly found. It cannot be overlooked that such invasions may prepare the way for infections of staphylococcus and streptococcus.

Eczematous otitis externa may be confused with true eczema. Dermatologists

Read before the Section on Eye, Ear, Nose and Throat, Annual Meeting, Oklahoma State Medical Association, Oklahoma City, May 3, 1939.

today generally agree that the majority of cases of so-called eczema of the external auditory meatus are really examples of infective meatitis. Mitchell, a dermatologist of Chicago, states that itching and scaling skin conditions of the ear are often termed eczema and mycosis, but in reality they are pyogenic infections caused by hemolytic streptococci. It has been shown that the eczematous reaction occurs when the tissue cells of the skin become sensitized to any of the infecting micro-organisms or their antigens. Hence, it may superimpose itself upon any of the simple infections such as are produced by pityrosporon, staphylococcus aureus, streptococci or even the tubercle bacillus. In passing it is well to m e n t i o n a few conditions which may be found, which are not of infectious origin, but which must be considered in differential diagnosis.

Malignancies are receiving a great deal of public attention today. It is of note that malignancies of the external a u d i t o r y meatus are of such rare occurrence that little reference is made to them in text books. In fact, it accounts for only 0.197 per cent of affections reported by the Eye, Ear, Nose & Throat department of the Edinburg Royal Informary. It is not usually difficult to diagnose, but it may be simulated by chronic inflammation with granulation tissue, by lupus of the ear or by rodent ulcer. Histological procedure should be resorted to in doubtful cases.

Ossification in the auricle is rare. It is usually observed in males past 50 years of age, and sometimes produces no symptoms. It may be c a u s e d by frost bite, syphilitic perichondritis and general debilitating disease.

Hand Schuller Christian's disease, which is a disturbance in the lipoid metabolism and characterized by the triad of symptoms (1) defects in the membranous bones,

(2) diabetes insipidus and (3) exopthalmus, frequently involves the parietal and temporal bones. Graufenstein found evidence of ear involvement in 50 per cent of the cases reviewed. Rosenberg reports a case of xanthoma of the external canal, the type of cell being the same as found in this disease.

In secondary lues, condylomata may occur in the external meatus. The discharge is usually serous and may have a foul odor.

Suppurating sebaceous cysts may occur, since the cutaneous lining of the external auditory meatus is well supplied with sebacious glands, and the signs and symptoms may closely resemble furunculosis.

PREDISPOSING FACTORS

1. *Trauma:* This is by far the most common predisposing factor, particularly in furunculosis. Any mechanical cause acting locally may accomplish this. Attempts to clean the ear by such objects as toothpicks, matches, hair-pins, ear-spuds, and so on, may result in the introduction of organisms and production of lesions; sea bathing or fresh water bathing and accidents of any nature may be factors.

2. When trauma is absent, there may be found to e x i s t *debilitating disorders* lowering the general resistance to infection, such as tuberculosis, diabetes, cardiac disease, trophic nerve changes and rheumatism. Or there may be chronic skin disorders of the face and ears, such as seborrheic tendency, eczema or other scaly affections. Excessive use of bromides has been mentioned as a predisposing factor. Occasionally one will see infections accompanying or following an acute head catarrh.

3. *Acute infections* may be primary invaders, and thus serve as predisposing factors, chief of which are s c a r l e t fever, measles, pneumonia, diphtheria, influenza, typhoid, variola, varicella, pertusis and cerebrospinal diseases.

4. Age and seasonal effects may be important, the majority of ear infections occurring in childhood and during the cold season of the year, the period from the middle of January until the middle of May showing the largest incidence.

5. The infective organism or virus may reach the ear by way of the blood stream producing eruptions that can be recognized as exanthematous, syphilitic or influenzal.

6. In passing we must mention such obscure etiological factors as heredity, environment, immunity, c e l l sensitization, the allergic condition and the virulence of the invading organism and its saprophytic or parasitis qualities.

SYMPTOMS

Furunculosis: Furuncles in the ear do not differ essentially from furuncles in any other part of the body, except that due to the thinness of the lining membrane the swelling is more diffuse, covers a larger superficial area, and frequently almost occludes the canal in the early stages, but they are more painful. They sometimes offer difficulties in diagnosis; the anomilies which they s i m u l a t e being principally aural polypi, perichondiritis of the auricle, granulations of the external canal, exostoses, paratid abscess, carious teeth, mastoiditis and middle ear conditions.

The earlier signs are itching and discomfort in the canal, due to the congestion of the perichondrium. Discomfort is experienced in mastication. Undue motion of the auricle elicits considerable pain.

Subjectively there is itching, fullness, heat and pain in the order of their development. Objectively, there may be impairment of hearing, tinnitus, redness of the canal, swelling of the canal, and finally suppuration.

The most important thing from the patient's standpoint is pain. It d e v e l o p s about 48 hours after the initial itching, of all degrees of severity depending upon whether the furuncle involves only the superficial layers or involves the deeper cartilaginous structure of the canal. It may be entirely out of proportion to the pathology found, becoming so severe as to be unendurable. In some cases it is excrutiating, radiating to the face, head and neck, and may be aggravated by pressure over the tragus or any movement of the mandible, such as mastication or yawning, which necessarily increases the pressure against the e x t e r n a l fibro-cartilaginous canal.

Ispection of the canal during the early stages may fail to disclose any objective finding whatsoever; or, at b e s t, a small reddened elevation may be discerned at times. The point of distinction between otitis externa and otitis media lies in the pain and tenderness of the f o r m e r on manipulation of the auricle. The slightest attempt at lifting the auricle to straighten the canal for examination with a speculum causes exquisite pain. This is due to the associated perichondiritis. Due to the unyielding c h a r a c t e r of the cartilaginous frame-work, pressure on one point is communicated throughout its whole extent. In doubtful cases, observation over a day or so may still be necessary for accurate diagnosis. If the canal is not occluded, and it can be ascertained that the tympanic membrane shows little or no acute signs of inflammation, the diagnosis is certain.

Discharging ears may be the result of infection with a number of organisms other than staphylococcus or streptococcus, but which present similar symptoms. Laboratory procedures will point out the differential diagnosis.

Mycosis: Mycotic infections often give a sensation of intense itching, as though a foreign body were present. This is sometimes responsible for the trauma given by the patient himself, with a resultant pyogenic infection of the irritated canal, and pain becomes a prominent symptom.

During the beginning infection the skin of the canal becomes desquamated and exfoliated, with the production of a mass of debris, and may be at times so extensive that the canal becomes more or less occluded and the hearing of the patient impaired. Let us digress for a moment to consider briefly the anatomy of the ear canal. It is of irregular contour with a pocket like pouch near the drum, which makes for an ideal place for moisture and debris to collect. The skin is thin, with a small amount of subcutaneous tissue and is not very vascular. Thus accumulating moisture and heat predispose to the rapid and toxic growth of the fungi. As regards climatic conditions, it is therefore apparent that the incidence is greater in the temperate zones than in colder regions, accounting for the fact that it is a common condition in this part of the country during the summer season.

Mycosis is not a serious disease, but it is an annoying condition, and particularly in the summer, is responsible for many patients seeking relief for itching ears.

THERAPY

The treatment of ear infections must be directed not only against the present attack, but also recurrences. When they occur as a result of a primary infection, or as a result of debilitation for any reason, systemic alleviation and improvement are the sine qua non, and presage the prognosis; this in addition to local therapy.

Heat: Heat is a great alleviative, and not only influences the status quo but relieves accompanying pain. Hot water bottles, the electric pad, diathermy and hot douches are all in order. The instillation of warm drops of glycerine or sweet oil and laudanum also accomplish the purpose, as well as such homely remedies as blowing smoke into the ear and breathing into the ear. Any procedure which influences the vaso-dilator mechanism brings into play such natural body defenses as exist. It will be recalled that there is a relatively impoverished supply of blood to the middle and inner ear.

Chemo-Therapy: The choice of a suitable non-irritating germicide to be applied locally may sometimes present a difficult problem. Drugs which prove efficacious in some instances may not produce comparable results in others, and the etiological factor is of cardinal concern. The literature reveals multitudinous therapeutic procedures, each authority advocating his favorites, all of which have indubitably proved of value.

Pyogens: In infections of p y o g e n i c origin, the insertion of a small wick of gauze along the length of the canal permits continuous application of soothing medications. Spirits of boric or iodine in glycerine or aluminum acetate may be employed in this manner. From three to five drops are instilled every two hours. These have been found to be satisfactory alleviates of both pain and swelling.

As r e g a r d s the external ear, we find mention in the older literature of many therapeutic agents, chief of which are:

1. Aq. opii 4.0., aq. dest. 12.0
2. 5% cocain solution
3. Burow's solution (argill. acet. solution Burowii aq. dest., aa 15.0, cocain muriat 1.0)
4. The insertion of a long piece of solid fat

(hog's), covered with a morphin-boracic acid salve (acid boric 1.0, vaseline 20.0, acet. morph 0.2)

5. Carbolic acid 0.5, glycerin 15.0
6. Boric acid 1.0, alcohol 20.0
7. Argill. Acet. Burowii and aluminum aceti-cotartaricum
8. Sublimate alcohol (hydr. muriat. corros 0.05-0.1, spirit vini rectif 50.0)
9. A cotton tampon, dipped in pure alcohol, or hot Billroth solution (lead acetate 1.0, alum 10., water 100.0)

Kerrison advises preparation of the canal prior to instituting treatment, by cleansing of all extraneous material by warm boric acid irrigations and scrubbing with applicators dipped in 95 per cent alcohol. He follows this preparatory treatment by pledgets of cotton saturated with phenol 1:100 dilution, which are allowed to remain one or two minutes. A wick of gauze is then inserted dipped in phenol 1:3000 dilution, which is allowed to remain 24 hours.

Phillips advocates a tampon of cotton dipped in either a 50 per cent boroglycerid solution or preferably a 12 per cent solution of phenol in glycerin, allowing it to remain 12 to 24 hours.

Turner believes the instillation of menthol in liquid paraffin (10 per cent) or of acetotartrate of aluminum (eight per cent) on a gauze wick, to be of value. He also used 10 per cent ichthyol in glycerine.

Hays cleanses the canal thoroughly, swabs with tincture of iodine and then packs the ear with a strip of gauze saturated in 4 per cent aluminum acetate solution.

Barnhill relies on sterilizing and cleansing the meatus with alcohol and then painting with tincture of iodine, and believes this will suffice in incipient cases.

Odeneal heartily criticizes phenol, and prefers a 5 to 10 per cent solution of aluminum acetate on a gauze wick within the canal.

Beck contributes the suggestion of dilute acetate of aluminum solution as a dressing within the canal.

Keeler first sterilizes the canal with applications of boric acid solution and then applies 70 to 95 per cent alcohol. He then inserts a gauze drain impregnated with camphorphenol (camphor gum 55 parts, phenol 45 parts). Ichthyol tampons are also applied.

Ballanger, in addition to the aforementioned carbolated glycerine and aluminum acetate solutions, also avails himself of the gentian and acriviolet dyes.

Gleason advocates the use of cotton tampons with yellow oxid of mercury ointment (six grains to an ounce of vaseline). He syringes the canal with warm 1:5,000 bichloride solution and paints the canal walls with 12 per cent silver nitrate.

Kerrison and Odeneal have raised valid objections to the long continued use of phenol as tending to macerate the skin and prolonging staphylococcus infections. Gidoll has found the same to be true of the excessive use of aluminum acetate, and advances his opinion that alcohol and glycerine answer every purpose in the abortive treatment of boils, setting forth their effectiveness in allaying pain and arresting the progress of infection. In any case, it should be reiterated that care must be taken that none of the mendicants employed trickle down the canal and touch the membrana tympani.

Of the many ointments suggested, Brown believes those of a zinc base to be preferable, and advocates cream of zinc and Lassar's paste. He admits their chief function is probably protective in nature rather than germicidal. Sulphur and mercury ointments more often than not appear to be too irritating, however, three per cent amon. mg. has been highly recommended by Mitchell of Chi. When a stimulating ointment is required it will be found convenient to add liquor carbonis detergens (or its successor, liquor picis carbonis) to the zinc preparation. When desquamation is present, salicylic acid, 10 grains to the ounce, is essential.

In treating infections of the middle and inner ear, mechanical cleansing of the recesses is always impossible, and the procedure painful. Harris and Mertins have reasoned that if all the dead tissue in a suppurating ear could be dissolved, digested or cleaned away, the majority of these cases would heal spontaneously. For this purpose Mertins advances the use of a urea solution. Harris advocates powdered extract of carica papaya as a digestant, and his protocol is as follows: 3 drops of glycerine are placed in a medicine glass, together with 2 droppers or 2 c.c. of water, and about 15 gr. of the above named powder. Mix quickly with a metal applicator and instill enough to be plainly seen in the canal when the patient is in a prone position with the infected ear toward the ceiling. After 1 or 2 minutes, dry with cotton. Repeat this procedure o n c e or twice a week. The solution deterioates in five minutes, and application must be immediate. If redness and swelling are profuse, this must subside before repetition of the treatment.

Bacteriophage: Bacteriophage was discovered independently at about the same time by D'Herrelle and Twort about 20 years ago. They demonstrated that bacteria possess a l y t i c substance filtrable through the Bergfeld or other filters, and that this substance is. able to ingest and destroy other bacteria of similar strains. It has been proven a valuable agent in aborting as well as curing furunculosis. Freund has had such striking success with this agent that he recommends the procedure before attempting any other form of t r e a t m e n t . Squibb & Co. and the Franco-American Co. have on the market, phage in 20 c.c. vials, which can be used either for t o p i c a l application or hypodermic injection. It is also obtainable in ampules of 2 c.c. for injection purposes.

The staphylococcus phage yields better results than the streptococcus phage. It must be. borne in mind that this agent is highly specific, and has no effect on unrelated organisms.

BACILLUS PYOCYANEUS INFECTIONS

In infections of the ear arising from pyocyaneus, M o r l e y advocates syringing with boric lotion as hot as the patient will tolerate. After this the meatus is allowed to drain by posture for a few minutes. He makes no effort to cleanse the meatus, as the pain is exquisite. The ear is next filled with warm one per cent marboglycerin drops and a hot boric foment is applied, large enough to include the pre and postauricular glands. This treatment is carried out four-hourly, and is combined with initial purging by four grains of calomel in split dosage followed by salts. Incision is contra-indicated, and it is best to allow the boil to burst under the conservative treatment described. For chronic cases, the meatus is cleansed and dried, and a small quantity of boro-iodine powder tapped in and insufflated with Siegle's speculum. Care must be taken that none of the

powder reaches the patient's or operator's eyes. Without delay the meatus is plugged with a firm pledget of wool and left undisturbed for 48 hours. It causes slight discomfort for the first hour or two, but is not intolerable. At the conclusion of this period the ear is gently syringed to clear away remains of the p o w d e r, the greater quantity of which has usually been dissolved, and the meatus filled with borospirit drops for a few minutes, afterward being drained by posture.

Hydrogen per oxide and ether as a cleanser, and the application of silver nitrate in spiritus aetheris nitrosi, have been used in pyocyaneus infections. Then spirit and biniodide of mercury, 1 in 4,000 was substituted for the ether. A r g y r o l (2 per cent), mercurochrome (1 per cent) and liquid iodex packs were given exhaustive trials, with disappointing results. Z i n c ionization promised well, but recurrences were numerous.

Fungi: Treatment of otomycosis from the first has consisted chiefly in mechanical removal with fine forceps or an applicator followed by thorough irrigation: secondly, destruction of the offending invader and thirdly a l l a y i n g the inflammation which their growth has caused.

If we can find an efficient agent fulfilling the second requirement without tissue damage, then nature will do much in the third instance towards a successful and satisfactory culmination.

Of the many fungicidal a g e n t s used, varying degrees of success have been obtained; that is, their use had allayed and not cleared up the condition; they have required multiple applications or they have acted as tissue irritants; they have been ideal in the hands of one worker and not with others.

Upon reviewing the literature dealing with otomycosis from 1844, when first described by Mayer, we find mention of some 60 different chemicals used since that time, either alone or in combination, in an effort to give relief or effect a cure. It is of historical interest to note that Schwartz in 1867 recommended cleansing with warm w a t e r, followed by application of two leeches inside the tragus. This was subsequently followed by an aqueous solution of lead acetate. The whole took six weeks to effect a cure.

From recent literature, it will be found that the following are the germicides in greatest favor:

Alcohol.
Salicylic acid 2 to 5% in alcohol.
Boric acid 2 to 5% in alcohol.
Zinc oxide.
Mercuric chloride.
Iodine dusting powder (Sulzberger).
Formaldehyde 2 to 5%.
Sodium borate.
Cresatin or metacresylacetate.
Tricresol 2% in glycerin.
Castellani's solution (saturated alcoholic solution of basic fuchsin to which 10% resorcinal has been added, with small amounts of phenol, boric acid and acetone).
Iodine in liquid petrolatum.
Phenyl mercuric nitrate 1/3,000 alcoholic solution.
Copper salts, such as copper sulphate, chloride and oleate.
Thymol. (Because of its tendency to produce a burning sensation, thymol is best mixed with oil, powder bases or diluted.)

Searcy and McBurney, who have done considerable experimental work on the efficacy of various germicides are of the opinion that metacresylacetate or cresatin heads the list in the degree of effectiveness as a fungicide in otomycosis. Wm. Gill, also an authority in this field, prefers a powder of the following formula:

Iodine 2.00 grams.
Tricresol—1.00 gram.
Thymol—1.00 gram.
Boric acid powder—100.00 grams.

Vaccines or filtrates from cultures of the responsible organisms have been used with varying degrees of success.

It is of interest that cerumen in the ear sometimes exerts a restraining influence against invasion with fungi, though it is true that instances have been encountered in which fungi were actually growing on a ceruminous plug.

Ultra Violet Ray: For the most part, the use of violet ray is mentioned in the literature in passing, but not advocated. However, Odeneal of Massachusetts in a resume of treatment of conditions of the ear, states that eczema of the canal can be relieved, but not cured, by its use. He does encourage it as a general radiation rather than a local application.

Shock Therapy: This therapy has its uses, but should be employed late in the disease. It is accomplished by the production of fixation abscess by injection of turpentine.

Insulin: D. C. Jarvis of Barre, Vt., has written glowingly in the literature of the use of small doses of insulin in ear disorders, as well as those of nose and throat.

The basis on which his recommendations are made is in part theoretical and in part his own clinical experience and that of a correspondence study group. One may of course not agree with theoretical considerations and still have to acknowledge the claims of the experienced clinician when these claims are based on careful study of patients. Knowledge gained this way is frequently discovered in later years to have a sound basis in fact, even though the theory proposed may be found faulty. The curative value of small doses of insulin in cases of chronic otitis media in which the usual methods of treatment have failed, is attested by a number of competent observers. The usual dose is three units given subcutaneously daily, with a lengthening of the interval as clinical improvement takes place. Eventually the insulin may be given no oftener than once a week and continued for months.

Surgical Intervention: There is a growing tendency to withhold surgical intervention in every infection where other means are available, and it has come to be the court of last resort. There are numerous articles in the journals of the last few years, dealing entirely with the inadvisability of such procedure. The cardinal rule is: "Incise inflammation and spread infection; drain pus and hasten healing." However, it is very difficult to determine when the animal body has successfully walled off infection, as regards infections of the ear canal. Too, care must be taken in making incisions; for example, too deep an incision on the posterior wall may penetrate the mastoid cells, as this forms the anterior boundary of the mastoid bone. The facial nerve is located immediately below the articulation of the lower jaw, anterior to the cartilagenous meatus. Also the paratoid gland lies in close proximity. These structures must be kept in mind constantly. In infants the facial nerve is more exposed to danger, lying immediately below and internal to the attachment of the lobule; hence the greater danger of severing this nerve. Carelessness in the direction of the knife may sometimes cause the severance of the ligaments of the temporomaxillary joint and thus cause permanent facial disfigurement.

The use of anesthesia when surgery is resorted to, is generally recommended. As a rule the patient has undergone several days and nights of unceasing and sometimes excrutiating pain, and it is brutal to subject him to additional torture. A whiff of ether or gas or ethyl chloride or nitrous oxide is both merciful and desirable. Local anesthetics are almost useless.

It is best first to probe for the most tender point or the point of fluctuation. If superficial, the i n c i s i o n is made simply through the swelling; if deep, it must be continuous down through the perichondrium. In some severe cases where the canal is completely occluded by swelling, parallel incisions of this kind may be made to advantage around the whole l u m e n. They radiate from the latter like the spokes of a wheel from the hub. They may be aptly called the "wheel-spoke incisions."

General Considerations: Looking at the picture as a whole, it is essential to contribute as much as possible to the comfort of the patient. Sedatives for sleep are indicated. It is a matter of choice whether morphia, barbiturates, amytal, amidopyrin or other sources are used. Diet should be restricted to liquids particularly in cases where mastication is quite painful. Fluids should be given in large quantities, not forgetting fruit juices.

In conclusion it should be called to your attention that there is nothing new mentioned, not even the new drug sulphanilamide. This paper is a resume of the literature and the purpose was to stimulate a little discussion in order to bring out your

methods and your ideas. Therefore, we welcome your discussion.

BIBLIOGRAPHY

Urea Solutions in Treatment of Otitis Media, Martins, Arch. Otolaryngol. Vol. 26, No. 5, Nov., 1937.
A Clinical Note on the Treatment of Chronic Suppurative Otitis Media, Harris, Laryngoscope, No. 48, 276, 1938.
Furunculosis of the External Auditory Canal With Special Reference to Treatment by Bacteriophage, Freund, Laryngoscope, Vol. 46, 419, 1936.
Furunculosis of External Auditory Canal Gidoll, California and Western Medicine, Vol. 42, 378, 1935.
Otitis Externa, Morley, British Medical Journal, Feb. 19, 1938.
Otitis Externa, Brown, British Medical Journal, Oct. 9, 1937.
Furunculosis of the External Auditory Canal, Effler, Ohio State Medical Journal, Vol. 25, 546, July, 1929.
Otomycosis: An investigation of Effective Fungicidal Agents in Treatment, McBurney and Searcy, Vol. 45, No. 4, 988, Laryngology, Dec., 1936.
Archives of Otolaryngology, 28:10, July, 1938.
Insulin in Otolaryngology, A.M.A., 112:355, Jan. 28, 1939.
Etiology of Influenzal Otitis, Pirodda, Giornale di Batteriologia e Immunologia, Turin 21:657, Nov., 1938.
Diseases of the Ear, Griffith, Saunders & Co.
Otomycosis: Some remarks concerning its Prevalence, Symptomatology and Treatment; Gill, Annals of Atology, Rhinology and Laryngology; Vol. 47, 189, March, 1938.
Mycotic Infections in Otolaryngology; Gill, Southern Medical Journal, Vol. 31, 678, June, 1938.
Index of Differential Diagnosis, French, Wm. Wood & Co.
Cholesteatome-like Accumulations in the External Auditory Meatus, Lois D. Greene, Archives of Otolaryngology, August, 1933.
Allergic Diseases of the Ear, L. W. Dean, J. S. Agar & Lloyd D. Linton, Laryngoscope, Oct., 1937.
Primary Carcinoma of the External Auditory Canal and Meatus, Otto C. Risch & James R. Lisa; Laryngoscope, Sept., 1938.
Tuberculous Papillomatos Cutis of the Ear, Frank L. Dennis, Archives of Otolaryngology, July, 1930.
Otitis Externa Mycotica, King Gill, Archives of Otolaryngology, 16:76-82, July, 1932.
Vincents Infection of the Ear, L. H. Barenberry & J. M. Lewis, Journal of the American Medical Association, April 5, 1930.
Diseases of the External Ear, C. N. Dezer, Journal of the Medical Society of New Jersey, March, 1935.
Physical Therapy in the Treatment of Diseases of the Ear, Nose & Throat. T. H. Odneal, Archives of Otolaryngology, July, 1931.
Aspergillis Infection as the Cause of External Ear Disease, Reben F. Simms, Southern Medical Journal, Dec., 1937.
Fungus Infection of the External Ear, Edqard J. Whalen, Journal of the American Medical Association, Aug. 6, 1938.
The Pharmacopia and the Physician, Clyde A. Heatly, Journal of the American Medical Association, Dec. 5, 1936.
Streptococci Dermatoses of the Ears, James R. Mitchell, Journal of the American Medical Association, May 14, 1936.

---o---

The Use of X-Ray in Obstetrics*

P. N. Charbonnet, M.D.
E. O. Johnson, M.D.
TULSA, OKLAHOMA

With the improvement in equipment, the development and d i s c o v e r y of new technics and methods of X-ray diagnosis using different opaque medias, the use of X-rays has not only become a necessary adjunct to the teaching of obstetrics but also to the practice. Because of the many

*Read before the Section on Obstetrics and Pediatrics at the Annual Meeting of the Oklahoma State Medical Association in Oklahoma City, May 3, 1939.

uses for X-rays in obstetrics several of the obstetrical clinics are equipping their own department with units instead of relying on the central X-ray department of the hospital. Even the most enthusiastic exponents of the clinical approach to obstetrics and the most critical of the laboratory methods welcome the aid a radiograph can give in the obese patient, where the question of hydramnios, multiple pregnancy, abnormal position and presentation of the fetus, and abnormalities of the fetus are often determined with difficulty if only the examiner's senses are relied upon.

In addition to the above uses of X-ray, the obstetrician often finds that they are of great value in the study of his sterility cases to determine an obstruction in the genital tract. They are often of value in the establishment of a diagnosis of early pregnancy, and in the differential diagnosis of pregnancy and tumors[20]. In cases of disproportion, p e l v i c contracture or bony deformity, X-ray cephalometry and pelvimetry may often be of great value in determining the conduct of labor. The diagnosis of death in utero, placenta previa, extra genital pregnancy can be demonstrated with X-ray. In some instances the age of the baby as determined by X-ray is of value. A well identified radiograph showing the fetal bony parts is indisputable in court, where the question is whether the patient has ever had a baby.

Obstetricians o f t e n have therapeutic abortions to perform and the use of X-rays to produce these is often the ideal way, especially in the patient that can take an anesthetic only with a grave risk to her life. Also X-rays are occasionally used for the purpose of sterilization in the female.

Many immediate problems which arise in the newborn are often the obstetrician's concern. X-rays will often aid materially in diagnosing congenital pneumonia, atelectasis, congenital syphilis, enlarged thymus, fractures, and other pathology of the newborn.

Besides these definite obstetrical conditions, there are the many other associated conditions from fractures to cancer which can occur in the pregnant woman where X-rays are of great value, both from the diagnostic and therapeutic standpoint.

It is not advocated that the use of X-rays should supplant any portion of the routine clinical obstetrical examination. Rather should they be used as an aid in corroborating a point in question which is first discovered by the clinical examination.

Two very r e c e n t experiences of the author impresses one with the value of X-ray studies of the obstetrical patient. Had a very c a p a b l e internist directed the cathode rays into the pelvis instead of running repeated G. B., G. I., and chest films on a p a t i e n t already in her fifth month of pregnancy, he could have diagnosed the cause of her gastric symptoms before her friends sent her to the obstetrician. Pelvic examination in this instance was not particularly easy. A Friedman test had not been run. The legal question of whether a certain patient had ever had a baby would have been facilitated by an X-ray, which is often more convincing to a jury than the testimony of many doctors.

Let us consider some of the indications for X-ray studies in obstetrics.

USE IN STERILITY STUDIES

Uterosalpingography[1-2-3-7] is effected by the injection of 5 to 8 cc. of opaque media such as Skiodan, Lipiodal and Hippuram into the uterine cavity with a tight fitting cannula using enough force to send the media into the tube and taking an X-ray film at periodic intervals thereafter. In obstetrics its c h i e f use is to determine patency of the genital tract in sterility. Some have advocated its use to determine an extrauterine pregnancy in which case it is always well to rule out a coexisting intrauterine pregnancy. Before making a uterosalpingo gram all cases should be free of genital tract infection, bleeding, an intrauterine pregnancy and have had previous Rubin tests. In interpreting the X-ray, if there is an obstruction present one must always remember that the condition of the remainder of the tube is not known. This procedure is not without d a n g e r. Some cases of pelvic infection[4], abdominal and tubal pregnancies[5] have been reported following the oil injection. Several cases of the oil gaining entrance into the venous system of the uterus[6-8] have been reported. Violent rupture of the cervix[9] and oil embolism where the oil was found in the pulmonary vessels at autopsy have also been reported. However, in careful hands in selected cases uterosalpingography is a very valuable aid in sterility studies.

DIAGNOSIS OF EARLY PREGNANCY, AND AGE
OF FETUS IN UTERO

Ossification of the fetal skeleton does not occur until the seventh week of gestation. Therefore the diagnosis of pregnancy by X-ray at present is not theoretically possible until at least the second month of pregnancy. However, practically the diagnosis of pregnancy by X-ray cannot be accomplished before three and one-half months gestation where the bony skeleton has to be depended upon. Perhaps with the development of amniography[28] a technique may be devised where the fetal soft parts can be seen earlier. The value of X-ray for this purpose is little when one considers that a diagnosis can be made only three to six weeks before quickening. Other clinical and laboratory tests are of greater practical value.

The age[16] or maturity of the fetus in utero has been determined by roentgenological studies of the points of ossification of the fetal bones, measuring the f e t a l length, and by measuring a fetal bony part, such as the femur and tibia, or occipitofrontal diameter and computing its relationship to the length (Thoms).

Reed feels that since the weight of a full term fetus is so variable ranging from five to ten pounds that the most constant factor is the length which varies from only 48 to 53 centimeters. Thus, he doubles the length from the vertex to the buttocks to estimate the age of the fetus. Duvoir estimates the age of the fetus in days by multiplying its length in centimeters by the factor 5.6. He also determines the length of the fetus by multiplying the length of the diaphysis of the tibia and or humerus by 6.5 and added eight centimeters.

Thoms[11] u s e s the relationship of the occipto-frontal diameter to the fetal length to determine fetal maturity. Hess says that fetal maturity is indicated by complete ossification of the hyoid bone, presence of an ossifying center in the distal epiphysis of the femur, ossification of the transverse and articular processes of the vertebral arches, ossification of the first segment of the coccyx, and all bones of the hand but not of the carpus.

It would be very helpful if X-ray studies could determine post maturity of the fetus. Christie, a research fellow at Johns Hopkins is working on this problem at present.

Concluding one can readily see that the use of X-ray for this purpose is still academic.

ABNORMALITIES OF THE FETUS AND DEATH IN UTERO

In the obese patient with a thick pendulous abdomen the question of hydramnios and multiple pregnancy can easily be differentiated, often, but not always, by a single X-ray film. In the case of hydramnios abnormalities of the fetus should always be looked for. Some of the frequent anomalies are absence of clavicles, portions of the skull, and the radius. Also the presence of extra fetal bony parts can often be seen readily, such as extra digits, decephalus, etc. Hydrocephalus[12] is characterized by wide suture and fontanelles. Here the r a d i o g r a p h is of indisputable value since often if the condition is known one can determine the conduct of labor early.

An excellent rule is to examine by X-ray all patients with multiple pregnancies, and all patients who are to have an abdominal delivery (Caesarean section), if the clinical examination is in any way doubtful. It is unfortunate to do a Caesarean section to obtain a monster, unless it cannot be delivered otherwise because of its size or shape. And occasionally a clinical multiple pregnancy will prove to be a monster by X-ray.

Fetal death in utero can be diagnosed by X-ray examination by finding overlapping (Horner[13-14]) of the fetal cranial bones in the radiograph. Lordosis of the caudal half of the fetal spine (Jungmann) due to the loss of muscular tone in the lumbosacral muscles is also supposed to be a sign of death in utero. Other signs of fetal death are collapse of the thoracic cage, decalcification of the bones, and abnormally small fetus in proportion to the duration of gestation. However, most clinical evidences of fetal death in utero are satisfactory without corroboration of the r a d i o g r a p h, inasmuch as Dipple[19] has shown that the management of the patient is conservative anyway. After sufficient time has elapsed there is no doubt clinically of the death of the fetus (except possibly where it occurs early in pregnancy).

PLACENTA PREVIA

Roentgenological diagnosis of placenta previa by use of a cystogram has been accomplished by Ude and Urner[15-30] and corroborated by Wells[16], McIvor[19], and others. The cystogram is made by injecting 30 to 40 cc. of 12½ per cent sodium iodide with a catheter into the bladder followed by an X-ray film in the supine position. Normally, there is a distance of one centimeter between the fetal head and the u p p e r margin of the bladder, and a separation greater than this is indicative of placenta previa. The advantage of an X-ray diagnosis in this condition lessens the chance of introducing an infection by a pelvic or rectal examination, and the chance of separation by this manipulation. One disadvantage is that it is of little or no value (Robecchi) before the seventh month of pregnancy.

W. Snow was able to demonstrate the placenta in the routine roentgen examination of pregnant women in a high percentage of cases without the use of contrast media. Dr. A. L. Dippel is to demonstrate the placenta in X-rays in the coming meeting of the A.M.A.

The indications for X-ray in this condition are clear cut, and certainly any diagnostic aid which is of value without risk to the patient or fetus deserves frequent usage.

CEPHALOMETRY, PELVIMETRY, AND DISPROPORTION[22-23-24-29-32-33-35-36-37]

In all previous conditions discussed the indications for the use of radiography are generally quite definite, since they may be based on a condition which arises during the course of the pregnancy. The measurement of the obstetrical pelvis immediately confronts the obstetrician when the patient first presents herself. The extreme a c c u r a c y with which Thoms, Hodges[33], Caldwell, Dippel[34], and others have measured the pelvis with the use of X-rays, and checked them subsequently with an a c t u a l measurement during a laparotomy suggests that this is the ideal method of mensuration. Both Thoms' and Hodges' method have been shown to be within two millimeters of accuracy. This almost exceeds the limit of accuracy in a c t u a l measurements. Also, Caldwell's classification[21] of the various shapes of pelves based on radiographic s t u d i e s is considered by many to be the b e s t yet available. Thus, the question arises whether or not at least every primipara should not have X-ray pelvimetry, since this is an ideal m e t h o d of mensuration. This would mean that at least 600,000 women annually would receive this added attention at quite an additional expense. If this is a necessity then those who cannot af-

ford it should be provided for by some means.

One must remember, however, that the bony pelvis is not the only important factor in the passage of the fetus through the birth canal. Many of us have seen a large fetus come through a small pelvis, so that clinical judgement, soft tissue resistance, adaptation, etc., are still important in deciding this problem. It seems then that even though radiographic mensuration of the pelvis of each woman would be ideal, as well as cephalometry at term, that other factors such as soft tissues, stretching of ligaments, etc., p r e c l u d e and make unnecessary its routine use at present. However, a step forward in the care of our obstetrical patients would be the use of X-ray pelvimetry in all patients that have contracted or border-line pelvic measurements as taken during a clinical examination. Also, X-ray of the pelvis is indicated in all abnormally shaped pelves from whatever cause, trauma, disease, birth, etc.

The question of cephalometry[26-27] and disproportion[25] can be considered together. Obviously if there is a definite clinical disproportion there is no need of X-ray confirmation. However, with the use of technics of Ball[31] and others cephalometry and pelvimetry is of great aid in the determination of disproportion in the borderline cases, that cannot be determined clinically.

Discussion of uses in sterilization and abortion may be checked in the literature as listed[39-40].

CONCLUSION

Concluding, one can say without fear of contradiction that X-rays are fastly assuming a more and more important role in o b s t e t r i c s, and that every obstetrician should stay well acquainted with its development in order to offer the best and most intelligent care to his patients.

BIBLIOGRAPHY

1. S. G. and O., 60:224, Feb. 1, 1935.
2. Radiology, 21:568, Dec., 1933.
3. Am. J. Obst. and Gyn., 33:164, Jan., 1937.
4. Gynec. et obst., 31:852, June, 1935.
5. Am. J. Surg., 29:244, Aug., 1935.
6. J.A.M.A., 104:545, Feb. 16, 1935.
7. Am. J. Obst. and Gyn., 29:100, Jan., 1935.
8. Am. J. Obst. and Gyn., 28:568, Oct., 1934.
9. Zentralb f. Gynak, 60:1154, May 16, 1936.
10. Curtis Textbook "Obstetrics and Gynecology," Vol. III.
11. Am. J. Obst. and Gyn., 29:876, June, 1935.
12. Bull. Soc. d'obst. et de gynec. 24:625, Dec., 1935.
13. S. G. and O. 35:67, 1922.
14. Am. J. Obst. and Gyn., 32:67, 1936.
15. Am. J. Roentgenology, 31:230, 1934.
16. J. Okla. State Med. Assoc., Aug., 1937, page 285.

17. Texas State J. Med., 32:471, Nov., 1936.
18. Am. J. Obst. and Gyn., 33:436, March, 1937.
19. Bull. Johns Hopkins Hospital, 54:24, 1934.
20. Am. J. Surg., 18:270, 1932.
21. Am. J. Obst. and Gyn., 28:482, Oct., 1934.
22. Am. J. Obst. and Gyn., 28:497, Oct., 1934.
23. J.A.M.A., 102:2075, June 23, 1934.
24. J.A.M.A., 102:602, Feb. 24, 1934.
25. Ill. Med. J., 66, 171, Aug., 1934.
26. S. G. and O. 58:721, April, 1934.
27. Am. J. Obst. and Gyn., 27:691, May, 1934.
28. Am. J. Obst. and Gyn., 27:894, June, 1934.

29. West J. Surg., 43:84, Feb., 1935.
30. Am. J. Obst. and Gyn., 29:667, May, 1935.
31. Am. J. Obst. and Gyn., 32:249, Aug., 1936.
32. S. G. and O., 61:735, Dec., 1935.
33. Am. J. Roentgenol., 37:664, May, 1937.
34. S. G. and O., 68:642, March, 1939.
35. Am. J. Obst. and Gyn., 34:150, July, 1937.
36. N. Y. State J. Med., 38:83, Jan. 15, 1938.
37. Am. J. Obst. and Gyn., 35:938, June, 1938.
38. Jour. Okla. State Med. Assoc., p. 236, July, 1938.
39. Amer. J. Obst. and Gyn., 34:507, Sept., 1937.
40. Amer. J. Obst. and Gyn., 32:945, Dec., 1936.

---o---

Infection in Extremities of Diabetics

W. D. HOOVER, M.D.

TULSA, OKLAHOMA

Infection and gangrene, in extremities, accompany each other with such frequency in diabetic individuals that it is almost impossible to discuss one group without the other. For this reason both are included in this paper. Surgical conditions in extremities of diabetics are becoming more numerous in recent years. Increased longevity as a result of insulin therapy accounts for this rise due to the vascular changes attending long standing diabetes. This fact together with the great use of machinery in our age bring many diabetics with injuries, infections and gangrene to the surgeon. This paper is limited to the extremities and the usual surgical conditions of the abdomen, chest or neck can be more fittingly discussed when those regions are discussed from a surgical standpoint.

Diabetics notoriously have great susceptibility to infection as well as poor resistance to them. Infections occurring in unrecognized diabetics often become advanced conditions before reaching the surgeon. Arteriosclerosis, which is a gradual process characteristic of this disease, contributes greatly to surgical affections of the extremities in the later years of life. Accidental injury, either in the course of daily pursuits or in industry, is an etiological factor of major importance in these cases. Especially is it becoming important from a medico-legal and insurance standpoint. Many of that type of cases are of the untreated and unrecognized diabetic.

In reviewing the literature on this subject it is surprising to note the extremely high mortality rate which attended these cases in the years previous to 1924. The rate at present remains rather high but previous to 1912 the rate was 80 per cent. From 1895 to 1926 in a group of 1,864 operations the mortality rate was 25.6 per cent. McKittrick recently reported operations on extremities in 807 cases with a mortality of only 8.4 per cent. Walters, Meyerding, Judd and Wilder of the Mayo Clinic report a group of this type of cases of recent years. There were 226 in the group and in 155 without surgery the mortality rate was 23 per cent while in 71 with surgery the rate was seven per cent. The mortality rates become very impressive when viewed from the standpoint of previous diabetic management. Standard, Ralli, and Brandaleone in 1938 report 343 cases of infection or gangrene of the extremities only 141 of which had had previous diabetic management and the mortality rate in this group was 10.6 per cent. The remaining 192 who had received no previous diabetic care had a mortality rate of 35.4 per cent. Of a small group of cases in St. John's Hospital in Tulsa, Oklahoma, from 1934 to 1939 the mortality rate was close to this. The mortality rate in the untreated was 41.6 per cent while in the treated it was 10 per cent. The average age was 61; the youngest being 41 and the oldest 78.

In considering the diagnosis in these cases one must not undervalue the simple test for sugar in the urine. This test should be made on any patient who presents himself for treatment of infections of the extremities or any suspicious lesion of the extremities. Often it is neglected for several visits so if it is made when these cases are first seen much time may be saved because the infections will not improve if the diabetes is unrecognized and untreated. If sugar is present in the urine the blood sugar determination should be made to clinch the diagnosis of diabetes.

The treatment of this condition requires, always, prompt surgical procedures. Before these measures are undertaken, however, the patient must be carefully investigated and meticulously prepared for operation. This must be done as quickly as possible but nevertheless very thoroughly.

In the treatment, bed rest, proper diabetic diet, adequate insulin and large quantities of fluids are of prime importance in preparation for surgery. Many v a r i e d opinions exist with regard to diabetic diet but the diet my associate and myself have found most beneficial in the surgical diabetic is one high in carbohydrate with a moderate amount of protein and low in fat. Diets consisting of 180 to 250 grams of carbohydrate, 70 to 80 grams of protein and 60 to 70 grams of fat in 24 hours seem to be the most satisfactory. Insulin should be given f r e q u e n t l y and in sufficient amounts to render and maintain a sugar free urine and a blood sugar level near normal. Fluids should be given freely by mouth and glucose in normal saline must be given intravenously at times before operation to be governed by the individual case as to frequency and amounts. Some insulin is given at the same time the intravenous glucose is given but not with the p u r p o s e of completely neutralizing the sugar. It is unnecessary and sometimes dangerous to attempt to completely neutralize the glucose g i v e n intravenously. Careful preparation as described here is designed for the chief purpose of obviating acidosis which is so often disastrous in diabetes. If possible the patient should be under the care of an internist for as one can readily see, medical supervision here is tantamount to surgical success. Supervision of an internist is often impossible, hence the surgeon must be prepared to render this service himself.

For anaesthetic the spinal is the anesthesia of choice, unless rapid incision only, is to be done in which case short inhalation anaesthesia such as ethylene oxygen may be used. Ether disturbs the patient's metabolism and leads to acidosis, thus it should be avoided.

Surgical measures should be instituted as early as possible after proper preparation of the patient has been rapidly accomplished. The exact type of procedure to be undertaken depends upon the condition present. In infections this depends upon the circulation of the extremity and the depth of tissues involved in the process. Superficial infections in extremities with adequate circulation may be treated by wide incision. If this is done early enough often gangrene is prevented because gangrene is usually secondary to local thrombosis resulting from infection. If cellulitis extends to deep tissues amputation is indicated. Amputation is also indicated with gangrene of any degree where sepsis is present. Gangrene with apparent advanced i m p a i r m e n t of circulation, evidenced by absence of dorsal pedis pulse and lowered temperature, should also be treated by amputation. Whatever procedures are employed should be as simple as possible and consume as little time as possible.

Amputations of infected extremities are done without the use of the tourniquet and those of the lower extremities are in most cases above the knee. This depends, however, much on the individual case taking into consideration the extent of circulatory impairment. A circular amputation, with little regard for flap, is done and the stump closed with drainage or left open entirely. Amputations where infection is absent and the patient is in satisfactory general condition may be of the flap type with more concern for the stump. Complete c l o s u r e may be made in this instance without drainage. In cases with gangrene only more time may be spent in completing the preoperative preparation.

Post-operatively the same measures are instituted as pre-operatively. The treatment is greatly individualized, however, and much depends upon the general condition of the patient and the amount of sugar in the urine. Intravenous glucose in normal saline should be given in large amounts with sufficient insulin to utilize the major portion of the sugar. In the experience of my associate and myself 1,500 to 2,000 cc. of 10 per cent glucose in normal saline each 24 hours, for the first few days, seems adequate to supply fluids, nourishment and prevent acidosis post-operatively. Of course the usual postoperative routine must be carried out including sufficient opiates to r e l i e v e pain and good nursing care. The urine must be examined frequently for sugar to help in determining the insulin dosage. Acidosis, manifested by the presence of acetone and diacetic acid in the urine, is more important and more to be prevented at this time than the presence of sugar in the urine. The removal of an infected area or proper drainage of abscessed regions soon increase the sugar tolerance of the patient so that less insulin is needed than before operation. This must be kept in mind and reductions in insulin dosage should be made as indicated to prevent hypoglycemic reactions. Oral feeding should begin as early as possible.

In diabetic surgery of the extremities aside from the local lesion much attention must be given the patient with regard to the disturbed metabolism peculiar to the diabetic and the treatment must be highly individualized. Short anaesthesia, expeditious surgery and close medical supervision are necessary for best results.

I wish to acknowledge my indebtedness to Dr. Thos. J. Lynch, my associate, for his counsel and advice which have been of great value in preparation of this paper.

BIBLIOGRAPHY

1. James E. Paulin. S.G.O. Feb. 15, 1939.
2. Leland S. McKittrick. S.G.O. Feb. 15, 1939.
3. F. M. Allen. Cyclopedia of Medicine. 1933.
4. Standard Brandaleone and Ralli. J.A.M.A., 1938, 110-627.
5. Rabinovitz and Weisman. New England Journal of Med., 1938, Vol. 219, p. 428.
6. Stanbro. J. Okla. State Med. Assn., Feb., 1939.
7. Walters, Meyerding, Judd and Wilder, Minnesota Medicine, 17:517-526, (Sept.) 1934.
8. Leland S. McKittrick and H. Root. Diabetic Surgery. Lea & Febiger, 1931.

---------------------0---------------------

Renal Emergencies*

ALFRED R. SUGG, M.D.
ADA, OKLAHOMA

In a sense any renal disease is an emergency, and a full discussion on any one of the major renal emergencies would consume all of the time allotted. The purpose of this paper then is not to go into a detailed discussion, but rather to call to your attention s o m e practical suggestions in connection with serious disturbance of the urinary tract which are common and for which immediate diagnosis and p r o m p t treatment is imperative if the patient is to survive. These every day emergencies are both surgical and non-surgical.

Anuria is one of the most dramatic and trying of these emergencies. It generally follows trauma, injection of poisons, or surgery, though it also follows burns, transfusions or even bacterial invasion. The actual production of the anuria is probably due to arterial congestion and swelling in-

terfering with normal venous return. But w h e t h e r it is secretory, obstructive or transitional in origin nothing is more disconcerting to the physician than to discover the patient has a large amount of albumin, casts and blood and that edema and blood urea are on the increase and in the later stages that no urine at all is passed.

This generally means that p r e v i o u s damage to the kidneys (or at least to the vascular system) has existed—as a postoperative condition it often means that a more careful study before operation would have served notice to abandon or postpone surgery or at least to have forewarned the surgeon. Often a trace of albumin was present—or there was a history of edema or of albuminuria or hypertension, either of which is a danger signal. Even a history of previous infectious disease especially of scarlet fever, septic t o n s i l s, etc., should suggest estimation of blood urea,

*Read before the Section on Genito-Urinary Diseases and Syphilology, Annual Meeting, Oklahoma State Medical Association, May 3, 1939, Oklahoma City.

determining the CO2 combining power as well as renal function tests. The sick kidney is unable to concentrate solids and a test for this function is of great importance.

Post-operative anuria therefore, about adds up to preventing it rather than curing it. But if it slips up on us, a usually effective procedure is administration of concentrated glucose, or there is little doubt that sucrose in like amounts is more effective—200-500 c.c. of 20 per cent can be given at one time. Strohm says that twice as much urine is passed if sucrose is given first followed by fluids as the other way round. The diet should be low in salts and condiments with moderate reduction of protein, say to 50 gm. per day. If edema is present limit fluids to one liter until water balance is obtained and then gradually increase them. If no edema is present simple forcing of fluids by mouth or parenterally is o f t e n sufficient though there is danger of cell edema interfering with metabolism before clinical edema is in evidence.

If the patient is able to take fluids by mouth mild diuretics may be tried. Potassium nitrate in enteric coated pills after meals is the most effective.

There is much difference of opinion regarding the use of strong organic mecurial diuretics of which salyrgan is perhaps best known. Many men are dreadfully afraid of them and they may be harmful but I have never seen any apparent damage done by their use. Binger suggests a practical method for their use. If the output of urine is 300 c.c. or more per day and if the blood urea is below 50 mg. per cent, one c.c. of salyrgan can be given in the vein. If no toxic effects are produced such as diarrhea, hematuria, etc., develop two c.c. can be given the following day and two c.c. each third day as long as indicated. One of the safest and most effective drugs to stimulate urinary output is aminophylin and five gr. added to your intravenous solution may help. Urea itself is a valuable diuretic and should not be overlooked.

If cardiac weakness is a factor or if hypotension exists these factors should be treated, for the arterial tension must be 50 before any urine is secreted and anything below 100 renders the formation of urine difficult. If anuria is due to an obstructive lesion it goes without saying that re-

moval of the obstruction is mandatory and that in a hurry. The obstruction need only be on one side as there is such a thing as reflex anuria. Surgery may help in some cases of anuria. Decapsulation undoubtedly does some of them good and should be tried when everything has f a i l e d. Whether it gives relief from the compression as some say or a disturbance of the enervation of the capsule is of no practical importance.

Nephrosis is a renal disorder which is an emergency, for failure to recognize and treat it promptly is serious. Whether it is a form of nephritis or not is beside the point. Edema is the outstanding characteristic. The urine is loaded with albumin and casts but R.B.C. are never present. The PSP test is normal. The serum protein is low and the albumin globulin ratio is reversed. It is considered that the fall in serum to a point so low that the osmatic pressure is below that of the capillary arterial pressure is the cause of the edema. If the protein of the blood goes to less than 4.5 grams, edema will develop. The osmatic pressure can be increased at least temporarily by blood transfusions or by intravenous acacia. Five hundred c.c. of a five per cent solution can be given every day or so. There is a concentrated blood serum which is reported to work well if available.

There has existed a time honored edict for many years that no meat, eggs, or other protein food could be allowed when albumin is present in the urine. For the past few years some literature has appeared to the contrary but the discussions have sometimes been more confusing than enlightening. Here then in nephrosis is one indication where the loss of protein through the kidneys is so severe that edema will soon put out of business other vital organs and it depends for its existence upon a minimum level of protein in the blood. The diet should contain not less than 75 grams of protein daily and even then you may have to resort to transfusions or acacia. If fluids are not restricted and salt withheld pulmonary edema is in the offing.

Uremia is classed as a renal emergency and it often is dramatic enough. If decreased (or absent) urinary output remains very l o n g this symptom-complex will surely be manifested. It is not an entity and is not due solely to an excess of urea. Cases with urea above 300 have been reported with little or no e v i d e n c e of uremia. Furthermore kidneys will continue to handle urea until they are almost completely destroyed. A low NPN is not an absolutely safe criterion of impaired function. Creatinine will begin to accumulate earlier and its increase is often the first sign of damage. Uremia sometimes develops when there is a fair output. That is the kidneys can put out water but cannot concentrate solids, hence the urine is clear and has a low fixed specific gravity—1004 to 1007. It is especially u n a b l e to eliminate properly the normally produced acid products of metabolism. Also the impaired function interferes with the production of ammonia from urea, one of the mechanisms by which the normal organism compensates for a c i d o s i s. The increased acids in the blood stimulates the respiratory center and increases pulmonary ventilation thus tending to eliminate the excess acids in the form of CO_2 through the respiration. This rapid respiration is the most valuable clinical sign of impending uremia. The other item of physiology which is effective is that the excess acids are combined with soda, thus if the CO_2 is below the normal of 55 the alkali reserve is diminished. If the patient is too ill to take soda by mouth, Hartman's solution intravenously is ideal. It is much safer than soda bicarbonate and even the lactate is of value as it is either oxidized to produce energy or is synthesized to glycogen by the liver.

The treatment of the hypertension and increased intra-cranial phases of uremia is necessarily empirical since the cause of these phases is unknown. The dyspnoea, edema, and heart pain is cardiac failure and should be referred to the cardiologist or treated as any other heart failure.

The muscular twitching, itching, fetid breath, coma and convulsions are the results of dehydration and r e n a l failure. Make up for the loss of power to concentrate by increasing the quantity of urine. The skin cannot eliminate solids, hence sweating is of little or no value. If aminophylin is added to intravenous fluids more can be given without producing pulmonary congestion or edema.

Hematuria is an emergency that the patient rarely neglects, especially a man. He gets scared and if he is not scared the doctor should be and should let no grass grow under his feet until a diagnosis is made. Bleeding from a b l a d d e r lesion with obstruction by clots is seen. If the clots are washed out and a large retention catheter left in place the bleeding will usually stop for it is the distention that keeps up hemorrhage. As soon as possible cystoscopic examination s h o u l d be done even if the hemorrhage has stopped. If hemorrhage cannot be controlled by catheter then most of it can be by fulguration. Only occasionally is it necessary to do a supra pubic cystotomy. Culture of the urine (and often biopsy) at first cystoscopic is desirable. We want to know what bacteria are there at the onset not what we carry in with our manipulations.

Acute retention brings them in without urging and it is a real emergency. The patient is wild with pain and back pressure can easily produce reflux infection in the kidney not to mention reflex anuria and death. Much harm is frequently done the patient in this condition by the physician. Strictures and prostatic hypertrophy being usually the cause. Catheterization is not easy. The doctor often grabs a catheter of questionable sterility and with unwashed hands and no preparation proceeds to torture the patient with no visible results and with increasing discomfiture to himself. If a catheter won't pass when properly inserted it won't and it responds poorly to strong armed methods and woe be unto the patient when a careless doctor resorts to a metal catheter. The trauma, hemorrhage, infection, false pockets, extravasation, etc., f o l l o w i n g unskillful catheterization are legion. Cleanliness, gentleness and an assortment of instruments are all that are necessary. If one won't pass, try another, but if force is necessary then quit. Striking water is not the end of the danger for an over-distended bladder suddenly released may produce severe hemorrhage, shock, or even death. Decompress slowly; suprapubic cystotomy is much more desirable than forceful catheterization.

Renal colic is almost always due to obstruction which if not relieved will result in disaster. It should be remembered that morphine actually stimulates ureteral peristalsis and only when enough is given to act through the central nervous system is the pain relieved. This demonstrable physiologic fact has been known for sometime now but it will be another generation before the doctor will stop going for the morphine pellet when a man is passing a gravel down his ureter. Atropine, nitroglycerin, amyl nitrite all tend to relax smooth muscle and should at least be given in conjunction with morphine. Pancreatic tissue extract, now available, will according to recent reports relieve ureteral pain presumably by counteracting the epinephrin in the tissues. If cystoscopic manipulation is necessary, I feel certain the special brand of Avertin put out for the purpose will relax a spastic ureter very well.

The chief surgical emergencies are due to obstructions, trauma and operative accidents. The obstruction demanding emergency attention would fill a book and will be passed here with the single phrase: Relieve the obstruction.

It is something of a paradox that the kidney injured by trauma is not as frequently an emergency as many other conditions. A patient who has received an injury to a kidney if it is not too severe will recover spontaneously with rest and time much more certainly than with ill considered s u r g i c a l interference. This does not imply that every effort should not be made to determine the exact situation. Rupture of a kidney sufficient to produce extravasation is certainly surgical and the sooner operated the better. The kidney should be exposed in all suspected cases with a rising pulse (Wesson), falling blood pressure, anemia and bad general state though the shock should be treated first. They never bleed to death. It is infection of the blood clots and traumatized tissue that kills. For this reason catheterization should be avoided and if done only under the strictest asepsis. The diagnosis can usually be made by intravenous pyelograms and physical examination. Senger and Bottone report good results in a large series with ultra conservative measures. I recently saw a young w o m a n who, while slightly inebriated, d r o v e her car into a d i t c h. She was brought to the office at 7 p.m. The only c o m p l a i n t was pain in the right chest which was thought to be a fractured rib. She refused examination and seemed to be alright, so she went home 10 miles distant. At 2 a.m. she was brought to the hospital in grave shock. The bladder was f i l l e d with blood and blood was seen coming from the right ureter. In this case a retrograde pyelogram was made which showed severe damage to the kidney with a large hematoma between the kidney and the spinal column. As soon as the shock had abated a bit the kidney was exposed and the upper pole was found crushed beyond r e p a i r, so nephrectomy was done.

The point in reporting this case especially is to point out that irremediable trauma to the kidney can take place with absolutely no external evidence of injury and furthermore that the evidence of severe injury may be delayed for several hours.

The operative accidents producing urological emergencies are not often found in the literature but we all know they occur. In a single week last summer I saw two women with both ureters either cut or tied off and by surgeons of wide experience and high standing. I mention them here indirectly to call attention to two facts: first the true situation was not suspected for a much too long interval though there was anuria and rapidly developing signs of uremia. Second: In one case apparently in extremis a bilateral nephrostomy not only proved to be a life saver but in a few days the sutures were absorbed, the ureteral patency became re-established and in a few weeks normal kidney function returned, the nephrostomy sinus closed and the patient was discharged cured.

I was called sometime ago by one of our best surgeons to see a patient he had operated—bilateral ovarian tumors had been resected—the most difficult to remove being on the left side. A few days postoperative the abdomen became distended on the left side especially, with a dull percussion note and e v i d e n c e of toxemia— suspecting a cut ureter he aspirated and removed a large quantity of urine. Thinking to relieve both himself and his patient he decided on a left nephrectomy. Imagine his chagrin when this procedure dried up the bladder completely but decreased by not a drop the output of urine from the abdominal urinary sinus. He had removed the wrong kidney.

These are but a few of the renal emergencies but they call for training, judgment and equipment with about equal division between decisive action and masterful inactivity.

New Books

NEW AND NONOFFICIAL REMEDIES, 1939, Containing Descriptions of the Articles Which Stand Accepted by the Council On Pharmacy and Chemistry of the American Medical Association on January 1, 1939. Cloth. Price, postpaid, $1.50. Pp. 617-LXVII. Chicago: American Medical Association, 1939.

Each year a revised list of the articles which stand accepted by the Council on Pharmacy and Chemistry of the American Medical Association as of January 1 is published in book form under the title of "New and Nonofficial Remedies." The book contains the descriptions of acceptable proprietary substances and their preparations, proprietary mixtures if they have originality or other important qualities, important nonproprietary nonofficial articles, simple pharmaceutical preparations, and other articles which require retention in the book.

A list of articles and brands accepted by the Council, but not described, is included in the book to cover simple preparations or mixtures of official articles (U.S.P. or N.F.) marked under descriptive, nonproprietary names for which only established claims are made. Diagnostic reagents which are not used in or on the human body, and protein diagnostic preparations are not included in New and Nonofficial Remedies unless the determination of the status of these products by the Council has been requested by the distributor: If such products are found to be marketed in accordance with the Council's rules, they may be included in the list of undescribed, but acceptable articles.

A supplement to the annual volume of New and Nonofficial Remedies is published twice a year to bring up to date such current revisions and additions as have been necessary since its last publication. Every product included in the book is subject to the official rules of the Council. The comments on rules are changed occasionally by way of clarifying interpretation to insure fair consideration of all submitted preparations as new standards are recognized. Such constant and critical consideration of its contents provides the physician with a valuable reference list of acceptable new preparations on which to base his selection for use in treatment according to the established current practices of the profession.

New and Nonofficial Remedies for 1939 omits many articles which appeared in the publication for 1938. A few of these have been omitted by action of the Council because they conflict with the rules that govern the recognition of articles or because their distributors did not present convincing evidence to demonstrate their continued eligibility. Among these are: biliposol, serobacterins and suppositories salyrgan. A considerable number of others have been omitted as being off the market.

The 1939 New and Nonofficial Remedies, of course, contains the revisions which appeared in the supplements for the 1938 edition, and continues the plan of grouping together articles having similar composition or action under a general discussion. These discussions have undergone considerable revision in the 1939 edition. Further revision of statements regarding the actions, uses, dosage, composition, purity, identity, strength or physical properties of many of the articles has also been necessary in some cases. Noteworthy revisions are: anesthetics, local; bismuth compounds, organs of animals; vitamins and vitamin preparations and liver and stomach preparations.

The indices of the new volume of New and Nonofficial Remedies are of the same order and plan as in previous editions. A general index lists accepted articles, including those not described. This is followed by an index to distributors in which appear all the Council accepted articles listed under their respective manufacturers. Finally, a bibliographical index is added for listing proprietary and unofficial articles not included in N.N.R. This includes references to the Council publications concerning each such article as has appeared in The Journal of the A.M.A., reports of the Council on Pharmacy and Chemistry, Propaganda for Reform, Vol. 1 and 2, or Reports of the A.M.A. Chemical Laboratory.

ANNUAL REPRINT OF THE REPORTS OF THE COUNCIL ON PHARMACY AND CHEMISTRY OF THE AMERICAN MEDICAL ASSOCIATION FOR 1938. Cloth. Price, $1.00. Pp. 120. Chicago: American Medical Association, 1939.

This volume as usual contains noteworthy examples of the various kinds of reports made by the Council on Pharmacy and Chemistry: (1) preliminary reports; (2) supplemental reports on therapeutic or pharmacologic problems; (3) reports on the rejection of preparations offered for the Council's consideration.

Among the preliminary reports in this volume that on sulfapyridine, which carries a special article by Dr. Perrin H. Long, a Council member who has been much concerned with the work on this drug, is perhaps of greatest interest. After the Food and Drug Administration had released the drug for the use of physicians early in 1939, the Council accepted various brands for inclusion in N.N.R. and in connection with the published descriptions issued another status report (J.A.M.A., 112:1830, May 6, 1939) based on a questionnaire sent to men who had been prominent in the experimental use of the drug. This report, no doubt, will appear in the next volume of reprinted Council reports. Other preliminary reports are the following: Allantoin, a preparation of glyoxyldiureid purposed to supersede the use of surgical maggots; and Sulfapyridine, published shortly before the Council acceptance of this new chemotherapeutic drug.

Among the supplemental (or status) reports are those on Colloidal Sulfur in the Treatment of Chronic Arthritis, showing that much confirmatory evidence is needed to establish the value of this therapy; on Ergonovine, a careful study of the relation of this newly discovered principle to ergot therapy in general; and on Picrotoxin in Poisoning by the Barbiturates, showing the promise and the present limitations of this antidotal therapy.

Among the reports of rejection the following are noteworthy: Collodaurum, a "colloidal gold" preparation, promoted with unwarranted, exaggerated and misleading claims for its use in the treatment of cancer; Dermo-G, stated to be a mixture of Spermaceti, White Wax, Oil of Sweet Almonds, Sodium Borate, precipitated Sulphur and Water, an unscientific and superfluous mixture marketed under a therapeutically suggestive name with exaggerated, unwarranted claims; Fru-T-Lax, a needlessly complex and unscientific mixture advertised to the public under a misleading and inadequately descriptive name with claims which are unwarranted; and Hyposols Sulisocol, claimed to be "Sulphur Colloid" in 2 cc. of "Autoisotonized Solution," exploited for use in arthritis with inadequate evidence of its therapeutic value. Other rejections are explained in the reports on Map and Myoston, Nupercainal-"Ciba," Pulvoids Sulfanilamide and Sodium Bicarbonate (The Drug Products Co., Inc.), Quinoliv, Sedormid, and Tri-Costivin,

THE JOURNAL
OF THE
Oklahoma State Medical Association

Issued Monthly at McAlester, Oklahoma, under direction of the Council.

Copyright, 1939, by Oklahoma State Medical Association, McAlester, Oklahoma.

| Vol. XXXII | OCTOBER | Number 10 |

EDITORIAL BOARD

Dr. Ned Smith..Tulsa
Dr. L. J. Moorman..Oklahoma City
Dr. L. S. Willour, Chairman and Editor-in-Chief...McAlester

Entered at the Post Office at McAlester, Oklahoma, as second-class matter under the act of March 3rd, 1879.

This is the official Journal of the Oklahoma State Medical Association. All communications should be addressed to The Journal of the Oklahoma State Medical Association, McAlester Clinic, McAlester, Oklahoma. $4.00 per year; 40c per copy.

The editorial department is not responsible for the opinions expressed in the original articles of contributors.

Reprints of original articles will be supplied at actual cost provided request for them is attached to manuscripts or made in sufficient time before publication.

Articles sent this Journal for publication and all those read at the annual meetings of the State Association are the sole property of this Journal. The Journal relies on each individual contributor's strict adherence to this well-known rule of medical journalism. In the event an article sent this Journal for publication is published before appearance in The Journal the manuscript will be returned to the writer.

Failure to receive The Journal should call for immediate notification of the Editor, McAlester Clinic, McAlester, Oklahoma.

Local news of possible interest to the medical profession, notes on removals, changes of addresses, births, deaths and weddings will be gratefully received.

Advertising of articles, drugs or compounds unapproved by the Council on Pharmacy of the A. M. A., will not be accepted.

Advertising rates will be supplied on application.

It is suggested that wherever possible members of the State Association should patronize our advertisers in preference to others as a matter of fair reciprocity.

Printed by News-Capital Company, McAlester.

EDITORIAL

HIGHWAY FIRST AID

In 1933 through the efforts of Dr. E. Payne Palmer of Phoenix, Arizona, the American Red Cross became interested in the establishment of Highway First Aid Stations and while there has been considerable activity in Oklahoma in the development of this project there are still all too few of these stations along our highways.

Today we are spending millions in improving our highways and more millions in buying machines with greater speed and power. A million and a quarter people were injured in automobile accidents last year. Many of these accidents occur in the areas where there are no hospitals or facilities for their care. Consequently before trained assistance can be secured there is a considerable period when complications may develop. These complications may take the life of the injured person or lay the foundation for sequelae which will retard recovery or cause permanent deformities.

The establishment of these Stations should be encouraged by each County Medical Society. Proper locations should be selected and the training of the personnel supervised. Day and night service should be maintained where possible. There is no personnel cost in connection with this work as the entire service is on a volunteer basis from the time that first aid is given until the injured person is delivered to a physician or hospital.

The cost of operation is consequently slight and can be easily financed from the proceeds of the annual Red Cross roll call.

Accidents resulting in sprains, lacerations and bruises can be given first aid easily. Fractures can be handled so as to avoid further injury to the bones or soft tissues and prepared for transportation by fixed traction.

These stations are all properly marked and as they are established some publicity should be given as to their location.

Not only will such stations provide a much needed service but will be an ever present warning to the careless driver.

Will your County Medical Society help through the American Red Cross to develop this system along the highways of Oklahoma?

THE MEMPHIS MEETING OF THE SOUTHERN MEDICAL ASSOCIATION
NOVEMBER 21-24

Those who were privileged to attend either one or both of the previous meetings of the Southern Medical Association in Memphis (1917 and 1927) will remember the manifest charms of that city.

DATE OF THE MEETING

For some 30 years it has been the policy of the Association to meet between election week and Thanksgiving week. In determining the date for the Memphis meeting, the officers of the local society expressed a preference for the third week of November, November 21-24. And since

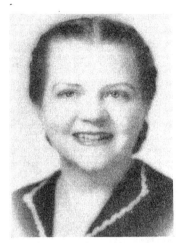

DR. EMMA JEAN CANTRELL

A unique position is that held by Dr. Emma Jean Cantrell (above) of Healdton, this year's president of the Carter County Medical Society.

Files of the Oklahoma State Medical Association show that Doctor Cantrell is the first woman to hold the presidency of such a group in a long series of years. She was elevated this year to head of the Carter county group from the secretary-treasurer position last year, an office not so uncommon for women physicians.

Doctor Cantrell moved to Healdton with her husband, Dr. David E. Cantrell, Jr., in January of this year. They practice with her father-in-law, Dr. D. E. Cantrell.

Dr. Cantrell was graduated from the Oklahoma school of medicine in 1933. After receiving her internship at the University and Crippled Children's hospitals in Oklahoma City, she spent the following year in Boston doing clinical work. With her husband, whom she met at Oklahoma university and married in 1927, at which time he was a pre-medical student, she moved in 1935 to Wilson, Okla. They practiced medicine there until their moving to Healdton.

Before her marriage, Doctor Cantrell was Miss Emma Jean Anthis, daughter of Mr. and Mrs. James M. Anthis of Muskogee.

that date did not interfere with either election or the traditional Thanksgiving, it was selected as the meeting date.

The announcement of President Roosevelt suggesting that Thanksgving this year be a week earlier caused considerable concern. Numerous obstacles stood in the way of any change of date for the convention. A large obstacle was the fact that engagements for the use of the necessary meeting place, the Municipal Auditorium, were completed nearly a year ago by the Southern M e d i c a l Association, and for other groups at other times. The officers of the Association, therefore, unanimously decided to hold to the original date. The Governor of Tennessee has announced that Tennessee will observe the traditional date, November 30, so the meeting will not be on Thanksgiving Day in Tennessee, even if it should be on Thanksgiving in some other s t a t e s. Governors of Oklahoma, Alabama, Arkansas and other Southern states have also indicated that they will observe the traditional date of November 30.

PROGRAM

The program for Memphis will follow in general the plan of recent meetings. Tuesday will be "Memphis Day," a program of short clinical presentations by physicians of Memphis. A General Clinical Session, a program arranged by the President, will be conducted on Wednesday morning. Beginning Wednesday, the 19 sections of the Association and the three conjoint meetings will convene. A General Session featuring the address of the President, Dr. Walter E. Vest, of Huntington, West Virginia, followed by the President's Reception and Ball, will be on Wednesday evening. As usual, the alumni reunions will take place on Thursday night. On Tuesday evening there will be a public session, a program arranged for the laity.

The programs of the section and general meetings in Memphis are complete and promise g e n e r o u s and stimulating discussions of many phases of medical progress.

---o---

Group Hospitalization

On September 21 in Oklahoma City, Mr. Walter R. McBee of Group Hospital Service, Inc., of St. Louis was the guest of the committee on group hospitalization of the Oklahoma State Medical Association. He spoke to a large and enthusiastic crowd of doctors, hospital representatives, and laymen on the subject of group hospitalization.

This was the first step in presenting this topic as an anticipated project of the Oklahoma State Medical Association.

The following night Mr. McBee apepared on a program in Tulsa sponsored by the Tulsa County Medical Society.

---o---

Cancer Program

Dr. W. F. Keller, chairman of the cancer committee, has outlined a most extensive program to be operated in cooperation with the women's field army for the coming year. Any County Cancer Committee desirous of sponsoring a program of this nature in their county should write the offices of the association, 210 Plaza Court, Oklahoma City. Speakers and diversified material will be supplied upon request.

Clinical Conferences This Month

Of the various obligations which exist between the doctor and his patient, and which are assumed by everyone in the practice of medicine, two are outstanding. These are: first, to continue the study of medicine in order to be familiar with the advances which are constantly being made; and second, to keep one's self as physically perfect as possible in order to be able to continue under the constant strain of modern-day practice. It is rather a rare and unusual experience when one has the opportunity of developments along both these lines at the same time. This unusual situation is offered to the doctors of Oklahoma and surrounding states during the Fall Clinical Conference, October 30 through November 2.

For the past year committees of the Oklahoma City Clinical Society have been working long hours to perfect a program which would meet the requirements of the high standards, which have been set by this particular meeting in the past. This work has been, through the year, motivated not by any purpose of self-aggrandizement or the advancement of any particular group but rather entirely for the benefit of the busy men who make up the profession in this area.

The opportunity for study and for entertainment is offered with only one idea in mind; to-wit, the benefit of the medical profession. Each individual can, therefore, select for himself what he most desires to study and to learn, and he is assured of authoritative opinions on the subjects presented and at the same time a release from the turmoil and strain which is characteristic of medical practice. Round-table discussions give him the opportunity to hear discussed any topic in which he may be interested and which may not be included in the formal program.

More particularly than ever, is this year one in which such an opportunity should be utilized in order that our patients have the utmost in examinations and the best advice based on most recent advances. It will accomplish a great deal in the proper relationship of the physician and the patient, which relationship, always a great help to the physician, has to some extent been lost in recent years.

It is for these various reasons that the Oklahoma City Clinical Society invites the attendance of all doctors for the benefit of their patients and themselves.

―――――o―――――

Malpractice Insurance

With the season for renewal of malpractice insurance by the doctors of Oklahoma almost at hand, a great number of inquiries relative to the Oklahoma Group Malpractice policy are being received by the executive secretary's office.

This policy, which is written only for doctors who are members of the Oklahoma State Medical Association, is now carried by approximately 250 members of the state society. Insurance coverage in this policy, which is written by the Houston Fire and Casualty Company, is for minimum limits of $25,000 for any one claim and maximum limits of $40,000 for any one policy year.

Application forms have just been mailed to every member of the state organization and anyone desiring information is invited to write the state society office, 210 Plaza Court, Oklahoma City.

―――――o―――――

Locations

Of recent date, the office of the executive secretary has received numerous requests for physicians to locate in cities of Oklahoma.

Anyone desirous of investigating any of these locations please write to the office of the association, 210 Plaza Court, Oklahoma City.

―――――――――――――――

Editorial Notes—Personal and General

The Tulsa city commission approved late in September the appointment of Dr. R. M. Adams of Ada as Tulsa city health superintendent. Doctor Adams, formerly a state health department officer, assumed his duties October 1.

―――――

Approximately 60 members of the four-county medical society, composed of medical groups of Pottawatomie, Seminole, Pontotoc and Hughes counties, attended the fall quarterly meeting recently in Shawnee at the home of Dr. J. A. Walker. Following a barbecue supper, a program was presented by the Hughes county medical society.

―――――

Construction of a much-needed ward building at the Western Oklahoma hospital, Supply, is expected to begin soon. Bids for construction work were to be received by the state board of affairs October 4.

―――――

Dr. O. E. Templin, Alva, has received his commission of a lieutenant-colonel in the medical reserve corps of the United States army for five years. Doctor Templin entered the war as a captain, and has been in the reserve corps since 1928.

―――――

Appointment of Dr. C. C. Gardner, Ponca City, as temporary superintendent of health of Kay county has been announced by the state health department. Doctor Gardner has been city physician at Ponca City for a number of years.

―――――

DR. D. W. BRANHAM wishes to announce the removal of his office from 514 to 502 Medical Arts Building, Oklahoma City, Oklahoma.

―――――

Appointment of Dr. Claude Bloss of Okemah as American Red Cross roll call chairman of Okfuskee county has been announced by G. W. McCoy of the national organization.

―――――

Visiting Oklahoma City physicians presented two medical papers at the Caddo county session of the Tri-County Medical society in Anadarko recently. Dr. Rex Bolend, presenting a paper on "The Male Climacteris," was followed by Dr. Wilbur F. Keller, who spoke on the same subject. Dr. R. Q. Goodwin gave the second paper, "The Anemias."

―――――

DR. W. P. LONGMIRE and family of Sapulpa are leaving for the East, October 12. The doctor will attend the meeting of the American College of Surgeons at Philadelphia. From Philadelphia he will go to Baltimore to visit his son who has a residency in Johns Hopkins Hospital.

―――――

Members of the Women's Auxiliary of the LeFlore County Medical Association held their first regular meeting recently at the Judkin-Forbes hotel in Poteau. Following presentation of the constitution and by-laws, Mrs. Wayne Lowrey discussed the Southeastern medical meeting at Poteau and Mrs. W. L. Shippey talked on philanthropic work.

―――――

Dr. John F. Hackler, Stillwater, has completed his enrollment in the School of Hygiene and Public Health, Johns Hopkins university, and expects to receive the Master of Public Health at the close of the school year.

―――――

Dr. Troy F. Long and Dr. John Davenport, two newcomers to Holdenville's medical fraternity, were guests at the September meeting of the Hughes County Medical Society. Discussion of various problems and developments of interest to the profession made up the program.

New county health officer of Nowata county is Dr. S. P. Roberts of Nowata, according to an announcement by the state health department.

Dr. Ray H. Lindsey of Pauls Valley was engaged in a few weeks post graduate medical course last month at the Cook County hospital in Chicago.

DR. GEORGE H. KIMBALL gave a talk on Plastic Surgery showing slides of same, at the Woods County Medical Society meeting at Altus on September 25, 1939. Dr. Algood was Chairman at Altus.

OBITUARIES

Dr. W. S. Stevens

Death came Monday, September 11, to Dr. Walter S. Stevens, first superintendent of the Choctaw-Chickasaw sanitarium at Talihina and for the last 14 years medical director of district five, U. S. Indian service. Doctor Stevens died at St. Anthony hospital in Oklahoma City following an extended illness.

Born in Pike county, Illinois, he studied medicine at Barnes university, St. Louis, returning to his home county in 1914 to begin the practice of medicine at Hull. He entered the Indian service and came to Oklahoma as first superintendent of the Choctaw-Chickasaw sanitarium at Talihina in 1919.

When the district five medical setup was made in 1925, he was named director, with offices in Shawnee. In 1932 the office was moved to the federal building in Oklahoma City, and Doctor Stevens had lived there since.

Doctor Stevens is survived by his wife; a sister, Mrs. R. F. McCallister; and his parents, Mr. and Mrs. William Bell of Rockport, Ill.

The body was sent to Springfield, Ill., for interment.

Dr. V. M. Wallace

Dr. Virgil May Wallace of Morris, Oklahoma, died August 22, 1939, at his office, following a stroke of paralysis.

A native of Cleveland, Ark., Doctor Wallace was graduated from the medical school at the University of Oklahoma in 1911. He began the practice of medicine in Allen, Pontotoc county, moving to Morris in 1914. He had been there continuously since that time. He was a member of the Masonic lodge, and a Shriner.

Surviving are his widow; two sons, a brother and three sisters.

Funeral services were conducted from the home August 24, with the Rev. L. L. Shaw, pastor of the Christian church at Morris, officiating.

Dr. L. A. McComb

Dr. L. A. McComb, Tulsa surgeon, died at his home in Tulsa September 2.

Private funeral rites were held in the chapel of the Fitzgerald funeral home September 4, with Dr. Golder Lawrence, pastor of the First Methodist church, officiating. Interment was in Memorial Park.

Doctor McComb is survived by three children, Mrs. Howard Gooden of Tulsa, and Virginia and Martha Ann of the home; his parents, Dr. and Mrs. J. W. McComb of Jacksboro, Texas; three sisters and three brothers.

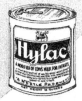

Resolutions

Whereas: Virgil M. Wallace, M.D., earned the love and respect of the people of Morris, Okla., and its surrounding territory by his many years of service as their family doctor, as well as by his cheerful, and friendly personality; and

Whereas: He was ever faithful and loyal to the best interests of his fellow practitioners of medicine, serving actively in any positions of honor and trust, to which he was called by the Okmulgee Medical Society; and

Whereas: He has now been called to his eternal reward;

Therefore: Be it resolved, that the Okmulgee County Medical Society, in regular meeting, assembled, this 18th of September, 1939, do hereby express their deep regard and respect for Dr. Wallace, and their sympathy for his bereaved family; and

Do direct a copy of these resolutions be sent to the family, be placed in the archives of the society, and be published in the Journal of the Oklahoma State Medical Association.

S. B. Leslie, M.D.
T. C. Carloss, M.D.
M. B. Glisman, M.D., Chm.

Whereas: Loyal B. Torrance, M.D., served the people of Okmulgee faithfully and well, throughout his whole active medical life, from 1909 to the time of his last illness; and

Whereas: He always was interested in the affairs, activities, and interests of the medical profession, of this County and State, as well as in the progress of medical science, serving faithfully and well in every position of honor and responsibility to which his colleagues called him; and

Whereas: He has now been called to his eternal reward;

Therefore: Be it resolved, that the Okmulgee County Medical Society, in regular meeting, assembled, this 18th of September, 1939, do hereby express their deep regard and respect for Dr. Torrance, and their sympathy for his bereaved family; and

Do direct a copy of these resolutions be sent to the family, be placed in the archives of the Society, and be published in the Journal of the Oklahoma State Medical Association.

S. B. Leslie, M.D.
T. C. Carloss, M.D.
M. B. Glissmann, M.D., Chm.

Examinations—American Board of Obstetrics and Gynecology

The written examination and review of case histories (Part I) for Group B candidates will be held in the various cities of the United States and Canada on Saturday, January 6, 1940, at 2 p.m. Formal notice of the place of examination will be sent each candidate several weeks in advance of the examination date. No candidate will be admitted to examination whose examination fee has not been paid at the Secretary's Office. Candidates who successfully complete the Part I examination proceed automatically to the Part II examination held in June, 1940.

Candidates for re-examination in Part I (written paper and submission of case histories) must request such re-examination by writing the Secretary's Office not later than November 15, 1939. Candidates who are required to take re-examinations must do so before the expiration of three years from the date of their original examination.

The general oral and pathological examinations (Part II) for all candidates (Groups A and B) will be conducted by the entire Board, meeting in Atlantic City, N. J., on June 8, 9, 10, and 11, 1940, immediately prior to the annual meeting of the American Medical Association in New York City.

Application for admission to Group A, Part II examinations must be on file in the Secretary's Office not later than March 15, 1940.

After January 1, 1942, there will be only one classification of candidates, and all will be required to take the Part I and Part II examinations.

For further information and application blanks, address Dr. Paul Titus, Secretary, 1015 Highland Building, Pittsburgh (6), Pennsylvania.

Tri-County Health Unit Program

Approximately 2,200 typhoid fever immunizations have been given in 22 schools in Bryan county in early fall operations of the extensive program of the tri-county health unit, composed of Bryan, Marshall and Love counties.

The clinics were held in school buildings in each community, while in some cases transportation was arranged with several schools meeting at a central point.

Central headquarters for the unit are at Madill, the staff including a doctor, Dr. William Mead; a sanitarian, Mr. New; a clerk, and three nurses.

The program will include immunization for typhoid, smallpox and diphtheria, prevention and spread of contagious diseases where follow up work may be arranged, examination of water and milk supply, and any other problems of sanitation.

How To Give Cod Liver Oil

Some authorities recommend that cod liver oil be given in the morning and at bedtime when the stomach is empty, while others prefer to give it after meals in order not to retard gastric secretion. If the mother will place the very young baby on her lap and hold the child's mouth open by gently pressing the cheeks together between her thumb and fingers while she administers the oil, all of it will be taken. The infant soon becomes accustomed to taking the oil without having its mouth held open. It is most important that the mother administer the oil in a matter-of-fact manner, without apology or expression of sympathy.

If given cold, cod liver oil has little taste, for the cold tends to paralyze momentarily the gustatory nerves. As any "taste" is largely a metallic one from the silver or silver-plated spoon (particularly if the plating is worn), a glass spoon has an advantage.

On account of its higher potency in Vitamins A and D, Mead's Cod Liver Oil Fortified With Percomorph Liver Oil may be given in one-third the ordinary cod liver oil dosage, and is particularly desirable in cases of fat intolerance.

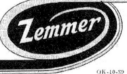

ABSTRACTS : REVIEWS :.COMMENTS
and CORRESPONDENCE

SURGERY AND GYNECOLOGY
Abstracts, Reviews and Comments from
LeRoy Long Clinic
714 Medical Arts Building, Oklahoma City

Carcinoma of the Breast. End-Results: Massachusetts General Hospital 1930, 1931, and 1932. By Channing C. Simmons, M.D., F.A.C.S., Grantley W. Taylor, M.D., F.A.C.S., and Claude E. Welch, M.D., Boston Massachusetts. Surgery, Gynecology and Obstetrics, August 1939, Volume 69, Page 171.

This paper is the seventh in a series of reports on the end results of operation for carcinoma of the breast at the Massachusetts General Hospital. This paper covers the three year period 1930 to 1932. There was an operable rate of 80 per cent and this report is on 185 patients who had operations performed during this three year period.

"Five to eight year cures were obtained in 70 per cent of the cases in which disease was confined to the breast, in 31 per cent when the axillary nodes were involved, and in 45 per cent of the entire group." The end results were known in every case that was operated upon.

All of the breast tumors were graded pathologically and the results indicate that the pathological index of malignancy was of great significance in prognosis. Those classified as grade I showed cures in 86 per cent. Those classified as grade II showed cures in 51 per cent. Those classified as grade III showed cures in 31 per cent. By reviewing their record, these authors feel "the age of the patient is of prognostic importance only in so far as younger patients tend to present higher grades of malignancy and earlier metastasis to the axilla."

It is therefore felt that the most important basis for prognosis in a given patient lies in the extension of the disease and the pathological index of malignancy which is to say whether it is limited to the breast or whether it has extended to the axilla and whether pathological index is grade I, II, or III.

Their series shows that the clinical diagnosis of axillary lymph node involvement is highly fallible. Nearly half of the cases in which no nodes could be felt clinically, had axillary lymph node involvement. Incidentally, two-thirds of the entire group proved to have axillary lymph node involvement. Incidentally, two-thirds of the entire group proved to have axillary node involvement at the time of operation.

This difficulty in determining clinically the involvement of the lymph nodes in addition to the advisability of radical surgery in any type of malignancy, has led to the radical operation in all of these patients with removal of considerable subcutaneous fat, the breast, both pectoral muscles and the axillary contents. R e a s o n a b l y large amounts of skin were excised but the wounds were able to be closed in practically all cases.

No preoperative X-ray was employed in this series and only a very few patients had postoperative X-ray.

The sites of recurrences are tabulated and the most common site is found to be lungs, although bone metastasis was nearly as frequent. Only 10 recurrences in the operative field were found.

They believe the improvement in curability in this series as compared with their previous series may be based upon standardization of radical operation and to better selection of patients. They feel that there may be some improvement due to shortening of preoperative duration of the disease as the result of educational programs but they cannot attribute any of the improvement in results to radiation therapy which was not employed.

They have established certain criteria for operability of carcinoma of the breast. "Carcinoma of the breast is operable when the disease is confined to the breast, or to the breast and axilla. The primary tumor must be movable in relation to the chest wall, and must not present extensive skin involvement, skin metastases, or the subepidermal infiltration known as 'inflammatory' carcinoma. The axillary nodes must be movable in relation to the chest wall and great vessels, and these nodes must be few in number. There must be no evidence of disease in the supra-clavicular areas or in the opposite axilla, nor of metastatic disease in the lungs, pleura, liver or skeleton. Patients in the last two series have had pre-operative X-ray studies to rule out the presence of skeletal and pulmonary metastases."

Even with this more careful selection of patients for operation and with their belief that many of the advanced patients are being sent directly to radiation institutions, the operability rate has still remained 80 per cent. This, together with the fact that the average duration of the disease before consultation has reduced to 2.8 months in the cases in which the disease was limited to the breast and to 5.3 months in the cases in which disease had extended to the axilla, lead these authors to believe that the educational programs of the past 13 years have been of distinct advantage in assisting their excellent results.

Comment: This is an excellent report showing splendid end results in a series where every patient had been followed. It is equally important that it represents a series which has been treated surgically only and offers good comparison with those series reported with combination radiation therapy. Preoperative radiation has not yet become fully established as offering advantages over the radical operation alone, and it is by comparison of series such as this one and those in which preoperative radiation has been employed that we may arrive at a correct conclusion.

It is also noteworthy that these authors have carefully selected their cases and established criteria for doing so and have employed almost the identical type of operation.

Wendell Long.

What is the Value of Appendicostomy in Grave Peritonitis of Appendicular Origin? (Que Vaut L'Appendicostomie Dans les Peritonites Graves d'origine Appendiculaire?) By Paul A. Poliquin, F.A.C.S., Chirurgien-adjoint a l'hopital Saint-Francois-d'Assise, Assistant-chirurgien a l'hopital Saint-Luc et a l'hopital de l'Enfant-Jesus (Quebec). L'Union Medicale du Canada, September, 1939; page 949.

The author directs attention to the fact that

surgeons have observed for a long time that in the case of perforation of the appendix with peritonitis there is an occasional patient who, after operation, develops a fecal fistula, and that in those cases developing a fecal fistula the patients have usually progressed in a very much more satisfactory way than those who did not develop a fistula.

From time to time surgeons have made practical application of this clinical observation by providing for drainage from the intestinal tract itself in the immediate neighborhood of the appendix at the time of operation. The author refers to this procedure as "primitive derivation," and he gives credit to Dr. W. E. B. Davis for formally advising it in a statement at a meeting of the Southern Surgical Association in 1890. The author quotes Dr. Davis as follows: "We are very rarely called before the third day after the rupture (apparently referring to perforation of the appendix). Before this time the patient has had all sorts of treatment, and is then sent to us for operation." This is a very free translation of the quotation in French by Dr. Poliquin. Poliquin's statement in French being as follows: "Nous sommes tres rarement appeles avant le troisieme jour de la rupture. Avant ce temps on a eu recours a toutes sortes de traitement, cest alors qu'on s'adresse a nous pour operer." The author quotes Davis to the effect that in such a situation he advised opening of the intestinal tract for the purpose of securing "primitive derivation." "Open the abdomen, incise the intestine, irrigate with warm water and make an artificial anus. This will relieve the patient of his distention and give him the best chance of recovery," is the statement attributed to Davis. In speaking of this statement by Davis in 1890, there is a reference to an article by Edgar P. Hogan, entitled "The Appendix Problem" appearing in the Annals of Surgery, May, 1937, page 815.

In 1805 Mixter established a technique in which a cecostomy was performed at the time of operation for appendicitis, followed by extensive peritonitis.

In 1910 C. B. Keetly of London recommended appendicostomy. The question was studied more completely by Patry in 1916. Statistics were reported by Jackson in 1917. This was followed by another report in 1920 by A. Caucci of Milan, these statistics being the first in connection with the procedure.

According to the author, appendicostomy as a treatment of appendiceal peritonitis has been the subject of many articles contributed by numerous surgeons in both the United States and Europe.

In connection with technique, the author advises as follows: "Place a purse-string suture around the base of the appendix, remove the appendix without ligating it, introduce into the cecum by way of the lumen of the stump of the appendix a No 16 Neladon catheter, the end of the catheter being cut off, taking care to pass the catheter through omentum; fixation of the catheter to the margin of the stump, followed by tying the purse-string suture, the stump of the appendix being inverted at the same time. In addition, the author advises two drainage tubes, one of them extending into the pelvis, and the other to the space on the outer side of the cecum. Close the abdomen, and fix the catheter to the skin so that it will not be displaced.

Comments: When one takes into consideration the inhibition of peristalsis in the presence of peritoneal inflammation, one can understand the value of a "vent" for the escape of gas and toxic liquid material from the intestinal tract. One understands, also, why intestinal incompetence (so-called "ileus," a term that has neither anatomical nor pathological foundation—is developed. "Ileus" is derived from a verb that means to twist. There is not, necessarily, any twisting in connection with so-called "adynamic ileus." The difficulty is due to the temporary reduction and disturbance of function of the intestinal musculature—hence, in our judgement, the appropriateness of the term "intestinal incompetence.")

Between 25 and 30 years ago we were impressed with the remarkable improvement immediately after the development of a fecal fistula following appendicectomy in the presence of spreading peritonitis. It was observed that nausea, vomiting, and abdominal distention, with pain, were relieved. About that time we inaugurated the treatment of appendiceal peritonitis that we have followed ever since — that is, nothing by mouth, morphin as necessary to keep the patient comfortable, the end of a colon tube introduced just well beyond the sphincter for the escape of gas, proctoclysis, large, moist, hot packs over the abdomen, to be changed frequently. At that time the chief difficulty was to give the patient as much water as he ought to have, together with sodium chloride. Some years later the parenteral administration of normal saline solution and of dextrose solution became feasible, and gradually, in our service, the administration of fluid per rectum has been discontinued as a routine measure.

While I was preparing to dictate the abstract of this article by Poliquin, Dr. Earl Garside, Chicago, came in to visit us. I spoke to him about the article by Poliquin, and then he told me that he and his associates had written an article on the conservative treatment of appendiceal peritonitis. The article is by A. T. Lundgren, Earl Garside, and William A. Boice, Augustana Hospital, Chicago, and was published in the June number of Surgery, page 813. It is a splendid review of the conservative management of appendiceal peritonitis, and in connection with it the authors speak of deliberate cecostomy, the technic indicating that a catheter is introduced into the cecum by way of the stump of the amputated appendix.

In the article by Poliquin, abstracted above, it is advised that about 100 c.c. of warm water or normal saline solution be instilled into the catheter entering the cecum about every two hours.

In addition to the performance of the appendicostomy, and its subsequent management, the author (Poliquin) advises the Fowler position with inclination to the right side, the parenteral administration of fluids if necessary.

Poliquin reports a series of 80 cases of grave peritonitis in which appendicostomies have been done. There were 63 recoveries and 17 deaths, being a mortality of 21.3 per cent.

We had not deliberately performed an appendicostomy at the time of operation, because we have been quite satisfied with the management that I have briefly indicated above. We believe that the management that we have indicated above is applicable in the average case of appendiceal peritonitis as a pre-operative procedure. It has been our experience that our plan of treatment is just as applicable before operation as it is after operation. Notwithstanding these statements, I regard the article by Dr. Poliquin as being a very valuable contribution.

LeRoy Long.

Conservative Myomectomy. By Professor Bernhard Zondek, Jerusalem, Palestine. Surgery, Gynecology and Obstetrics, August, 1939, Volume 69, Page 214.

Since he has been in Jerusalem, Zondek has performed 82 myoma operations. Of these, 67 were performed in women sexually mature up to an age of about 40. Of these 67, 40 were operated upon conservatively with the removal of the tumors by myomectomy and conservation of the uterus, 59.7 per cent of the 67 in the sexually mature age. He reports in the last 10 cases nine were operated upon conservatively.

"The size, the number, the site or even benign degenerative changes in the myoma do not contraindicate the use of conservative operative methods."

After his conservative operation conception took

place in seven patients in which the pregnancy as well as the parturition and puerperium were normal.

He states that he has been led to this extremely conservative treatment of fibroid tumors since going to Jerusalem because the women there are willing to take risk of recurrences in order to preserve menstruation and the possibility of conception.

In the direction of possible recurrences, it is not only interesting to know that he has had two cases but that Victor Bonney, of London, who uses the conservative operative method chiefly, reports that in many years he has had only 2.3 per cent of recurrences. Zondek emphasizes the fact that this operation can be only successful and recurrences reduced by removing every perceivable and palpable myomatous nodule.

Comment: One of the interesting features of this article is the change in the author's approach to the treatment of fibroid tumors since he has been located in Palestine, following a long period of practice in Germany. There is little question that the attitude of the patient has considerable bearing upon the choice of operative procedure for fibroid tumors where there is a distinct possibility of recurrence, and it is interesting to note that in different parts of the world fibroid tumors are treated more conservatively or more radically to a considerable degree dependent upon the wishes and the character of the people so treated.

Myomectomy is a valuable procedure and should probably be employed much more extensively than is at present the case. Though one would hardly endorse such a high percentage of myomectomies in the treatment of fibroid tumors, it may well be emphasized that myomectomy should be employed more frequently especially in younger women who have not had children or who have not been married. The t e c h n i c a l difficulties are somewhat greater than hysterectomy but despite the additional technical burden and the slight additional mortality risk it is an extremely desirable procedure in many instances.

Wendell Long.

A Simple, Efficient Method to Diminish the Instances of Primary and Secondary Infection in Surgical Wounds. By Reginald H. Jackson and Reginald H. Jackson, Jr. Surgery, September, 1939, Page 398.

The authors felt that there was a potent source of direct infection in clinical wounds in addition to the following long recognized potential factors of infections of clinical wounds.

They enumerate the long recognized factors as (1) contact infection from defectively sterilized hands, gloves, instruments, skin in the field of operation, sutures, ligatures, dressings; (2) faulty hemostasis; (3) rough handling of tissues; (4) mass ligature necrosis; (5) excessive bulk of catgut in ligatures and sutures; (6) suturing which interferes with proper blood supply; (7) use of strong antiseptic solution with resulting necrosis or diminished functional repair ability of cells.

They felt that in addition to the above, long recognized, potential factors that there actually exists today in every operating room a most potent source of direct infection, one which strikes with a frequency and viciousness directly related to the following factors:

1. The number of human beings present in the operating room.

2. The frequency with which the room is used.

3. The time of year, the highest incidence of such clinical wound infection being coincident with high rate respiratory infection of humans.

4. That there are nearly always in the room carriers of staphylococcus aureaus or hemolytic streptococcus.

5. That the surgeon, himself, unwittingly may be the carrier.

6. That it is practically impossible to guard against droplet infections without the use of impossible face and nose masks.

7. That practically all operating rooms contain, in the air, and on the floor, walls and ceilings, more staphylococci and, at times, hemolytic streptococci, than any other department in the hospital except the nose and throat department.

8. That staphylococcus aureaus is the principal and general source of infection of clinical wounds.

9. That these infecting agents gain direct entrance to the wound by precipitation from the air overlying the wound and by droplet infection.

10. That every wound made by the surgeon is contaminated and potentially infected in direct proportion to its size and the length of time of its exposure.

11. That a run of such cases always means that the air in the room contains, as proved by culture, a higher percentage of these organisms than normally.

12. That the percentage of viable bacteria reaching the wound may be greatly diminished, almost to the vanishing point, through appreciable continuous special ultraviolet radiation of the air and field of operation, with a resultant marked percentage reduction in the incidence of infected wounds.

13. That while the average incidence of such baleful clinical wound infections is from four to six per cent (heretofore recognized as an irreducible minimum) it at times rises to 18 to 20 per cent.

14. That a scientific bacteriologic checkup on every link in the so-called aseptic chain may achieve a 100 per cent credit, and yet the incidence of clinical wound infections continue at two to three times the average.

They were primarily, before experimental work again, interested in the statement of Mason of Northwestern Medical School who emphasized that it is within the power of the surgeon to change a contaminated, traumatic wound into a surgically purified one which generally will heal per primam without the use of any antiseptic whatever, provided soap may be so classified.

The authors then reasoned that in as much as every operative wound is contaminated and potentially infected, why should they not cleanse it in the same way?

They set up their experiment on the basis of the following two questions:

1. Will the same thorough cleansing with soap and water used in accidental wounds militate in any way against ideal healing if applied to clinical surgical wounds before closing them?

2. In a clinical wound proved by culture to be contaminated, what percentage of success in debacterialization may be expected by cleansing with soap and water?

In their work they proved to themselves that (a) However clean and aseptic an operating room appears, wound infecting organisms are always present in the air and on the walls.

(b) Gentle scrubbing of a surgical wound with soap and water before closure does not militate in the slightest degree against ideal healing.

(c) In a surgical wound proved to be contaminated, soap cleansing will debacterialize it.

The method of preparation of the soap mixture used by the authors is given in detail. They also explain in detail their exact technique in scrubbing out the wound with this soap mixture.

Their conclusions are as follows:

1. The air of every operating room is practically always badly contaminated with staphylococci and streptococci. The incidence of primary wound infection with these organisms averages four to six per cent, but at times may be as high as 20 per cent.

2. Every surgical wound develops a sticky fibrinous nutrient film which catches and holds bacteria and dust as would flypaper.

3. The amount of contamination and potential source of wound infection is directly proportional to the size of the wound and the length of time the air exposure continues.

4. Mechanical cleansing with soap and water just before closure of wounds very efficiently and harmlessly removes this chance of primary wound infection with staphylococci, streptococci, etc.

5. The method they describe is said to actually aid in ideal wound repair as evidenced by the very high per cent of wounds healing with "complete placidity," no redness, induration, or irritation such as is often seen and noted in wounds which just manage to pass muster as healing per primam.

LeRoy D. Long.

----------------o----------------

EYE, EAR, NOSE AND THROAT
Edited by Marvin D. Henley, M.D.
911 Medical Arts Building, Tulsa

Choroidal Angino-Sclerosis with Special Reference to its Hereditary Characters. Arnold Sorsby, London. The British Journal of Ophthalmology, July, 1939.

This is an original communication accompanied by numerous pictures of the fundus, colored and otherwise. A review of the literature is given quite completely. Aetiological considerations enumerated are as follows:

1. Age.—Most patients with choroidal sclerosis, no matter of what type, were elderly. But in some cases the history was of long duration, as in Harman's case; Bednarski's patient was aged 23 years and developed night blindness at eight years; Knapp's patient was aged 11 years.

2. Syphilis.—In a case of rather patchy distribution illustrated Oeller (b), and in one of Di Marzio's patients, syphilis appears to have been present. In another case of Oeller (a) (1899) and was assumed by Guglianetti for a case of generalized choroidal sclerosis.

3. Tuberculosis.—Pulmonary tuberculosis was assumed to be the cause in one of Di Marzio's cases.

4. Cardio-vascular disease.—Only in one case (Harman 2nd case) was there a definite heart lesion. Most reports speak of the patient's good health. Morton reported of his patient that seven years later the general condition had deteriorated and that there was albuminuria.

5. Familial Incidence.—Most case reports give a negative family history; a familial factor is suggested, but not conclusively, in four case histories.

6. From reporting cases there is no question but what there is a definite relationship between choroidal sclerosis and retinitis pigmentosa.

The summary of the literature shows:

1. It would appear that three clinical forms of choroidal sclerosis have been described.

(a) "Central senile areolar choroiditis." (Nettleship, Retze, Thompson). In this type a more or less regular oval area extends from the disc temporally and engulfs the macula.

(b) Peripapillary type (Haab, Harman, Cuperus, Guglianetti, Di Marzio, Pillat). Here the choroidal sclerosis radiates from the disc to a variable but considerable extent peripherally in all directions.

(c) Generalised sclerosis (Morton, Frost, Harman). In Morton's and Frost's cases the macula was spared allowing good central vision, with fields of a tubular type. In Harman's case the macula was engulfed.

2. Evidence of syphilis was present in four cases (Oeller, Frost, Guglianetti, Di Marzio); and of tuberculosis in one (Di Marzio). Otherwise the case reports were negative, except that remote consanguinity is noted by Knapp and a possible familial factor is suggested by Holloway and Fewell, by Cuperus, Guglianetti and by Wilmer. In practically all cases, those of Pollot and of Di Marzio excepted, the diagnosis of "atypical retinitis pigmentosa" could be ruled out.

(In this review the limited peripapillary choroidal sclerosis sometimes seen in myopia and the patchy secondary sclerosis following inflammatory lesions in the choroid have not been considered.)

There are case reports of familial choroidal sclerosis given.

Night blindness and undue contraction of the field was not a feature in any of the patients reported in the present study—clinically some cases of retinitis pigmentosa show considerable choroidal sclerosis with relatively little retinal involvement—the distinction between a peripapillary type and a central and peripapillary type of choroidal sclerosis has some justification—the nature of choroidal sclerosis requires elucidation—the present case reports establish its familial character and the fact that the lesion develops in adult life—presumably the choroidal circulation earlier in life was normal —in so far as the lesion appears to develop in post-natal life in fully differentiated tissue, and is of hereditary character, it may be regarded as belonging to the group of heredo-degenerations or abiotrophies."

Subconjunctival Injections of Neoprontosil in the Treatment of Ocular Infections. R. Townley Paton, M.D., New York. Archives of Ophthalmology, September, 1939.

In a detailed and comprehensive communication Paton gives the results obtained in the clinic of the Manhattan Eye, Ear, and Throat Hospital. Loe, Rychener, Lian, Kirk, McKelvie, Hussein and Thygeson have reported on sulfanilamide in treatment of trachoma and gonococcic infections of the eye. Newman, Perry, Willis, Goldenbury, L. J. and R. Fernandez have written on cases of gonococcic infections of the eye which have been cured with sulfanilimide or neoprontosil.

Loe has reported successful treatment of trachoma among the Sioux Indians with sulfanilimide. He gives ⅛ gr. of sulfanilimide per pound of body weight per day, in divided doses, with an equal amount of sodium bicarbonate. Gradle has also done some work with trachoma. Heinz is the only reference in regard to the use of subconjunctival injections of neoprontosil. Brav used 2.5 per cent solution of neoprontosil topically in corneal ulcerations with good results. In addition Glover used the oral administration with corneal ulcerations with equally good results.

In the discussion of toxic reactions we are reminded that there is no specific therapeutic test available to determine idiosyncrasies. It is recommended that small doses be given at first and then larger ones later with a hematologic follow-up. Where large numbers are dealt with daily in a clinic this follow-up is almost impossible, so the subconjunctival injections were inaugurated. Thus far no reactions have been observed.

In regard to dosage "the total amount required over the first 24 hours of treatment is calculated on the basis of one cc of a 2.5 per cent solution for each pound of body weight up to 120 pounds." The total daily amount is divided into six parts and given every four hours subcutaneously.

For the subconjunctival injections there is no available data but at the Manhattan Eye, Ear and Throat Hospital they give 0.3 to 0.5 cc. of a 2.5 per cent solution every two days for quite a number of doses without apparent injury to the surrounding tissues. The purpose of giving the neoprontosil in this manner was to give it in a safe way when there was no follow-up possible. It also gives a more concentrated effect at the site of the infection. Patients who cannot tolerate the drug by mouth may possibly take it better subconjunctivally. According to Loe, and with which the author agrees, this method in trachoma produces the following result:

"Improvement of objective symptoms included paling of the conjunctiva and paling of the trachomatous patches and flattening of the granules and follicles. The blood vessels of the conjunctiva become more visible on the fifth and sixth day of treatment and daily thereafter they become more normal."

The method of administration is first thorough anaesthesia with 0.5 per cent pontocaine hydrochloride. The first injection is 0.3 cc. neoprontosil in either the upper or lower cul-de-sac with a tuberculin syringe. There follows a stinging sensation which lasts about three minutes for which gentle massage is done. If there is much scar tissue numerous small injections may be used instead of the one of 0.3 cc. Iritis, scleritis and interstitial keratitis have responded well and shown good results. The author's own conclusions are as follows:

Neoprontosil when administered subconjunctivally in small doses has been well tolerated by the eye in the presence of certain severe intraocular and extraocular infections.

For ambulatory patients, especially clinical patients, for whom a daily blood count and determination of the hemoglobin and sulfanilamide concentration of the blood cannot be performed, the combined oral and subconjunctival injections lessen the danger of severe toxic effects.

Otogenic Meningitis. Terence Cawthorne, London. The Journal of Laryngology and Otology, August, 1939.

Since 1935 when Domagk introduced prontosil into the treatment of this disease, the author has collected records of 194 recoveries from otogenic bacterial meningitis. For 34 years previous to 1936, Gray was able to find records of only 27 recoveries of otogenic streptococcal meningitis. Neal, Jackson and Appelbaum in a report of 2,674 cases determined that 67 per cent occurred under the age of 10 years. In 623 cases these same men determined that the leading organism was pneumococcus, then streptococcus and in order B. Influenza and staphylococcus.

The method of spread of the infection is by one of the following routes: by the spaces already present naturally formed by injury, long standing disease or previous operation; along vascular channels; or by actual destruction of intervening bone. The author says: "Acute suppurative otitis media may cause meningitis within hours by s p r e a d through certain preformed spaces, within days by spread through veins, and within weeks by direct destruction of intervening bone."

The cerebrospinal fluid is likened to a mirror of meningeal behaviour. It shows the serous, cellular and bacterial stage in addition to giving other valuable information. The clinical features of this disease are discussed thoroughly under the stage of onset, the stage of established disease and the stage of paralysis. A cerebrospinal fluid is necessary for a definite diagnosis.

Under avoidable factors that the author in his own experience has found to lead to meningitis are mentioned and discusses premature surgery (wait until the second or third week to operate), incomplete surgery (all cells have not been completely exenerated and inadequate drainage), excessive surgery (accidental injury during operation). In addition there is the neglected aural suppuration, both acute and chronic as well as an acute upper respiratory infection (where nasal douches have spread the infection to the middle ear).

The treatment is discussed in order of importance according to the author's opinion. Sulphanilimide is of the most importance. The history of sulphanilimide is discussed. He says in regard to this treatment: "In dealing with a dangerous disease such as meningitis, the only justification for discontinuing the drug before the patient is cured would be the onset of a complication that might prove fatal unless the drug were stopped." The cerebrospinal fluid should be drained as often as necessary to keep the pressure normal. It may be done two or three times in the first 24 hours if necessary and about once daily thereafter until the pressure remains normal. The eradication of the primary focus should be undertaken with as little delay as possible. Anti-sera, vaccines and blood transfusions are also recommended. The general treatment consists of rest, suitable diet, alkalinazation with sodium bicarbonate and adequate conservative treatment of the ear (mopping and keeping clean). A table of cases are reported. A bibliography is appended.

Nasal Allergy in Children. E. J. Barnett, M.D., and H. D. Carnahan, M.D., Spokane, Washington. Archives of Otolaryngology, August, 1939.

"It is reported that 44 per cent of patients with chronic nasal complaints seen in routine otolaryngologic practice have nasal allergy." One of the most common complaints of the parents is that the child "has one cold in the nose after another." Some common symptoms are sneezing, sniffling, nasal itching, obstruction, and discharge. In between attacks the nose feels stuffy. Tonsillectomy and adenoidectomy are done ineffectually and the parents may say that the child even has more colds than before the operation or that the adenoids have recurred. The appearance of the nasal mucous membrane is characteristically pale and edematous; the secretion serous or mucoid. The presence of eosinophils in the smear is indicative of the allergic condition; a negative smear does not exclude allergy. If both eosinophils and neutrophils are present in large numbers, there is undoubtedly allergy plus an infection present. If neutrophils alone are present in the smear, then it is infection alone or an infection so severe that the allergy is overshadowed, in which case repeated smears must be made.

"In an allergic child hypersensitiveness to inhalents, contactants, pollens and foods is the rule. The child's allergy is rarely due to a single cause; multiple and mixed factors are involved. "Prophylactic measures include exclusion of pets from the house followed by a thorough cleaning, elimination of feather pollows or covered with cellophane slips, enclose the mattress with rubberized sheeting, a plain bare sleeping room — floors waxed—no dust, during the sweeping and dusting of the house the child should be kept out doors, avoid insecticides or sprays, use unscented soaps and nonallergic cosmetics, avoid the presence of smoke."

When the prophylactic measures do not give sufficient relief then it is advisable to carry out skin testing and hyposensitization. About 50 scratch tests are made with pollens, with all epidermal substances and with such foods as eggs, milk, wheat, chocolate, nuts and cottonseed. Then about 200 allergens are used to test intradermally. All foods that produce a reaction are removed from the diet. Hypersensitization of the offending allergens is also carried out. Foods are cautiously added to the diet from time to time to determine the tolerance.

This is a very worthwhile paper for both pediatrician and rhinologist. The author's conclusions are as follows:

1. Allergy should always be suspected as the cause of rhinitis in children.

2. Cytologic examinations of the nasal secretions with predominance of eosinophils offer confirmatory evidence.

3. Routine repeated cytologic examinations for all patients with chronic nasal symptoms are important.

4. Local treatment for nasal allergy must be conservative.

5. Disappointments in rhinologic practice often result from failure to recognize and relieve associated allergy.

6. Prophylactic allergic measures are often sufficient to give relief from nasal allergy.

7. Allergic testing and hyposensitization may be reserved for unrelieved or complicated conditions.

8. The importance of allergy to the rhinologist cannot be overemphasized.

--------o--------

PLASTIC SURGERY
Edited by
GEO. H. KIMBALL, M.D., F.A.C.S.
404 Medical Arts Building, Oklahoma City

Repair of Large Defects After Removal of Cancer of the Lips: Ernest M. Daland, M.D., F.A.C.S., Boston, Mass. S.G.&O., September, 1939.

The author calls attention to the fact that small carcinomas of the lip may be repaired by a "V" shaped incision. He states that this operation is not satisfactory for lesions over two centimeters in diameter since it makes the lip so narrow that secondary procedures may be necessary. He refers to a previous article by himself for a total restoration of the lower lip by using flaps from the nasolabial folds. This operation, he states, is unsatisfactory functionally because it is devoid of muscle and serves only as a dam for food and saliva but does give a fairly acceptable cosmetic appearance when total removal is necessary.

In this paper the discussion is confined to the problem of reconstruction when the removal of from one-third to two-thirds of the lip is necessary. Discussion of the muscular structure of the mouth is undertaken in which the author shows that the orbicularis oris is a muscle or group of muscles which is a sphincter, is therefore circular and forms the oral opening and commissures due to the lateral pull placed on this circular muscle from the other muscles of the face. He calls attention to the fact that the skin and mucous membrane have the same attachment in all portions of the lip and thus the commissure is formed by extra oral muscular pull and shows that in reconstruction operations the extra oral musculature may be detached and the commissures shifted. Thus in the reconstruction the shape of the mouth is not changed leaving a larger overhanging upper lip but that the entire opening is made smaller with reconstruction of the commissures.

The technique of the operation is one of a rectangular excision of the new growth including at least one centimeter of normal tissue and extends down to the fold between the lip and the chin. The corresponding mucous membrane is also removed, but it is not necessary to remove so much as is removed from the skin. The mucous membrane is separated from the muscle and skin for a distance of about two inches out on the cheek. Lateral incisions are made from the angle of the defect; the musculature is separated from the mucous membrane leaving as much fat as possible to insure nutrition, then the orbicularis oris is separated from the other muscles of the face. Closure is then made, using cat gut for the mucous membrane and deep structures, and black silk for the skin. Hemostasis is accomplished by packing and pressure.

The author states that the patient's appearance as the operation is finished is almost alarming, but within a few days rotation has been effected; commissures have reformed and that what is really accomplished is a narrowing of the entire mouth. He states that in none of his 23 cases has this been too small for functional results. The orbicularis oris is innervated by the facial nerve and because of the multiple origins of the fibers which make up the nerve, the cutting of a few fibers does not seem to interfere with the innervation. This was proved by the first patient in the series who could whistle normally a few days after the operation.

Treatment of the lymph nodes of the neck closely follows that of the other facial carcinomas in that glands which remain palpable after their reaction subsides are widely dissected. The results of the treatment as reported by this author are excellent.

In two tables he gives 23 cases, six of the upper lip and 17 of the lower lip which have been treated in this manner. He reports three, four year cures; six, three year cures; one, two year cure; and one cure, one year or less. There are four cases of recurrence in metastatic areas and three cases of local recurrence. Because of the short time that he has attempted this operation he draws no conclusion of permanent cure but his figures show that he has a fair percentage of temporary cures without recurrence at the site of the operation. His case histories show good percentage on his 23 cases and give a very interesting study of this condition.

Comment: The author here has reviewed an operation which is similar to some of the older works but does give a method of repairing large defects of the lips which is a one stage procedure and leaves a functioning os to the mouth which is not devoid of muscle in its circumference and is adequate. The cosmetic results of the operation as shown by pictures in the article are very good although there is a comparatively short follow up and a comparatively small series of cases.

As a curative operation this seems to be adequate when combined with lymphatic gland dissection in this series of cases.

Treatment and Management of Burn Cases. H. Jerry Lavender, M.D., Cincinnati, Ohio.

The author begins the article with a discussion of the eschar method of treating burns. He states that advocates of this method claim that it is a big factor in reducing shock, relieving pain, preventing loss of tissue and body fluids, helping to minimize the toxic stage, controlling sepsis, and speeding recovery. But without exception these men emphasize treatment for shock and relief of pain. Quote: "It would appear then, that the crust-forming method affords the patient a protective or leathery coat in the burned areas, but that the fluid loss, pain, toxemia and sepsis have to be met with other measures to enhance restitution and recovery."

He calls attention to the difference between scalds and burns produced by fire, stating that he believes that fire burns are much deeper than scald burns and that the depth of burned tissue must of necessity play a large part in the recovery from the burn. He points out that where there is burned tissue that the tissue which is dead must slough, separate and be removed before healing takes place. He also feels that escharing only forms a coat over the burned tissue and for this reason cannot coagulate the entire depth of the burned tissue, therefore does not prevent toxic absorption but merely acts as a coagulum to seal the toxic materials and pyogenic organism. He further states that most fluid loss is controlled by coagulation in a very few hours after a burn.

The first treatment is for shock by common methods of relief of pain, restoration of body fluids, blood transfusions and stimulating drugs.

The local burn is not treated for from 10 to 12 hours, the patient in the meantime being wrapped in a sterile sheet. Treatment is to place patient in a warm bath which contains about a pint of aqueous solution of green soap, allowed to soak for a few minutes and then removed from the bath. The time of the bath is increased as the patient's condition permits until it reaches one hour daily. The advantage claimed for such a method of treatment is that the burned tissues are removed more rapidly and with less harm to the patient and that the toxic materials are removed as they are formed. The contractures are less apt to develop and are recognized earlier and that the granulating beds are prepared for skin grafting at an earlier stage.

Comment: This article is a plea for a modification of the eschar treatment of burns in that many deep burns do not seem to be practically treated by escharring since the eschar does not reach to the depth of the burn. This fact has been previously observed in several cases and it is usually necessary in these cases to remove the eschar with the slough at an early date. Personal experience in the treatment of burns by daily bathing has been gratifying where the condition in the bath tub can be well controlled and the burned areas not contaminated from the tub.

Separation of slough is effected somewhat earlier by bathing patient in the tub and in most instances is very acceptable to the patient. Release of contractures has been noted in this manner and an early preparation of the area for skin grafting is probably effected although we do feel that the eschar treatment has a place in a good many instances because of its simplicity.

———o———

ORTHOPAEDIC SURGERY
Edited by Earl D. McBride, M.D., F.A.C.S.
717 North Robinson Street, Oklahoma City

"The Treatment of Volkmann's Ischemic Contracture," Henry W. Meyerding and Frank H. Krusen, Annals of Surg., Vol. 110, No. 3, September, 1939.

Volkmann's ischemic contracture consists of a contraction and fibrosis of the flexor muscles of the forearm and produces flexion deformity of the wrist and fingers. A partial permanent disability is always produced once it is definitely established.

It occurs most frequently in children as a result of injury to the lower humerus.

The authors consider physical therapy to be the most valuable single method of treatment. Surgery alone is entirely without value.

Causes of the contracture are described as being due particularly to hemorrhage, pressure on blood vessels and injury to the nerves in the ante-cubital fossa.

It is advised that to treat such fracture of the lower humerus early may result in a contracture, and in some cases it is advisable to defer reduction of the fracture for several days. The arm should be elevated in bed or in an airplane splint. Division of the fascia and drainage of the hematoma may be necessary.

Physical therapy methods of correcting this severe deformity consists of stretching with proper splinting, heat, massage and proper manipulation. Usually the fingers are first corrected; pulled into complete extension. Later the wrist is straightened again by similar splinting. Occasionally Banjo type splints are of distinct value in loosening the joints of the fingers, thumb and wrist. Old cases occasionally require plastic procedures on the contracted joints, but this is not the rule.

Following correction of the position, circulation usually improves. Splinting is then augmented by radiant heat, contrasting baths and general massage and occasionally electric stimulation of the muscles. Splints are worn at intervals between treatments. The whirl-pool bath seems to offer the best method of administering heat.

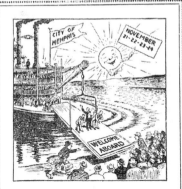

WELCOME to MEMPHIS to the outstanding medical meeting of the year—the annual meeting of the Southern Medical Association, November 21-24. In the nine general clinical sessions, the nineteen sections, the three independent medical societies meeting conjointly and the scientific and technical exhibits, every phase of medicine and surgery will be covered —the last word in modern, practical, scientific medicine and surgery. Addresses and papers will be given by distinguished physicians not only from the South but from all over the United States.

REGARDLESS of what any physician may be interested in, regardless of how general or how limited his interest, there will be at Memphis a program to challenge that interest and make it worth-while for him to attend.

ALL MEMBERS of State and County medical societies in the South are cordially invited to attend. And all members of state and county medical societies in the South should be and can be members of the Southern Medical Association. The annual dues of $4.00 include the Southern Medical Journal—the equal of any, better than many.

SOUTHERN MEDICAL ASSOCIATION
Empire Building
BIRMINGHAM, ALABAMA

Manual manipulations are occasionally of great value after correction has been obtained sufficiently with mechanical splints. Active exercise is the final curative measure and occupational therapy is brought into use here; using the hand loom, weaving, basketry, block printing and occasionally a large floor loom.

To the abstractor the most important thing about Volkmann's contracture is its prevention. With proper care there should be practically no cases ever develop. Once it has developed, the proper follow-up care as described by the authors is then certainly necessary to reduce the existing disability.

"Local Implantation of Sulfanilamide in Compound Fractures," N. K. Jensen, Luverne W. Johnsrud, and M. C. Nelson, Surgery: 6:1-2 (July) 1939.

The authors have used sulfanilamide locally in some 39 compound fractures. They first debride the wound carefully, as is now customary in all well managed institutions, with saline irrigations. They feel that primary closure of the wound without tension is indicated.

Sulfanilamide has been used in amounts up to 20 grams; being instilled directly into the wound after thorough debridement.

It appears that the only definite advantage this offers over the usual method of treatment of compound wounds by thorough cleansing and removing devitalized tissue is that the local instillation of the sulfanilamide apparently holds any remaining organisms in check so that the local defense mechanism can become organized.

It goes without saying that the fracture should be reduced and held rigidly immobilized during healing of the skin as well as the fracture.

The authors report 39 fractures and two compound dislocations healing without a single instance of primary infection. Previous series of 94 cases show 27 per cent infection.

Sulfanilamide in these wounds does not protect against gas gangrene.

Comment by abstractor: We have certain rather fixed ideas by primary suture of compound fractures. We have obtained many successful and safe closures by thorough debridement and scrubbing, but have had no experience with instillation of sulfanilamide. This appears to offer a hope of improvement in the treatment of compound fractures, but it is not to be advised as a routine measure until further research has been done on this subject.

CARDIOLOGY

Edited by F. Redding Hood, M.D.
1200 N. Walker St., Oklahoma City

Outline of Lecture on "The Treatment of Congestive Heart Failure" by Dr. Samuel A. Levine, Given before Post-Graduate Class in Cardiology, Harvard Medical School.

The treatment of congestive failure is the treatment of an incurable condition, i.e., a progressive disease with an inevitable end. The aim is to prolong life.

Rest In Bed—This will save about 25,000 beats in each 24 hours and above all make the patient comfortable for to be in bed without comfort is not rest.

Sleep—Sleep is important since a sleepless night produces a restless day. Use sedatives, the smallest amount necessary, using bromides, barbitols, codeine, or morphine as needed.

Digitalis—Digitalis is the most important and potent drug in congestive failure regardless of the rhythm. It has been found better to use pills or capsules since the liquid preparations may vary greatly as to the drops in 15 M. and there is no way to know exactly how much of the drug the patient has taken. A digitalis preparation that won't produce nausea is of no therapeutic value.

In a patient who has not had digitalis before will require about 1.5 gr. per 10 pounds body weight given over several days time. It can be given in one dose for digitalization in eight to 12 hours. The difficulty is that different people will require different amounts. A general method, there can be no set rule, is to give ¼ of the estimated amount the first day and repeating it the second day. The third day reducing the amount to about 1/6 of the estimated total and judging from the condition of the patient the balance of treatment. We may follow the effect in auricular fibrillation by using the apical pulse, the optimum being 60-70. In a regular rhythm slowing is not indicative of the effect. The aim of treatment is to arrive at a maintainance dose probably about 1.5 gr. daily.

When a patient comes in with a history of having had digitalis and with failure so marked that large doses are indicated the above rule may be used but if not marked then start with 1.5 gr. T.I.D. and watch for results.

A patient may need digitalis and still be vomiting, it due to liver pathology as a result of the failure, then digitalis is not contra-indicated. If it can not be taken by mouth, then give it per rectum for a day or two, the dose being the same as per mouth. Give the daily ration in one dose.

Signs for omiting or lessening the dose: (1) When the desired results are obtained (like to have the apical rate in auricular fibrillation down to 60-70) (50 to 60 is better). (2) Signs of toxicity—subjective signs being nausea, anorexia, sick feeling, vomiting, or yellow-green vision. Or the objective signs of extrasystoles, coupling, or heart block in any degree. If a patient does not show subjective symptoms but has any of the objective signs except complete heart block no harm has been done, but it shows that digitalis cannot be pushed.

In treating auricular fibrillation with digitalis and a regular rhythm develops the possibilities are that there has been a return to normal rhythm or that complete heart block has set in. Any time under these conditions the heart becomes regular stop digitalis as it is either not needed or is dangerous.

Digitalis is not indicated for rapid rates per se.

The question of the use of digitalis in pneumonia has long been debated but digitalis is useless in the presence of fever except in the presence of auricular fibrillation or failure. Pneumonias with a compensatory hypertrophy of the heart will do better while digitalis makes for a small heart by increasing the tonus at the same time tends to diminish the output.

Diuretics—These are better given after digitalization and in acites will work better after tapping. The increased abdominal pressure bringing pressure on the renal vessels probably account for the failure in marked acites. Mercuric diuretics should be used cautiously and be preceded by digitalization and acidulation with ammonium chloride, then giving it intravenously in the morning so that the effect will occur during the day. Undesirable effects may occur in the presence of renal edema or from re-digitalization as the fluids contain digitalis that must again pass through the blood stream.

Phlebotomy has a place in cardiac failure when there is venous congestion, enlarged liver, or pulmonary edema due to hypertension. It should be done quickly to give the right side of the heart a chance to regain its tone.

INTERNAL MEDICINE

Edited by Hugh Jeter, M.D., 1200 North Walker,
Oklahoma City

**"A Critical Consideration of the Value of Post-
mortem Examinations." M. A. Blankenhorn,
M.D., Cincinnati. (Abstracted from Hospitals,
Vol. 12, April, 1938.)**

"To consider the value of the autopsy to medicine is a waste of breath or of printer's ink if the
consideration is to be what the autopsy has done
for medicine. It is common knowledge, even to
those outside of medicine, that the entire structure of medical practice is built on facts learned
from the dissection of the dead."

"At times and in certain isolated medical problems, one might question the wisdom of studying
the dead rather than the living. This question is
expressed in the old contention as to whether the
study of form outranks in importance the study
of function; and also, specifically in medical science,
as to the relative importance of pathology and
physiology. Regardless of these contentions, medical history is clear in that the modern procedures
of practice are founded on anatomy (normal and
morbid) and on physiology."

"In the first instance, the autopsy is done to
check the soundness of any particular medical procedure. In the second, the autopsy is performed to
advance medical knowledge. When the autopsy
is done at the request of the attending physician,
in most instances it is expected to accomplish both
these ends. Now one may suggest, for argument,
that the autopsy no longer is able to advance
knowledge because of its limitations and that
modern methods of diagnosis no longer require
the checking process of the autopsy. Whether the
ends are desirable is beyond criticism at this particular moment; but whether the autopsy actually
gains these ends is the object of this study."

"Does the autopsy advance medical knowledge?
The ink-wasting part of this question has to do
with the autopsy of the past. There can be no
denial of the debt medicine owes to those whose
bodies were dissected and to the dissector. But
now in our present state of knowledge, is dissection
outmoded because all mysteries are laid bare, and
is there nothing more to learn? Certainly no
understanding person claims that to be the case.
Also we may ask, is the autopsy outmoded because
it is supplanted by less gruesome methods to gain
the same ends? To advance this claim, one must
say that our instruments of precision applied with
high skill can explain all the hidden manifestations
of disease that lie beneath the surface. As one
who has devoted much time in applying these
methods for many years, I make no such claim,
nor do I know of any sound-minded person who
does. After all, there are few methods that are
truly precise and there are very few infallible
(pathognomonic) signs of disease."

"This uncertainty which dogs the steps of the
bedside doctor is overcome by faith and confidence
that within the limitation of his art the practitioner
does his best. But this best, at its best, is not
scientifically exact. There is always the modest
apology by which all bedside facts are qualified by
referring to them as "clinical." That is, that these
facts are limited in their value because other information is wanted which only the autopsy can
supply."

"It is no doubt true that the autopsy as done on
man now gives less to the advancement of medicine than it did formerly, but that is not because
there is no progress to be made. In the so-called
degenerative diseases (as Bright's disease of the
kidneys; diabetes; coronary, renal and cerebral
sclerosis) as well as other less common phases of
poorly understood conditions that resemble aging
processes, more autopsies in the early stages must
be done before one can say that the autopsy can
not advance the frontiers of medical knowledge.
Formerly, that is before the days of functional
testing of the living, the early stages of these diseases could not be recognized. The disease of "degeneration," both clinically and pathologically,
was seen only in severe form. The clinician found
only the end stages; and since the patients did
not die in early stages, the pathologist failed to see
their beginning. Now with functional testing to
make a clinical diagnosis and the zeal to "autopsy"
all deaths, especially those so-called accidental and
unrelated deaths, the early stages may thus be
seen in serial form in a manner now unknown."

"It is by no means fair in this criticism of the
value of the autopsy to assume that the autopsy
as now done is perfect, for such is by no means
true. On rare occasions the autopsy when thoroughly done finds no cause for death whatsoever;
in fact, it discloses a state of bodily perfection
consistent with life and vigorous health. This may
be the case in status thymolymphaticus or in status
epilepticus. Or the autopsy may disclose a disease,
or a condition not fairly called a disease, for which
no reasonable explanation is at hand (as, for
example, idiopathic enlargement of the heart, or
congenital cystic disease of the kidneys). The
whole category of congenital malformations is
unexplored as to cause—and they are important
diseases, even in adults."

"In most of the audits that have been made of
the accuracy of clinical diagnosis, usually the best
or better examples of medical practice are chosen,
as in Karsner's 600 cases and in those of Wilson.
Both these examples were in circumstances where
the effect of a high percentage of autopsied deaths
is felt. Even in such conditions Wilson says that
in the three principal causes of death, namely,
cancer, tuberculosis, and heart disease, the percentage of correctness is about 75, 50 and 40 per
cent, respectively."

"In practice, generally considered, of all reported
deaths that comprise our vital statistics, there is
about one in 100 checked by autopsy. In medical
teaching centers some hospitals manage to do as
high as 80 per cent autopsy and even higher on
all deaths. Seventy-five per cent is regarded as a
very good percentage; and hospitals approved for
internship must do a certain total number to guar-
antee the atmosphere necessary to an excellence
of practice that will be profitable to a beginner.
Sir Henry Christian in 1926 advised that the 'best
single index of selection' of a hospital for intern-

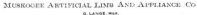
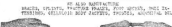

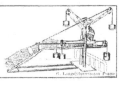

ship is the autopsy percentage, 25 per cent of 100 deaths being desirable."

"All things considered, it would be utterly futile to discuss further the idea that medical research, medical practice, or medical teaching has reached a stage that can even be maintained, much less progress, without the continued practice of post-mortem examinations."

Comment: This is an abstract of one of a series of articles written and recently published in the Hospitals. All of these are extremely interesting and worth reading.

---o---

UROLOGY

Edited by D. W. Branham, M.D.
514 Medical Arts Building, Oklahoma City

Retention of Urine and Residual Urine in Post-Operative and Postpartum Cases, Use of Catheter In. Thomas D. Moore, M.D. Urologists' Correspondence Club, August 28, 1939.

Urologists frequently are called in consultation in cases of so-called pyelitis, occurring following various surgical procedures and childbirth. Usually such patients have required catheterization and our confreres among the general surgeons and obstetricians are disposed to blame the use of the catheter for the urinary infection. Some years ago Curtis called attention to the common occurrence of residual urine in cases where there had been acute retention with apparent restoration of vesical function. In other words, when the act of voiding is resumed, it is inefficient and the bladder does not empty completely. He further demonstrated that the routine use of a catheter at least every 24 hours, until residual urine disappears, is a protective measure and that very few patients will develop a urinary infection if this precaution is taken. It is generally known that urinary stasis is fertile soil for infection and it seems that the bladder is primarily involved in these cases and that renal infection, characterized by repeated rigors and fever, appears later, probably by the ascending route.

In the routine testing for residual urine of patients who have undergone an operation, as well as postpartum cases, it has not been uncommon to find from 10 to 20 ounces of residual urine, although the patient may have passed eight to 10 ounces immediately before the catheterization. One of my obstetrician friends, Dr. Walter A. Ruch, recently has tested for residual urine 65 consecutive delivery cases who required catheterization for postpartum retention, and found that 58 (90 per cent) had residual urine in varying amounts on the third postpartum day; in 39 cases (60 per cent) there was from four to 50 ounces. Since he has adopted the precaution of daily catheterization of these cases until no residual urine is found, instances of so-called postpartum pyelitis and cystitis are practically unknown. Thus it may be seen that it is not the use of the catheter in such cases that brings about the trouble, but rather its non-use, and that the great fear of employing catheterization, so prevalent among general surgeons, is really ill founded. It behooves urologists to reeducate those in the profession who still cling to the idea that a catheter is a dangerous instrument and to teach them that its routine use for the drainage of residual urine will prove it to be not an object of fear, but a trustworthy friend.

Comment: Because urinary tract infections contribute too much of the morbidity of surgery it is well for every surgeon to digest the facts herein presented by Dr. Moore. An appreciation of the factors responsible for such infections together with appropriate treatment will make the post-operative course of many patients smoother.

Urethral Caruncle With Particular Reference to the Sessile Type. Philips J. Carter, M.D., F.A.C.S., New Orleans, Louisiana. The Urologic and Cutaneous Review, September, 1939.

An excellent essay on this most common and distressful ailment of women. Because they are persistent growths that tend to recur, the ordinary mode of treatment; local fulgeration, cauterization, etc., are frequently followed by recurrences. The author feels that his therapeutic results have improved since he has performed surgical removal of the growth in toto together with its base of normal urethral tissue.

---o---

Combination of Treatments Effective In Peritonitis Morphine, Decompression of Duodenum, Use Of Fluids and Blood Transfusion Cut Death Rate Two-Thirds

Widespread peritonitis (inflammation of the membrane lining the abdominal wall), a dire complication often following perforation of the appendix, is best combated, and its mortality rate is reduced by two-thirds, through the intelligent use of morphine, fluids administered under the skin or by vein, decompression of the duodenum (the intestine adjoining the stomach) and blood transfusion, Thew Wright, M.D., A. H. Aaron, M.D., J. S. Regan, M.D., and Elmer Milch, M.D., Buffalo, declare in The Journal of the American Medical Association for September 30.

The authors believe that the death of patients with this complication is primarily due to two factors: shock and intestinal obstruction. They do not operate on any such patient until shock, abdominal distention and the diminished water balance of the body are combated.

By using the above four factors of treatment and then operating on 60 cases of diffuse peritonitis caused by a perforated appendix, the Buffalo physicians reduced their average mortality rate to 11.7 per cent, as compared with the United States average of 33 per cent and their former hospital rate of 45.4 per cent.

The days of life of the patients who finally died were thus lengthened to an average of 13.8 days instead of the usual three or four days. Therefore this combined preparatory treatment, by prolonging the life of a patient with peritonitis, provides the time necessary to increase the body's protective mechanism, a vital factor in recovery.

The patient with diffuse peritonitis on the fourth or fifth day of illness has blue lips and finger nails, falling blood pressure and increased respiratory rate. These are manifestations of the large amount of blood stagnated in the abdominal vessels and not available for surface circulation. The rise in the pulse rate is a compensatory effort of the heart to bring the blood, which it is receiving in a markedly diminished amount, to the tissues of the body.

By means of continuous duodenal decompression, gas and fluid are removed from the stomach and intestine, and the high elevation of the diaphragm, with the consequent compression of the overlying lungs, is partially overcome. This removes a contributory factor in the production of a terminal pneumonia. In addition, the effects of a high intestinal obstruction are decreased.

All one can possibly hope to do with the administration of fluids is to meet the increased metabolic needs and endeavor to keep the patient as nearly as possible in a normal water balance.

By the use of morphine, pain is relieved and the patient is kept quiet. If the drug is administered properly after several large initial doses at comparatively short intervals, the patient may get along without any morphine for from six to eight hours.

Transfusion increases the volume of circulating blood, attempts to restore the blood pressure, and supplies blood to the exterior tissues.

Riboflavin Added to Squibb Vitamin Line

Riboflavin (vitamin B2 or G) is now being supplied by E. R. Squibb & Sons, New York, in synthetic form for oral use in capsules containing one milligram, or approximately 400 Bourquin-Sherman units each. The capsules are packaged in bottles of 25.

Necessary for animal growth, a deficiency causing loss of hair, dermatitis and sometimes cataract in rats; in humans a lack of which has been reported to cause a chapped condition of the lips (cheilosis), a contributing factor in the development of pellagra, Riboflavin is said to be "a component of an oxidation enzyme" which performs a ver yvital function in the body of every animal—that is, it takes an active part in tissue respiration.

Riboflavin was isolated some time ago in pure crystalline form from liver, yeast and milk. It appears in the dry state as a yellow, water-soluble powder, very stable to heat and oxygen but rather unstable to exposure to direct light. Because of the cost of separating it from its environment, Riboflavin produced from natural sources is rather costly. The synthetic product, such as now being marketed by Squibb, is much less expensive.

The average daily requirement of Riboflavin for an adult is estimated to be from two to three milligrams or more, as prescribed by a physician. Riboflavin Squibb is biologically standardized, assayed by the Bourquin-Sherman method.

---o---

Operating Risk In Heart Disease Not So Great As Many Believe

That the operating risk for those who have a severe heart disease is not as great as many people think, is indicated in a report by Harold J. Brumm, M.D., and Fredrick A. Willius, M.D., Rochester, Minn., in The Journal of the American Medical Association for June 10.

Reporting on a study of the surgical risks in patients with heart disease, the two Rochester men say they found a death rate of only 4.3 per cent among 257 persons with severe heart disease who underwent imperative major operations.

Pointing out that they believe the mortality in the group of cases studied was remarkably low, the authors say this should encourage the sufferers from heart disease when surgical intervention is necessary.

"However, it must not instil false optimism into the clinician or the surgeon," they warn, "for he must realize that this accomplishment is not of casual origin but one resulting from the coordination of careful preoperative study and judicious selection, expert administration of anesthetic agents and skilful surgical technic and judgment. Operation must be confined to those cases presenting unmistakable indications.

"Likewise, gentleness in the manipulation of organs and tissues lessens the dangers of surgical shock, which in itself may tilt the balance away from recovery in these patients. Of paramount importance is the surgeon's determination to limit the operation to the procedure planned in advance and to avoid undertaking additional operative steps that might be indicated in the patient without heart disease."

---o---

Bacon Not Recommended For Infants

There is no rational basis for the common practice of giving bacon to babies, the October issue of Hygeia, The Health Magazine declares.

The practice apparently originated from the belief that the fat contained in bacon carried with it some valuable nutritional element. Since it is now known that the vitamin content of bacon is practically negligible, there is no obvious reason why bacon should be given.

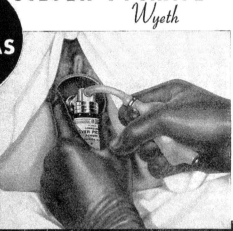
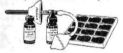

A.M.A. Journal Refutes Charges of Unnecessary Surgery

"Much of the propaganda devoted to breaking down public confidence in the American medical profession in recent years has been devoted to an attack on the medical profession because of fee splitting and because of the performance of unnecessary surgical operations," an editorial on "Unnecessary Surgery" in The Journal of the American Medical Association for September 30 says.

"Obviously, this kind of propaganda is never supported by actual facts or figures but is largely devoted to what has come to be called 'a smearing campaign.' In contrast is a report recently made available of surgery performed in a Brooklyn hospital. According to figures supplied by Dr. S. S. Goldwater, major surgical operations were performed in that hospital on 979 patients, exclusive of bones and joints, and fractures and other lesions of bones and joints were treated to the number of 788. At the same time in this institution 68 patients with possible surgical conditions were treated conservatively without operation, and 117 patients who came into the hospital with surgical diagnoses were not operated on because further study failed to confirm the diagnosis.

"The Journal ventures to say that this type of figures would be duplicated in the vast majority of hospitals in this country and particularly in those institutions approved by the Council on Medical Education and Hospitals of the American Medical Association as institutions suitable for the training of interns."

Rabbit Serum Valuable In Pneumonia

A reduction of almost 25 per cent in the pneumonia mortality rate, with a minimum of serum reaction or sickness, by the use of specific concentrated rabbit serum is reported by Italo F. Volini, M.D., and Robert O. Levitt, M.D., Chicago, in The Journal of the American Medical Association for September 30.

The mortality in their 153 pneumonia patients who were treated with the serum was 9.8 per cent as compared to 38.4 per cent in 164 patients not given serum.

The authors state: "Sensitivity to rabbit serum is rarely encountered. It is remarkably free from immediate reactions and produces fever in a relatively small percentage of patients. Delayed serum reactions are also infrequent. Serum lends itself to the concentrated single total dose administration, which procedure saves much time and probably enhances its curative efficiency."

Potassium Chloride For Allergy

When potassium chloride, alone or in conjunction with insulin, was given allergic patients with acute and chronic urticaria (severe hives) and bronchial asthma, definite relief occurred, Howard A. Rusk, M.D., T. E. Weichselbaum, Ph.D., Michael Somogyi, Ph.D., and Ernest Simms, St. Louis, report in The Journal of the American Medical Association for June 10. These patients showed a high increase of potassium in the blood serum during an attack.

The authors assumed that the increased blood potassium indicated a depletion of the normal potassium of the tissue cells. They were of the opinion that any substance that would decrease the blood potassium would drive the potassium back to the cells and thereby reestablish a state of balance. They found this true in that the patients were relieved when given insulin and potassium salts.

With further studies, now under way, the authors hope to determine criteria for selection of patients.

Proper Canning Will Help Retain Much Vitamin C In Fruit Juices

Commercially canned fruit juices retain considerable quantities of vitamin C when proper precautions are taken during the canning process, the July issue of Hygeia, The Health Magazine states.

The conservation of vitamin C is generally accomplished by raising the temperature of the juice rapidly, in order to drive out dissolved air and to destroy the "oxidase," which destroys vitamin C. Further conservation of vitamin C is made possible by performing the canning operations under reduced pressure or in an atmosphere of steam.

Citrus fruit juices are acid in reaction, and it has been found that vitamin C activity is retained much better in such a medium than in a neutral or alkaline medium.

Index to Advertisers

THE JOURNAL

OF THE

OKLAHOMA STATE MEDICAL ASSOCIATION

| VOLUME XXXII | McALESTER, OKLAHOMA, NOVEMBER, 1939 | Number 11 |

The Toxic States Seen in Urology*

BASIL A. HAYES, M.D., F.A.C.S.
OKLAHOMA CITY, OKLAHOMA

The purpose of this paper is to list the various toxic states which occur in patients suffering from damage to the urinary tract and to give as nearly as possible the diagnostic criteria by which they may be identified. I shall discuss them as follows:

Renal—
1. Uremia
2. Acidosis
3. Encephalopathy
4. Dehydration
5. Edema

Cardiovascular—
6. Shock
7. Hemorrhage
8. Anemia
9. Myocarditis

Gastro-Intestinal—
10. Starvation
11. Alkalosis
12. Hepatic Insufficiency

Unclassified—
1. Sepsis
2. Cachexia

Taking up these subjects in the order of their listing, uremia naturally appeals to us as being the one of major importance. Its cause is renal failure, which may be due to back pressure from any cause or to parenchymal damage. Parenchymal dam-

*Read before the Section on Genito-Urinary Diseases and Syphilology, Annual Meeting, Oklahoma State Medical Association, May 3, 1939, Oklahoma City, Oklahoma.

age in turn is caused by three main agencies:

a. Defective blood supply
b. Infection
c. Toxins of any kind

This subject is well known to all of you, and I will waste little time upon it. It might be interesting to recall that the mechanism of the production of uremic symptoms has been fairly well worked out by Becher and other biological chemists, being about as follows:

The end products of protein metabolism in the intestinal tract give rise to aromatic substances such as phenol, p-kresol, thyrosin, tryptophane or indican. These are absorbed into the blood stream where they are detoxified by the liver adding sulphuric or glukuronic acid and eventually appear in the urine as phenolsulphuric acid or indoxylsulphuric acid, these latter two being relatively harmless compounds. If the kidney cannot eliminate these substances or if the liver cannot detoxify them, they accumulate in the blood. When they accumulate in the blood in large enough amounts, they break over into the spinal fluid. Up to that time they give rise to no symptoms but when they appear in the spinal fluid, the symptoms of uremia begin. Babies and Torok have shown that the Xanthoproteic test is positive in the blood stream long before it is in the spinal fluid; but that when it does appear there, uremia invariably begins. On the other hand, the Xanthoproteic test is never positive in the spinal fluid unless uremic symptoms exist. The symptoms are oliguria with a urine of low specific gravity, w h i c h eventually leads to the retention of nitrogenous products in the blood. Following this there may be pruritis, delirium, coma, muscular twitching, convulsions, hiccoughs, reflexes lively or normal, subnormal temperature, diarrhea or blood stools, a yellowish tint to the skin with occasional deposits of white urea crystals on the skin, and an increase in the amount of nitrogenous substances in the blood. The supreme laboratory test which reveals the presence of impending uremia is high blood chemistry such as high NPN, blood urea, or creatine. The final and absolute test of uremia is a positive Xanthoproteic test in the spinal fluid.

The treatment of uremia consists of improving drainage from the urinary tract, not only from the bladder but from the kidneys themselves. I have saved the life of more than one moribund prostate case by getting a urethral catheter up to the kidney. Besides urinary drainage, colonic lavage, lumbar puncture, blood transfusion, and intravenous fluids are all measures of importance which are well known.

Another toxic condition which is sometimes confused with uremia is acidosis. In fact, it often accompanies uremia and is responsible at times for more symptoms than the actual uremia. It is seen in various conditions such as starvation or diabetes, asphyxiation, ketosis, severe fevers (caused by decomposition of proteins), and nephritis (lack of excretion of the phosphates).

The symptoms of acidosis are three in number:

1. Acid urine, which remains persistently so regardless of administration of large amounts of alkali.

2. Air hunger.

3. Coma.

Some years ago a test was d e v i s e d known as Sellard's Test, in which a patient was given five grams of sodium bicarbonate e v e r y three hours until his urine became alkaline. The u r i n e was boiled each time before testing. On the basis of this test a tolerance of 20 to 30 grams of sodium bicarbonate indicated a moderate acidosis, and 75 to 100 grams indicated a severe acidosis. This test really is of very slight practical value except where laboratories cannot do a CO_2 combining power test. The modern laboratory is able to do this test, in w h i c h a figure of 60 indicates a normal reaction of the blood whereas a figure of 50 or less indicates acidosis, 30 being severe.

The treatment of acidosis is quite simple. In mild cases intravenous glucose will suffice. In severe cases of coma or impending coma, Hartman's solution (Sodium R-Lactate diluted to isotonicity) is given until the CO_2 combining power reaches the normal figure of 60.

The third toxic syndrome to be mentioned is encephalopathy, whose classic form resembles epilepsy and consists of a prodrome followed by clonic and tonic convulsions with coma continuing after the convulsions. In toxemias of pregnancy we call it eclampsia. D u r i n g the prodromal period there may be sensory phenomena such as a dead feeling in the right hand, a bad smell, pallor of the skin, increased blood pressure, decreased urinary volume, or paroxysmal dypsnea. Lumbar puncture at this time will as a rule show increased cerebral p r e s s u r e. The eye grounds will occasionally show papilledema; vomiting is common; blindness may occur in both eyes. The onset is usually sudden but may be g r a d u a l. Mental changes may occur, especially delirium. Such attacks may occur with no change in kidney function. Blood chemistry may reveal no retention of the urinary constituents, all findings being normal. As a rule, blood pressure is quite high. It may occur in diffuse glomerulonephritis, pregnancy, or lead poisoning. It is rarely seen in prostatic cases though I have seen it in two that I now recall. At necropsy the brain shows only anemia and sometimes edema.

The treatment is as follows:

1. Venesection. Four or five hundred ccs. of blood may be removed from an a d u l t and proportionate amounts from children. The result is often striking.

2. Lumbar puncture and dehydration is very valuable and on occasions spectacu-

lar. When the fluid is found under pressure, it should be removed slowly.

3. Intravenous administration of 200 ccs. of one per cent magnesium sulphate may be found to lower the blood pressure and act as a diuretic. Along with any or all of these treatments, sedation is the rule.

4. Fluids without salt.

5. Better kidney d r a i n a g e. This is based upon the work which I have done in toxemias of pregnancy, in which eclampsia is invariably relieved when the pelvis of each kidney is drained by urethral catheters. The stoppage of convulsions by this procedure is spectacular and has b e e n described by me in papers which I have written on toxemias of pregnancy.

The next state to be mentioned is dehydration. It is particularly important in the treatment of prostatism and many of these patients go without sufficient water for days, even in a hospital. It should be remembered that the normal output of water consists of the following:

Feces	200 ccs.
Lungs	300 ccs.
Insensible evaporation	1,200 ccs.
Total	1,700 ccs.
Add 1,500 ccs. of Urine	1,500 ccs.
Total	3,200 ccs.

This is assuming that the urine has a normal specific g r a v i t y and can carry away 30 to 35 grams of solids.

This 3,200 ccs. is normally replaced by the following:

Water of oxidation from food	200 ccs.
Water drunk as such	3,000 ccs.
Total	3,200 ccs.

If we calculate how much water 3,000 ccs. is, it may be enlightening to consider that if we drank one glass of water per hour from 7 a.m. to 10 p.m., we w o u l d drink 15 glasses. Assuming that we take as much as six ounces in each glass, we have still only drunk 90 ounces or 2,700 ccs. of water, leaving us 300 ccs. short. The only reason why healthy people are not chronically dehydrated is that we do not evaporate quite as much as is herein listed although a sick man might lose that much or more. Also an inactive person will in many instances not pass out a total of 1,500 ccs. of urine. If the specific gravity of the urine is 1,010, the patient must excrete 3,500 ccs. of urine to carry off 35 grams of waste; and when we consider that the average urological patient is excreting a urine of low specific gravity, we must realize that his total urinary output should be g r e a t e r than 1,500 ccs. This calls for a greatly increased i n t a k e of water to balance his increased output. If in addition to having urine of low specific gravity the patient does not eat, he will miss the water of oxidation which he normally takes in with food, thus adding another 100 ccs. or more to his r e q u i r e d amount. If he is also septic, he is forced to excrete and burn more tissue, which raises the total amount of metabolic end products he must excrete, hence he will require another 500 to 1,000 ccs. of urine to carry it off, making a necessary increase of 3,000 to 3,500 ccs. above the normal 1,500 ccs.

By considering these facts, we may calculate and find what the patient should have. If aseptic or with poorly functioning kidneys, he will need a fixed output of 1,700 ccs. plus 3,500 to 4,000 ccs. of urine, making a total of 5,200 to 5,700 ccs. output. Against this we may assume that he will oxidize enough water out of his ingested food to account for 100 ccs., leaving a net of 5,100 to 5,600 ccs. to be replaced through the mouth, skin, or veins.

On the basis of these figures, I fancy that most of us are guilty of allowing our patients to become dehydrated.

Just here I wish to say a word about salt. Water will not remain in the tissues unless held by salt, hence we may give all this fluid and still have a p a t i e n t dehydrated. If we give distilled or tap water, it pours right through, taking along a part of the chlorides that are already in the tissues. Since the blood remains tonic with a fixed chloride content, the water of the tissues will move into it by osmosis, thus further dehydrating the tissues but leaving them isotonic. This will go on indefinitely unless salt is ingested in order to replace that lost in the urine and in perspiration. For this r e a s o n corporations give salt to their men in the summer to prevent them from greater fatigue due to dehydration. Also it should be remembered that hypertonic salt solutions pull water from the tissues in order to dilute salt for excretion through the glomeruli, hence both hypotonic and hypertonic solutions tend to dehydrate the tissues regardless of how much water is g i v e n. Therefore, for dehydration give only isotonic salt solution or drugs in this solution. Five per cent glucose is isotonic on administration but the glucose burns up into CO_2 and water, leaving a hypotonic solution which will dehydrate the tissues. It should, therefore, in dehydration be given in i s o t o n i c salt. If on the other hand diuresis is desired, use glucose in distilled water or use five per cent salt solution which is hypertonic.

The symptoms of dehydration are dry tongue, shrunken lips, sunken eyeballs, and loss of skin elasticity. The only laboratory test of any value consists of a rise of the total red count and hemoglobin in the absence of anemia or polycythemia. It should be remembered that hemorrhage, on the other hand, would cause a lowering of the count so that if we have a dehydrated patient who is suffering from hemorrhage, the blood count will be of little or no value in diagnosis.

The treatment of dehydration is to replace the fluids by isotonic solution, not all at once but about 3,500 ccs. per day plus six per cent of the body weight (Standard). This 3,500 ccs. represents 2,000 ccs. for insensible loss plus 1,500 ccs. for urine. All intravenous fluids should be given at the rate of about 300 to 400 per hour, even slower than this in the aged and in those who are suffering from myocardial damage.

Edema is of three main types: first, that due to plasma protein loss; second, from salt retention; third, from capillary paralysis. The first type is seen in persistent albuminuria, hemorrhage, or in primary anemia from any cause. It causes a swelling of the tissues due to osmotic attraction of the tissues for thinned out blood serum. The only laboratory test of value in this condition is a blood albumin determination, which is rarely done owing to the technique being somewhat difficult. Normal plasmaprotein is 6.3 g r a m s per cent in women and 8 grams per cent in men. This will increase with the loss of water into the tissues. This test is hardly

necessary, however, because edema due to other conditions can clinically be ruled out.

The treatment consists of transfusion in order to increase the amount of protein in blood plasma. If this is not possible, six per cent acacia solution in normal saline should be given, 300 to 500 ccs. at a time. An eastern surgeon has recently recommended the use of ascitic fluids to replace protein loss in blood plasma. P o s s i b l y this method will soon be worked out so as to be of great practical value.

The second type of edema due to salt retention is caused by the failure of kidneys to excrete sodium chloride, which is retained and in turn holds water with it. This is seen especially in arteriosclerotic kidneys where infusions are given. The treatment consists of leaving salt out of the diet, giving intravenously five per cent glucose in distilled water or 50 per cent glucose, 50 ccs. at a time.

The third type of edema is that usually seen in terminal condition and is caused by a capillary paralysis due to anoxia seen in prolonged s h o c k or very debilitated states. All internes will recall that when p a t i e n t s are extremely low and going downhill, there comes a time when veins cannot be found due to slight swelling of the skin. This is the type referred to under this heading. The best treatment consists of transfusion, which takes oxygen to the capillaries and which likewise draws fluids from the tissues back into the blood stream by osmosis.

While discussing toxic conditions, I must m e n t i o n circulatory disturbances. Of these there are four general kinds

1. Shock.
2. Hemorrhage.
3. Anemia.
4. Myocarditis.

Shock and hemorrhage are sometimes confused in postoperative states because their symptoms are quite similar, consisting of low blood pressure, rapid pulse, air hunger, and a pale color. It should be remembered, however, that in shock there is rapid loss of fluid into the tissues whereas in hemorrhage the opposite occurs; that is, there is a rapid loss of plasma and red cells due to the bleeding. This fact brings about a normal or high blood count in a case of shock whereas in hemorrhage the red count would be low. The treatment for these two conditions is the same, consisting of transfusion, heat, and fluids. In shock, transfusion tends to bring fluids back from the tissues into the blood stream by raising the osmotic tension of the fluids circulating in the vascular system. In hemorrhage the blood is simply replaced.

Anemia results from a condition which destroys the blood cells or which causes their loss over a long period of time. This is easily determined by a blood count. The clinical symptoms consist of paleness of the patient's skin and mucous membranes, and in aggravated cases a slight edema of the tissues.

In myocarditis it is unnecessary to point out that the pulse will be weak or irregular. Sometimes there will be edema of the feet and dyspnea, blood pressure may drop low from a previous high and sometimes the heart dilates. The proper remedy for this is caffeine for quick stimulation, digitalis to tolerance, glucose intravenously, and the use of other stimulants such as may appeal to the fancy of the attending physician.

Even the gastro-intestinal system does not escape when we consider the toxic states of urinary disease. Many times the patient will come in suffering from muscular weakness, low or normal blood sugar, acetone in the urine, and with a history of poor appetite and little food for weeks past. In the absence of sepsis, dehydration, uremia, circulatory failure or any of the previously mentioned conditions, we are justified in considering this patient to be suffering from starvation, the proper remedy for which is to give him glucose intravenously until he builds up to the point where he can take food and digest it.

Another condition which is sometimes seen without being recognized is alkalosis. In severe vomiting, particularly in pregnancy or uremia, the patient loses enough chlorides that he or she develops a state of alkalosis. This is also seen in excessive breathing while at rest, and some of our uremic cases suffer from this. Exposure to high temperature, pyloric or high intestinal obstruction will also give rise to alkalosis. The symptoms are dehydration, persistent vomiting or tetanic contraction of the muscles, particularly of the hands and feet. If alkalosis c o n t i n u e s long enough, it occasionally ends as a uremia, the reason for which is not clear. The one definite test which establishes alkalosis is the CO2 combining power in which a normal figure is 60, 50 or less indicating acidosis, and 70 or more indicating alkalosis. The treatment is to give ammonium chloride or calcium chloride until the urine becomes acid.

The most important toxic c o n d i t i o n arising in the gastro-intestinal symptom is hepatic insufficiency. It is seen in toxemia of pregnancy, nephritis, and in certain prostatic cases. It is well, therefore, to cover the salient points in this paper. The liver has the following p r i n c i p a l functions:

1. It regulates blood sugar (glycogen mechanism).

2. It de-amidizes amino acids.

3. It synthesizes urea.

4. It helps destroy uric acid in metabolism.

5. It excretes bile constituents.

6. It removes micro-organisms from circulation and excretes them through bile.

7. It removes particulate matter and colloidal material by phagocytosis.

8. It protects body from anaphylactic reactions of foreign proteins.

9. It detoxifies certain poisons—chloroform, benzoic acid, strychnine, phenol. It does this detoxifying at the expense of its own tissues, hence it is a question whether hepatic cirrhosis, hepatitis, or the toxemias of pregnancy may not sometimes be a result of repeated attacks of toxicity. The liver regenerates rapidly after injury, after chloroform poisoning, and after surgical removal of any part of its lobes. Seventy per cent of the organ may be taken and will regenerate in a few weeks. It is interesting to note that the liver will perform adequately all its functions even though markedly disabled by disease. Its functions are sometimes damaged selectively as when the excretory functions are d a m a g e d yet carbohydrate metabolism goes on.

The symptoms of disturbed function of the liver consist primarily of jaundice, of which there are three main types. First, obstructive, which indicates a blockage of the biliary passages. The bile is reabsorbed into the blood stream, giving rise to jaundice. A good example of this is carcinoma of the head of the pancreas, which blocks the common bile duct. Second, hemolytic jaundice, wherein due to blood destruction, there is too much bilirubin in the blood, thus giving rise to jaundice. This is seen in anemias, blood dyscrasias, large hemorrhages in the thoracic cavity, etc. The third type of jaundice is that due to intrahepatic damage by toxins or infections. In this there is an injury to the parenchyma of the liver, possibly obstructing its discharge of bile high up before it enters the duct. To this class belongs the jaundice seen in uremia or renal sepsis. Babies and Torok think that we can assume with correctness that the accumulated t o x i c metabolic products in uremia lead to a disturbance of the liver function, whereby the severity of the clinical picture is at t i m e s definitely made worse in addition to the already bad function of the kidneys. In some cases they think the disturbance of liver function can dominate the picture. McKay has reported three cases with severe liver complications following the removal of ureteral stone by operative cystoscopy. He states that the patients were desperately sick and that he has seen other cases of the kind. The disease came on about a week or ten days following removal of the stone, and he says that the laboratory tests gave definite indications of the obstructive type of jaundice. It was his impression, however, that the condition was a cholemia, using this term to mean an overloading of the blood by reabsorption of performed biliary constituents. In his experience the condition followed urinary sepsis such as chills and fever with no laboratory evidence of blood stream infection. I have seen a mild jaundice follow urethral chill and have seen it on more than one occasion in patients who were suffering from severe toxemia due to prostatic obstruction. I have also seen cases of severe pyelitis of pregnancy in which the patient was markedly jaundiced, but the jaundice disappeared after proper drainage of the kidneys had been instituted. I have seen a similar mild jaundice in a woman who was suffering from total anuria as a result of accidental injection of an irritating chemical into the pelvis of the kidney. It seems there is no doubt that liver cells are definitely damaged by the accumulated toxic products arising from a state of uremia or urosepsis, and the only remedy consists of relieving the primary condition.

Finally may be mentioned two unclassified toxic states which are quite common. One of these is s e p s i s, the symptoms of which are elevation of the leukocyte count, fever, chills, pyuria, delirium, and sometimes positive blood culture. The treatment consists of tonic and supportive treatment, drainage of abscesses where feasible, and in selected cases the use of drugs such as intravenous mercurochrome, sulfanilamide, or vaccines. I have recently had a case of renal abscess in a polycystic kidney. I could not remove the kidney because the opposite side was also polycystic. I drained a large abscess but the patient remained septic for a period of two months, during which time I saturated her with sulfanilamide and gave her intravenous injections of one per cent mercurochrome every other day until she made an ultimate recovery and is today well. I recently saw a ten-year-old girl who had been operated upon by another surgeon for a perirenal abscess and who drained for three or four weeks, then stopped draining but continued to run chills and high fever. A diagnosis of renal carbuncle was made, and I was c a l l e d in consultation. Owing to the weakness of the patient and the danger of starting a possible septicemia, I preferred to take the conservative course and began giving the child intravenous mercurochrome. She showed an immediate improvement, recovering completely on no other treatment. These and other cases have convinced me that sepsis can be handled conservatively in m a n y cases with less risk than would be produced by additional surgery.

Cachexia can be produced by any one of many things, such as cancer, tuberculosis or syphilis. In hopeless cachexia where the condition cannot be remedied by urinary drainage, tonic treatment or upbuilding foods, it has been my habit to give the patient intravenously 10 ccs. of one to 500 dilute h y d r o c h l o r i c acid every second day. I have found it to be of considerable value in relieving the patient's cachexia and general weakness. It makes him feel better and is something to do. I first used it in a case of carcinoma of the uterus a few years ago. X-ray treatment had been given to the limit of tolerance and the vagina and r e c t u m were simply a cloaca of sloughing material, the patient bedfast, and in a t e r r i b l e state. Intravenous hydrochloric acid b r o u g h t about a magic change. Her appetite immediately picked up, her color improved, and best of all the sloughing area cleaned up. She thought she was getting well. I knew she was not but preferred to leave her thinking so because up to the day of her death she felt good and even got out of bed and began to move a r o u n d the house. She finally died of intestinal obstruction due to progressive infiltration by the malignancy, but the case taught me that sometimes very simple drugs are valuable. I have used this treatment in malignancies of the bladder, not once but several times, helping these poor people into a better feeling, less nausea and weakness, more spirit and courage in eating, and consider it to be very valuable as a palliative remedy in hopeless cases.

SUMMARY

In this paper I have attempted to outline the various conditions which produce a state of low vitality in a patient who may be suffering from s e r i o u s urinary tract disease. Many of these conditions are susceptible of considerable relief if they are definitely diagnosed. The remedies to be applied are quite different in each condition, and it is of great importance that the attending surgeon be thoroughly cognizant of each state and with the diagnostic tests by which it may be established. This knowledge will give a much more accurate prognosis and will in many cases assist the patient to a quicker recovery.

--------O--------

Gall Bladder Surgery*

F. A. HUDSON, M.D.
ENID, OKLAHOMA

Some time ago I received an a r t i c l e from the Wesley Hospital in Chicago, a review of gall bladder surgery in that institution, calling particular attention to the evolution of surgery of the gall bladder. It was particularly interesting to me because it covered about the same time that I have had an opportunity to observe this type of surgery.

Thirty years ago most gall bladders were drained, and the article I have referred to, describes how an attempt was made at that time to suture the gall b l a d d e r to the parietal peritoneum and then to pack the upper abdomen full of gauze drainage. I can remember very well when the padded

*Read before the Section on General Surgery, Annual Meeting, Oklahoma State Medical Association, Oklahoma City, May, 1939.

drainage tube was first used and what an improvement it seemed to be, since by the use of such a tube the gall bladder could be closed around the tube so as to probably prevent leakage when the gall bladder was dropped back into the peritoneal cavity, and some of the other drainage could be dispensed with. I can also remember the a r g u m e n t s for cholecystotomy and for cholecystectomy, and I can r e m e m b e r hearing one of the great surgeons in Chicago state that even if the gall bladder had to come out, he thought it much safer to drain it first and remove it later, and that the death rate from the primary removal of the gall bladder was at least 15 per cent. Today, diseased gall bladders are mostly removed, unless there is some definite reason for not doing so, such as the condition of the patient; the difficulty of the surgical procedure due to the condition in the operative area; obstructions in the common bile duct, which cannot be r e l i e v e d, in which case the gall bladder may be utilized as a duct by anastomosing it into the duodenum or into the stomach, and certain cases of empyema of the gall bladder.

I had hoped to be able to report a thousand cases and think probably I should be able to report that many, but farther back than about 15 years our records are not available, or are of such character as not to admit of analysis.

The disease is very common, particularly among women, and I think, especially common among w o m e n who have had children, and more common after the age of 35 or 40. The youngest one in this series was a girl 16, and the oldest, a man, 88.

The symptoms are very variable, depending upon whether there are stones, or not; whether there is infection present, or not; whether the gall bladder alone is involved; or whether the liver, pancreas, or bile ducts are involved, and whether or not there is obstruction, and where. The most common symptom is that of indigestion. If a woman, 40 years old, or thereabouts, who has had children, complains of indigestion or discomfort in the upper abdomen, gas, belching, etc., it is quite likely that she has trouble about her gall bladder. The ordinary case, after a little study, is not difficult to diagnose. A case with small stones, who passes one occasionally, gives a different picture—severe attacks of colic, often followed by some jaundice, and p e r h a p s no symptoms between attacks other than a vague indigestion. Cases with obstruction of the common duct, due to stone or otherwise, give a different picture entirely, but they usually have a suggestive history, often over a long period of time. Cases with obstruction of the cystic duct give another picture, and if this is complicated by secondary infection of the gall bladder, still a n o t h e r one. These cases with infection throughout the biliary tree are different again. In some of them the symptoms are more general than local. Some few c a s e s have very vague symptoms, or no symptoms pointing to the gall bladder, as for instance, one case who complained of severe pain under the shoul-

der, never in the epigastrium, no dyspepsia, just the pain under the shoulder. The diagnosis in this case was made by elimination of other possible causes of the pain and by radiographs of the gall bladder. Another case, with an intractable diarrhea of several weeks duration was promptly relieved by removal of the gall bladder. We had a recent case in which the predominating symptom was a tachycardia, who had had a pulse of between 180 and 200 most of the time for three months, which nothing relieved. His heart was apparently normal. He had some vague history suggestive of gall bladder disease. There was tenderness in the epigastrium, and radiographically, he had a diseased gall bladder. He was in the hospital a long time under observation. Removal of the gall bladder was followed by a p r o m p t cessation of the tachycardia, and he has not had any recurrence, since.

Radiography of the gall bladder, in a case where the diagnosis is at all obscure, is of very great value. Sometimes stones show. Usually not. Sometimes, when the gall bladder visualizes fairly well, they will produce a reverse shadow; but, generally speaking, if the patient retains the dye and the gall bladder is not visible in the films, it proves to be diseased. Also, if the gall bladder visualizes fairly well but empties very slowly after taking the fat meal, it usually proves to be diseased. On the other hand, a gall bladder, which fills well and empties promptly, should be considered as not causing trouble, unless there is a great deal of evidence to the contrary.

There is, of course, a great deal of argument about the treatment of these people with diseased gall bladders. There are various diets and drugs, and drainage by stimulation with the duodenal tube advocated. I think that some of these things possibly help some of them. I don't know whether they do or not. Most people with diseased gall bladders have periods—sometimes long periods—during which they are not bothered very much. Possibly the patient and the doctor are a little prone to think the medication has benefited the patient, when he has really just been having one of his intervals between attacks. We know that many people go through life with a d i s e a s e d gall bladder, or with stones, and live to a good old age. We also know that too many of them go to the surgeon when they are old and in such a condition that something has to be done for them, with a damaged liver, a pancreatitis, a nephritis, and perhaps a chronic myocarditis. I think gall bladder disease is very conducive to all of these conditions. However, there cannot be any particular argument between the surgeon and the internist about gall bladder disease, because the case that comes to the surgeon has almost always been elsewhere. She has been dieted and has been given bile salts and various other drugs, usually for a long period of time, and when she does come to the hospital she is suffering either from a very acute attack or has had trouble so long that she had become disgusted with it. It takes a good deal of discomfort and time to get the patient in this frame of mind, however. It is not unusual to see cases who have had trouble any place from 15 to 30 years. The i n t e r m i t t e n c y of the trouble encourages the patient to procrastinate in the hope that maybe this spell will be the last one. You can be very sure that the individual with the diseased gall b l a d d e r, with some exceptions, of course, is going to go to some doctor, or maybe several of them, in hopes of curing the condition before he contemplates surgery, and that a considerable per cent are going to be poor risks because of age, or conditions secondary to the diseased gall bladder.

This report is based on 771 private cases.

TABLES

Number of cases in this report _____771
Men—188 or 24.4%
Women—583 or 75.6%
Almost exactly 1 man to 4 women.

AGES
None in First Decade
Youngest—16   Oldest—88

Age	Men	Women
10-20	3	15
20-30	23	101
30-40	41	164
40-50	51	143
50-60	43	102
60-70	20	47
70-80	6	11
80 plus	1	0

TYPE OF OPERATION

	Men	Women	Total
Gall bladder removed	129	405	534
Gall bladder drained	42	125	167
Anastomosis between gall bladder and stomach or between gall bladder and duodenum	17	53	70
Duct drainage where gall bladder was removed	26	89	115

Number cases having other surgery—509

	Men	Women	Total
Stomach	29	18	47
Pelvic	—	81	81
Appendectomy	92	271	363
Herniotomy	4	14	18

DEFINITE COMPLICATING FACTORS

	Men	Women	Total	%
Stones	56	278	334	43.
Duct stones	4	33	37	—
(% of those having stones)				11.
Ruptured gall bladder	9	20	29	2.6
Gangrenous gall bladder	6	4	10	1.3
Empyema of gall bladder	39	69	108	14.
Total of those which ruptured, would have ruptured, or were apt to rupture, 138 cases or				18.
Definite liver pathology	63	264	327	42.
Definite pancreatic pathology	21	72	93	12.
Carcinoma	4	9	13	1.7
Gastric or duodenal ulcer	29	27	56	7.4
Previous drainage	4	22	26	3.3
Jaundice	21	61	82	10.6

TOTAL NUMBER OF DEATHS, 70

Of the fatal cases, there were—
3 cases of nephritis
13 cases of pneumonia
3 cases of embolus
2 cases of fat embolism
4 cases of so-called liver shock
1 case of suppurative parotitis
3 cases of septicemia
3 cases of peritonitis and
3 cases of cardiac complication, or
35 cases in which the surgery probably had some bearing upon their deaths, but over half of these cases were known to be poor risks. In fact, an analysis of these cases which did not recover would rather emphasize the danger of delayed surgery than the danger of the operation, itself.

There were—
9 deaths from peritonitis following a ruptured gall bladder
4 from carcinoma of the gall bladder
2 from acute pancreatitis
6 from cancer of the pancreas
6 from inanition
1 case 88 years old, with empyema of the gall bladder
1 case of cancer of the colon, with common duct obstruction and jaundice, and

6 cases which were violently jaundiced, and had been jaundiced for a long time, who just kept on dying. Most of these can be described as exploratory operations in hopes that we might be able to do something in an apparently hopeless situation.

This latter fact is especially brought out by an analysis of the last 100 cases operated.

ANALYSIS OF LAST 100 CASES OPERATED
6 DEATHS

One was an old man, 54, with cirrhosis of the liver, ascites, and an empyema of the gall bladder.

One was a woman, 68, who had been previously operated for ruptured gall bladder, who came into the hospital extremely ill and jaundiced. She was in the hospital 15 days before the operation during which time attempts were made to improve her condition by blood transfusions, etc., and who lived two and a half months after she was operated.

One was a young man, 26, who entered the hospital starved, with an enormously dilated stomach as the result of a pyloric stenosis. His gall bladder was removed because it was amalgamated into the mass of scar tissue around the pylorus. He lived some weeks after surgery and died of inanition.

One man, 66, and another one, 65, both had cancer of the pancreas.

One woman, 49, died of peritonitis, which we think was due to leakage of a suture line in the stomach.

None of these deaths certainly could be attributed to the surgery of the gall bladder, and only one of them could possibly have had any connection at all with the operative procedure.

IMPRESSIONS

Diseased gall bladder, or what somebody called cholecystic disease, referring to the biliary system, is a very common affliction, and is about four or five times as common among women as among men, and apparently more common among women who have had pregnancies than others. It affects people of all ages, but is more prevalent after the age of 35. Not nearly all of them have stones, and many of the worst cases with most extensive damage to the liver and other organs do not have stones. Some of these cases can be helped by diet and medication—that is, without surgery, but there is no reason for any argument between the internist and the s u r g e o n about this, because cases are not coming to the surgeon until they have tried something else, usually many things. The cases that do come to the surgeon are usually cases who have had trouble for any place from five to 30 years, and of whom a large per cent are poor risks, because of age and o t h e r conditions secondary to the prolonged trouble about the gall bladder and the biliary tree. Many of them, in fact, are in such a condition that surgery is attempted because it is quite evident that something has to be done or the patient cannot survive, and often in these very desperate cases, the results are very gratifying, too.

Results in gall bladder surgery, taking into consideration the length of time these people have been afflicted, and the condition they are in when they come to the surgeon, are astonishingly good, and the death rate is very low. It is much easier for me to understand why a good many of these cases do not obtain complete relief, than it is to understand how so many of them do. The ability of the liver and the pancreas, especially the liver, to recover, must be enormous. I think the death rate from gall bladder surgery, if done reasonably early on people who are not too old, who still have fairly good hearts and kidneys, and not too much liver damage, is very low—probably not more than one or two per cent. I also feel that although many cases will go through life and live their normal length of time with trouble in the gall bladder, if all cases of gall bladder disease, that is, those with gall bladder disease who have been given a reasonable chance to recover, were operated while they are still in good condition, that the average length of life would be much increased and the average health much better. I think the chances of the patient with a diseased gall bladder developing a cancer of the gall gladder, if he tries to keep his gall bladder, are about as great as the operative risk, if surgery is done early before there is too much secondary damage, to say nothing of the other risks he runs by trying to avoid removal of his gall bladder.

I have had my share of people who have come back complaining of t r o u b l e, and quite a few of them do have somewhat the same symptoms they had before the operation, though very rarely as severe. We have found that a large per cent of these cases have an achylia, and in the last few years I have determined this fact in all cases, and if they do, have put them on hydrochloric acid. If they do not get acid, they are liable to have a good deal of flatulence and discomfort. Also, some of them, I think, have trouble due to infection in the liver, which does not always clear up.

I believe these cases with liver damage should be kept under observation for some time, their diets regulated, and an attempt made to improve their general condition as much as possible. Some of them seem to have symptoms due to a spasm of the sphincter, and, of course, some of them have trouble because stones are overlooked in the ducts, or because an infected biliary tree was not drained. I think, however, that some of the reports in recent literature in regard to the high percentage of these cases of common duct stone, and of cases requiring common duct drainage, are too high, and that like other classes of people, we sometimes go to extremes.

I believe it is s a f e r to prepare these cases for operation by putting them to bed and seeing that they are well fed, giving them a few days' rest, pushing fluids, and saturating them with glucose. I believe that this will eliminate a large per cent of those cases who d e v e l o p what was formerly called liver shock—that is, a high temperature, rapid pulse, vomiting, and even evidence of nephritis—some of whom die. I think it is better, also, to allow the patient to recover from his attack if he will, and certainly a very large per cent of them will.

I think it is s a f e r to remove the gall bladder from the fundus downward than from the duct upward. In this manner, very good peritoneal flaps can usually be obtained for suturing over the raw surface on the liver. The cystic artery can be better visualized, and if it should be cut accidentally, it can be picked up easier; and, since there can be any conceivable anomaly of the ducts—the hepatic duct can even wind around the cystic duct—this type of removal makes duct i n j u r y much less likely.

I am of the opinion that it is better to use drainage. It is certainly not always necessary, and I have closed some of them myself without having any trouble, but quite a few of these cases have an astonishing amount of drainage for about a day or two, and it would appear to be better to allow this to escape on the dressings than to be retained. I think it is also a very good thing to tuck the omentum in between the liver and the duodenum following the operation. If there are stones in the c o m m o n duct, the duct should be d r a i n e d. If there are no demonstrable stones in the duct, whether or not it should be drained, depends probably more upon the symptoms the patient had before he was operated, than upon what is found at the time of the operation. The glucose should be continued postoperatively until the patient can take fluids freely.

I am under the impression that there are too few gall bladders treated surgically; that the number of these c a s e s is very much greater than the number who are operated without sufficient justification; also, that the tendency is to be operated too late, rather than too early; that the disease can be diagnosed very accurately, and that postoperative symptoms are much more apt to be due to secondary damage and to co-existing disease, or conditions acquired subsequent to the surgery, than to error in the diagnosis.

ANALYSIS OF REPORTS

CHOLECYSTECTOMIES

Total Number—280

Complete relief	169 or 60.3%
Almost complete relief	54 or 19.2%
Partial relief	52 or 18.5%
No relief	5 or 1.7%

COMPLICATING CONDITIONS PRESENT AT TIME OF OPERATION

Gall stones	89	Kidney stones	3
Stone in duct	11	Gastric or	
Hepatitis	39	duodenal ulcer	10
Pancreatitis	9	Gangrenous G. B.	2
Ventral hernia	1	Lues	1

TROUBLE DEVELOPED SINCE

Asthma	1	Female trouble	3
Low blood pressure	1	Neuritis	1
Nervousness	2	Headaches	3
Malta Fever	2	Heart trouble	2
Constipation	2	Lues	1
Diarrhea	1	Colitis	1
Rheumatism	6	Insane	7
Arthritis	2	Diabetes	1

1 died later of cancer of the liver.
1 died 4 years later of brain tumor.

CHOLECYSTOTOMIES

Total number—48

Complete relief	29 or 60.4%
Almost complete relief	7 or 14.5%
Partial relief	12 or 25. %

1 woman, 78, stones, still living and in good health 5 years later.

COMPLICATING CONDITIONS PRESENT AT TIME OF OPERATION

Gall stones	17	Empyema	6
Stones in duct	5	Rupt. g. b. with	
Pancreatitis	1	abscess	1
Hepatitis	1	Jaundice	1

TROUBLE DEVELOPED SINCE

Hernia	4	Rheumatism	2
Constipation	4	Diabetes	2
Hemorrhoids	2	Biliary fistula	1

1 had relief 6 months, anastomosis later.
1 had relief 1 year, anastomosis later.
1 had relief 4 years, anastomosis later.
   All have complete relief since.
1 had partial relief 2 years, anastomosis. Still has trouble.
1 died of a stroke, 8 years after operation.

ANASTOMOSIS
Total Number—34

Complete relief	18 or 52.9%
Almost complete relief	5 or 14.7%
Partial relief	11 or 32.3%

COMPLICATING CONDITIONS PRESENT AT TIME OF OPERATION

Gall stones	13	Pancreatitis	2
Stone in duct	7	Jaundice	7
Kidney stone	1	Cancer of liver	1
Previous drainage	6		

TROUBLE DEVELOPED SINCE

Diabetes	1	Parkinson's	1
Malta Fever	1	Pancreatitis	1

1 patient age 41. Cancer of liver, lived 3 years.
1 patient 70. Stones. Degenerative disease of liver, heart, and kidneys—lived 3 months.
1 patient 66. Empyema. Stones. Stone in cystic duct. Died a few years later of pneumonia.

We were able to trace 362 cases. Of the cases reporting, a much larger percentage of the cholecystectomies reported than the other cases, which can be explained by the fact that a large per cent of the drainage cases were operated years ago, and more of them have died since or moved away, and could not be reached. There are so few of the drainage cases that reported that it is not possible to make much of a comparison between the two types of cases. My impression is that there were somewhat better results in the cholecystectomies than in the cholecystotomies, but the majority of the drainage cases were cases in whom there was more pathology than in the cholecystectomies, and in the last half of the period covered by this report, the gall bladder was almost invariably removed, except in such cases, who because of their age, or because of the condition found at operation were not considered safe cases for removal of the gall bladder. These tables are made out as reported by the patient, but I am convinced that they are not very accurate.

One question in the questionaire was in regard to other diseases since the operation which the patient may have had, and there was also a place for remarks. Those cases who say they are completely relieved probably are. Unquestionably, a great many of the cases who reported that they were not completely relieved, were relieved, but were having ill health from some other reason. It was rather the rule for those cases reporting partial relief to recite a list of afflictions which were causing them trouble at the present time, and not mention their liver area at all. I also noticed in comparing the questionaires with the records, that a very large per cent of those cases who did not report complete relief had a great deal of secondary pathology, particularly marked hepatitis, quite a few of them gastric or duodenal ulcer, and some of them chronic pancreatitis. I am convinced that a great many cases which have some symptoms after removal of the gall bladder have them as a result of liver damage before the surgery. In fact, it is hard to understand, after inspecting some of these livers how the patient can ever be well at all.

There was a greater per cent of complete relief in cases where the information was obtained from the doctor than where it was obtained from the patient. If the patient was not enjoying good health at the time of the report, the doctor stated the reason why he was not. There was frequently something quite foreign to his gall bladder condition in which we were interested, while a large per cent of the patients seemed to be unable to make this differentiation.

There was a somewhat greater percentage of complete relief in those cases who had stones than in those who did not. This could be explained, of course, in a good many ways. One could be that where there are stones present in the gall bladder there is not much chance of the diagnosis having been incorrect, while in the absence of stones perhaps the diagnosis might be incorrect, and the patient might have been operated and his gall bladder removed when the cause of his ill health was elsewhere. However, I think that the explanation is more likely to be this—that a great many cases have stones in a gall bladder which does not appear to be very abnormal, and a great many with a liver which does not show much evidence of damage, while in those cases which have gall bladders which are markedly pathological, there would seem to be a greater percentage of abnormal livers. Or, to put it in another way, if the symptoms are not due to stones, they are more likely to be due to an infection, and infection in the gall bladder is liable to be attended by infection in the biliary tree, etc.

There were 34 reports from cases in which there was an anastomosis made between the gall bladder and the stomach, or between the gall bladder and the duodenum. Eighteen, or 52.9 per cent reported themselves as completely relieved; five, or 14.7 per cent, as almost completely relieved, and 11, or 32.3 per cent reported themselves as having obtained some relief. Two of the cases which were not completely relieved had very serious liver damage. One had cancer of the liver, and one states she had relief for eight years. Two, under remarks, explained their present ill health by something entirely foreign to the gall bladder condition. This operation, of course, is done only in cases in which there is rather excessive pathology. One case had relief for a time and then had a recurrence of symptoms. She was re-operated. It was found that the os between the stomach and the gall bladder was closed. The gall bladder was removed and the common duct drained, and she has been quite well ever since. There was another case which was operated in 1923, at which time she had an empyema of the gall bladder with stones. The stones were removed and the gall bladder drained. She was operated again in 1929. She again had stones and an empyema of the gall bladder. The stones were removed and an anastomosis was made between the gall bladder and the stomach. She was operated again in September, 1938. She was jaundiced and the os had closed between the gall bladder and the stomach, and the gall bladder contained one fairly large stone. At this operation, the gall bladder was removed and a T-tube was placed in the duct. It has been there now for seven months.

The replies to t h e s e questionaires are

very interesting. Of course, some just answer the questions and let it go at that. Some of them under remarks go into considerable detail of how much better they are now, and how thankful they are for the relief they have obtained, and how much they think of us, and others are rather sarcastic. One woman stated that a b o u t the only difference as far as she could see in her condition now and before the operation was as to who had the $150. Another one cursed me in considerable detail and ended up by saying, "You asked for it, so here it is." One lady said I was a long time showing any interest in her, but that she was willing to forgive me if I would ask her up to tell me all about herself. About the time I was beginning to feel right good, I usually ran onto a report that was not conducive to my self-esteem. Some of these cases, instead of filling out these reports came in to see me. One lady told me she did not think she was at all better, and after examining her I found she was suffering from hives and varicose veins. Another one said she had been considerably better for some time, but that now she was having just as much trouble as she ever had. Examination in this case revealed an achylia and an active undulant fever.

There is certainly a very strange tendency among a large per cent of our people who have had surgery to blame almost anything that happens to them at any period thereafter, to the operation. It is true that we had quite a number of reports in which the patient specified definitely that his present condition was not due to his gall bladder, but then also definitely specified the ailments he had at this time and what he thought they were due to. For instance, we have one report which I will quote: "I seemed to be in perfect physical condition for about a year and a half after my operation. Then a condition arose which was diagnosed by one doctor as a kidney ailment. A recurrence of the same ailment was diagnosed by another doctor as heart trouble. Frankly, I do not know which, if either, was correct, and I hope to be able to return for examination."

The way these reports are coming in, we

expect to receive them in dribbles for the next six months, and hope to be able to investigate these cases who do not report at least almost complete relief. I imagine that if we are able to accomplish this, that it will be very instructive. I think I shall ask the Journal to publish this later, as a sort of post-script on this report.

------o------

Repeated Convulsions in Children*
The Relation of Demonstrable Organic Pathology in Twenty-Two Consecutive Cases

JESS D. HERRMANN, M.D.
OKLAHOMA CITY, OKLAHOMA

Within recent years the term "idiopathic epilepsy" has lost favor in clinics where the problem of repeated convulsive seizures has been encountered. This change is largely due to the increase in understanding of the underlying pathologies associated with this condition. It has been accepted that all true convulsions are a manifestation of cortical irritation whether due to a primary cerebral lesion or secondary to systemic disease. I fear that we are all prone to make such a diagnosis without obtaining a careful history and without thorough examination of the patient. Because we are unable to find the cause for many of these convulsive disorders it does not follow that they arise spontaneously nor that the problem will not be well understood in years to come.

As surgeons we are often disappointed, sometimes to the point of being discouraged, in finding so few children out of the many studied who have a correctable lesion. We have, however, been interested in the rather large number that has shown evidence of gross organic pathology. It is through a better understanding of the pathology found and its role in producing the convulsions that eventually we hope to aid more of these unfortunate children.

It has been our observation that the results obtained by the continued administration of sedatives of varied types have

not been generally satisfactory. Fay and McQuarrie have advocated dehydration therapy in these cases. There are many instances of unquestioned benefit from the use of such measures but it falls short of solving the problem. The same can be said of the therapeutic effect of ketogenic diet. Each of these methods of treatment is directed at preventing the "cerebral explosion" and in most cases decreases the number of severity of the attacks for a time. The many instances of continued attacks in spite of all forms of conservative management, however, should stimulate us to further efforts instead of causing us to admit defeat.

We are concerned in this review of cases not with etiology or treatment directly but in the demonstration of gross pathologies made during the investigation of 22 consecutive cases of repeated convulsive seizures in children seen at the Crippled Childrens' Hospital during the year 1937. We do not presume that the pathology shown in each case is the cause of the convulsions but we do feel that in many instances there is a definite relationship between the two.

Each of the children selected for this review has as a chief complaint "convulsive seizures" or "fits." The descriptions of the attacks varied somewhat but were of general epileptiform nature, either grand mal or grand mal plus petite mal. There was one exception in which the seizure was of a tonic type. Occasionally

*Read before the Section on Obstetrics and Pediatrics, Annual Meeting, Oklahoma State Medical Association, Oklahoma City, May 2, 1939.

there was a history of a focal origin of the attack. Some of these children had associated complaints and in some there were physical findings indicating organic cere-

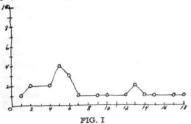

FIG. I
Age at Time of Investigation.
Horizontal—Age in Years.
Vertical—Number of Patients.

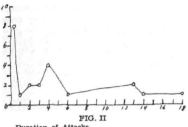

FIG. II
Duration of Attacks.
Horizontal—Number of Years.
Vertical—Number of Cases.

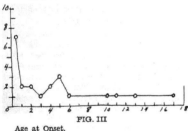

FIG. III
Age at Onset.
Horizontal—Age in Years.
Vertical—Number of Patients.

bral lesions. The children ranged between the ages of one and 18 years at the time of their investigation (Fig. 1). The duration of the attacks was from one month to 18 years with the majority being less than five years (Fig. 2). We are struck with the large number that began having attacks before the age of one year (Fig. 3).

The pathologies demonstrated in 15 of the 22 cases were as follows:

Condition	Incidence
Intestinal Parasites	2
Diabetes	1
Hyperinsulinism	1
Telangiectasis of Parietal Bones	1
Fracture of Skull with Extra-dural Hemorrhage and Pontine Hemorrhage	1
Right Frontal Lobe Neoplasm	1
Cerebellar Neoplasm	1
Cortical Atrophy, Internal Hydro-cephalus or Porencephaly as Demonstrated by Encephalograms	10

Pendergrass, Southard and Thom, and others have demonstrated gross cerebral pathologies by encephalographic s t u d i e s and post-mortem examinations. E v e r y neurosurgeon has seen gross changes in the brain, its vessels or coverings while attempting to r e l i e v e a convulsive disorder of focal nature.

As we have said before, we are discouraged at times because so few of the patients investigated have lesions even when demonstrated that are amenable to treatment. You will probably ask: "What has been gained as far as the individual patient is concerned even though a probable organic cause for the convulsions has been found, if the attacks cannot be relieved?" In diseases as in most other things we fear most that about which we know l e a s t. Each time I hear the diagnosis of Idiopathic Epilepsy I am reminded of the definition of idiopathic which the late Dr. M. Smith made while in a facetious mood— "Idio—I don't know; pathic—a damn thing about it." It has been our experience that the parents of these children can much better accept the situation if some tangible condition is explained or demonstrated to them as to the cause of their child's attacks, than to supply a diagnosis the meaning of which they obtain chiefly from the lay press or the family medical book.

BIBLIOGRAPHY

Fay, Temple: Generalized Pressure Atrophy of the Brain Secondary to Traumatic and Pathologic Involvement of the Pachionian Bodies. J.A.M.A., 94:245, 1930.

McQuarrie, T.: Experimental Studies of the Acid Base Equilibrium in Children with Epilepsy. Am. J. Dis. Child. 37:261, 1929.

Pendergrass, E. P.: Interpretation of Encephalographic Observations; Comments on those Found in Convulsive States. Arch. Neurol. & Psychiat., 23:946, 1930.

Southard, E. E., and Thom, D. A.: Contributions from the State Board of Insanity, Mass. No. 46. 1915.

Second Year of Survey of Type Incidence of Pneumococcal Infections in Oklahoma

H. D. MOOR, M.D.
IDA LUCILLE BROWN, M.S., M.T.
University of Oklahoma School of Medicine
Department of Bacteriology
OKLAHOMA CITY, OKLAHOMA

During the period of May 1, 1938, to June 1, 1939, we had reported to us or typed by us a total of 518 cases of clinical pneumonia or pneumococcic meningitis. In 357 cases the causative agent of the pneumonia was proven by cultural and serological methods. Of these 357 cases, 339 were definitely proven to be pneumococcal in origin with the following distribution of types.

Type I	56
Type II	51
Type III	34
Type IV	9
Type V	14
Type VI	10
Type VII	48
Type VIII	28
Type IX	3
Type X	5
Type XI	7
Type XII	5
Type XIII	2
Type XIV	9
Type XV	9
Type XVI	4
Type XVII	0
Type XVIII	6
Type XIX	4
Type XX	4
Type XXI	2
Type XXII	2
Type XXIII	4
Type XXIV	1
Type XXV	0
Type XXVI (no typing sera)	
Type XXVII	1
Type XXVIII	3
Type XXIX	4
Type XXX (No typing sera)	0
Type XXXI	1
Type XXXII	1
Mixed Types I & II	3
Mixed Types II & V	1
Mixed Types III & XI	1
Mixed Types X & XX	1
Mixed Types III & VIII	2
Mixed Types IV & VI	1
Mixed Types XXI & XXII	1
Mixed Types VII & XIX	1
Mixed Types II, V & XIX	1

Of the 18 other cases in which the causative agent was determined, 13 were streptococci, three were caused by the influenza bacillus and one by Friedlander's bacillus and one staphylococcus.

Types found to be most prevalent this year were I, II, VII, III, VIII, V, VI, XIV and IV in the order of their prevalence. We were not able to learn the age and sex of the patients in all cases but there was apparently no difference in type incidence between males and females though a much larger number of cases in males than in females was reported. The types most prevalent in children from the data at hand were found to be I, V, VII, VII and XIV for this year. Some of the higher types such as XIX, XXII, and XXIX were encountered more often in children than in adults.

The months in which pneumonia was most prevalent this year, according to the typings done, were December, January, March and April. There was a sharp decline in February. In fact in May of this year we had as many typings reported or done by us as in February.

In 298 of the 339 cases we have records of the month in which typing was done. In some cases records were sent in for three or four months at one time so we were unable to determine in which month the case occurred. The following chart shows the typings reported or done here, by months, also the incidence of all cases of pneumonia from all causes as reported to the State Health Department.

Typings done or reported	Cases of Pneumonia Reported to the State Health Department
August, 1938, 2	26
September, 1938, 3	29
October, 1938, 7	71
November, 1938, 12	100
December, 1938, 42	322
January, 1939, 58	408
February, 1939, 32	317
March, 1939, 58	261
April, 1939, 48	278
May, 1938, 32	119
June, 1939, 4	43

Mr. J. C. Rose, the State Statistician, reports that the total number of cases of pneumonia, all types, was 1,805 for the months of May 1, 1938, to June 1, 1939. During the period December 1, 1937, to May 1, 1938, the most prevalent t y p e s were I, VII, II, III, V, IV, and VIII, in the order of their prevalence.

For the two-year period during which we have been determining the type incidence, we have a total number of 606 cases of pneumococcal pneumonia in which the type was definitely determined. The distribution is as follows:

Type I	133
Type II	88
Type III	67
Type IV	17
Type V	24
Type VI	13
Type VII	98
Type VIII	34
Type IX	6
Type X	7
Type XI	9
Type XII	6
Type XIII	2
Type XIV	14
Type XV	9
Type XVI	5
Type XVII	2
Type XVIII	7
Type XIX	8
Type XX	6
Type XXI	7
Type XXII	5
Type XXIII	9
Type XXIV	1
Type XXV	1
Type XVI (No typing sera available	—
Type XXVII	1
Type XXVIII	3
Type XXIX	5
Type XXX (No typing sera available)	—
Type XXXI	0
Type XXXII	2
Mixed Types	17

We have reviewed approximately 100 papers during the past year dealing with typing of the pneumococci, serum therapy, and chemotherapy in pneumococcal infections. These p a p e r s were distributed among the following Journals—Journal of the A.M.A., Southern M e d i c a l Journal, American Journal of Public Health, Journal of Medical Sciences, Journal of Laboratory and Clinical Medicine, and American Journal of Medical Technology.

It is not the purpose in this report, nor is it possible to review the results of all these investigations. It does seem important to briefly point out the general conclusions to date.

I. The Neufeld rapid method of typing pneumococci is established as a reliable time saving laboratory test for making a specific diagnosis in pneumococcal infections, especially pneumonia and meningitis.

II. Types most prevalent in Oklahoma as shown by the two-year survey to date are I, VII, II, III, VIII, V, IV, and XIV.

III. Every case of suspected pneumococcal infection should be typed as early in the course of the disease as possible. The typing should be done before serum ·or chemotherapy is started. This applies especially to chemotherapy, particularly sulfapyridine. This drug has been f o u n d by numerous investigators to have a dissolving effect on the capsules surrounding the pneumococci. Others claim that it does not dissolve the capsule. (MacLeod, Journal A.M.A., October 7, 1939.) However that may be, our experience as well as the experience of others has been that its use before typing renders the procedure difficult, prolongs the t i m e required, and may result in failure to type at all. It is now definitely established that sulfapyridine is not equally effective in all types of pneumococcal pneumonia, for e x a m p l e Dr. D. Seargeant Pepper and others in the July, 1939, issue of the American Journal of Medical Sciences report the use of sulfapyridine therapy in 400 cases of typed pneumococcal pneumonia. Eighty-four per cent of these cases were caused by Types I to VIII and Type XIV. They report a mortality of 5.8 per cent in Type I treated with sulphopyridine, 6.7 per cent in Type II and 16.4 per cent in Type III. Dr. L. H. Schmidt in the Procedings of the American Society of Biological Chemistry for July, 1939, reports as follows: "Treatment with sulfapyridine seemed to show the greatest efficiency in Types I and VII infections, next in IV, V, VI, XI, XXII and XXIX. On types II, III and VIII it had little curative action although it did prolong life."

Williams and Morgan writing in the Southern Medical Journal for June, 1939, and Dr. Colin M. MacLeod in the Journal of the American Medical Association for October 7, 1939, sum up the sulphopyridine pneumonia situation in harmony with the great majority of investigators. Williams and Morgan say: "Since the available evidence s u g g e s t s that sulfapyridine and specific aintipneumococcus serum e x e r t their favorable influence upon pneumococcic infections through distinct and, possibly, altogether unrelated mechanisms, it appears reasonable to hope that a combination of the two agents will give better results than have been obtained when one only is utilized." Dr. MacLeod writing on the chemotherapy of pneumococcic pneumonia states: "Sulfapyridine gives promise of reducing the death rate from pneumococcic pneumonia and present indications make it seem probable than an even greater reduction in the mortality rate can be accomplished if the drug is used in conjunction with type specific antipneumococcus serum."

Practically all the investigators agree that the introduction of s u l f a p y r i d i n e and sulfanilamide is in all probability the g r e a t e s t contribution to chemotherapy since the introduction of the arsenicals in the treatment of syphilis. They are very definite in their statements that it will require a great deal more study and investigation of these compounds before we will have an a d e q u a t e knowledge of their pharmacology, toxicology and therapeutic value. It therefore follows as a final conclusion that every infectious disease treated with sulfanilamide, sulfapyridine, or any of the various preparations containing them or their derivatives should have an early accurate and specific diagnosis. It is only by so doing that we can arrive at a scientific evaluation of the effects of treatment. I wish to stress this final conclusion b e c a u s e when sulfapyridine was first introduced a great many thought that at last a chemical c o m p o u n d had been found that was effective in pneumococcal infections regardless of the type. I am sure that as a result of this belief although there were 1,805 cases of pneumonia reported in the state last year, in only 518 cases was an effort made to determine the cause of the pneumonia, in fact we received reports from several sources that they had discontinued typing of pneumococci, or trying to discover the etiological agent because they were now using sulfapyridine.

We wish to continue this survey for a third year, so again we are asking the cooperation of the doctors, hospitals and laboratories throughout the state in reporting typings to us and sending us specimens from such places in the state where facilities for typing are not available. We wish to thank the following institutions for their excellent co-operation during the past two years:

OKLAHOMA CITY—
    State Department of Health (also their related laboratories)
    University Hospital
    Crippled Children's Hospital
    St. Anthony's Hospital
    Wesley Hospital
    Samaritan Hospital
    Oklahoma City General Hospital
    Polyclinic Hospital
    McBride's Reconstruction Hospital
    Hubbard Hospital
    Medical Arts Laboratory No. 1
    Medical Arts Laboratory No. 2
TULSA—
    St. John's Hospital
    Nelson Clinical Laboratory, Medical Arts Building
MUSKOGEE—
    Musogee Baptist Hospital
    U. S. Veterans' Administration Facility
ENID—
    Enid General Hospital
SHAWNEE—
    A. C. and H. Hospital
McALESTER—
    Lattimore Laboratories
CHICKASHA—
    Chickasha Hospital
GUTHRIE—
    Cimmarron Valley Wesley Hospital
    Louis L. Share Laboratory
PONCA CITY—
    Ponca City Hospital
NORMAN—
    University of Oklahoma Infirmary
DUNCAN—
    Weedn Hospital
FORT SILL—
    Station Hospital, Field Artillery School
EL RENO—
    El Reno Sanitarium
    Fort Reno Remount Station
        In addition we had reports from private physicians in Blackwell, Lawton, Pawhuska, Chickasha, Cromwell, and Commerce.

This investigation was made possible by funds appropriated by the State Legislature for research purposes.

———o———

Children's Food Dislikes

"There is no one food, with the possible exception of milk, which is absolutely essential in the child's diet," William I. Fishbein, M. D., Chicago, declares in the October issue of Hygeia, The Health Magazine.

It is not necessary, he believes, to force a child to take any food which he dislikes, inasmuch as satisfactory substitutes are available. As the child grows older food dislikes often disappear, although many persons carry some of them over into adult life with no harm to themselves.

Asphyxia of the Newborn*

W. M. TAYLOR, M.D.
Emeritis Professor of Pediatrics, School of Medicine,
University of Oklahoma
OKLAHOMA CITY, OKLAHOMA

For a pediatrician to offer suggestions for the resuscitation of the infant, is real temerity, as perhaps less than half of one percent of the newborn have the services of a pediatrician available. Nevertheless with closer cooperation of the pediatrician and obstetrician each may learn something from the other and therefrom contribute something which may reduce the high mortality of fatal first 14 days of life. This is too high, and though much has been said about it not much has been done about it in the past 20 years.

The term "asphyxia" is used to describe all cases in which spontaneous respiration is not established with sufficient promptness to or sufficient force to m a i n t a i n life[1].

Clinically the distinction between asphyxia livida and pallida is easily made: The practical factor is that the differential diagnosis suggests the management to be followed as it is in the latter that prompt and efficient treatment is imperative.

Eastman finds no fundamental difference between clinical livid and pallid asphyxia other than the degree of changes in the blood[2]. In livida the predominating symptoms and signs are those of good muscular tone, forceful heart beat and cord pulsation, generalized cyanosis, response to external stimulation as from the air and mild stimuli of a more direct nature.

In the condition of asphyxia pallida one notes the flaccid muscles, the presence of blue lips with a waxy palor of the cold skin. Heart action is weak and usually slow. Apex beat cannot be felt. Pupils dilated. The jaw falls, the spinctor relaxed. The condition c l o s e l y resembles shock and should be treated as such. It is not infrequently associated or due to intracranial hemorrhage.

*Read at the Meeting of the Southern Medical Association, Oklahoma Day, Oklahoma City, Oklahoma.

ETIOLOGY OF ASPHYXIA OF THE NEWBORN

Asphyxia may be of central or peripheral origin. Any forces which interfere with the free exchange of the placental fetal circulation or the oxygen carrying power of the maternal blood are factors:

1. Disproportion between the pelvis and presenting parts.

2. Premature separation of placenta.

3. Trauma with its danger to the respiratory center from pressure as in hemorrhage.

4. Depression of respiratory center from injudicious use of drugs such as morphine, barburates, anesthetics or other analgesics. One of the first effects of all drugs used to produce analgesia in labor is the depression of the respiratory center. This is especially true of the premature infant. The ideal anesthic for labor has not yet been found.

5. Toxemia of the mother.

6. Obstruction of air passages by mucus and other fluids.

7. Developmental defects.

Intrauterine asphyxia should be expected with the passage of meconium with the vaginal discharge and with weakness or absence of heart sounds previously heard.

In a clinical and statistical study on "Apnea of the Newborn and Associated Cerebral Injury" read before the Section of Obstetrics and Gynecology of the A.M.A., San Francisco, in June, 1938[3], Dr. Frederick Schreiber of Detroit, presented a schematic diagram showing the relationship between the stages of oxygen deficiency and results of that deficiency and the possible degrees of cerebral damage from a deficient supply of oxygen. In his closing summary of this study as published in Jr. A.M.A. of October 1, 1938[4], Dr. Schreiber remarks:

"The depressing effect, on the respiratory center, of birth analgesics given in greater than pharmacologic doses bears a direct relationship to the degree of apnea. The extent of the apnea has a direct relationship with the severity of the cerebral symptoms after birth. The severity of the cerebral symptoms is in direct relation to the amount of damage to the brain tissue. From these relationships it appears that analgesics given in greater amounts than the pharmocologic dosage may in many instances be the causative factor of fetal anoxemia, with resultant cerebral damage in the infant."

TREATMENT

The prophylaxis of asphyxia as far as such is possible, is an obstetrical problem, and in each delivery which is prolonged for any reason, if instrumental or if the mother is narcotized to the degree of cyanosis, evidence of fetal distress, or in the premature, preparations should be made for prompt and efficient care for an asphyxiated infant, instead of the last minute rush which often happens in a busy delivery room.

A well trained interne or nurse who is able to direct the resuscitation in an intelligent way should be available, even to pass a tracheal catheter if there is evidence of obstruction by fluids, for which but little practice is necessary, though a delicate procedure. Good judgement and skill are required in management of such a situation.

McGrath and Kudor, Jr. A.M.A., March 14, 1936[5], suggest and I believe advisedly, the administration of oxygen and $CO2$ to the mother early in the progress of labor, as a prophylactic measure.

1. Immediate clearance of the upper air passages, nose, mouth and t h r o a t of mucus and other fluids should be routine, even in normal deliveries of the full term baby; for as too often happens with the first respiratory effort there is aspiration of fluids followed by a cyanotic attack. This can best be accomplished by posture and suction by means of bulb syringe, preferably with a hard rubber point; by inverting the baby and gently stroking the neck toward the chin. This last procedure is advised against if meningeal hemorrhage is suspected.

2. The cord is immediately cut and tied which may stimulate a respiratory act. This is also advisable if the mother is narcotized by morphine or ether, thus preventing further respiratory depression. Even in some instances the release of blood from cord may be beneficial.

3. If muscular tone is good, heart beat forceful, with deep cyanosis, which at this stage of asphyxia livida is normal, the infant should be wrapped in warm blanket, placed in a warmed bassinett and observed, not handled for a few minutes. Thus giving him an opportunity to initiate his own respiratory acts through natural channels which he usually does. If not, the very gentlest peripheral stimulation may be instituted as: (1) Contact of air with the skin. (2) Gentle pinching of the skin.

(3) Slapping soles of the feet.

If cyanosis continues or changes to a palor and with no respiratory effort, heart sounds grow weaker and slow, dilated pupils and flaccid muscles, the infant is approaching the stage of asphyxia pallida. This clinical picture c l o s e l y approaches that of the baby delivered with an already existing intracranial hemorhage.

TREATMENT OF ASPHYXIA PALLIDA

1. The upper air passages should again be cleared as above and the introduction of the tracheal catheter with suction applied to assure a clear air passage, thus permitting interchange of gasses by the pulmonary alveolar capillary system.

2. Whole blood 10 to 20 cc. should be given intramuscularly, and maintenance of normal body heat.

3. Clinical stimulation is on the whole disappointing t h o u g h metrozol, epinephrine, caffein sodium benzoate, may be used. Physiologic stimulation by the use of $CO2$ is the important method, if possible.

I am indebted to Dr. Gerry Rogers, member of the Obstetrical Staff of St. Anthony's Hospital, for the following suggestions in the technique of passing the tracheal catheter.

4. If child is very apnic, insert finger into pharynx and palpate epiglottis. The glotteal reflex is the best index of the d e g r e e of asphyxia or narcotization. Prompt r e m o v a l of accumulation of mucus in the larynx may be done with tracheal catheter. By introducing the finger far enough to plug the pharynx the glottis and tracheal opening may be palpated with the palmer surface of the finger and the catheter is guided into the trachea. He follows with this advice — "Practice on the stillborn. Never lose this opportunity until the technique is mastered." The use of a h e a d stethroscope as a prophylactic measure cannot be over emphasized. This requires ausculation of the heart tones at 10 to 15 minute intervals during the second stage of labor; the obstetrician's duty unless another dependable attendant is present. He believes that 50 per cent of asphyxia (not narcotization) may be diagnosed prior to delivery, and delivery, p r o v i d i n g of course, that conditions for extraction are present, a high percentage of these babies may be saved.

5. Tracheal catheter inserted just inside the trachea, aspirate mucus, reinsert to end of trachea, retract about one-fourth inch and reaspirate mucus. This should be repeated until air passages are clear (usual care to avoid trauma).

6 Gentle insufflation of lungs—mouth to catheter. Do not do this unless definitely indicated by deep asphyxia with evidence of circulatory failure as evidenced by brady-cardia. Then only if operator has no respiratory infection.

7. Insufflation of CO_2-O_2 (30-70 mixture); when respiration is established mixture is reduced to five per cent CO_2—95 per cent O_2.

8. Stimulants only when e v i d e n c e of medullary pathology.

A Few Points to Remember

1. The baby with asphyxia pallida should be treated as for shock and with the same gentle care as any other "head injury." Do not traumatize to stimulate respiration. Maintain body heat.

2. Gaseous exchange is possible only when the air passages are clear.

3. Insufflating mucus into the lung after cord is severed can drown infant.

4. Once the air passages are clear, one need not fear narcotization except in the premature. There is a d e f i n i t e ration in the amount of trauma incident to labor and delivery and the degree of asphyxia.

5. Do not insufflate forcibly into the fetal lung, nor attach any apparatus for administering gas into lung in a direct closed system.

6. Traction on tongue will help keep glottis open in deep asphyxia.

As Flagg has expressed it[6] "In the management of the asphyxiated newborn infant it has become increasingly clear that the primary indication is not for vigorous external stimuli, but rather to provide and maintain a clear air passage, and to supply oxygen in some way to the circulation. Whether this be accomplished by mouth to mouth technique or by several of the more elaborate mechanical devices is of secondary importance." To substantiate this a few citations may be of interest and stimulate persistence in efforts at resuscitation even with the most discouraging outlook.

The recent acquisition of the new modified Drinker respirator and incubator combination by the St. Anthony Hospital Obstetrical and Newborn service, has added a new impetus to observe this method of mechanical artificial respiration in the asphyxiated infant.

Tow mentions[7] several cases of recovery having been reported after continued efforts at passive artificial resuscitation lasting from 20 to 64 minutes before any evidences of breathing were perceptible.

On our service we have had opportunity to observe two similar instances in infants born in the stage of asphyxia pallida, having all the appearance of a dead baby with only a weak heart beat to suggest it was alive. In both infants the mucus and fluids were first removed from nose, pharnyx and mouth by methods as above advised.

Case Report—No. 113307. Evans: . Born February 14, 1938—St. Anthony's Hospital, Oklahoma City. Spontaneous delivery, full term, short labor. Ether anesthesia given m o t h e r the last 30 minutes. Morphine grs. 1/6, five hours before delivery. Born in state of asphyxia pallida. Heart sounds weak and slow, no other signs of life. Fluids r e m o v e d from nose, throat and mouth. Placed in modified Drinker respirator; artificial resuscitation attempted by positive and negative pressure method. Baby was in respirator 24 minutes before first effort at breathing. Oxygen 95 per cent and CO2—5 per cent was supplied intermittently by the ether mask from oxygen tank. Remained in warmed incubator respirator for 24 hours, receiving CO- and O2 as needed for cyanosis.

Perfect recovery and baby taken home on the fourteenth day. Since leaving hospital have had no report of child's condition relative to remote effects of prolonged anoxemia.

Case Report — No. 114062. Chandler — Born March 31, 1938, at St. Anothony's Hospital, Oklahoma City. Born at full term of a primipara. Labor eight hours. Ether anesthesia given mother last 35 minutes before delivery. Morphine grs. 1/8, three hours previously. Baby in incubator resuscitator 30 minutes before first visible efforts at breathing. During resuscitationO—95 per cent and CO2—5 per cent was given intermittently with the idea of stimulating respiratory effort. Baby left hospital on the fourteenth day; condition good. At seven m o n t h s the baby shows normal gain and normal mentality. No effort was made at tracheal insufflation while in respirator.

SUMMARY

1. Gentleness and judgement must be the key note in management of asphyxiated infant.

2. The ideal anesthetic or analgesic has not been found.

3. Tracheal catheter insufflation in competent hands is the safest procedure, though prolonged passive mechanical resuscitation may be in some desperate cases, a life saving measure.

REFERENCES

1. Holt and McIntosh—10th Edition—"Diseases of Infancy and Childhood."
2. E. P. Eastman—"Fetal Blood Studies," Am. Jr. of Obstetrics and Gynecology, 31-563-1936.
3. Dr. Frederick Schreiber—"Apnea of the Newborn and Associated Cerebral Injury,"—Jr. A.M.A., October 1, 1938.
4. Dr. Frederick Schreiber—Jr. A.M.A., October 1, 1938.
5. McGrath and Kudor—Jr. A.M.A., March 14, 1936.
6. Flagg—Treatment of Postnatal Asphyxia. Am. Jr. Obstetrics and Gynecology, 21-537-1936.
7. Abraham Tow—Diseases of the Newborn. Oxford Press.

---o---

ARCH FOE OF YOUTH

By Anthony M. Lowell, Assistant Statistician
New York Tuberculosis and Health Association

Over half the tuberculosis deaths in the United States occur in the age period 15 to 45, the main ages at which the individual is economically most productive and socially important to his family and the community. Tuberculosis strikes down those who are young and those in whom their elders have invested long years of cherishing care. This peculiarity, that it kills in the young adult years, makes tuberculosis a far greater social evil than those illnesses which take lives at later years when family responsibilities are less heavy.

Although tuberculosis is the seventh leading cause of death at all ages, it ranks first in number of deaths from 15 to 45 years. In 1937, of the more than 250,000 deaths from all causes in this age group, tuberculosis accounted for 15 per cent, heart disease 11 per cent, pneumonia nine per cent, cancer six per cent, kidney disease four per cent and cerebral hemorrhage two per cent.

It is interesting to note that between the ages of 15 and 45 the tuberculosis death rates for both the male and female colored population are three to six times those found among the white.

An unusual characteristic of tuberculosis in the 15 to 30 age group is that in the early years it is of greater danger to the young woman than to the young man. During these years tuberculosis kills about 50 per cent more women than men. In this period tuberculosis may well be called a young woman's disease. After this age the number of male deaths exceeds that of the female.

No specific reason is assigned as the sole cause for the high rates among young women; however, these years are the strenuous years of a woman's life. The physiological, as well as the psychological, changes that take place in the growing female tend to make her unusually susceptible to tuberculosis. Childbearing and care of the child by the young mother are additional hazards that may contribute to an elevation of the tuberculosis death rate. It has been shown that this variation of tuberculosis mortality rates is essentially biological. After the age of 30 there tends to be a change in the woman's manner of living. The frequency of childbearing is less and in the main the woman's life takes on a more leisurely tempo.

Among males the situation is reversed. It is after 30 that greater demands are made upon the physical reserve of the young man. As the provider for the family his efforts are expended upon holding his job. The demands of his work, continued physical and mental strain, combined with the fact that he too often is unwilling or unable to keep in optimum physical condition, tend to decrease his power of resistance to disease. At this time of life he fails to heed the subtle signs of approaching illness.

Tuberculosis creates the greatest havoc among those least able to afford prolonged illness and results in a lowered standard of family life. Statistical studies show that the highest tuberculosis rates are found among the lower economic groups. If the patient is a dependent, it means hardship to the parents to bear the heavy expense of prolonged periods of invalidism. The tangible effect is reflected in the fact that there is a curtailment of earning power during the years when under normal conditions this earning power should be greatest. For those in the younger age group it brings about a drastic alteration in the manner of living, as the entire social aspect of life must be abruptly reversed. Preventable tuberculosis deaths among young people are a devastating and unnecessary blow to social morale.

THE JOURNAL

OF THE

Oklahoma State Medical Association

Issued Monthly at McAlester, Oklahoma, under direction of the Council.

Copyright, 1939, by Oklahoma State Medical Association, McAlester, Oklahoma.

Vol. XXXII	NOVEMBER	Number 11

Entered at the Post Office at McAlester, Oklahoma, as second-class matter under the act of March 3rd, 1879.

This is the official Journal of the Oklahoma State Medical Association. All communications should be addressed to The Journal of the Oklahoma State Medical Association, McAlester Clinic, McAlester, Oklahoma. $4.00 per year; 40c per copy.

The editorial department is not responsible for the opinions expressed in the original articles of contributors.

Reprints of original articles will be supplied at actual cost provided request for them is attached to manuscripts or made in sufficient time before publication.

Articles sent this Journal for publication and all those read at the annual meetings of the State Association are the sole property of this Journal. The Journal relies on each individual contributor's strict adherence to this well-known rule of medical journalism. In the event an article sent this Journal for publication is published before appearance in The Journal the manuscript will be returned to the writer.

Failure to receive The Journal should call for immediate notification of the Editor, McAlester Clinic, McAlester, Oklahoma.

Local news of possible interest to the medical profession, notes on removals, changes of addresses, births, deaths and weddings will be gratefully received.

Advertising of articles, drugs or compounds unapproved by the Council on Pharmacy of the A. M. A., will not be accepted.

Advertising rates will be supplied on application.

It is suggested that wherever possible members of the State Association should patronize our advertisers in preference to others as a matter of fair reciprocity.

Printed by News-Capital Company, McAlester.

EDITORIAL

THIS CHANGING WORLD

Fortunately, medicine has not only met the demands of a rapidly changing order, but it has often anticipated the progress of civilization. It is doubtful if advances in any other field of medical endeavor has equaled those in the diagnosis, treatment and prevention of tuberculosis. It is also doubtful if changes in the management of any other disease have placed such heavy demands upon the family physician.

A few decades ago, the treatment was relatively simple. The family physician understood that an early diagnosis was important, but early or late, he was comforted by the fact that the treatment remained the same. Today, the f a m i l y physician who makes a diagnosis of pulmonary tuberculosis faces a most difficult task. He is immediately confronted with the grave responsibility of determining whether the case is minimal, moderately advanced, or advanced; whether it is acute or chronic; whether predominantly unilateral or bilateral. He must also recognize the presence or absence of cavities, and, if cavities are present, he must determine their size and location, the character of their walls, and the condition of the surrounding tissues. He must consider the pleura, and, if possible, determine the presence or absence of adhesions; he must ascertain the position and mobility of the diaphragm and the mediastinal structures; he must at least attempt a clinical estimate of the vital capacity of the lungs; he must appraise the cardiovascular system, with particular reference to the integrity of the heart muscle; he must recognize serious complications when present, as well as other associated pathological conditions.

These demands require unusual knowledge of the anatomy and physiology of the intrathoracic organs; an appreciation of the pathology of tubercle from early proliferation to cavity formation; also special skill in physical diagnosis, plus the wisdom of clinical experience. F i n a l l y, fluoroscopic service and good stereoscopic X-ray films are indispensable. Other laboratory facilities and occasionally highly technical procedures are necessary in certain cases.

There must be a choice between home treatment and institutional treatment. In those chosen for institutional treatment, there must be a choice between r o u t i n e management and surgical collapse; in those chosen for surgical collapse there must be a choice between artificial pneumothorax, intrapleural and extrapleural pneumolysis, phrenic-nerve interruption and thoracoplasty. Often there must be a decision with reference to simultaneous bilateral or successive bilateral pneumothorax; also with reference to cautious combinations of the various surgical procedures mentioned above.

It is obvious that modern advances in the treatment of pulmonary tuberculosis have brought a multiplicity of problems. It is equally obvious that the family physician working alone cannot adequately meet all the above requirements. Even those who specialize in d i s e a s e s of the chest must resort to team work in order to accomplish the best results.

While there has been no change in our opinion with reference to the efficacy of the fundamental principles of treatment, rest, diatetic and hygienic; and while in certain cases these principles can still be successfully applied in the home environment; modern therapeutic advances, which have proved such a boon to those suffering from tuberculosis, require the equipment and facilities of the sanatorium and hospital. The minimal and moderately advanced cases not responding to r o u t i n e management, and all advanced cases, require special diagnostic consideration in order to determine appropriate therapeutic measures. With rare exceptions, such diagnostic studies cannot be successfully pursued in rural communities. Neither is it possible to apply the respective modern therapeutic measures o u t s i d e the well-ordered institution.

The above discussion makes obvious the fact that the difficulties are not only professional, but environmental as well. If these difficulties are not overcome, many of those suffering from tuberculosis will be denied the opportunities for recovery and many, who are not yet obviously tuberculous, will be unnecessarily exposed to infection.

The effective application of ever-increasing knowledge in the field of pulmonary therapy demands intensive cooperative professional efforts, with increasing emphasis upon the patient's individual needs. In this cooperative program, the position of the family physician is very important. He should never lose touch with his patient, and consultants and s p e c i a l i s t s participating in the management of the case should help maintain a close relationship between the patient and his family physician. After the active therapeutic program is completed, the family physician should d o m i n a t e the follow-up period which demands years of close observation.

Medical Defense Rules

Recently the office of the Executive Secretary mailed to all of the county societies the rules under which members of the Association might receive aid from the Medical Defense Fund. Since that time, there have been numerous requests that these same rules be published in the Journal so that each member of the Association might have a chance to review them.

The present rules governing the Medical Defense Fund are the same rules that were adopted at the time of the establishment of the Fund and are interpreted by the Committee on Medical Defense, appointed by the President of the Association. At the present time, this committee is composed of O. E. Templin of Alva, J. S. Fulton of Atoka, and L. C. Kuyrkendall of McAlester.

The rules governing the funds are as follows:
1. Suit must be reported as soon as service is received.
2. Report must include copy of petition and answer, if one is made.
3. Member is not subject to coverage if he carries other liability insurance.
4. Assistance will be given up to the amount of $100.00 toward attorneys' fees. If the fee is less than $100.00, the full amount will be paid.
5. No protection is given in cases of criminal malpractice or where the physician is under the influence of alcohol or narcotics.
6. Contact immediately the office of the Executive Secretary, 210 Plaza Court, Oklahoma City, as per the above rules, in order that consideration of your request can be brought at once to the attention of the Medical Defense Committee.

Should these rules not be clear to any member of the Association or should you desire further explanation of any particular rule, feel free to address an inquiry on the point in question to the office of the Executive Secretary, and every effort will be made to give you the proper interpretation.

———o———

Board of Ophthalmology Announces Examinations

From the offices of the American Board of Ophthalmology comes this announcement:
WRITTEN EXAMINATION, March 2, 1940, in various cities throughout the country. This will be the only written examination in 1940.
All applications for this examination must be received before January 1, 1940. All applicants must pass satisfactory written examination before being admitted to oral examination.
ORAL EXAMINATION, New York City, June 8 and 10. Fall examination to be announced later.
CASE REPORTS: Candidates planning to take June examination must file case reports before March 1.
For application blanks write at once to Dr. John Green, 6830 Waterman Avenue, St. Louis, Missouri.

———o———

Fourth Assembly, United States Chapter of the International College of Surgeons

The officers of the United States Chapter of the International College of Surgeons cordially invite all physicians and surgeons in good standing to their Fourth Assembly, to be held in Venice, Fla., February 11-14, 1940. There is no registration fee.
For general information please address Dr. Fred H. Albee, Chairman, 57 West 57th Street, New York City. For information about the presentation of scientific papers or exhibits, query Dr. Charles H. Arnold, Secretary of the Scientific Assembly, Terminal Building, Lincoln, Nebraska.

Clinical Society Meeting Attracts Record Number

Widely acclaimed by attending physicians as the outstanding program ever achieved by the organization, the Oklahoma City Clinical Society concluded its four-day meeting in the capital city November 2.

With a registration of 714, the Clinical Society marked up the largest attendance of both city and out-of-city physicians in the history of the society, maintaining a record of attracting greater numbers with each annual meeting. Random comments from those in attendance were unanimous in acclaiming the 1939 affair as one of the best rounded programs for practitioners yet held in the nine years the group has been steadily growing.

Of great interest was the appearance of Dr. Rock Sleyster of Wauwatosa, Wis., president of the American Medical association, whose interesting and valuable address on the economic as well as other sides of modern medical problems was well received.

Among the guest lecturers were Dr. A. Graeme Mitchell of Cincinnati, professor of pediatrics at the Cincinnati University school of medicine; Dr. Edgar G. Ballenger of Atlanta, urologist with the Crawford W. Long hospital; Dr. Albert H. Aldridge, New York physician and professor at Columbia University; Dr. Emil Novak, associate professor of gynecology at Johns Hopkins Medical College; Dr. Marion B. Sulzberger of New York City; Dr. William A. Wagner of New Orleans; Dr. Hobart A. Reimann of Philadelphia; Dr. Frank H. Lahey of Boston; Dr. Erwin R. Schmidt, professor of surgery at the University of Wisconsin; Dr. John A. Kolmer, professor of medicine at Temple University school of medicine; Dr. Lewellys F. Barker of Baltimore; Dr. Joe Vincent Meigs of Boston; Dr. Herman C. Schumm of Milwaukee; Dr. Lowell S. Goin of Los Angeles; Dr. Harry S. Gradle of Chicago.

In addition to formal lectures, group meetings and round-table luncheons, the program included a dinner honoring Doctor Sleyster; the annual dinner-dance at the Chamber of Commerce; a dinner for women physicians; annual smoker for the men at the Oklahoma Club; a golf tournament at the country club, won by Dr. E. S. Edgerton of Wichita, Kans., with Dr. Roy Emanuel of Chickasha a close runner-up; and a complete program for wives of visiting doctors, arranged by the ladies auxiliary of the county society.

Texas led the out-of-state attendance, with Kansas and New Mexico in second place. Other states well represented were Colorado, Arkansas and Missouri. The meeting attracted doctors as well from Arizona, Montana, Pennsylvania, California and Louisiana.

Officers of the Clinical Society are: Dr. H. Dale Collins, president; Dr. Wendell Long, director of clinics; Dr. Basil A. Hayes, vice president; Dr. W. F. Keller, secretary; and Dr. J. H. Robinson, treasurer.

Editorial Notes—Personal and General

Dr. R. N. Holcombe was elected president of the Oklahoma Baptist hospital medical staff at the annual banquet and election meeting in mid-October. He succeeds Dr. H. A. Scott. Others elected on the staff were Dr. I. B. Oldham, Jr., vice president; Dr. S. D. Neely, secretary. Re-elected as executive committeemen were Dr. I. B. Oldham, Sr., Dr. J. H. White and Dr. W. P. Fite.

McAlester will be the meeting place for the next gathering of the Southeastern Oklahoma Medical Association, it was decided at a district meeting in Poteau in late October.

New president of the Pawhuska city hospital, elected at a staff meeting October 26, is Dr. Roscoe Walker. Other officers elected are Divonis Worten, vice president; and George K. Hemphill, secretary. Preceding the meeting, the doctors were entertained with a dinner.

Members of the Hughes County Medical Society, at their October meeting, passed a resolution asking the newspapers of Hughes county to refrain from use of hospital or clinic names in reporting receipts of patients. The resolution asked that any newspaper mention of patients be confined to statements that they had been treated by local doctors, or at local hospitals.

Appointments of new county superintendents of health within the past month, as announced by Dr. G. F. Mathews, state health commissioner, include: Dewey county, Dr. W. E. Seba of Leedey; Ottawa county, R. H. Duewall of Miami; Mayes county, Leo Evans of Pryor; Muskogee county, J. T. McInnis of Muskogee; Creek county, Dr. O. H. Cowart of Bristow; Pontotoc county, Dr. Ivan E. Bigler of Ada.

Dr. Rex Bolend of Oklahoma City announces that his offices have been moved from 1010 Medical Arts Building, Oklahoma City, to 1205 Medical Arts Building.

Three state surgeons, members of the Oklahoma State Medical Association, were among 496 on whom the American College of Surgeons conferred fellowships at its annual meeting in Philadelphia. They are: Dr. Clifford C. Fulton of Oklahoma City, Dr. Raymond G. Jacobs of Enid, and Dr. Oscar Clarence Newman of Shattuck.

---o---

OBITUARIES

Dr. W. A. Aitken

Dr. W. A. Aitken, 62, well-known Enid physician and surgeon for many years, World War veteran and widely known in medical and social circles, died October 15 at an Enid hospital.

Doctor Aitken received his medical degree from Washington University at St. Louis, coming to Enid in 1904, where he engaged in the practice of medicine and surgery until he volunteered for service in the Medical Corps of the United States army in February, 1918.

Dr. C. E. DeGroot

A medical career 35 years old was ended October 26 with the death of Dr. C. E. DeGroot, 60, of Muskogee, pioneer member of the medical profession in eastern Oklahoma. Death resulted from a heart attack.

Doctor DeGroot was a former president of the Muskogee County Medical Society, and last May was appointed federal jail physician at Muskogee, succeeding Dr. John Reynolds, former Muskogee mayor.

Dr. James B. Lightfoot

Dr. James B. Lightfoot, longtime Miami physician, died October 5 at the Baptist hospital in Miami, at the age of 74 years. He had been ill for several months.

Doctor Lightfoot received his medical degree at a Memphis college. After practicing for a time in Texarkana, Ark., he moved to Muskogee in Indian Territory. He went to Miami in 1917.

Dr. Thomas Owen Crawford

Dr. Thomas Owen Crawford, Dewey, Okla.; Gross Medical College, Denver, 1910; former member of Oklahoma State Medical Association; Superintendent of Health of Dewey, Okla.; aged 66; died, October 20, of pneumonia.

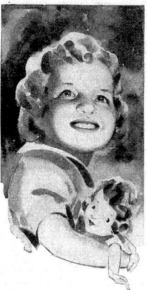
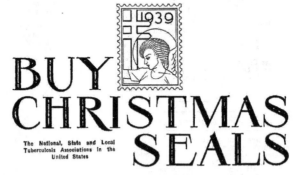

ABSTRACTS : REVIEWS : COMMENTS
and CORRESPONDENCE

SURGERY AND GYNECOLOGY

Abstracts, Reviews and Comments from
LeRoy Long Clinic
714 Medical Arts Building, Oklahoma City

"The Value of Cecostomy as a Complementary and Decompressive Operation," by Fred W. Rankin, M.D. Annals of Surgery, September, 1939, page 389.

One of the most important factors in the development of colonic surgery has been acceptance of the thesis that decompression either by surgical procedures or medical means is a highly important aid in returning a devitalized and desiccated patient, suffering from malignant disease, to a status approaching physiologic equilibrium.

When surgery is indicated, decompression may be easily accomplished in many cases by the employment of cecostomy. However, this procedure is frequently desirable both as the first stage of a graded operation, and as a complement to an offensive for extirpation of the colon. The indications given by Rankin for cecostomy he summarizes as follows:

"1. A complementary measure following:
   a. Obstructive resection;
   b. Resection and anastomosis of the intestine, end-to-end, or lateral;
   c. Exteriorization of a segment of the colon.
2. Decompression for intestinal obstruction:
   a. In acute obstruction secondary to cancer of the left colon or rectum;
   b. In subacute or chronic obstruction secondary to cancer of the colon or rectum unrelieved by medical measures.
3. A planned first-stage of a graded operation."

The author concludes that "(1) Cecostomy is a valuable adjunct to any type of resection of the colon. It prevents distention, moderates peristalsis, and promotes a smooth convalescence."

"(2) Its usefulness as the first-stage of a graded operation for radical removal of rectal cancer has been demonstrated."

"(3) Blind cecostomy for acute intestinal obstruction localized to the large bowel is a useful and often a life-saving operation."

"(4) It is desirable to use different technics to perform cecostomy for its several indications. Complete by-passing of the fecal current by bringing out a loop of the cecum or right colon is superior as a means of decompression and irrigation prior to resection. For complementary cecostomy, however, where relief of distention by gas is the paramount factor, a wing-catheter introduced into the cecum by Witzel's technic is very satisfactory."

LeRoy D. Long.

"Warm Moist Air Therapy for Burns," by Sidney Smith, M.S., Roy Rish, M.D., and Charles Beck, M.S. Archives of Surgery, October, 1939, page 686.

Modern therapy for burns attempts to alleviate the subsequent toxemia and secondary shock of severe burns by rendering any supposed toxins arising from the heat-killed tissue insoluble. For many reasons, the conditions for healing under the coagulum of chemically coalesced debris do not approach the optimum conditions existing under the natural fibrin eschar.

The possibility of obtaining more rapid healing by providing a more nearly ideal physiologic environment for the wounded area led to the study on rats, in which a comparative evaluation of various therapeutic agents and methods used as controls was undertaken.

Deep cutaneous burns were inflicted on etherized rats. Studies of recovery with various types of therapy or lack of therapy were undertaken. The speed of healing constituted the criterion of recovery. The results of the experiments were as follows:

1. The cutaneous burns of rats receiving the warm moist air therapy healed faster than those of controls living in ordinary air at room temperature, even when the controls received in addition typical treatments with well known therapeutic agents (butesin picrate and tannic acid).

2. The use of tannic acid and surgical excision in addition to the warm moist air therapy did not produce significant differences in the rate of healing in the experimental rats.

3. Surgical excision of the debris in the control group of rats was better than no therapy but was inferior to the chemical coagulants present in tannic acid or butesin picrate ointment.

Among the many physiologic factors which might account for these results may be listed the following:

1. Healing processes are markedly slowed in the presence of debris (Bauer; Hauberisser; Dressel). In the humidity chamber the moisture of the air kept the entire body wet, and this soaking action softened the debris, which was sloughed off the wound or picked off by the rats within the first five days.

2. Increase the local temperature by thermal application increases the rate of healing in rats (Fuke). Ebeling, using the alligator, made the same observation. In the humidity chamber the warmth provided exceeded the normal temperature of the skin.

3. Epithelial proliferation is faster in the presence of moisture (Burrows, 1924). The saturated air of the humidity chamber not only provides moisture but permits retention of water, for evaporation is minimal in saturated air.

4. Chief among the many factors that delay wound healing is infection (Carrel; Kiser). According to a report by Schade and Calussen, the ph of tissue may be a prime factor in the incidence of pathogenic invasion. These investigators, working with the quinhydrone electrode, found that healthy granulating tissue had a ph of 5.6 but that if the tissue became dry the ph rose to 8.3. If the alkalinity persisted, infection and sloughing occurred. Reimers and Winkler reported that carbon dioxide escapes from the surface of wounded tissue 30 times as fast as from uninjured skin. The fact that Reimers and Winkler reported a rising ph coinciding with drying of the tissue suggests the possibility that moisture may act as a vehicle in the retention of the acid radicals responsible for the lowered ph.

As for the tannic acid or butesin picrate ointment the authors believe that these substances possess no specific accelerating healing action. It would seem that their main function is to provide an insoluble coagulant over the wound. The incidence of infection under the coagulant produced by tannic acid has been reported many times and constitutes the chief objection to the use of the medicament.

LeRoy D. Long

Treatment of the Menopause with Estradiol Dipropionate. Edward M. Dorr and R. R. Green, Chicago, Illinois. American Journal of Obstetrics and Gynecology, Vol. 38, September, 1939, page 458.

"An estrogenic substance is any substance which has activities similar to those exhibited by the hormone of the ovarian follicle. In the human being, three clinically distinct and biologically active estrogenic substances have thus far been isolated." These are estrone (theelin), estriol (theelol) and estradiol. "Various observers do not agree as to the exact potency of these three compounds, but do agree that estradiol is more potent than estrone and that estriol is the least potent of the three substances." It has been demonstrated that esterification of estradiol or estrone leads to a more prolonged physiological effect, presumably due to slower absorption. Such a preparation is estradiol dipropionate which was used in these studies.

Sixty-two menopausal patients were treated with estradiol dipropionate in an attempt to determine whether the substance would be clinically valuable or not when given in moderate doses at infrequent intervals. It was found that the substance had a prolonged effect and that patients could be given dosages of from one to five milligrams at two to four week intervals with relief of symptoms.

They found that estrone, a substance that is supposed to have the same minimal effective dose, has been subjectively and objectively inadequate when substituted for estradiol dipropionate.

Eleven patients in this series whose maintenance dosage of estradiol dipropionate had been determined, were given the same amount in milligrams of strone at the same time intervals. The patients were not informed of this substitution. Ten of the 11 patients had a recurrence of symptoms under treatment with estrone and when estradiol dipropionate was again given the symptoms disappeared.

Comment is made in the article to stilboestrol, a drug discovered by Dodds of England, effective by mouth, and having a remarkable estrogenic effect. These authors have not had experience with it.

The conclusions of the authors of this article are to the effect that estradiol dipropionate has a prolonged effect in human beings and that it is of unusual clinical value in that injections may be given at infrequent intervals. Their comparison with estrone has shown estradiol dipropionate to be clinically more effective.

Comment:

This is an article with practical significance and it is unquestionably true that the various estrogenic substances have different clinical effect, both qualitatively and quantitatively.

It is therefore important that the doctor know the most effective estrogenic substance to employ in therapy as well as to know the patient and the time in which it should be used.

I have used a certain amount of stilboestrol and, as all others who have employed it, I am markedly struck by its potency and efficiency. Stilboestrol or a modification of this drug will probably supplant most of the commercially available estrogenic substances.

Wendell Long

The Changes of the Urinary Tract Associated with Prolapse of the Uterus. By Arthur J. Wallingford, M.D., Albany, New York. American Journal of Obstetrics and Gynecology, Volume 38, September, 1939, Page 489.

This author is forcibly calling attention to the fact that neglected cases of uterine prolapse frequently have changes in the urinary tract as a result of the prolapse. These changes are hydroureter, hydronephrosis, and eventual renal insufficiency, probably caused by obstruction of the lower end of the ureter in the sling-like position of the uterine artery as it is pulled over the ureter.

Complete histories and laboratory findings in five cases of prolapse of the uterus and postmortem findings in one other case are fully reported.

It is pointed out that replacement of the uterus by pessary or operation relieves the obstruction upon the ureter and consequently prevents the pathological changes in the urinary tract.

Comment: I am sure that most of us have had the unpleasant task of seeing these neglected instances of uterine prolapse with consequent urinary changes. It would, therefore, seem unnecessary to add the admonishment that all instances of uterine prolapse be corrected.

Wendell Long.

"The Evaluation of the Human Vaginal Smear in Relationship to the Histology of the Vaginal Mucosa," by Samuel H. Geist, M.D., and Udall J. Salmon, M.D., New York, N. Y. American Journal of Obstetrics and Gynecology, September, 1939, Vol. 38, page 392.

In their work, the authors felt the need for a simple method of estimating ovarian function. Papanicolaou had demonstrated changes in the cytology of the human vaginal secretion corresponding to the follicle changes in the ovary. Subsequently, Papanicolaou and Shorr reported striking cystological characteristics in the human vaginal smear after the menopause or castration. Since the preparation of smears by Papanicolaou technique was complicated and long, Salmon and Frank simplified the procedure by diluting a little of the vaginal secretion with normal saline, spreading it upon a glass slide, allowing it to dry in the air and staining it for one minute with fuchsin. The smear was then washed with tap water and ready for examination.

These authors studied a group of 60 women with various degrees of estrogen deficiency, both menopausal and surgical and X-ray castration. Vaginal biopsies were taken and the degree of regression or regeneration was compared with vaginal smears before and after treatment with estradiol benzoate.

The vaginal smears and vaginal mucosa were classified into four groups, representing various degrees of estrogen deficiency. Because of their practical importance, the findings in each of their reaction groups of vaginal smears is quoted.

"Reaction I—(Advanced estrogen deficiency.) The characteristic features of this type of smear are the complete absence of squamous epithelial cells and the presence of small, round or oval epithelial cells with rather large, darkly-staining nuclei (atrophy cells). These are the cells which Papanicolaou and Shorr have described as 'deep cells.' Leucocytes and erythrocytes are present in varying numbers."

"In some smears the epithelial cells are few in number and associated with large numbers of leucocytes; in others, particularly in very old women, the epithelial cells are very small, few in number and are associated with a scattering of leucocytes and erythrocytes."

"Reaction II—(Moderate degree of estrogen deficiency.) There is a variable number of large, epithelial cells many of which are irregular in shape. The nuclei are relatively large. Interspersed among these cells is a varying number of 'atrophy cells' and leucocytes. The relative proportion of the large epithelial cells to the 'atrophy cells' is variable. What distinguishes this smear from the I and III is the association of the 'atrophy cells' with the larger epithelial cells."

"Reaction III—(Slight degree of estrogen deficiency.) Predominance of rather large irregular epithelial cells is the striking feature of this smear. The cells vary in size and shape, their edges are somewhat irregular and frequently indistinct in outline. They frequently occur in clumps; a few 'atrophy cells' may be present."

"Reaction IV.—The smear consists of large, flat, clearly-outlined, squamous epithelial cells with s m a l l, deeply-staining nuclei. These cells are larger, more clear-cut and the nuclei relatively smaller than those in the III smear. No 'atrophy cells' and usually no leucocytes are seen."

The vaginal smears classified by these criteria were found to correspond with graded degrees of atrophy of the vaginal mucosa.

It was their finding that after treatment with estradiol the changes in the vaginal smear reflected clearly the regenerative changes in the mucosa. The vaginal smears prepared by the fuchsin method were entirely satisfactory and reflected the degree of regression as well as of regeneration. These authors therefore recommend it as a method which is simple and reliable for determining the presence of normal ovarian activity or estrogen deficiency as well as an indicator of the efficacy of administered estrogens in cases of estrogen deficiency.

Comment; At the present time, all quantitative methods for the determination of estrogen are moderately inaccurate and the interpretation of estrogen excretion in relation to ovarian function is not upon a stable basis. However, interpretation of qualitative tests is much more sound and of more clinical value at the moment.

The vaginal smear examination, so ably investigated by Papanicolaou, is purely qualitative and there has been a good deal of question as to its reliability. However, those who have carefully studied the smears and have religiously followed the criteria laid down by Papanicolaou, have found them to be of reliable qualitative clinical significance.

Wendell Long.

EYE, EAR, NOSE AND THROAT

Edited by Marvin D. Henley, M.D.
911 Medical Arts Building, Tulsa

Ulcus Rodens Mooren. Original paper by Dr. Esther Dalsgaard Nielsen and Dr. G. Osterberg, Copenhagen, Denmark. Published in Digest of Ophthalmology and Otolaryngology, October, 1939. Volume 1, Number 12. Digested from Acta Ophthalmologica, Copenhagen, Volume 17, Fasc. 1, pp. 28-37.

"This disease was described first by Mooren in 1867 as a chronic superficial ulceration, beginning at the margin of the cornea and extending irregularly over the entire cornea, characterized by the sharply defined, undermined, line of infiltration between abnormal and apparently normal tissue and by pronounced superficial vascularization of the area involved. This disease does not stop till the entire cornea is involved, and it is accompanied by very severe pain. It preferably attacks elderly persons.

"The etiology of this lesion is as yet unknown. Various hypotheses have been advanced as to the cause of this lesion. Some authors have thought it involved an infection, and in some cases they have demonstrated the presence of Grampositive diplobacilli. Koeppe thinks that some cases are

due to tuberculosis and that they respond favorably to treatment with tuberculin. Heintz attributes this ulceration to nutritional disturbances in the cornea; Junius and Triebenstein attribute it to trophic disturbances owing to pathological changes in the trigeminus. According to Junius and Triebenstein, these trigeminal disturbances would be apt to arise in various diseases, and thus the Mooren rodent ulcer would be the end-result of many lesions differing essentially as far as their etiology is concerned. In this connection it may be mentioned that the sensibility along the infiltration line is lowered in some cases, while in other cases there is an increased sensibility corresponding to the entire area affected.

"In itself the disease is so characteristic that it presents no differential-diagnostic difficulties; when less pronounced the lesion may be mistaken for rosacean keratitis, certain forms of corneal herpes, or neuroparalytic keratitis. It is to be kept in mind, however, that not all cases of ulcus rodens Mooren present all the characteristics described by Mooren. Thus, Axenfeld has described one case in which the lesion looked for a long time like any ordinary marginal keratitis. Salus has described one case in which the only sign of this lesion consisted in episcleritis; then an epithelial vesicle was formed on the limbus, and this was followed by a Mooren ulcer with the characteristic undermined line of infiltration and the marked vascularization of the whitish-grey area involved.

"In spite of the severe condition associated with the clinical picture,, the lesion keeps localized to the cornea, without complications from the deeper layers of the eye. Thus, when Feingold has reported a case of this lesion, associated with hypipyon, other authors have interpreted the occurrence of this phenomenon as a sign of secondary infection.

"According to Duke-Elder, 25 per cent of the cases are bilateral, even though the eyes need not necessarily be affected at the same time. Thus, in Wiedensheim's case the interval between the bilateral appearance of the lesion amounted to four years.

"In the course of years, various therapeutic measures have been tried, often rather radical, with internal medication as well as local surgery—but, on the whole, with rather unfavorable results, as the process keeps on progressing, albeit with periodical pauses; and generally the prognosis must be said to be poor."

Dr. H. Okkels of the University Institute for Pathological Anatomy is quoted as saying, "There is found an ingressive infiltration of vessels with concomitant perivascular cellular infiltrations circularly in relation to cornea. The vessels in question, mostly concentrically along the corneal periphery, present an outer diameter of about 30 microns and are fairly radially arranged, so that in the sections we may see them cut lengthwise to a considerable extent. The endothelium is normal, and the elements of the vascular wall itself show no signs of degenerative changes. Adventitiously, on the other hand, serial, ovoid, easily stainable elements are found, corresponding in shape and size to the adventitious cells which frequently occur in certain chronic productive inflammations. Centrally (in the direction towards vertex cornea) the said vessels are transformed into more sinuous stretches of capillary dimensions, but the concomitant cellular infiltrations constantly retain the character of adventitious, proliferous cells.

"Peripherally, in the voluminous infiltrations by the corneoscleral junction, lymphocytic elements as well as plasma cells and mast cells are found. There are also here vessels, which show signs of obliteration in different stages, rising to a completely structureless, detritus-like transformation. Further, in these infiltrations there are found groups of cells of a type similar to those described in connection with the adventitious cellular infiltrations. A few of these elements contain particels which convey the impression of undergoing phagocytosis; if this conception is correct, we should be justified in supposing the cellular types in question to be histiocytes.

"Among the various theories on the etiology of the affection, chiefly the neurotrophic one is based on pathologic-anatomical arguments. According to Junius, the simultaneous occurrence of necrosis vesication and edema are characteristic of trophoneurosis. The adherents of the theory point out that the violent pain which is characteristic of the disease, occurs in connection with hypotension (Ahlstrom, Dormalgen, Junius; and the fact pointed out by Heintz, that the thinning of cornea in ulcus rodens does not involve the formation of a staphyloma).

"The old vascular theory unconstrainedly explains the predilection of the disease for elderly individuals, its bilateralness, its peculiar impassivity to treatment that induces destruction, such as corrosion and cauterization. It is possible that several forms of ulcus rodens exist; both clinical and histologic evidence might seem to suggest this. The vascular genesis, however, can hardly be rejected, and no doubt ought to be still taken into consideration in each separate case."

The Treatment of Cancer of the Larynx with Comparison of Results Obtained by Surgery and Radiation Therapy. M. F. Arbuckle, M.D., St. Louis. Southern Medical Journal, October, 1939.

A short series of intrinsic and extrinsic cancers are presented. Cancer is second in cause of death in the United States; that of the larynx constitutes about 1.8 per cent. Various opinions of men throughout the world who have had extensive experience along this line make up a large part of the paper. Two tables are included showing the results obtained by the author. A long bibliography is appended. The author's own summary and conclusions are as follows:

1. Cancer occupies second place in the list of causes of death in the United States. Cancer of the larynx constitutes about 1.8 per cent of these.

2. The site of origin of cancer of the larynx most often is the true vocal cord.

3. The lymphatic supply to the true vocal cord is practically nil, therefore metastases do not occur while the tumor is still actually confined to the true cord. For the above reason surgical removal by laryngofissure, when the cancer is truly cordal, with lasting cure and without loss of function, is possible in over 80 per cent of cases.

4. The suffering and inconvenience to the patient after laryngofissure is comparatively little and the mortality rate is very low. Reported results of treatment of cordal cancer by radiation alone do not equal those obtained by surgical treatment.

5. In extrinsic cancer the results of treatment by radiation alone have, in the last ten years, shown tremendous improvement both in palliation and in cure. With further improvements in technic of administration, I feel that we may confidently expect still greater developments. It is my belief that this is the treatment of choice either alone or combined with surgical approach in this type of cancer.

6. Treatment must be selected to meet the particular requirements of each case.

7. The universal cry is for early diagnosis and treatment. The universal practice, almost, is late diagnosis and delayed treatment.

8. This situation will be corrected and the mortality rate from laryngeal cancer decreased if and when the medical profession as a whole becomes actively aware of these facts.

The Symptoms, Signs and Treatment of Nasal Sinusitis in Children. S. E. Birdsall, London. The Journal of Laryngology and Otology, September, 1939.

Eighty cases occurring two consecutive years are reported. There were 36 boys and 44 girls, ranging in age from two to 13 years.

The symptoms in order of their frequency are as follows:

	Cases
1. Nasal obstruction	39
2. Cough	33
3. Frequent colds	32
4. Rhinorrhoea	21
5. Pain	14
6. Throat symptoms	12
7. Anorexia	8
8. Otorrhoea	7
9. Bronchitis (confirmed)	6
10. Listlessness	5
11. Post-nasal discharge	4
12. Asthma	4
13. Epistaxis	3

There is a detailed analysis of these symptoms as elicited from the history and examination.

Probably the common cold is the most common aetological factor, therefore it is suggested by the author that colds in children always be treated, preferably by nasal alkaline lotions or with ephederine to relieve the obstruction. In 13 cases a definite specific illness was found to have preceded the symptoms of sinusitis, seven of these being a sequalae of pertussis. Thirty-three of the children of this series had undergone tonsillectomy and adenoidectomy without benefit—in contradistinction to the theory that such operations will favorably influence the course of a sinus infection.

Anterior and posterior rhinoscopy, translumination and X-ray of the sinuses showed muco-pus present in the anterior portion in 42 cases, significant changes in the appearance of the nasal mucous membrane in 34 cases. There was an excessive pallor present in 12 cases, hyperemia in 10 cases, and atrophic change in 10 cases. Muco-pus, or mucus in excess, was present in the nasopharynx in 27 cases, of these nine had muco-pus which must have originated in the posterior sinuses. The anterior group of sinuses appear to be much more commonly involved in childhood.

Translumination in 11 cases showed opacity of the antra, in six cases unilateral, and in five cases bilateral. In unilateral sinusitis translumination is of distinct value but when there is present a bilateral infection it is of little value because there is always doubt as to the degree of transradiancy to be expected in children. Twelve cases showed enlarged or inflammed tonsils. In 10 cases after treatment of the sinusitis the condition of the tonsils improved. There was a dermatitis of the upper lip and anterior nares observed in five cases. This was not an eczematous condition so frequently associated with a watery rhinorrhoea. Two of the cases were pustular, in one a lesion resembling herpes and in one the lip was greatly swollen and everted with ulceration of the mucous membrane.

Thirty-seven cases were X-rayed. In 35 of the cases the pictures showed the antra as the predominantly affected sinuses. In 22 cases the opacity showed involvement of the ethmoid cells as well as the antra. Both antra were equally diseased in 24 cases, and one side predominantly in nine, but in only two cases was the infection strictly unilateral.

The cases reported are those in which simple conservative methods of treatment have failed. There is given a discussion regarding the rationale of the treatment of sinusitis in children, as to how the infection occurs and why and how it gets well. The nasal blockage the author takes care of by means of ½ per cent solution of ephederine in normal saline and removal of the secretions by sniffing or syringing with some alkaline lotion. He has demonstrated to his own satisfaction that this solution of ephedrine can be introduced into the sinuses of children, even when their linings are grossly swollen, by the Proetz displacement method.

The majority of this series of cases were so treated at weekly intervals. If the cases were advanced the treatments were given twice weekly. With this treatment 34 cases were completely relieved of their symptoms and signs of infection in the average time of one month. The results showed to be lasting over quite a period of time (months). If no improvement was noted with the replacement treatments, then antral lavage was carried out (in 16 cases). Improvement was immediately noted and the replacements effected the cure. The conservative treatment failing in nine cases then antrostomy was performed. The intranasal route was used in seven cases and the Caldwell-Luc in two cases.

The summary shows that about one-half of the cases responded well to the replacement treatments, and that the majority of the remainder responded to lavage plus replacement treatments.

Some Phases of Tuberculosis of the Larynx. Mervin C. Myerson, M.D., New York. Annals of Otology, Rhinology and Laryngology, September, 1939.

This is a valuable discussion of this troublesome subject, viewed from many different angles. It is about 40 pages in length and include many excellent drawings, microphotographs and tables. There is a lengthy bibliography. Practically all the different phases of the pathology, classification, methods of treatment, etc., are discussed in full. It does not lend itself well to abstracting. One of the opening statements: "Tuberculosis of the larynx is always secondary to disease of the lung."

According to the experience of the author the electrocautery is the best single weapon available to the laryngologist. With it the edema is reduced as well as searing the active and inactive ulcers. It should be applied with great precision and not used to destroy diseased tissue. His experience shows that it should be applied to from one to four places at a sitting with probably a week interval. Indirect laryngoscopy with 10 per cent cocain was used routinely. If the pain cannot be controlled by the electrocauterization then the superior laryngeal nerve should be injected with novocain followed by alcohol. In this manner the patient is able to keep up his nourishment where otherwise swallowing would be so painful that he would refuse to take nourishment. These injections give relief of varying periods of time, sometimes lasting only a few days. Although X-ray treatments are advocated by some the author thinks that acute and active cases will be made worse by X-ray therapy.

In conclusion the author says:

"An analysis of the 145 larynges which were healed reveals that 87 received no therapy except silence, which is routine for all cases. Nothing was used in these larynx, some of which healed, even though the patient died. This confirms the opinion I have long held, that the value of local therapy in tuberculosis of the larynx is greatly overestimated. The larynx will heal if the tissues can undergo fibrosis. If such fibrosis cannot occur, no therapeutic measure will be of value. In conclusion, it behooves the laryngologist to understand the significance of the pulmonary disease and its many phases when he is treating laryngeal tuberculosis. With this understanding he can more properly treat the larynx and evaluate the future course and outcome of the disease.

PLASTIC SURGERY
Edited by
GEO. H. KIMBALL, M.D., F.A.C.S.
404 Medical Arts Building, Oklahoma City

Correction of Congenital Deformations of the Hand. Henry W. Meyerding, M.D., and Douglas D. Dickson, M.D., Rochester, Minn. American Journal of Surgery, April, 1939.

The authors have gone into the congenital deformities of the hand and have attempted to classify these deformities broadly and to give some method of correction of the various deformities. With such a wide subject and variety of congenital anomalies it is obvious that any method of repair or reconstruction is general and every case must be studied individually. The procedure carried out in each instance must give the best functional results as well as the best cosmetic appearance. It is pointed out by the authors and we should like to emphasize the point that function should never be sacrificed for cosmetic result. A practical or working classification of congenital malformations is difficult because of the multiplicity and variance and because so many will occur in various combinations.

The basic approach to the study of these congenital malformations is through etiology. Hypotheses too numerous to mention in a paper of this kind have been put forth. Similar congenital malformations of the hands and feet frequently are encountered in examining the same individual; this fact together with the high incidence of a history of similar malformations in forebears, suggests the possibility that the germ plasm hypothesis of origin of the condition is correct. The work of Bagg demonstrated that congenital deformities may be produced by insult to the germinal cells, that these deformities may manifest themselves in the progeny.

Syndactylia: Web Fingers

Syndactylia is a congenital anomaly perhaps most often met with in the hand and it may be present in all degrees. A great many operations have been described for its correction and in the very mild cases some of these procedures may be applicable. But a case of any severity especially for those cases in which the fingers are fused in their entire length, should be separated without flaps except that a triangular flap should be left on the dorsum of the hand to form the web. The remaining denuded area should be closed with a thick split graft as described by Blair and Brown.

Polydactylism: Supernumerary Digits

A great many supernumerary digits are seen. These may be marginal or central. Those on the thumb or little finger are seen most commonly. These may have any degree of fusion from many soft tissue attachments to the fusion of the phalanx. Polydactylism is frequently bi-lateral and frequently involves the feet. Before any surgical procedure is carried out a complete study of the relationship of the extra digits should be made and a plan of reconstruction made so that injury will not result to the normal digit. An extra digit to the thumb may be better left alone in some instances since an effort at removal frequently disturbs nerves, vessels and joints, so that the main digit may be made useless. In the simple polydactylism, simple amputation usually suffices. Bilhout-Cloquet plastic procedure has the advantage in caring for bifurcated distal phalanges, of preserving the attachment of the tendon.

Ectrodactylia: Cleft Hand, Lobster Claw Hand, Crab Claw Hand

The classical claw hand is one in which the middle finger is missing. This may or may not extend into the palms of the hand or involve the third metacarpal. In either case the primary object in correction is to obliterate the cleft with removal of the rudimentary third metacarpal if necessary.

Clinodactyly, Dactylogryposis: Flexion of Fingers

This deformity may exist in any finger and in any degree. Those of milder degree seen early may be splinted and thus correct the effection. The more severe conditions seen later in life may be corrected by division of contracting bands, possibly lengthening of the tendon and closure of the defect with a split graft.

Megalodactylia, Macrodactyly: Giant Fingers

Hypertrophy of the digits, a rare entity, usually affects the thumb, index finger or middle finger. Giant fingers result from one of two causes: 1. Bony growth. 2. Lymphatic and neurofibromatous hyperplasia. If overgrowth is the result of neurofibromatous tissue, a plastic procedure, in the course of which the hyperplastic tissue is removed, can be carried out in an attempt to improve the appearance of the hand. When the gigantism is a result of bony overgrowth as well as of hypertrophy of the soft tissues, both function and appearance of the hand can be improved by amputation.

Vascular Lesions: Arteriovenous Fistula

Arteriovenous aneurysms and the various vascular nevi are frequently seen in the hand. Diagnosis is frequently aided by arteriography and may be surgically treated in some cases. The vascular nevi are treated here in accordance with the general principles of management.

Talipomanus: Club Hand

The normal axis of the hand usually parallels that of the forearm. Disturbance in the relationships of these axes results in the deformity denoted clubhand, either congenital or acquired. Congenital clubhand is commonly associated with defects of one of the two bones of the forearm. Bilateral clubhand is seen about as often as is the unilateral variety. Other congenital malformations frequently are associated with clubhand. Congenital absence of the radius frequently is associated with absent or rudimentary thumb and carpal bones on the radial side, atrophy of the forearm and an enlarged and curved ulna. Correction is carried out by physiotherapy and stabilization of the hand. Club hand with contracture is analagous to congenital club foot. In the treatment of contracted club hands, without bony defects, plastic procedures on the fascia and tendons usually are sufficient. These procedures are to be followed by adequate immobilization and proper physiotherapy.

Malformations With Extensive Maldevelopment

These may exist in any degree from an absence or malformation of the entire extremity to the smallest part of the extremity. These conditions must be corrected according to the individual case.

Malformations With Mild Development

Congenital contraction rings or so-called amniotic furrows are deformities of milder degree. These contraction bands consist of dense fibrous tissue and may encircle the extremity at any level. That portion of the extremity which is distal to the contraction ring may exhibit any degree of maldevelopment and may determine the advisibility of surgical removal of the contraction furrow.

Congenital Variation In The Carpal Bones

Supernumerary carpal bones are not uncommon. Numerous types have been described. These are not important except those cases which might be traumatic and comparison with the opposite wrist may aid in treatment.

Symphalangism: Congenital Fusion of the Interphalangeal Joints

This condition is extremely rare. It is a hereditary anomaly characterized by fusion of the interphalangeal joints. It is frequently associated with other congenital lesions. Genealogic investigations have demonstrated that this anomaly is inherited according to Mendel's law. Drinkwater has traced the condition back 14 generations. Should the function of the hand be seriously impaired the only applicable surgical procedure would be arthroplasty.

Miscellaneous

Under these congenital variations may be mentioned brachyphalangia and brachydactylia, hyperphalangism, arachnodactylia, which are described as abnormal shortness or abnormal length of metacarpals and phalanges. Another is multiple exostosis which is a hereditary condition characterized by more or less symmetrical bony or cartilaginous overgrowths occurring at the disphyseal extremities. The hands may be involved as well as other parts of the skeletal system. Because of the proximity of the abnormal tissue to the epiphysis, disturbances of growth frequently are encountered. The cortex of the diaphysis may have irregular instead of regular margins. Of the bones of the hands, both phalanges and metacarpals may be involved but the carpus and epiphysis escape.

Comment. It is observed from the foregoing article that the multiplicity of congenital lesions presents problems in treatment which require accurate knowledge concerning which of the bones and soft tissues are involved. One attempting to treat these anomalies must of necessity study each individual case thoroughly and draw up a plan of correction which will give the best function and cosmetic result remembering never to sacrifice function for cosmetic reasons. In only a few of these conditions can any definite rule for correction be laid down and each must be treated on its own merit.

---o---

ORTHOPAEDIC SURGERY
Edited by Earl D. McBride, M.D., F.A.C.S.
717 North Robinson Street, Oklahoma City

Oklahoma City, Oklahoma,
605 N.W. 10th St.,
October 19, 1939

Dr. L. S. Willour,
McAlester, Oklahoma.
Dear Dr. Willour:

Instead of sending in abstracts for the next issue of the Journal under the Orthopedic Section, I am submitting a resume of the recent meeting

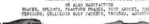

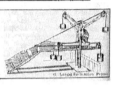

of the Clinical Orthopedic Society which met in Oklahoma City and Little Rock, Arkansas, on October 13 and 14. I hope this will be satisfactory:

* * * *

The orthopedic surgeons of Oklahoma City considered it a great honor to be hosts to the Clinical Orthopedic Society on October 13. This is an organization of national scope. There were approximately 100 orthopedic surgeons in attendance. Many distinguished surgeons from Chicago, Detroit, Rochester and other cities were here to take part in the meeting.

The program of the meeting was conducted entirely by local orthopedic surgeons. It is the policy of this Society to visit annually two different cities and review the work of the local orthopedic surgeons. The morning meeting was held at Crippled Children's Hospital and the afternoon meeting at the Municipal Auditorium. The following day the Oklahoma City Orthopedic men accompanied their guests to Little Rock for the second day of the meeting.

The morning session was called to order by Dr. Wallace Billington of Nashville and Dr. H. Earle Conwell of Birmingham. The resident orthopedic surgeons began the work.

Dr. Klein demonstrated fractures of the spine.

Dr. Swenson discussed luetic lesions of the long bones and presented a number of cases.

Dr. Sell demonstrated the treatment of congenital club feet by the Kite method of checking the deformity with X-ray until the astragalus is well reduced before forcing the foot up into dorsiflexion.

Dr. Bishop demonstrated vertebral lesions in undulant fever and severe gunshot wound of the foot.

Dr. VonSall presented cases of idiopathic scoliosis. He demonstrated post-operative results of fusion of the spine following forcible plaster correction.

Dr. Paul C. Colonna demonstrated post-operative cases of arthroplasty of the hip and presented a case in which he had used the Smith-Petersen Vitallium cup over the head of the femur.

Dr. Howard B. Shorbe presented cases showing results after shortening the femur of the well leg for equalization of leg length.

Dr. Chas. Rountree showed an unusual case of paralysis of both shoulders following poliomyelitis in which he had done a bilateral flexorplasty of the elbow with shoulder fusion.

Dr. R. L. Noell demonstrated the operative treatment of pronated feet, showing cases where the anterior tibial tendon was transferred in a position to correct the deformity.

Dr. John Burton explained his method of treatment the wide ulcerations over the tibia following osteomyelitis. He showed cases in which the skin had been shifted over this region by · plastic methods.

Dr. Earl D. McBride presented a number of post-operative cases which had been treated by his original operation for bunion and hallux valgus deformity.

Dr. W. K. West and Dr. Colonna discussed benign and malignant bone tumors.

Dr. D. H. O'Donoghue demonstrated his method for medial osteotomy for correction of resistant club foot deformity.

The afternoon session also proved very profitable in the demonstration of many post-operative results.

Dr. Elias Margo presented cases of fracture of the upper end of the tibia treated by open surgery, and cases where the head and neck of the humerus were excised.

Dr. West demonstrated end-result of fractures lower end of radius and ulna; Dr. Shorbe discussed old unreduced dislocations of the elbow; Dr. McBride showed several cases of fracture-dislocation of the cervical spine, reduced by closed manipulation under anesthesia. Dr. Rountree demonstrated results in reconstruction of the lower extremity and equalization of leg length following multiple fractures. Dr. Noell closed the program with discussion of the treatment of paralysis valgus deformity of the foot by tendon transplants.

After the guests were taken on an automobile trip through the oil fields and an oil well in the operation of drilling was demonstrated, a banquet was held at the Oklahoma City Golf and Country Club. The group then left by special train for Little Rock where Dr. F. Walter Carruthers of that city carried on the meeting in a very successful manner.

It was a pleasure to have so many distinguished orthopedic surgeons visit Oklahoma and express satisfaction in respect to the professional conduct of the practice of orthopedic surgery.

Yours very truly,

EARL D. McBRIDE, M.D.

———————o———————

INTERNAL MEDICINE

Edited by Hugh Jeter, M.D., 1200 North Walker, Oklahoma City

The Vitamins: A Symposium Arranged Under the Auspices of the Council on Pharmacy and Chemistry and the Council on Foods of the American Medical Association. (Published by the American Medical Association, 1939).

This is undoubtedly one of the most important, if not the most important recent contribution to medicine and particularly to those of us who practice internal medicine. It is a 637 page book covering all phases of the work which has been done on vitamins, setting forth the reliable claims for vitamins and their uses in various diseases for which they have been used; going thoroughly into the chemistry of vitamins; the physiology and pathology concerned in the diseases which are considered to be vitamin deficiency types; all of the important reports by various investigators are given including reports on all of the vitamins; knowledge concerning the effect of vitamin deficiency and also vitamin therapy in various types of animals; laboratory tests for vitamin deficiency; assays; sources; human requirements and many other interesting and extremely important problems are thoroughly reviewed.

The work of the most important contributors is given.

An abstract of the contents is, of course, impossible. The following paragraph, however, is a summary of one of the chapters, the one pertaining to the granulocyte and vitamin A.

"It may be concluded that no very striking effect of vitamin A on the cellular elements of the blood has been discovered."

Such pertinent facts as this are set forth throughout the book.

Many of the common vitamin deficiency diseases are also analyzed in a very satisfactory manner. For example, the Pathology of Beriberi and Vitamins in Relation to the Prevention and Treatment of Pellagra.

It may be said that this book is not only thoroughly scientific, but also equally practical and, as I see it, meets a much needed demand at this time.

---o---

UROLOGY

Edited by D. W. Branham, M.D.
514 Medical Arts Building, Oklahoma City

Carbuncle of the Kidney. George A. Ingrish. Journal of Urology, September, 1939.

Carbuncle of the kidney is sufficiently common and the treatment so definite, that unless it is recognized and properly handled an untoward mortality can result.

A summary of the article is as follows:

Eleven cases of metastatic staphylococcus infection of the kidney, proven by operation, have been reported. From review of these cases, I find several certain facts regarding the etiology, symptoms, diagnosis and management which I consider worthy of special emphasis.

The primary focus in each of the 11 cases was a cutaneous supurative lesion of no certain location. The organism isolated from the involved kidney was a staphylococcus aureus.

A rather diagnostic physical sign demonstrated by Dr. Frank M. Phifer, which has not been emphasized by other writers, is stony hard costovertebral rigidity on the affected side. This is due to a tremendous perinephric reaction and marked thickening of the fatty capsule which becomes leathery in character. Fullness over the renal angle is characteristically absent except in cases associated with perinephric abscess.

The urine in the majority of the cases was characteristically normal except for a slight trace of albumin which was undoubtedly on the basis of toxic nephritis.

Intravenous urography in conjunction with the careful interpretation of a flat X-ray film, when localizing symptoms are present, and a history of a recent cutaneous lesion, will usually suffice to make a diagnosis. Cystoscopy is seldom indicated.

Inasmuch as the pyelographic findings in two of the 11 reported cases could not be differentiated from that of a neoplasm, it is important to include carbuncle in the differential diagnosis in which a diagnosis of tumor of the kidney is made when the patient is showing evidence of sepsis.

Lesions of the anterior surface of the kidney are associated with abdominal symptoms which at times lead to an erroneous diagnosis of intra-abdominal diseases.

Considerable confusion and differences of opinion exist in the literature as to treatment. Inasmuch as conservative treatment with incision and drainage failed to effect a cure in two of these cases, it is felt that the toxic patient, especially if more than one lesion on the kidney is present, should be subjected to nephrectomy rather than to some form of conservative surgery.

The postoperative management of these patients is important inasmuch as they show evidence of myocardial damage due to the prolonged, severe sepsis and for that reason they should be kept at bed rest until the pulse approaches normal. Also, general measures to increase the resistance of the patient should be carried out.

Elusive Ulcer of the Bladder. A Report of 138 Cases. Herman L. Kretschmer, Urologist to Presbyterian Hospital. Journal of Urology, September, 1939.

A comprehensive survey of this most distressing bladder disease, almost totally confined to the female sex. Dr. Kretschmer particularly emphasizes the importance of recognization of the disease because from his series, many have gone undiagnosed for years.

Patients who present the history of painful and frequent urination without the presence of pus in the urine should be suspected of having elusive ulcer of the bladder.

He has found from the wide variety of treatments suggested that a combination of water dilation of the bladder in conjunction with simple fulguration of the ulcer area the most promising of theraputic benefit. He mentioned that perforation or rupture of the bladder wall is an accident that can should be taken in such procedures.

Summary and conclusion:

The ideal method of treatment is not yet at hand.

The most widely used measure and probably the most satisfactory is fulguration, either alone or with water dilatation.

The number of cures is still relatively low (20.37 per cent).

The number of greatly improved cases is more encouraging than one is apt to think (36.11 per cent).

The longer the duration of symptoms the less favorable the outlook.

Contrary to the prevailing opinion, the possibility of malignancy is one to be reckoned with. (One case in a series of 138 cases.)

---o---

New Books

SURGERY OF THE EYE: By Meyer Wiener, M.D., Professor of Clinical Ophthalmology, Washington University School of Medicine, St. Louis, Missouri; and Bennett Y. Alvis, M.D., Assistant Professor of Clinical Ophthalmology, Washington University School of Medicine, St. Louis, Mo. 445 pages with 396 illustrations. Philadelphia and London: W. B. Saunders Company, 1939. Cloth, $8.50 net.

It is the intention in bringing out this book to supply a handy atlas that the practicing ophthalmologist and student of ophthalmology can quickly refer to for information on the surgical correction of ocular defects and disease.

In this work not only is found the descriptive material but serial drawings illustrating the technic. These drawings which have been in many instances amplified by the addition of schematic inserts make all steps in the operative procedure very clear and will supply the ready reference for which the book is intended.

THE JOURNAL
OF THE
OKLAHOMA STATE MEDICAL ASSOCIATION

| VOLUME XXXII | McALESTER, OKLAHOMA, DECEMBER, 1939 | Number 12 |

Present Status of Active Immunization in Prevention of Disease*

JOHN A. KOLMER
Professor of Medicine, Temple University;
Director of the Research Institute of
Cutaneous Medicine
PHILADELPHIA, PENNSYLVANIA

PRINCIPLES INVOLVED

1. Vaccination or *active immunization* depends upon the capacity of vaccines for stimulating the body cells to actively produce specific antibodies. Non-specific effects w h i c h may be helpful in the treatment of disease do not appear to have much immunizing value.

2. Unfortunately and for reasons not understood at present, the *dead* vaccines of some pathogenic organisms l i k e those of *Sp. pallida,* the tubercle bacillus and gonococcus, are w i t h o u t these specific vaccinogenic effects.

3. As a general rule vaccines of *living* but *attenuated* organisms are more effective than dead vaccines as shown in vaccination against smallpox, rabies, poliomyelitis, tuberculosis, psittacosis, etc., but cannot be used on account of the dangers involved.

4. Vaccines of the exotoxins or their toxoids are usually highly e f f e c t i v e against diptheria, t e t a n u s, scarlet fever, etc. In vaccines of staphylococci and streptococci for therapeutic purposes they should always be included.

*Presented before the Oklahoma City Clinical Society, November 1, 1939.

5. Bacterial dissociation has an important influence upon the effectiveness of active immunization. Smooth, virulent and completely antigenic strains should be employed whenever possible because of higher vaccinogenic activity.

6. In some diseases like syphilis and tuberculosis the antibody appears to remain in or upon the cells instead of being in the blood. In these immunity is best produced by the establishment of foci of infection as depots of antibody production.

7. Those infectious diseases known to produce a lasting immunity are the ones in which vaccination is most likely to be successful.

8. It is likely that vaccination in diphtheria, tetanus, scarlet fever, typhoid fever, pertussis, etc., sensitizes the body cells so that immunity is prolonged t h r o u g h clinically unrecognized exposures and minor infections sufficient f o r stimulating antibody production.

9. Some of the greatest triumphs in preventive medicine have been due to the discovery of methods of vaccination and doubtless more will follow in time.

VACCINATION AGAINST SMALLPOX

1. In the United States alone there are reported annually about 50,000 cases of smallpox due to negligence in vaccination, despite the fact that it is one of the safest and most effective methods known for the prevention of a dreadful disease. During the 18th century o v e r 60,000,000 people succumbed to the disease.

2. Only a few cases of postvaccinal encephalomyelitis have been reported in the United States. Cowpox vaccine is not the specific cause and the etiology is unsolved.

3. Tetanus is almost always due to secondary infection of the v a c c i n a l lesion, as cowpox virus is rigidly examined for bacilli and spores before use.

4. Children should be vaccinated six to 12 months after birth and again at six years. Immunity may last for the the balance of life, but revaccination is desirable every seven to ten years and *always* in the presence of an epidemic.

5. Use only fresh virus; a l w a y s keep virus in a cold place as heat is destructive; vaccination d u r i n g cold months is preferred; keep children away from horses and stables after vaccination; advise against scratching; do not use shields; if a dressing is necessary use sterile gauze.

6. Acetone is preferred for the cleansing of the skin; antiseptics kill the virus

7. The multiple pressure method is preferred. Vaccinate in two areas in c a s e of: exposure to smallpox; in case of failure of previous vaccinations; in case of doubt as to potency of virus.

8. Daily applications of one per cent solutions of picric acid and iodine in alcohol to papule and vesicle reduces secondary infection (Schamberg and Kolmer).

9. Vaccination in the lower t h i g h s of girls is not recommended because of the increased risks of tetanus infection.

10. Calf lymph virus by the multipressure method is preferred. The intracutaneous injection of the Goodpasture chick vaccine is probably next best with slightly less s e v e r e local and constitutional reactions. The Rivers culture vaccine by intracutaneous inoculation gives a higher percentage of severe reactions.

* * *

VACCINATION AGAINST DIPHTHERIA

1. Has proven highly effective and all children should be immunized in the pre-school period, preferably at eight to 12 months of age.

2. Widespread immunization is gradually but definitely eradicating diphtheria and greatly lowering its mortality. It is believed that the disease can be as thoroughly eradicated as smallpox by immunization.

3. Diphtheria, h o w e v e r, can and does s o m e t i m e s occur (rarely) in immunized and Schick-negative individuals exposed to heavy, virulent infection.

4. The duration of immunity after vaccination is variable and probably not over five to eight years but may persist for the balance of life when reenforced by n a t u r a l immunization from c l i n i c a l l y unrecognized exposures.

5. The Schick test is not required in children under six years of age as at least 80 per cent are positive and all should be immunized.

6. The Schick test is advisable in older children and adults and only positive reactors should be immunized.

7. Children immunized at eight months to two years of age should have a Schick test at six years of age and given one or two additional doses of toxoid if positive.

8. Older children and adults should have a repeat Schick test about six months after immunization and given one or two additional doses of vaccine if still positive.

9. Even if a Schick-negative reactor later becomes Schick - positive the ability to produce antitoxin r a·p i d l y̅ upon

subsequent stimulation apparently lasts for the balance of life.

10. For infants and children under six years of age a *single* dose of 0.5 to 1.0 cc. of *alum-precipitated toxoid* usually suffices. It is highly and rapidly antigenic and immunizes at least 90 per cent within two to three months but immunity is less lasting. Local nodular reactions may persist for several weeks with danger of abscess due to the alum.

11. The author prefers two injections of *soluble toxoid* three weeks apart for infants and Schick-positive children under 12 years of age. Antitoxic immunity results in about 95 per cent, is more durable and produces less local reaction.

12. Children over 12 years of age and adults may be allergic to diphtheria bacillus protein and give severe local reactions to toxoid (Maloney reaction).

13. It is advisable to do the Schick test and at the same time a second test for allergy consisting in the intracutaneous injection of 0.1 cc. of 1:20 dilution of toxoid. Only Schick-positive reactors require immunization.

14. If the individual is not allergic the author recommends 0.5, 1.0 and 1.0 cc. of *soluble toxoid* at intervals of two to three weeks.

15. If the individual is allergic (positive Maloney reaction) the author recommends 0.1 or 0.25 cc. of soluble toxoid followed by two additional doses of the same or increased amounts or three injections of T-A (1 cc. each) at intervals of two weeks. The former is preferred because more antigenic without danger of serum sensitization.

* * *

VACCINATION AGAINST TETANUS

1. Natural antitoxic immunity to tetanus doubtless occurs but there is no skin test available for its detection.

2. Vaccination with alum precipitated *toxoid* is of proven value and deserves general adoption.

3. It is free of spores and perfectly safe. Local and general reactions are usually trivial and negligible.

4. At least two and preferably three doses of 1 cc. each by subcutaneous injection are given three to four weeks apart; for children 0.5 cc. For persons who are frequently injured one dose annually thereafter apparently gives sufficient protection.

5. Antitoxic immunity develops slowly and requires at least several months; apparently 0.1 unit of antitoxin per cc. of blood suffices for protection. It is of no value in the treatment of tetanus.

6. The duration of immunity is variable; it lasts at least one to three years and probably for the balance of life in a high percentage.

7. If a *vaccinated* person is injured it may suffice to give only 1 cc. of toxoid for additional protection since antitoxin production is rapid under these conditions. If, however, the chances of infection are great 1,500 units of antitoxin should be given at the same time.

8. If an *unvaccinated* person is injured give 1,500 units of antitoxin immediately and at the same time 1 cc. of toxoid. In severe injuries contaminated with dirt a second dose of 1,500 units of antitoxin is advisable five to seven days later to prolong passive immunity followed one month later by a second dose of toxoid.

9. Vaccination is now compulsory in the English, French and Italian armies and widely used in the U. S. army.

10. It is highly advisable among civilians including even children and especially among adults whose occupation exposes them to frequent injuries, as farmers, mechanics, truck drivers, miners, railroad employees, etc.

* * *

COMBINED IMMUNIZATION

1. Ramon and other investigators have found that the combination of diphtheria and tetanus toxoids gives better results than the use of each toxoid separately.

2. Many physicians now believe that the r o u t i n e immunization of children against tetanus is desirable. For this purpose two or three doses of combined diphtheria and tetanus alum-precipitated toxoids may be given.

3. In the Italian army tetanus toxoid is combined with typhoid-paratyphoid vaccine for simultaneous immunization.

* * *

VACCINATION AGAINST SCARLET FEVER

1. From 45 to 70 per cent of children under five years of age give positive Dick reactions; about 25 to 35 per cent of older children and about 15 to 20 per cent of adults.

2. The test may be omitted, therefore, in children under five years of age but should always be done in older children and adults as only positive reactors require immunization.

3. In contacts and during epidemics it is excellent practice to give the first dose of toxin in one arm and a Dick test in the other; if positive the remaining four doses are given (Park).

4. Vaccination deserves wider use than at present and is especially advisable in institutions for children, for physicians, medical students and nurses in scarlet fever hospitals and to check epidemics.

5. At least five subcutaneous injections of toxin are advised at weekly intervals: 500, 2,500, 20,000, 40,000 and 80,-000 skin test doses (Dick).

6. Severe local and general reactions may occur due to toxin, allergic sensitization to bacterial protein or to broth constituents. The author uses 250, 2,000, 10,000, 20,000 and 40,000 skin test doses with fewer reactions and satisfactory results.

7. Three intradermal injections of 1,600, 4,000 and 10,000 skin test doses have been advised but value is uncertain at present.

8. Immunity develops in about 90 per cent of susceptible individuals (Dick negative reactions). The duration is unknown but probably three to eight years. It may possibly last for balance of life through reenforcement by clinically unrecognized exposures to hemolytic streptococci.

9. A recent change by Dick in the broth medium employed for the preparation of toxin has greatly reduced the incidence of reactions and it is likely that one or two doses of this new toxin will suffice in the future.

10. Immunization by toxoid or oral administration of toxin is not satisfactory.

11. The author believes it is advisable to use a mixed vaccine of t o x i n and chemically-killed *streptococcus scarlatinae* to p r o d u c e antibacterial as well as antitoxic immunity.

* * *

VACCINATION AGAINST WHOOPING COUGH

1. Whooping cough ranks third among the destroyers of children with an incidence averaging about 200,000 and a mortality of about 5,000 yearly in reported cases.

2. There is apparently no natural immunity with greatest susceptibility from six months to five years of age.

3. The Sauer vaccine is recommended prepared of freshly isolated and completely antigenic smooth strains of B. *pertussis* carrying 10 million per cc., suspended in saline s o l u t i o n and sterilized with phenol.

4. The total amount injected is 7 cc. divided into four doses at weekly intervals. At present double-strength vaccine may be employed (20 million per cc.) in total amount of 5 cc. (1, 2 and 3 cc.) for children under two years and 6 cc. (1, 2 and 3 cc.) for older children at weekly intervals.

5. Immunity d e v e l o p s in one to three months but its duration is uncertain although apparently l a s t i n g about four years and sufficient for protection over the age of greatest susceptibility when reenforcement by clinically unrecognized exposures apparently prolongs the immunity.

6. The incidence in all types of exposure

has been reduced from about 80.2 to about 16.7 per cent by vaccination.

7. Even if vaccination fails to prevent the disease it greatly reduces the severity of the attack in about 40 per cent with less chances of the d r e a d e d bronchopneumonia.

8. The best time for vaccination is about six months to two years of age and the a u t h o r recommends its widespread use. Its value in treatment has not been determined.

* * *

VACCINATION AGAINST THE COMMON COLD

1. The infectious "common cold" is a disease of great economic importance as well as one predisposing to chronic sinusitis, pneumonia and tuberculosis.

2. It is due primarily to an ultramicroscopic virus which appears to lower resistance to bacteria in the respiratory tract resulting in an important secondary infection.

3. The virus has been cultivated but vaccination with it has y i e l d e d disappointing and inconclusive results.

4. Immunization against t h e secondary bacterial infection, however, is apparently e f f e c t i v e in about 50 per cent of individuals and is apparently worth while.

5. Of little or no value in the presence of purulent sinusitis and adenoids for the prevention of so-called "colds" due to exacerbation of such chronic infections.

6. Stock vaccines may be used but the author p r e f e r s a mixed stock and autogenous vaccine carrying a total of 1,000 million per cc.; for adults 0.2, 0.4, 0.6, 0.8 and 1 cc. at weekly intervals; children one-half these amounts.

7. Immunity u s u a l l y lasts four to 12 m o n t h s but sometimes for several years.

8. Oral immunization is still in the experimental stage but has given promising results and is certainly worthy of trial. The vaccine is prepared of d r i e d organisms in capsules one of which is taken with a glassful of cold water 30 minutes before breakfast for seven days in succession followed by one per week for a total of 20 doses. It is likely that the results are improved by u s i n g organisms with a high heterophile antigen content.

9. The author recommends g i v i n g a m o n t h l y subcutaneous injection of mixed autogenous and stock vaccine following the five initial injections or following with oral vaccine, to reenforce immunity and p r o l o n g the period of protection.

* * *

VACCINATION AGAINST INFLUENZA

1. Influenza is due to an ultramicroscopic virus; *Bacillus influenzae* is an organism of secondary infection. "Grippe" is mild or sporadic influenza.

2. The v i r u s has been cultivated artificially and some attempts made to actively immunize against it but the results have been inconclusive or disappointing.

3. Immunization with vaccines of *B. influenzae* alone have given little or no evidence of protective value.

4. Immunization with mixed vaccines of *B. influenzae*, streptococci, staphylococci, pneumococci, etc., are of doubtful value but may give some protection against secondary pneumonia.

5. There is, therefore, no m e t h o d of proven value at present for vaccination against sporadic or epidemic influenza.

* * *

VACCINATION AGAINST LOBAR PNEUMONIA

1. The author calculates that the yearly incidence is about 267 per 100,000 population and that a b o u t 335,000 whites and 67,000 negroes over one year of age contract pneumonia yearly with the great majority due to pneumococcal infections.

2. About 50 to 60 per cent among adults are due to Types I and II, about 12 per cent to Type III and the balance to Types IV to XXXII. This multiplicity of t y p e s complicates, therefore, the problem of active immunization.

3. The r e s u l t s of vaccination against Types I and II with single subcutaneous injections of 1 to 2 mg of Felton's water-soluble antigen have indicated that it may reduce the incidence of the disease.

4. The duration of immunity after immunization is unknown but probably q u i t e brief and not over 4 to 12 months.

5. Vaccination against Types I and II is worthy of further trial in epidemics and especially in camps; also in those individuals whose occupation exposes them greatly to the disease.

* * *

VACCINATION AGAINST TUBERCULOSIS

1. The possibilities of effective immunization with killed vaccines of B. tuberculosis in combination with other antigens is highly problematical although such may be elaborated in the future sufficient for reducing tuberculosis in infants and children.

2. Living non-virulent bacilli have been given in the form of the B C G vaccine to about 1,500,000 infants without a single death (the Lubeck disaster being due to an accident).

3. It is best given orally shortly after birth and has apparently reduced the tuberculosis mortality among exposed infants in the first years of life.

4. The duration of the immunity is undetermined but may scarcely be expected to protect against marked exogenous reinfection during adult life.

* * *

VACCINATION AGAINST TYPHOID FEVER

1. Vaccination against typhoid and paratyphoid fevers along with the filtration or disinfection of drinking water and other hygienic measures have undoubtedly greatly reduced the incidence and mortality of these enteric diseases.

2. Not all strains of typhoid and paratyphoid bacilli are suitable for the preparation of vaccine. It is important to use "s m o o t h," virulent and completely antigenic s t r a i n s. At present the Panama carrier strain No. 58 of B. typhosus is employed.

3. The vaccine carries 1,000 million typhoid and 750 million paratyphoid A and B bacilli per cc.; three doses of 0.5, 1.0 and 1.0 cc. are given by subcutaneous injection at i n t e r v a l s of seven to ten days.

4. Tuft has shown that the intracutaneous injection of 0.1, 0.15 and 0.2 cc. at weekly intervals may give a better immunity response with lesser reactions.

5. Oral immunization is possible but not advisable.

6. While the immunity is not complete it usually protects against ordinary chance i n f e c t i o n for two to three years. It may be reenforced thereafter by a single dose of 1 cc. subcutaneously or 0.1 cc. intracutaneously. The mouse serum protection test is a better index of acquired immunity and the need for revaccination than the agglutination test.

7. Vaccination is especially recommended in localities where typhoid fever is endemic, in the case of all contacts and those exposed to the d i s e a s e, during epidemics, in c a m p s, those traveling to foreign countries, etc.

* * *

VACCINATION AGAINST BACILLARY DYSENTERY

1. The high toxicity of vaccines of B. dysenteriae (Shiga) has made active immunization difficult.

2. Sero-vaccine (mixture of 0.5 cc. immune serum and 0.5 cc. of killed bacterial suspension) has been used by Shiga with a lowering of mortality but with practically no e f f e c t on morbidity.

3. Dysentery toxoid has been employed as likewise oral vaccines but with uncertain and poor results.

4. At the present time dysentery immunization cannot be recommended as a general prophylactic measure.

* * *

VACCINATION AGAINST ASIATIC CHOLERA

1. Ferran f i r s t employed vaccination

against cholera in 1885, and since then many different vaccines of living but attenuated or dead cultures have been used. At the present time, vaccination against this disease is believed to have distinct value.

2. The method is similar to vaccination against typhoid fever. Three injections are usually given at weekly intervals.

3. O r a l administration of vaccine has been t r i e d but subcutaneous injections are believed to give better results.

4. The immunity probably lasts only two years.

5. During the W o r l d War, vaccination appeared to reduce both the morbidity and mortality from cholera.

* * *

VACCINATION AGAINST UNDULANT FEVER

1. The incidence of undulant f e v e r is progressively i n c r e a s i n g in the United S t a t e s and is an important public health problem.

2. Killed vaccines and filtrates of brucella have largely failed to effectively immunize cattle and goats.

3. Some success has been attained with vaccines of living brucella but these are too dangerous for human beings.

4. Killed v a c c i n e s and glucidolipoid fractions may, however, e n g e n d e r sufficient immunity in human beings for protection against ordinary chance infection and are being tried to a limited extent in the immunization of veterinarians, meat handlers and laboratory workers. F r o m his experimental work the author believes the prospects are promising for ultimate safe and effective immunization.

* * *

VACCINATION AGAINST RABIES

1. One of the most mortal of diseases, since recovery is almost unknown, and of increasing frequency urgently requiring the wholesale vaccination of dogs and especially the rigid enforcement of other p u b l i c health measures.

2. Fortunately o n l y from 6 to 16 per cent of human beings bitten by rabid animals develop the disease. Vaccination has reduced the incidence to less than one per cent.

3. The saliva of rabid animals is infectious about one week before the onset of symptoms. If an animal shows no symptoms whatever for a week or two after a bite, the d a n g e r of rabies may be excluded.

4. In case of doubt it is always better to start vaccination and stop if subsequent examinations and observations show that the animal was not rabid.

5. Bites about the head and hands are particularly d a n g e r o u s; contamination of the hands with saliva alone is potentially dangerous.

6. Thorough cauterization of bites with fuming nitric acid within 12 hours is apparently of value.

7. The original vaccine of Pasteur has now been l a r g e l y replaced by the phenolized vaccine of Semple given by subcutaneous injection in dose of 2 or 2.5 cc. for 14 to 15 days in succession.

8. It is still doubtful if completely killed virus is sufficiently vaccinogenic; apparently a residue of living but attenuated virus in the vaccine is required for effective immunization.

9. The duration of immunity is variable but probably lasts only one to two years.

10. The incidence of treatment paralysis has v a r i e d with different vaccines but is ordinarily of rare occurrence (1:3538). It is unknown in children under five years of age and has never occurred during the first five days of treatment; it usually develops after 6 to 10 doses; the prognosis is good but never give the treatment unless the patient or family understands the slight risks entailed.

* * *

VACCINATION AGAINST ROCKY MOUNTAIN SPOTTED FEVER

1. A vaccine of the Rickettsia may be obtained from the U. S. Public Health

service field station at Hamilton, Montana.

2. It is given subcutaneously or intramuscularly in dose of 2 cc. for two or three injections, five to seven days apart; the dose for children under 10 years of age is 1.0 cc.

3. As a rule only local reactions occur; occasionally there may be a mild general reaction with urticaria in about one per cent (allergic).

4. The vaccine should be given before or shortly after the appearance of ticks, i.e., during the late winter or early spring.

5. The immunity lasts only one to possibly two years and is usually sufficient for protection against infection with strains of low virulence while greatly increasing the chances of recovery from infection with virulent strains.

6. Of no value in the treatment of the disease.

* * *

VACCINATION AGAINST EQUINE ENCEPHALITIS

1. Equine encephalitis in man presents a new and important clinical and public health problem. It is due to an ultramicroscopic virus which may be transmitted not only by horses but probably by pigeons, pheasants and other birds. The disease is severe in man with a high mortality; greatest incidence among children under five years of age.

2. The virus has been successfully cultivated in the chick-embryo medium and vaccines have been successful in the immunization of horses.

3. The vaccine is now being employed for the vaccination of laboratory workers, veterinarians and other exposed persons. Apparently safe and effective with no untoward reactions but its exact value cannot be appraised at the present time.

* * *

VACCINATION AGAINST INFANTILE PARALYSIS

1. The age of greatest susceptibility is from 1 to 15 years of age. The majority of adults are apparently immune but the disease may occur among them.

2. Completely killed vaccines of the virus from the spinal cords of monkeys are regarded as ineffective.

3. Only the living virus in vaccines is capable of producing immunity in monkeys and presumably in man but are regarded as too dangerous for use.

4. At present there is no known method of proven value for the prophylaxis of infantile paralysis. The author believes that safe and effective immunization may be ultimately accomplished with vaccines of living but attenuated non-infective virus.

* * *

VACCINATION AGAINST YELLOW FEVER

1. Killed vaccines of the virus have been found ineffective.

2. Some success has attended vaccination with mixtures of mouse virus and human immune serum.

3. At present a vaccine of living chick-embryo culture virus is being tried since it appears safe because of marked attenuation of its viscerotropic and neurotropic properties. Its value cannot be expressed at present but the results are hopeful and encouraging.

* * *

VACCINATION AGAINST BUBONIC PLAGUE

1. Vaccination against bubonic plague was first tried in 1877. Since then many different kinds of vaccines of B. pestis have been used, and especially that prepared by the Haffkine method.

2. One or two large doses, by subcutaneous injection, confer an early immunity of short duration (about three months).

3. Vaccination is of no value against the pneumonic type of plague but is regarded in India, China and elsewhere, as of distinct value in combating epidemics of the bubonic type.

* * *

VACCINATION AGAINST MENINGITIS

1. Vaccination appears to have some

value in epidemics of meningitis although the results have not been entirely convincing.

2. The vaccine should be freshly prepared of *strains producing the epidemic* which are virulent and completely antigenic. Three injections at weekly intervals of 500, 100 and 1,000 million are advised.

3. The author has found it possible to vaccinate the lower animals against pneumococcus and streptococcus meningitis and believes that when conditions permit it is advisable to vaccinate human beings with three to six weekly injections of autogenous vaccine before operations on the mastoid and nasal accessory sinuses (particularly in ethmoiditis and sphenoiditis) and especially if cultures show that infection is due to hemolytic streptococci and pneumococci. This procedure promises to reduce the chances of complications and particularly suppurative meningitis.

SUMMARY

Disease	Practical Value
Smallpox	Effective
Diphtheria	Effective
Typhoid fever	Effective
Pertussis	Effective
Scarlet fever	Effective
Rabies	Effective
Tetanus	Effective
Bubonic plague	Worthy of Use
Asiatic Cholera	Worthy of Use
Rocky Mountain Fever	Worthy of Use
Common cold	Worthy of Use
Equine Encephalitis	Worthy of Use
Yellow fever	Worthy of Use
Meningitis	Worthy of Use
Lobar pneumonia	Uncertain
Influenza	Uncertain
Tuberculosis	Uncertain
Bacillary Dysentery	Uncertain
Undulant Fever	Uncertain
Poliomyelitis	Not available

ADVISABLE ROUTINE IMMUNIZATIONS

Pertussis	9 months of age
Diphtheria or Diphtheria and Tetanus	12 months of age
Smallpox	2 years of age
Scarlet fever	3-4 years of age
Typhoid fever	8-12 years of age

---o---

The Private Physician's Part in a Public Health Program*

J. C. ROSE, Statistician

OKLAHOMA CITY, OKLAHOMA

As Public Health grew from a more or less temporary organization called into action to cope with an emergency and took on the aspect of planning and carrying on an active program for the reduction of unnecessary illness and death and for the improvement of health, record-keeping became an important phase of every service. Without the careful recording of circumstances under which a disease occurs, there would not be available for studying the splendid expositions on epidemiology which are available to us today. Only with careful recording of services and results over a long period of time can Public Health advance to a more exact science so that favorable results may follow the expenditure of funds and effort in accordance with a predetermined plan.

As the program of the local Health Service became less concerned with the present and began to carry on activities of a truly preventive nature, records became increasingly important as a measure to insure improvement in the service to individuals as well as an aid in sound planning of the program on a wide basis to the end that the expenditure of funds and effort may be justified by the results obtained. Life saving campaigns of the last few decades have borne fruit. The death rate has been lowered and the average span of life correspondingly lengthened.

*Read before the Section on General Medicine, Annual Meeting, Oklahoma State Medical Association, Oklahoma City, May, 1939.

As a matter of fact, since 1913—a short space of 25 years—the average age at death has increased 13 years. The amount of sickness, on the other hand, has not been reduced or controlled to the same degree. There still is too much sickness among us; i n d e e d, there are those who with some authority maintain that illness has actually increased in spite of *all the saving in mortality.*

The basis for any campaign against sickness must be an accurate knowledge of its prevalence. Just as the reduction of mortality is furthered by a complete registration of deaths and their causes, so are efforts to reduce the frequency of disease dependent upon machinery for reporting the cases of sickness, their causes and their duration for each group in the community. For this purpose, it is not sufficient to know only the number who died from any particular disease; emphasis must be placed upon the cases of s i c k n e s s themselves. They are s o c i a l l y more important than deaths and our program must more and more prevent their occurrence and effect their control.

The state must, therefore, in the first instance, see that all preventable diseases are recorded in order that we may lay a foundation for efficient sanitary administration. The health departments have always realized the importance of registering disease. The first laws required the reporting of plagues such as smallpox, yellow fever, cholera, etc.; later the list was extended to include the acute infections, especially those of childhood. Later diphtheria, scarlet fever and measles, first on a voluntary basis; later this was made compulsory. Finally, c e r t a i n non-infectious diseases, such as cancer, pellagra and even a few of the occupational diseases have been made reportable.

At the present time, all states of the Union have laws requiring the reporting of one or more of the preventable diseases.

Professor Irving Fisher of Yale University has estimated that about 3,000,000 people are seriously ill at any one time in the United States, about one-half of whom are suffering from preventable diseases. Faulk estimates that not less than 500 out of each 1,000 of the population suffers a disabling illness during any given 12-month period.

That means in Oklahoma 1,250,000 people suffer disabling illness annually. The average amount per capita cost is estimated at $30.00 per annum. It is further estimated that wage losses by employed persons amount to another $30.00 per annum per capita. That means $76,000,000.00 annually to our state. That is a tidy sum, is it not?

These figures, we believe, are conservative but it is obviously impossible to make an estimate which will approximate the truth in view of the lack of completely accurate i n f o r m a t i o n. Whatever be the exact amount of loss sustained, thorough effective registration will help to reduce it and it will thus yield a big return to the community on the relatively small investment required.

The effect upon the social welfare is far reaching. It makes possible the immediate and effective treatment of certain infectious diseases. In cases of tuberculosis, for example, an early report to the department of health puts at the disposal of the patient the advantages resulting f r o m the resources of the organization.

In the case of diphtheria, where success in the treatment depends so largely on an early and correct diagnosis, the registration of a suspected case enables the health authority to make a culture which settles the diagnosis. In positive cases, the information placed at the disposal of a physician in charge helps to make a cure almost certain. So, too, the reporting of eye-infections of new-born b a b i e s brings the nurse or medical inspector into the home who sees that the required treatment is given. As a result, many children now grow up with normal vision whose lives otherwise would have been shrouded in darkness.

The registration of all communicable diseases enables health officers to discover the foci of infection in time to prevent further spread of the disease. The early and complete reporting of typhoid fever at once puts the efficient health officer on the track of the infection.

It may be the sewage system or the water or milk supply which is at the bottom of the trouble. In any event, the location and sequence of the cases settles the questions and the epidemic may in this way be prevented from spreading to other sections. The reporting of preventable diseases enables the health authority to superintend the efforts of the state department of labor in following up cases to their sources. Thus, the compulsory reporting of blood poisoning puts the authority on the trail of the careless company or factory where other workmen may be finally exposed to possible poisoning. The health and labor departments can then bring to bear their facilities on the employers or employees and also further fulfillment of the various requirements of the law.

The reporting of occupational diseases can be made to serve as a most excellent check on the efficiency of the existing labor legislation. The registration of certain diseases such as cancer, and pellagra, throws much light upon the origin of these maladies. We have much to learn with regard to the frequency with which these diseases occur in the various social groups. There is already at hand sufficient evidence to indicate that their incidence varies greatly with regard to race, sex, age, occupation, personal habits and other conditions. Our advance, therefore, in the control of cancer will depend in a large measure upon the cooperation of the physician, the registrar and the vital statistician.

The registration of preventable diseases is furthermore the chief test at our disposal for measuring the efficiency of the community control over them. Millions of dollars are spent annually in campaigns to control their progress. There is, however, a considerable difference of opinion as to the best methods to pursue and the several communities are applying their appropriations in different ways.

It is clearly an advantage for every group to know the results obtained through the application of their special methods. In this way the recording of cases, together with a complete statement of their methods, will ultimately decide the fate of the methods employed.

In conclusion, I want to say just a few words about the recording of deaths and a completing of the medical certificate of death.

Every physician appreciates, in a general way, the importance of the collection, tabulation and assembling of mortality statistics. It is doubtful, however, if many of them realize the importance of care and judgment in making their statements. The achievement of accurate statements which reflect the physician's considered opinion depends first upon the physician understanding clearly the significance of the questions related to the cause of death and the general principles upon which the death certificate is based. Official records can never be more accurate than the statements of the medical practitioner, no matter what conventional treatment be employed.

What does the physician need to know to enable him to complete a satisfactory medical certificate?

He must, first, understand clearly what is meant by "cause of death" for statistical purposes. This is defined as "the disease or injury which initiated the train of events leading to death" and it is this entity of which a clear indication is desired. This information is designed so that medical records may serve to direct attention to the point at which preventable measures may be best applied.

Detailed statements are not desired. A single entry is preferable in all cases where this can be regarded as adequate. The physician's statement of the cause of death is not intended to be an abstract of the clinical history and pathological findings. Detailed studies in any case can and should always be made on samples where greater reliability may be attached to such details, as in hospitals.

Death certificates are supposed to contain merely a clear authoritative scientific and logical explanation of the medical officer as to the cause of death. An entry of several morbid conditions or states has of course no particular disadvantage from the medical or statistical standpoint, if they are presented in logical order and without ambiguity. As an example, from the statistical standpoint, the fact that the injured person in an automobile accident died as a result of concussion is not important. The important thing is *how the accident occurred.*

Terminal conditions are not satisfactory causes of death from the statistical standpoint for the reason that they do not give us the point from which to start preventive measures.

Peritonitis, without qualification given as a cause of d e a t h, practically masks many other of the communicable diseases and accidents and even suicides and murders.

————————0————————

Thiocyanates in the Treatment of Hypertension

W. TURNER BYNUM, M.D.
CHICKASHA, OKLAHOMA

Thiocyanates have enjoyed varying degrees of popularity and disrepute in the treatment of hypertension for a number of years, but it remained for Barker[†] in 1936 to explain the diverse results obtained by the different investigators. He believes that the thiocyanates are retained in the body to varying degrees in different individuals — they being a foreign substance in the body, each kidney eliminates them with varying facility; i.e., no definite dose will be effective in every individual —what is less than a therapeutic dose in one individual may produce toxic symptoms in another. Barker believes that the only safe method of controlling dosage is by the determination of the blood cyanate levels which, he states, should be kept between 8-12 mgm. per 100 cc. of blood. The method for determination is set out in his first article[†].

He believes that, if this method is followed, thiocyanates are an ideal medication for controlling hypertension and that the margin of safety in their use is sufficiently broad to warrant their more frequent and extensive use, as toxic symptoms usually do not arise before the blood levels have exceeded 30 mgm. per 100 cc.

I wish to report here a short series of cases in which I am in complete accord with Barker. My reasons for reporting this short series are the unusual nature of two of the cases, and the ideal circumstances these cases presented for such a study.

First let me state that I am not offering this method as a panacea nor do I believe that it is applicable to all cases, because of its untoward side actions; i.e., the frequent annoying sense of weakness and vertigo complained of by many even when thiocyanates are given in therapeutic doses.

All patients in this series have had a trial period of from several months to a year or more on sedatives and theophylin derivatives which failed to control either their blood pressure or their subjective symptoms.

Case No. 1. Miss R. W. P., Ph.D., professor of philosophy in a state college, was first found to have hypertension in 1920. At this time systolic pressure was 190/?. T h i s condition persisted unabated, the pressure gradually increasing until it was well over 200 in March, 1936, at which time she suffered a cerebro-vascular accident associated with a transient hemiplegia of the left side. However, she was able to carry on with her teaching the following year. In June, 1937, she had a s e c o n d cerebro-vascular accident, about a month following which she consulted Dr. Harvey Stone of Baltimore who found her blood pressure to be 260/?, and who, on July 14, 1937, performed a bilateral splanchnic resection. The following day, the b l o o d pressure was 135/90.

The patient states that for the following six weeks the blood pressure was very unstable, varying between this last figure and 200/130. On September 28, 1937, it was found to be 220/120. The patient was able to teach school for another year and felt

†Barker, M. Herbert: Estimation of Blood Thiocyanates in Hypertension, J.A.M.A., 106:762 (March 7) 1936.

"fairly well" although the blood pressure remained around 220/130.

I first saw the patient in September, 1938, following a rather extensive cerebro-vascular accident resulting in hemiplegia and aphasia. At this time her blood pressure was 276/160 and she was placed on bromides and phenobarbital, tissue extract by hypodermic, whiskey ounces one-half t.i.d., and aminophylin grains one and one-half t.i.d. However, her blood pressure remained at 260/150. She had another cerebro-vascular attack in November, 1938, and another light attack on February 1, 1939, when her blood pressure was 260/160. At this time she was placed on potassium thiocyanate grains five daily, and all other medication was discontinued. After one week her blood pressure was 188/130 and blood cyanate level 19 mgm. per 100 cc. The dose of thiocyanate was reduced to grains 3½ daily. The following week the blood concentration was 12 mgm. per 100 cc., the blood pressure 220/120, and the patient felt quite well. Since that time the blood levels have remained between 11-12 mgm. per 100 cc. and the blood pressure has been 190/100 for the past three months. The patient is up and around and perfectly comfortable but unable to carry on duties of teaching because of a speech disturbance and partial deafness which were present before institution of thiocyanate therapy.

Case No. 2. Mrs. M. E. A., age 53. A physician's wife with the history of having an exophthalmic goitre removed in 1912 and who was told at the Mayo Clinic in 1929 that she had a mild h y p e r t e n s i o n which was still present one year later. She was otherwise well until September 14, 1936, at which time she experienced an attack of coronary thrombosis verified by electrocardiogram. Since that time she has had a persistent blood p r e s s u r e of around 245/140—in spite of the taking of tremendous doses of sodium amytal (3 to 9 grains daily).

The patient first consulted me on December 10, 1938, b e c a u s e of weakness, nervousness, dyspepsia, and dyspnea on exertion. For these various symptoms she was taking some 17 different medicines; such as, alka seltzer, alkaroids, milk of magnesia, magnesium sulphate, bromides, caroid and bile, soda, etc.

Examination revealed the following essential findings: Bilateral exophthalmos; a dusky cyanosis limited to the head and neck; generalized arteriosclerosis, grade 2; blood pressure, 245/145; pulse, 120; temperature, 98.6; an old thyroid scar with no gland palpable; and moderate cardiac enlargement, associated with a definite gallop rhythm. The p a t i e n t weighed 183 pounds and was five feet two inches in height.

An electrocardiogram revealed a left axis deviation and presence of inverted T wave in lead 3. Urinalysis showed specific gravity, 1.018; slight trace albumin; and occasional granular casts. Non protein nitrogen was 22.5 mgm. per 100 cc. of blood.

The patient was advised to discontinue all medication, placed on a reducing diet and bowel management, and hospitalized. On January 4, 1939, the patient was discharged from the hospital feeling fairly well. Her blood pressure on dismissal was 210/120, and pulse 96. On January 23, 1939, the patient was re-admitted to the hospital with a mild congestive failure; pulse, 126; blood pressure, 190/110; hepatomegaly and edema of ankles. After four days in the hospital, and following digitalization, her blood p r e s s u r e was 230/124 which, on continued rest and administration of phenobarbital and aminophylin, was r e d u c e d to 210/120 in two weeks. At this point it persisted despite weight reduction to 137 pounds, continuous bed rest in hospital, and sedation, until April 10, 1939, when thiocyanate therapy was instituted and it was found necessary to give 10 grains daily to attain blood levels of 11-12 mgm. per 100 cc. This concentration, however, brought the b l o o d pressure down to 174/90 in two weeks time.

Since then the patient has remained in the hospital, principally as a matter of convenience, where she has had no medication other than the potassium thiocyanate, and where daily blood pressure determinations have varied between 184/106 to 148/84. The patient is up and around eight to ten hours daily, and comes and goes from the hospital at will feeling perfectly well save for a slight ease of fatigue.

Case No. 3. Mrs. J. Stinson, age 59, has had a known hypertension for four years and has been under constant observation for seven months. When first seen, January 10, 1939, her blood pressure was 260/100, which on bromides and theominal was reduced to 230/100 where it persisted for five months. Following the institution of thiocyanate therapy on May 24, 1939 (5 grains daily to sustain blood cyanates at 10 mgm.), her blood pressure has dropped to 180/80 and the patient states that she feels the best she has felt in many years.

Case No. 4. Mrs. W. W. W., a married woman, age 51, weight 155, first came to the clinic on March 28, 1939, complaining of headaches and vertigo. Her physical examination was essentially negative save for a blood pressure of 260/110. She was placed on a reducing diet, phenobarbital, bromides, and aminophylin, with added periods of rest. By December 13, 1938, her weight was reduced to 126, pulse 72, and blood pressure 230/110, the lowest it had been since under observation. The patient was advised to take thiocyanate therapy, but declined and continued the above treatment until May 4, 1939, when her blood pressure was found to be 240/120. At this time, the administration of potassium thiocyanate was instituted, grains 5 daily, which sustained blood cyanates between 11-12 mgm. per 100 cc. Her blood pressure at the end of one week was found to be 212/110; two weeks later 174/90, near which point it has remained to date. The patient complains of some weakness and occasional vertigo which she greatly prefers to her previous intense headache and nervousness.

Case No. 5. Mrs. R. L. B., age 31, who first consulted me on January 14, 1939, giving a history of repeated attacks of inflammatory r h e u m a t i s m and tonsillitis since childhood, and a history of intermittent edema of the feet and ankles since 1931. She had consulted her family physician some three weeks earlier, regarding a tonsillectomy, but he had refused to perform this operation at that time because of a marked hypertension, and had placed her on a starvation regime. She had had nothing but clear l i q u i d s for the week

prior to my first consultation with her, and had been at absolute rest in bed. Her blood pressure was found to be 165/118. Her urinalysis revealed a 3 plus albumin, occasional pus cells, occasional red blood cells, and alkaline reaction. Specific gravity 1.010, with the p r e s e n c e of many hyaline and granular casts. Her red blood count was found to be 3,330,000; hemoglobin, 11 gms.; white blood count, 4,550. She was placed on a 1,200 calorie, Sodium-free diet, and given a prescription for ferrous sulphate, grains 3½, four times a day. She was given calcium chloride, grains 20, four times a day, and potassium chloride, grains 60, once daily, a prescription containing bromides, bella donna, and phenobarbital, and advised not to be out of bed over ten hours a day. After one week on this regime her blood pressure was found to be 230/140, and at this time a concentration and dilution kidney function test was run, which revealed a maximum concentration of 1.014, and a maximum dilution of 1.002, and non protein nitrogen was 25.5 mgm. per 100 cc. of blood. Her urea nitrogen was 10.09 mgm. per 100 cc. She continued on this regime for four weeks with blood pressures c h e c k e d from once to twice a week, the readings being around 230/140 consistently. At this time she was advised to have a tonsillectomy, which was performed. Following this, her b l o o d pressure was lowered to around 194/120 for some three weeks, but returned to its previous levels in spite of the rest, sedation, and the other measures carried out. During all of this time her urine continued to show granular casts, pus, red blood cells, and albumin.

On March 9, 1939, she was placed on potassium thiocyanate, grains 5 daily, and all other m e d i c a t i o n was discontinued. After one week on potassium thiocyanate she was found to have a blood cyanate of 20 mgm. per 100 cc. of blood, and a blood pressure of 200/130, which one week later was found to be 190/110 with a blood cyanate level of 22.2 mgm. Her blood pressure remained at this point until May 12, 1939, at which time the dose of potassium thiocyanate was reduced to 2½ grains per day, which brought her blood c y a n a t e level down to 11 mgm. per 100 cc. and her blood pressure rose to 212/130. On maintaining her blood cyanate level between 10 and 12 mgm., her blood pressure rose to 230/130 where it was when the patient was last seen on July 6, 1939. She was advised to discontinue this medication as we felt it was not safe to carry her at the higher levels necessary to maintain a s y s t o l i c blood pressure under 200.

Case No. 6. Miss E. E., age 32. This patient had a history of acute glomular nephritis in 1931, and a history of rather intense anti-luetic treatment for four and one-half years following 1931. I first saw the patient in December, 1938, at which t i m e she was complaining of migraine headaches and nervousness. She had a 4 plus Kahn reaction at this time despite the prolonged treatment and was found to have a blood pressure of 210/120. Her urinalysis was a 1 plus albumin, occasional red cells, pus cells, and granular casts. Her physical examination was otherwise not remarkable. She was followed for five months on sedatives and was found to have a blood pressure fluctuating between 160/100 and 210/120. On May 14, 1939, she was placed on potassium thio-cyanate, and it was found necessary to give 10 grains a day in order to attain a blood level of 10 mgm. per 100 cc. On this her blood pressure was consistently around 170/90, but the patient discontinued the medication after four weeks because of the untoward symptoms of vertigo, weakness, and malaise.

SUMMARY

Reported here are six cases of hypertension due either to chronic glomular nephritis or to essential hypertension, with the results obtained by the use of potassium thiocyanate in doses sufficient to maintain the blood levels between 10 and 12 mgm. per 100 cc. The method was found effective in controlling the hypertension in all cases but was discontinued in one case because of the untoward side actions, and in another case of chronic glomular nephritis because it was felt that the blood levels necessary to satisfactorily reduce the hypertension; i.e., 20 to 23 mgm. per 100 cc.; was too high to warrant its continued use, although no toxic symptoms were manifest.

———o———

Cortical Hormone in the Treatment of Bromide Intoxication

COYNE H. CAMPBELL, A.B., M.D.
(From The Coyne Campbell Clinic and Sanitarium)
OKLAHOMA CITY, OKLAHOMA

This report is made upon seven patients with bromide intoxication. In six of these, cortical hormone (Eschatin)† was administered. The data presented would indicate that this substance is effective in the elimination of bromide from the tissues when given in combination with sodium chloride. There also appears to be a more rapid clinical improvement than in those cases in w h i c h only sodium chloride is used in treatment.

†Eschatin was supplied by courtesy of Parke-Davis and Company. Appreciation is acknowledged for the services of Dr. Charles A. Smith and Mr. Allen Bronston who executed the technical part of this experimental work.

Thorn[1] et al, and Hartman[2] et al, have reported that upon the administration of cortical hormone there is a definite reduction in the excretion of sodium and chloride. This information was the basis for the empirical usage of cortical hormone.

A recent study by Gundry[3] presents detailed information upon 15 cases of bromide intoxication and is an excellent summary of the etiology, symptoms, diagnosis, prognosis and treatment of this condition. In his article a correlation between the level of serum bromide and mental symptoms was pointed out. Mild nervous manifestations occurred in individuals in which the serum bromide content was between 50 and 150 mgms. per 100 cc. of blood. Cases in which the bromide content was from 150 to 250 mgms. presented mild intoxication, weakness, restlessness, thick speech, anxiety outbreaks, and hallucinations. When the bromide content exceeded 250 mgms. the clinical picture was dominated by the symptoms characteristic of a toxic psychosis. In 10 of his cases the serum bromide upon admission ranged from 196 to 555 mgms. per 100 cc. Under sodium chloride treatment (4 to 10 Gm. daily), upon an average of about two weeks after admission, the serum bromide level ranged from 85 to 244 mgms. This indicates the slowness with which bromide is eliminated.

The following table presents results in six cases treated by intramuscular injections of 5 cc. of Eschatin daily in combination with 6 to 10 Gm. of sodium chloride by mouth or parenterally. In one case, no cortical hormone was given. In another case, cortical hormone was given 12 days after sodium chloride treatment had been carried out.

Eschatin was given in doses of 2½ cc. twice daily. In two cases there was a temporary increase in mental symptoms, characterized by more confusion, and a tendency toward coma. This condition is analogous to that which occurs in some instances in which sodium chloride is given intravenously.

In severe cases, sodium chloride given intravenously or subcutaneously in the form of normal saline solution is advisable. Cortical hormone, when given in conjunction with this method of administration neutralizes the severe reactions formerly reported, evidently because of the fact that chlorides are being rapidly taken into the tissues. It is advocated that sodium chloride be given subcutaneously or intravenously in conjunction with cortical hormone.

Empirically, it is also recommended that cortical hormone be given in all other types of toxic psychoses.

CONCLUSION

Upon the basis of this empirical data, it would appear that cortical hormone is of definite value in the hastening of the recovery from bromide intoxication when given in conjunction with sodium chloride. Toxic levels of serum bromide can be rapidly reduced to non-toxic ones from within two to four days under the influence of cortical hormone in combination with sodium chloride. It is also recommended that cortical hormone be used empirically in treatment of all cases of toxic psychoses.

BIBLIOGRAPHY

1. Thorn, Geo. W., Garbutt, Helen R., Hitchcock, Fred A., Hartman, Frank A.; Endocrinology, 21:207-213, 1937.
2. Hartman, Frank A., Lewis, Lena A., Toby, C. Gwendoline; Endocrinology, 22:207-213, 1938.
3. Gundry, Lewis T.: Bromide Intoxication, J.A.M.A., 113; 446. August 6th, 1939.

Case	Condition Upon Admission	Serum Bromide Upon Admission	Sodium Chloride Given	Eschatin Given	Subsequent Serum Bromide	Number of Days After Admission	Condition At That Time
1.	Severe bromide intoxication	400 mgms.	8-10 Gms. daily	None	200 mgms.	18	Still confused
2.	Mild intoxication	150 mgms.	6 Gms. daily	5 cc. per day	50 mgms.	2	Relieved of bromide intoxication
3.	Severe bromide intoxication	360 mgms.	6-10 Gms. daily	5 cc. per day	115 mgms.	4	Normal
4.	Severe bromide psychosis	360 mgms. 360 mgms.	6-10 Gms. daily 6-10 Gms. daily	None 5 cc. per day	157 mgms. 63 mgms.	12 14	Still confused Practically normal
5.	Severe bromide psychosis	350 mgms.	8-10 Gms. daily	5 cc. per day	80 mgms.	4	Relieved of bromide intoxication. Epilepsy.
6.	Moderate intoxication	200 mgms.	6-10 Gms. daily	5 cc. per day	60 mgms.	2	Relieved of bromide intoxication. Involutional psychosis.
7.	Severe intoxication with general paresis	165 mgms.	8-10 Gms. daily	5 cc. per day	105 mgms.	1	Relieved of bromide intoxication.

Routine Laboratory Examinations for Typhoid Fever and Dysentery Organisms

WM. D. HAYES, Dr. P. H., Director
RITA ROBINSON, Bacteriologist
Laboratories of the
Oklahoma State Health Department
OKLAHOMA CITY, OKLAHOMA

In the past years large numbers of people have been immunized against typhoid fever in Oklahoma. In fact so many have been immunized against the disease that the Widal or agglutination determination is not of as much value in aiding in making an early diagnosis as it originally was, in that many individuals could not give their family doctor correct information as to when and how long since they had received the immunization. It would require examinations and d e l a y in many cases to determine the difference between the agglutination produced by t y p h o i d fever and immunization.

Our o w n experience and observation prompts us to s t a t e that the laboratory can and will aid in the diagnosis, release and detection of carriers, if blood and stool specimens are submitted for cultural determination. Hence, we suggest and highly recommend that one week after onset of typhoid fever, or suspected typhoid fever, that 5 cc. of the patient's blood be submitted for cultural determinations. In our hands it has been our experience, as our records will show, to demonstrate the organisms in better than 90 per cent of the cases during the first week.

During the second week of the illness of the p a t i e n t a specimen of blood and a small portion of stool (about one-half inch square) be submitted to the laboratory so that both blood and stool may be cultured. After the second week, for the diagnosis, release and detection of carriers, we desire to have stool and urine submitted for bacteriological growth and determinations.

STOOL AND URINE CULTURE FOR ENTERIC DISEASE

How stool and urine specimens are submitted: Specimen is submitted to the lab-oratory in a two ounce screw cap, round, glass jar, containing 10 cc. of glycerol-lithium chloride solution.

Sodium chloride	6 gm.
Distilled water	700 cc.
Glycerol	300 cc.
Lithium chloride	5 gm.

Added stool specimen size of almond or about one-half inch in dimension.

Method of Procedure:

First Day Planting: Two plates of Wilson Blair's Bismuth sulfite agar (Difco), one plate of Desoxycholate citrate agar (Baltimore Biologicals) streaked. Approximately 10 gms. of stool specimen in 50 cc. flask containing 12½ cc. of Selenite F. Enrichment broth (Baltimore Biologicals).

Second Day: Desoxycholate citrate agar plates read. Desired colonies fished to Russell's Double sugar agar (Difco) slants. Streak and stab method. Two plates of B. Sulfite agar streaked from Selenite F. Enrichment broth.

Third Day: B. Sulfite Agar plates from first day planting read and desired colonies fished to Russell's Double Sugar slants.

Russell's Double s u g a r reaction read. The culture is gram-stained and, if pure, it is examined for motility. The culture is fished to eight tubes of semi-solid agar m e d i a, one of which contains dextrose, maltose, mannitol, l a c t o s e, saccharose, xylose, rhamnose and dulcitol.

Fourth Day: The carbohydrate reactions are read. If these are typical a tube agglutination test with the indicated positive anti-sera is set up. The stool specimen is then reported "(indicated organism enciting the disease) present."

The Bismuth sulfite agar plates from the second day are read and if positive colonies have appeared which have not been confirmed from previous plates. These are examined as above shown. The specimen is reported as "No (   ) present," if second plate shows no growth. A known B. Typhosus control is used with each set of bismuth sulfite plates and one plate incubated uninoculated.

A known B. dysenteriae Sonne and Flexnor control is used with each set of desoxycholate citrate agar.

Extreme care should be exercised to prevent overheating of Bismuth sulfite agar e i t h e r in storage or preparation of the media.

The known cultures are carried through the entire procedure in confirming the organisms present.

SUMMARY

1. For first and second week after onset of suspected case of typhoid fever, submit to the laboratory 5 cc. of the patient's blood for cultural determination.

2. Seven days and after onset of suspected case of typhoid fever, submit stool to the laboratory for bacteriological growth and determination.

3. For release of patient and detection of carriers in typhoid fever, submit stool specimen to the laboratory for bacteriological determinations.

4. For the detection of bacillary dysentery, submit a stool specimen to the laboratory for bacteriological determination.

-----------------o-----------------

New Books

TREATMENT IN GENERAL PRACTICE: 259 pages. Little, Brown and Company, 34 Beacon Street, Boston, Massachusetts, 1939. Cloth, $7.50.

Recently the British Medical Journal carried out an interesting experiment. A series of articles on treatment was published, each article written by a well-known clinical teacher thoroughly familiar with his subject. Later the various articles were gathered together and published in book form. There were two volumes to the series. The first dealt with treatment of the acute infectious diseases and of cardio-vascular disease; the second with treatment of more chronic conditions such as diseases of the nervous system, diseases of the blood and blood-forming apparatus, rheumatism, diseases of metabolism, and kidney diseases.

For the first time these two volumes are published in the United States and will make valuable collateral reading giving to us clear cut phases of treatment as carried out in England and by some of the leading authorities.

CLINICAL DIAGNOSIS BY L A B O R A T O R Y METHODS: By James Campbell Todd, Ph.B., M.D., Late Professor of Clinical Pathology, University of Colorado, School of Medicine; and Arthur Hawley Sanford, A.M., M.D., Professor of Clinical Pathology, University of Minnesota (The Mayo Foundation); Head of Division on Clinical Laboratories, Mayo Clinic. Ninth Edition, Thoroughly Revised. 841 pages with 368 illustrations, 29 in colors. Philadelphia and London: W. B. Saunders Company, 1939. Cloth, $6.00 net.

Clinical pathology has become a recognized specialty in medicine. Every year new methods that have been developed in research laboratories are added to the facilities of the clinical laboratory; consequently, the worker in this field must constantly grow in his knowledge of diagnostic procedures. But old and tried methods must not be forgotten or discarded unless they become obsolete.

In the preparation of this edition many changes have been considered necessary in order to make the book more valuable to students, teachers, physicians, and laboratory workers.

The description of colorimetric methods is no longer considered properly placed in the chapter on urinalysis; therefore, it has been transferred to the chapter on clinical chemistry. Some of the obsolete procedures in urinalysis have been deleted.

Among the new tests should be mentioned the technic for the determination of serum lipase, the technic for the determination of cevitamic acid and sulfanilamide in blood and urine.

In this edition are many new illustrations and the work in every way brought up to date.

CLINICAL GASTRO-ENTEROLOGY. By Horace Wendell Soper, M.D., St. Louis, Missouri. With 212 Illustrations. C. V. Mosby Co., St. Louis, 1939.

I quote the following sentence found on page 195 in the chapter on Ulcerative Colitis. "So many 'treatments' have been employed that I shall not describe them here, but will proceed at once with my own method." This sentence characterizes the attitude and literary style of the author in presenting the multitude clinical conditions found throughout the tract from the mouth to the anus. Only the essential facts and rational of the treatment of each condition is presented. Some of the author's pet treatments discussed are:

1. 10 per cent mercurochrome swab for most oral lesions.

2. Levin tube for gastric hemorrhage.

3. 10 per cent sodium sulphate enemas for hypotonic type of constipation.

4. Bismuth subgallate-calomel insufflation proceedure for ulcerative colitis.

5. Stovarsal for Bacillary or unexplained dysenteries.

6. Mag. Sulphate for gall-bladder drainage.

7. His aversion for raw or pasteurized milk in all his diets for gastric and colonic lesions.

Another feature of this book that adds immensely to its value, are the profuse roentgen illustrations of the various gastro-intestinal lesions. The X-ray prints are conveniently placed at the end of each chapter discussed. The prints in general are good and are representative of the lesions discussed in the chapter; they are of distinctive aid to the general practicioner to visualize some of the gastro-intestinal pathology by roentgen methods. Roentgen technique and fluoroscopic studies in diagnosis of alimentary lesions are not discussed. Neither does histology or pathology have any place in this book, because of the author's desire to make this book essentially clinical.

THE JOURNAL

OF THE

Oklahoma State Medical Association

Issued Monthly at McAlester, Oklahoma, under direction of the Council.

Copyright, 1939, by Oklahoma State Medical Association, McAlester, Oklahoma.

Vol. XXXII	DECEMBER	Number 12

Entered at the Post Office at McAlester, Oklahoma, as second-class matter under the act of March 3rd, 1879.

This is the official Journal of the Oklahoma State Medical Association. All communications should be addressed to The Journal of the Oklahoma State Medical Association, McAlester Clinic, McAlester, Oklahoma. $4.00 per year; 40c per copy.

The editorial department is not responsible for the opinions expressed in the original articles of contributors.

Reprints of original articles will be supplied at actual cost provided request for them is attached to manuscripts or made in sufficient time before publication.

Articles sent this Journal for publication and all those read at the annual meetings of the State Association are the sole property of this Journal. The Journal relies on each individual contributor's strict adherence to this well-known rule of medical journalism. In the event an article sent this Journal for publication is published before appearance in The Journal the manuscript will be returned to the writer.

Failure to receive The Journal should call for immediate notification of the Executive Secretary, at 210 Plaza Court, Oklahoma City.

Local news of possible interest to the medical profession, notes on removals, changes of addresses, births, deaths and weddings will be gratefully received.

Advertising of articles, drugs or compounds unapproved by the Council on Pharmacy of the A. M. A., will not be accepted.

Advertising rates will be supplied on application.

It is suggested that wherever possible members of the State Association should patronize our advertisers in preference to others as a matter of fair reciprocity.

Printed by News-Capital Company, McAlester.

EDITORIAL

OKLAHOMA CITY CLINICAL SOCIETY 1939 MEETING

G u e s t Speakers, attending physicians and exhibitors, all proclaim the 1939 meeting of the Oklahoma City Clinical Society a decided success. Increased interest, as evidenced by a larger registration, and the distance from which the conference drew attendants, speaks well for the continued growth and success of the Society. Guest speakers had heard of the high academic quality and marvelous precision of the meeting as far east as New York, and as far west as California; Associate members travelled from such distant states as Montana, Pennsylvania and California in order to attend the sessions. This is an indication of the widespread reputation of quality enjoyed by the conference.

The Oklahoma City Chamber of Commerce and the Biltmore Hotel gave splendid cooperation, and much of the early growth as well as the later success of the meeting can be credited to their fine support. The exhibitors, as usual, were enthusiastic and cooperative, and extended every effort to make this an outstanding session.

There is an unusually fine feeling of fellowship which amalgamates these many different factors, the guest speakers, the exhibitors, the Chamber of Commerce, the Biltmore Hotel and the attendants, that inspires them to work in close unity for a single purpose. It is this fellowship and cooperative harmony that will make the Annual Meeting of the Oklahoma City Clinical Society one of the most outstanding medical meetings in the nation.

---o---

READ THE ADVERTISING SECTION

Again we must call your attention to our advertisers—in other words the people who furnish the Journal income or the people who make this Journal possible. Our annual financial report will show you the truth of the above statement.

Now in return just what does the individual subscriber give the advertiser?

There is some very valuable information, boiled down to a few words in these advertisements. There is much to learn as to the application of new products and the use of modern equipment. You can improve your efficiency by reading the advertising section of the Journal.

Perhaps the most important fact relative to the advertising is that each product presented is Council Approved. Our national advertising is procured through the Cooperative Advertising Bureau which you know is supervised by the American Medical Association and this Bureau will of course accept no product without Council Approval. Our position relative to acceptance of advertising has forced some firms to submit their products for Council action so that they might use our publication for advertising purposes. Their detail men become tired of being asked the question, "Is your product Council Approved?"

There are yet many firms who have not qualified and their detail men are calling upon the physicians of Oklahoma. We cannot be sure of the standard of the products they present and there is no good reason why we should accept them. It costs nothing to submit a product to the various councils of the American Medical Association and we feel their action or stamp of approval can be relied upon by our readers.

It is the same argument presented in previous editorials on this subject; read the advertisements and patronize our advertisers.

---o---

Group Hospitalization Committee Report

A Group Hospital service plan for Oklahoma on a mutual non-profit basis is rapidly approaching reality since the recent meeting of the Oklahoma State Hospital Association in Oklahoma City and its appointment of a committee composed of Dr. L. E. Emanuel of Chickasha, Sister Mechtildis Eickholt of Oklahoma City, R. L. Loy, Jr., of Oklahoma City, J. A. Bivins, Jr., of Ardmore, Dr. G. D. Funk of El Reno, and E. U. Benson of Cushing, to work with the committee from the Council of the Medical Association composed of Councilors V. O. Tisdal, A. S. Risser, Philip M. McNeill, James Stevenson, and J. A. Walker.

The n e c e s s i t y for such an organization was brought forcibly to the attention of the Council of the Association when, in June, it was discovered that there were more than 10 different plans of one type or another having a charter to do business in the State of Oklahoma under the Mutual Casualty Company Act of 1931. Section 10750, subsection 3 or 7 of this act allowed the forming of a mutual non-profit company upon the presentation to the Insurance Board of the proper legal documents, together with financial assets of five times the amount of a single liability under one contract. As an example, if a contract called for 30 days' hospitalization at $5 a day, the total liability under the contract would be $150. Five times this amount, $750, was then all that was necessary for the formation of a company. Investigation at the Insurance Department disclosed the astounding fact that the majority of the companies with charters were operating with an original capitalization of less than $1,000.

With these startling facts known, together with the increasing public demand for this type of coverage (and the majority of cases coming from groups that are in the income field most widely needing to have hospitalization), President W. A. Howard appointed a committee composed of V. K. Allen of Tulsa, John Carson of Shawnee, and John E. Heatley of Oklahoma City, to make investigations of other known group plans that had met with success and had been properly administered.

This committee made detailed study of the vast majority of plans in operation in the United States, and also gave extremely careful study to the recommendations of the American Hospital Association, the American Medical Association, and the American College of Surgeons. After careful deliberation of many weeks, the committee submitted its report to the Council of the Association. The present Committee of the Council was then appointed to continue study of the subject, as well as to consider the proper and most expedient way of organizing a plan that would eventually be statewide in coverage, have civic appeal, and be non-profit in every sense of the word.

This committee met numerous times, thrashing out many details, and on September 21 invited leading business men, members of the Council of the Association, officers of the Hospital Association, and other leading hospital owners, to a dinner and hear the subject discussed by Walter R. McBee, of St. Louis, associate director of Group Hospital Service, Inc., probably the most successful plan in operation today.

The following night Mr. McBee appeared before the officers, members of the board, and the Insurance Committee of the Tulsa County Medical Society. The response from these two meetings was so enthusiastic that, immediately, the Committee from the Council felt justified in requesting the officers of the Oklahoma State Hospital Association, that they be allowed to meet with them and discuss the advisability of working out together a plan of organization and a contract that would be acceptable to both organizations since it should have the support of both organizations.

This request met with enthusiastic approval from the officers of the Hospital Association, and from the meeting of the two Associations came tentative approval of the principles of the undertaking. However, the officers of the Hospital Association requested that, since the meeting of the State Hospital Association was only a few weeks away, no definite action be taken until after their meeting. Hence, on November 16 and 17, the dates of the Hospital Association meeting, the Council of the Association was called in session to consider any proposals that might come from the Hospital Association. The latter, after careful and lengthy deliberation, instructed its president to appoint a commitee to continue study with the Committee from the Medical Association on the organization of such a program.

These two committees are now in a position to work out final details for the formation of a program that will give hospitalization to the people of Oklahoma on a basis that they can afford to maintain. The final results of this six months' study will be announced as soon as possible.

A brief survey of the original recommendations of the first committee, and which no doubt the final deliberations will follow basically, are that the board of governors of the plan will have its representatives picked from the Hospital Association, the Medical Association, and the laity. The officers of the organization then will be picked from this board and will be men or women who are philanthropic and public-spirited, who will serve without pay, and who will, by virtue of their position in the business and civic world, lend honesty and integrity to the plan, as well as their proven ability in business judgment and management.

This procedure clearly takes the Medical and Hospital Associations out of the insurance business, as neither will invest any of their funds in the capitalization of the company. Neither will there be any members of either Association in its employment.

The entire program and the part played by the Association in giving impetus to the plan has always been and will continue to be the effort of the Medical Association to give to the people the most feasible and economical care from a medical standpoint that is in direct ratio with progressive medicine and business and financial stability.

Secretary-Editors Conference

This meeting held at A.M.A. Headquarters, Chicago, November 17 and 18, was attended by both the Secretary-Treasurer-Editor and Executive Secretary.

The time was largely taken up with discussion of two subjects. First—Distribution of Medical Care. Second—Legislative Problems.

Addresses of great interest and broad in scope were given by Dr. Rock Sleyster, President, and Dr. Nathan B. VanEtten, President Elect.

Medical service plans were presented from the states of New Jersey, Michigan, Washington and Pennsylvania. Following this presentation there was liberal discussion as to the strong and weak points of each plan, it appearing that no plan can be universally adopted as it takes a different pattern to fit different localities with their vastly varying conditions. Their presentation would be difficult to abstract in this report but will be available either in The Journal of the A.M.A. or in pamphlet form.

The Wagner Health Bill was discussed by W. C. Woodward, Director of the Bureau of Legal Medicine and Legislation, and he feels that there is no doubt about the consideration of this bill in the next session of Congress. We must be prepared for this and make our plans to do everything possible to see to it that the private practice of medicine is not destroyed. It means the expenditure of time and money to bring the true and correct information to the people of this country relative to the accomplishments and methods of the Medical Profession. It is not for the paid executives alone to carry on this work; each State and County Society must be properly organized and what is still most important, the individual physician must accept his portion of the responsibility.

At the Editor's Banquet Dr. Samuel J. Kopetzky of New York was the speaker and presented much food for thought to the Editors relative to the conduct of a Medical Journal. His address was liberally discussed and many valuable ideas were presented.

The Platform of the American Medical Association was presented to the conference and discussed by Dr. Fishbein. The Platform is as follows and the discussion will be published in the January issue of the Journal. This discussion is published in the November 25th issue of the Journal of the A.M.A.

The Platform of the American Medical Association
The American Medical Association advocates:

1. The establishment of an agency of the federal government under which shall be coordinated and administered all medical and health functions of the federal government exclusive of those of the army and navy.

2. The allotment of such funds as the Congress may make available to any state in actual need, for the prevention of disease, the promotion of health and the care of the sick on proof of such need.

3. The principle that the care of the public health and the provision of medical service to the sick is primarily a local responsibility.

4. The development of a mechanism for meeting the needs of expansion of preventive medical services with local determination of needs and local control of administration.

5. The extension of medical care for the indigent and the medically indigent with local determination of needs and local control of administration.

6. In the extension of medical services to all the people, the utmost utilization of qualified medical and hospital facilities already established.

7. The continued development of the private practice of medicine, subject to such changes as may be necessary to maintain the quality of medical services and to increase their availability.

8. Expansion of public health and medical services consistent with the American system of democracy.

———o———

Fellowships In the Medical Sciences of the National Research Council

These fellowships, administered by the Medical Fellowship Board of the National Research Council, are open to citizens of the United States or Canada who possess an M.D. or a Ph.D. degree, or equivalent experience and achievement. They are intended for recent graduates who, as a rule, are not more than 30 years of age.

The fellowships are designed to provide research discipline for men and women who are fitted for medical investigation. Fellows may choose any branch of medicine or public health for their ultimate career, but at present candidates (otherwise suitable) will be favored who plan to specialize in one of the preclinical sciences or to approach clinical medicine and surgery through identification with one of the sciences.

The fellowships are not granted to any institution or university. The choice of place to work is left to the fellow, subject to the approval of the Fellowship Board; but, as a rule, fellows will be expected to do their work in this country. The appointments are for full time and no other remunerative or routine work is permitted.

Ordinarily, before sending his application to the Board, a candidate should have assurance from the person with whom he wishes to work that he is acceptable. It is further requested that a fellow be charged no fees or tuition by the institution where he chooses to work.

The annual stipends are determined by individual circumstances and by cost of living in the location of study. The usual amount is from $1,600 to $2,400 per annum. The fellowships are usually granted for one year, but they may be renewed. Stipends may be increased on account of additional dependents, or for other cogent reasons, but only at the beginning of a new fellowship year. Fellows are chosen at annual meetings of the Medical Fellowship Board in February, and applications to receive consideration at these meetings must be filed on or before January 1. Appointments may begin on any date determined by the Board.

Further particulars concerning these fellowships may be obtained on request.

Address communications to the Secretary of the Medical Fellowship Board, National Research Council, 2101 Constitution Avenue, Washington, D. C.

———o———

Important Notice

Dr. J. E. McDonald, Chairman of the General Surgical Section for the State Medical Association, requests that members desiring to present papers before this section at the May meeting submit titles and short abstracts of the proposed papers.

Send these to Dr. J. E. McDonald, 309 Medical Arts Building, Tulsa, Oklahoma, not later than January 15, 1940. When these titles and abstracts are received, they will be reviewed by the General Surgical Section Committee, and a diversified program selected therefrom.

Those whose papers are selected will be notified shortly after January 15 so that they will have ample time to complete their material for presentation at the annual meeting to be held in Tulsa May 6, 7 and 8.

Physicians Attending the Meeting of the Southern Medical Association at Memphis

The following Oklahoma Physicians attended the Meeting of the Southern Medical Association at Memphis and report a splendid meeting with fine scientific and entertainment features:

Allen, Victor K., Tulsa.
Alexander, Robt. L., Okmulgee.
Anderson, Robt. M., Shawnee.
Andreskowski, W. T., Ryan.
Balyeat, Ray M., Oklahoma City.
Barnes, Harry E. (wife), Tahlequah.
Baylor, Richard A. (wife), Fairfax.
Bell, A. H. (wife), Oklahoma City.
Boadway, F. W., Ardmore.
Bondurant, Chas P. (wife), Oklahoma City.
Bonnell, W. LeRoy, Chickasha.
Byrum, James M., Shawnee.
Cameron, P. B., Tulsa.
Canada, Ernest A., Ada.
Chambers, Claude S., Seminole.
Collopy, Paul Jos., Oklkahoma City.
Cook, W. Albert, Tulsa.
Cooper, F. M., Oklahoma City.
Cotteral, John Robt., Henryetta.
Cottrel, John R., Oklahoma City.
Crawford, Paul H., Oklahoma City.
Curry, Jas. F. (wife), Sapulpa.
Darwin, D. W. (wife), Woowward.
Doler, Calhoun (wife, daughter and son-in-law), Clinton.
Denny, E. Rankin, Tulsa.
Drummond, N. Robert, Oklahoma City.
Dyer, Isadore (wife), Tahlequah.
Eastland, William E., Oklahoma City.
Ellis, Stephen S., Oklahoma City.
Emanuel, Roy E. (wife), Chickasha.
Ferguson, E. Gordon, Oklahoma City.
Fishman, C. J. (wife), Oklkahoma City.
Fite, W. Pat (wife), Muskogee
Foerster, Hervey, A. (wife), Oklahoma City.
Gibson, R. Berry (wife), Ponca City.
Gillis, Eugene A. (wife and daughter), Oklkahoma City.
Gentry, Raymond C. (wife), Bartlesville.
Glomset, John L. (wife), Oklahoma City.
Goldfain, E., Oklahoma City.
Harbison, J. E. (wife), Oklahoma City.
Haralson, Charles H., Tulsa.
Hasslser, F. (wife), Shawnee.
Hassler, Grace C., Oklahoma City.
Hazel, Onis G. (wife), Oklahoma City.
Hollingsworth, James I., Waurika.
Howard, R. M., Oklahoma City.
Hudson, H. Hackney, Enid.
Hudson, Walter Scott, Okmulgee.
Hull, Wayne M., Oklahoma City.
Jeter, Hugh G., Oklahoma City.
Keen, Frank M., Shawnee.
Lain, Everett S., Oklahoma City.
Lamb, Ellis, Clinton.
Lamb, John Henderson (wife), Oklahoma City.
Long, Wendell, Oklkahoma City.
Love, Robt. S. (wife), Oklahoma City.
McBride, Earl D., Oklkahoma City.
McBurney, C. H. (wife), Clinton.
McFarling, A. C., Shawnee.
McHenry, L. C. (wife), Oklkahoma City.
McKinney, Garland Young, Henryetta.
McKinney, G. Y., Oklahoma City.
Mechling, George S. (wife), Oklahoma City.
Messenbaugh, Jos. Fife (wife), Oklahoma City.
Moor, H. D., Oklahoma City.
Morrison, Henry C., Oklahoma City.
Morrow, J. A. (wife), Oklahoma City.
Munding, L. A. (wife), Tulsa.
Murdoch, R. L., Oklahoma City.
Osborn, Geo. R. (wife), Tulsa.
Pace, L. Rio, Seminole.
Patterson, Robert U., Oklahoma City.
Phelps, Malcom E. (wife), El Reno.
Pounders, Carroll M., Oklahoma City.

Renegar, J. Frank, Tuttle.
Ritzhaupt, Louis H., Guthrie.
Rollins, J. Stephens (wife), Prague.
Ross, Saml. P. (wife), Ada.
Salomon, Albert L., Oklahoma City.
Schreck, Philip M. (wife), Tulsa.
Shepard, Robt. M., Tulsa.
Showman, Winfred A. (wife), Tulsa.
Smith, Carlton E., Henryetta.
Smith, Ned R. (wife), Tulsa.
Stevenson, James, Tulsa.
Stough, Austin Robert (wife), Tecumseh.
Stuart, Frank A., Tulsa.
Trent, Robert I (wife), Oklahoma City.
Turner, Henry H. (wife), Oklahoma City.
Van Sandt, Max M., Wewoka.
Vernon, William C. (wife), Okmulgee.
Wails, Theodore G. (wife), Oklahoma City.
Walker, I. D., Tonkawa.
Watkins, Barton H., Hobart.
Weaver, Wm. Niebuhr, Muskogee.
West, W. K. (wife), Oklkahoma City.
Wickham, M. M., Norman.
Widener, Saml. Sherman, Pond Creek.
Wiley, A. Ray (wife), Tulsa.
Wilkins, Harry (wife), Oklahoma City.
Willie, James A. (wife), Oklahoma City.
Word, L. B. (wife), Bartlesville.
Worten, Divonis, Pawhuska.

---o---

Examinations
American Board of Obstetrics and Gynecology

The written examination and review of case histories (Part I) for Group B candidates will be held in the various cities of the United States and Canada on Saturday, January 6, 1940, at 2 p.m. Formal notice of the place of examination will be sent each candidate several weeks in advance of the examination date. No candidate will be admitted to examination whose examination fee has not been paid at the Secretary's Office. Candidates who successfully complete the Part I examination proceed automatically to the Part II examination held in June, 1940. Receipt of Group B applications for the current examination (January 6, 1940) closed October 4, 1939.

The general oral and pathological examinations (Part II) for all candidates (Groups A and B) will be conducted by the entire Board, meeting in Atlantic City, N. J., on June 8, 9, 10 and 11, 1940, immediately prior to the annual meeting of the American Medical Association in New York.

Application for admission to Group A, Part II, examinations must be on file in the Secretary's Office not later than March 15, 1940.

After January 1, 1942, there will be only one classification of candidates, and all will be required to take the Part I and Part II examinations.

For further information and application blanks, address Dr. Paul Titus, Secretary, 1015 Highland Building, Pittsburgh (6), Pennsylvania.

---o---

New Woods County Officers Reported First

First reports of newly elected county officers to reach the office of the Executive Secretary came from Dr. O. E. Templin, secretary of the Woods County Society.

They are as follows: President, Dr. Theodore D. Benjegerdes of Beaver; Vice President, Dr. Charles A. Royer, Alva; Secretary, Dr. Oscar E. Templin of Alva; and Delegate, Dr. Daniel B. Ensor of Hopeton. The officers were elected at the November 27 meeting.

Following the election, Dr. C. O. Von Wedel of Oklahoma City spoke on "The Role of Plastic Surgery in Injuries of the Face;" Dr. Paul Colonna of Oklahoma City, talked on "Acute Osteomyelitis;" and Dr. R. L. Noel of Oklahoma City used as his subject, "Fractures About the Elbow Joint."

State Licenses to Physicians

Physicians licensed during the period from January 10, 1939, to August 24, 1939, to practice in Oklahoma, and their present locations, are as follows:

Alwyn Travers Kornblee, Kansas City, Mo.; John L. Scott (colored), Boley; James France Shaw, Wetumka; George Warren Scott, Tishomingo; J. H. Blackburn, Denison, Texas; Howard C. Hopps, Fairview; Fred B. Cooper, McAlester; Thomas Taylor Beeler, Jr., San Diego, Calif.; Allen Grant Flythe, Durant; Clayton Hamilton Halverson, Tulsa; Stephen Stuart Ellis, Oklahoma City; Weldon Doak Blassingame, Ardmore; Dan M. Forbes, Texhoma; Paul B. Rice, Oklahoma City; Chester R. Seba, Oklahoma City.

Herbert Berzelious Shields, Wauwatosa, Wis.; William Henry Doyle, Louisville, Ky.; John Robert Davenport, Holdenville; Murble Henry Pearson, Perryton, Texas; John Williams Records, St. Louis, Mo.; Ray Ulman Northrip, Oklahoma City; T. Willard Pratt, Cheyenne; Rugie R. Coates, Duncan; William Randolph Cheatwood, Oklahoma City; Alexander Shadid, Elk City; Gervais Dean Smith, Picher; John Banner Terry, Wewoka; Warren Beall Poole, Oklahoma City; William Claude McCurdy, Jr., Purcell; Charles Earnest McArthur, Seattle, Wash.; John B. Rafter, Muskogee; Joseph Cannon Hibbett, Jr., Oklahoma City; Kieffer Dixon Davis, Nowata; William Polk Longmire, Jr., Sapulpa; Leslie Thompson Hamm, Oklahoma City; Bernard Eugene Bullock, Clinton.

John Russell Hubbard, Oklahoma City; Raymond A. Williams, Manhattan, Mont.; Earle W. Warren, Pasadena, Calif.; Dora W. Stevenson, Stillwater; Troy Frank Long, Okemah; Earl Morris Lusk, Tulsa; William Corder Alston, Jr., Vicksburg, Miss.; Meyer Kurzner, Oklahoma City; James Daniel Huskins, Oklahoma City; Sam T. Moore, Oklahoma City; Cecil Ewing Miller, Washington, D. C.; Hugh Malcolm Galbraith, Oklahoma City; David Shapiro, Tulsa; Frederick James Smith, Okeene; Percival LeMon Clark, Oklahoma City; Herbert Marvin Sanford, Perryton, Texas; John J. Cawley, Jr., Oakland, Calif.; Roy Junior Melinder, Claremore; Clyde Vincent Kern, Denver, Colo.; Clarence A. Buttran, Oklahoma City; James Ralph Ricks, Jr., Oklahoma City; Robert William Choice, Wakita.

Homer Clark Wheeler, Oklahoma City; Ivan Edward Bigler, Claremore; John Philip Haddock, Norman; Rheba LaLora Huff, Norman; Marvin Elkins, Orange, N. J.; Howard Angus, Lawton; Ernest A. Henderson, Birmingham, Ala.; Mack Irvin Shanholtz, Seminole; Rupard Glenn Smith, Minneapolis, Minn.; Victor David Mills, Portland, Ore.; Gilbert W. Tracy, Cheyenne; Rudolph Henry Duewall, Sentinel; Robert Milton Hall, Denver, Colo.; Robert Theodore Sturm, Detroit, Mich.; William Harrell Webster, Ada; Woodrow Louis Pickhardt, Chicago, Ill.; Eugene B. Ley, Detroit, Mich.; Murray Everette Gibbens, Oklahoma City; William Charles McClure, Oklahoma City; Elmon Laurence Collette, Dewey; Philip Crane Risser, Blackwell.

─────o─────

Commonwealth Fellowships

Announcement has been made by directors of the Commonwealth Fund of the eight fellowships which have been awarded for postgraduate work at Tulane University, New Orleans, La., beginning January 8, 1940.

The physicians receiving the fellowships are: Dr. William G. Dunnington of Cherokee; Dr. Ishmael F. Stephenson of Alva; Dr. Malcom E. Phelps of El Reno; Dr. Wendell L. Smith of Drumright; Dr. Hugh H. Monroe of Lindsay; Dr. Clella M. Hodgson of Kingfisher; Dr. Battey B. Coker of Durant; and Dr. George K. Hemphill of Pawhuska.

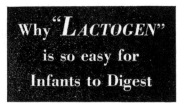
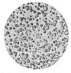

Southern Oklahoma Medical

The Southern Oklahoma Medical Association held its 45th quarterly session at Hotel Ardmore, Ardmore, Tuesday, December 5, under auspices of Carter County Medical Society. The association covers the counties of Caddo, Carter, Cleveland, Comanche, Cotton, Garvin, Grady, Jefferson, Johnson, Love, Marshall, McClain, Murray, Pontotoc, Pottawatomie, Seminole and Stephens.

Subjects featuring the program included: "The Relation of the Medical Profession to the Public," Dr. John L. Holland, Madill (with general discussion). "A Classification of Nervous and Mental Diseases Suitable to the General Practitioner," Dr. Charles L. Rayburn, Central State Hospital, Norman (general discussion). "Obstetrics," Dr. E. N. Smith, Post Graduate Instructor, American Medical Association. "Inhalation Therapy," Dr. Wayne M. Hull, Oklahoma City (general discussion). "Recent Development in Psychiatric Treatment," Dr. Arthur J. Schwenkenberg, Dallas, Texas (general discussion). "Interpretation of Heart Murmurs," Dr. George L. Carlisle, Dallas, Texas (general discussion).

Dinner was served at 6:30 at the Ardmore Hotel with entertainment by Douglas High School Quartette, and was enjoyed by all.

The sessions of the Southern Oklahoma Medical Association are always well attended and are a valued source of information and inspiration to its membership.

---o---

Basic Science Examinations

Examinations in the basic sciences are held twice a year, in the months of May and November, the dates being set by the state board of examiners, according to Dr. J. D. Osborn, Jr., secretary.

Those desiring to take the examination should apply for application blanks to the Secretary of the State of Oklahoma, the Hon. C. C. Childers, State Capitol, Oklahoma City.

Examination fees are $15, to be paid to the secretary, Dr. Osborn, at the time of entrance to the examination room. Personal checks will not be accepted.

---o---

Army Has Medical Post Openings

As a result of recent expansion of the United States Army, there is an opportunity for suitable young medical men to apply for reserve commissions as first lieutenants and obtain active detail at once, or for reserve corps officers to obtain extended duty.

They must be graduates of a Class "A" medical school and have had internship, or its equivalent in actual practice. At present, an opening exists for two men for duty at Fort Sill.

---o---

Editorial Notes—Personal and General

Members of the Woods County Medical Society furnished the program for Garfield county physicians in their late November dinner meeting at the Hotel Youngblood in Enid. Dr. D. B. Fensor of Hopeton presided, and talks were made by Dr. C. A. Traverse and Dr. C. A. Royer, both of Alva. Thirty-five doctors attended.

Organization of the medical staff of Stillwater's new $120,000 municipal hospital, which was opened in November, was near completion late last month. The newly elected executive board consists of Dr. C. E. Sexton, president; Dr. L. A. Cleverdon, vice president; and Dr. Powell E. Fry, secretary-treasurer.

Among the state doctors commissioned as first lieutenants in the regular army medical corps are Dr. Cannon A. Owen of Oklahoma City, who was assigned to Fort Crockett, Galveston, Texas; Dr. William H. Amspacher of Lawton, also assigned to Fort Crockett; and Dr. Glenn J. Collins of McAlester, to West Virginia.

Dr. David W. Gillick, superintendent and physician in charge of the Shawnee Indian Sanatorium, has been appointed district medical director for district No. 5 of the U. S. Indian Service, succeeding Dr. Walter S. Stevens, whose death occurred recently. Dr. Gillick's territory includes all of Oklahoma, Kansas, Mississippi, North Carolina and Florida, with offices in Oklahoma City. He will be succeeded at the sanatorium by Dr. Ralph M. Alley, formerly physician in charge of the Indian hospital at Pine Ridge, North Dakota.

Dr. Henry H. Turner appeared on the program of the Mid-Continent Dental Association meeting in St. Louis on October 4. He spoke on the "Role of Endocrinology in Dental Medicine."

Dr. Rex Bolend has recently moved his office from 1010 Medical Arts Building, Oklahoma City, to 1205, same building.

Dr. George H. Kimball was guest speaker at the Cleveland County Medical Society Meeting November 9, 1939. His subject was "Plastic Surgery."

---o---

OBITUARIES

Dr. George N. Bilby

Dr. George N. Bilby, who had served as state commissioner of public health for four years during the administration of William H. Murray, died November 26 in the Edward J. Hines Memorial Hospital for war veterans near Chicago. He was 71 years old.

Dr. Bilby came to Oklahoma in 1894 from Louisville, Ky., where he attended the school of medicine, and lived first at Cushing and later at Stroud. He moved to Alva in 1899, where he maintained his residence the remainder of his life.

During the World war, he served as a medical officer for 13 months. Surviving are his wife and a daughter, Miss Afton Bilby of Alva; and two sons, Lee and Paul, both of Pearidge, Ark.

Funeral services were held at Alva November 29, with the Rev. G. A. Parkhurst, pastor of the Alva Methodist church, officiating. Burial was at Alva.

---o---

Resolution

Dr. T. O. Crawford, Dewey, Oklahoma, born August 5, 1873, at Buckner, Illinois. Died Friday, October 20, 1939.

He attended the Southern Teachers College, Carbondale, Illinois, Washington University, St. Louis, Missouri, and University of Southern California at Pasadena. He was a graduate of the University of Colorado Medical School.

Dr. Crawford practiced medicine at Bay, Arkansas, Beggs, Bartlesville and Dewey, Oklahoma.

He is survived by his widow, Elizabeth Severns Crawford. His sons, T. O. Crawford, Jr., and Dr. G. W. Crawford preceded him in death.

Dr. Crawford specialized in the practice of Urology, and his ability was recognized by his fellow practitioners. He was a conscientious student of medicine.

Be it resolved by the Washington County Medical Society that a copy of the foregoing written expression of our esteem be placed in the minutes of the County Society and a copy be mailed to the office of the State Medical Association Journal and a copy be sent to the widow of the deceased.

Adopted unanimously.

Forest S. Etter, M.D.
E. E. Beechwood, M.D.

ABSTRACTS : REVIEWS : COMMENTS
and CORRESPONDENCE

SURGERY AND GYNECOLOGY
Abstracts, Reviews and Comments from
LeRoy Long Clinic
714 Medical Arts Building, Oklahoma City

The McClure-Aldrich Test in Water Balance Following Operation: Howard C. Hopps, B.S., M.D., Chicago, Illinois, and Frederick Christopher, B.S., M.D., F.A.C.S., Evanston, Illinois; Surgery, Gynecology and Obstetrics, November, 1939, Vol. 69, page 637.

There is a brief concise review of the excellent work done upon water balance by Coller and Maddock but these writers feel that the quantitative measurements of intake and output as described by Coller and Maddock are involved beyond the scope of the average hospital.

They point out that the usual guides in the management of water balance after operation are: (a) the clinical picture; (b) the urinary output; (c) quantitative measurements of intake and output; (d) the erythrocyte count; (e) the hemoglobin determination; and (f) the blood protein level. The clinical picture of the dry skin and dry tongue is unfortunately too familiar and should never be allowed to develop in the surgical patient to the point where it is clinically recognizable.

While sodium must be sufficiently replaced when lost by vomiting, its too liberal use in physiological saline or Ringer's solution as a routine fluid for intravenous infusion frequently brings about an oversufficiency of sodium, sometimes to the extent that edema is clinically evident.

With these thoughts in mind the authors have attempted a study on seven patients using the McClure-Aldrich test after operation in an effort to determine its value as a guide to the state of hydration.

This test consists of a measurement of the disappearance time of an artificial injected wheal of normal saline. The test was at first applied in cases of nephritis in an effort to determine the thirst of the subcutaneous tissue and thus estimate the severity, prognosis, and progress of the disease. Since that time it has received wider application and has been used in the study of vascular disease, cardiac failure, toxemia of pregnancy, scarlet fever, and other diseases. Until this time its use has been generally limited to those conditions in which edema plays a part, to measure the edema and detect it before it is clinically evident. The authors admit that there is considerable dispute about the mechanism of the test.

It is generally accepted, however, that disappearance of intradermal wheal is due almost solely to a dispersement of the fluid into the interstitial spaces and cells and that the length of time that this transfer takes, as measured by the disappearance of the wheal, is inversely proportional to the tissue avidity for water.

In the cases studied the management of water balance after operation was carried out independently of the McClure Aldrich test as a guide.

The test was made with an intradermal injection of 0.2 cubic centimeter of normal saline solution on the arms and chest with tests performed four to two hours before operation, two to four hours after operation, and thence every 24 hours at approximately the same time each day until a near normal fluid balance was considered established.

In their cases the test was found to be a sensitive and reliable index to the state of hydration. It was also found to be a useful guide to the optimal fluid administrations, provided the electrolytic balance was taken into consideration and in patients who were receiving large amounts of physiological saline solution and had developed slight edema from too much sodium, the test must be discounted.

"Although this series is too small to be conclusive, the McClure-Aldrich test appears to be a valuable adjunct to the clinical appearance of the patient, to the intake and output studies, and to the blood studies in the estimation of hydration after operation."

Comment: Water balance is recognized as of tremendous value in patients who are to be operated upon and those who are in their postoperative course. The extent of dehydration at operation was markedly demonstrated by the work of Coller and Maddock. All means which can give a more accurate idea as to the optimal fluid administration in order to overcome this dehydration are important.

While all of the usual guides of the management of water balance after operation cannot be neglected in any way, it is interesting to have the McClure-Aldrich test advanced as an additional simple means of directing our judgement as to the administration of fluids. As the authors have cautioned, the electrolytic balance must be duly considered in evaluating the results of this simple test.

Wendell Long.

"The Maintenance of Nutrition in Surgical Patients, With a Description of the Orojejunal Method of Feeding." By Alfred Stengel, Jr., A.B., M.D., and I. S. Ravdin, B.S., M.D., Philadelphia, Pa. Surgery, Vol. 6, October, 1939, page 511-519.

The nutrition of the surgical patient has become of increasing importance to the surgeon since it has been shown that a variety of complications following anesthesia and operation are the result of prolonged nutritional disturbances. It has been shown that the liver with a high carbohydrate-protein store is the one that is best prepared to withstand the insult of a volatile or lipid solvent anesthetic.

Ravdin and his co-workers have found by experimental and clinical studies that gastric emptying time is greatly prolonged in hypoproteinemia, even in the intact stomach and even though there is no deficiency of any known accessory foodstuff. They have also found that hypoproteinemia is associated with a delay in fibroplasia in the dog and have suggested that this condition may be a factor in wound disruption in surgical patients.

Not only is there frequently a deficiency in the primary foodstuffs, but many of the patients coming for operation also have a subclinical or clinical deficiency of certain of the vitamins. A deficiency in the B complex results in prolongation of the period of emptying of a water-barium meal from the stomach. The vitamin C deficiency results in a marked delay in wound healing. The use of vitamin K and bile salts in overcoming the prothrombin deficiency of patients with obstructive jaundice is still another example of the importance of nutrition in surgical patients. Hypoproteinemia may cause and accentuate the edema around a newly formed gastroenteric anastomosis, so as to mimic in every way a technical d e f e c t of the anastomosis.

These complications of surgical patients, many of which were previously explained on a mechanical basis, have greatly increased the interest of the surgeons in the state of nutrition of patients who are to be subjected to operation.

A high carbohydrate-protein dietary is the most satisfactory method of supplying the primary nutritional requirements of the surgical patient, without increasing the hazards of anesthesia and operation.

The oral method is not only the method of choice for the administration of carbohydrate, protein, and the necessary fat, but it is also a very satisfactory route for the administration of the accessory food-stuffs, the vitamins. Ravdin believes that a diet which contains 60 to 80 per cent carbohydrates, 20 to 30 per cent protein, and five to ten per cent fat in total calories is satisfactory. He believes that the level of fat in the diet should be kept as low as possible, for a supply of hepatic glucogen is effective in preventing necrosis of the liver only if the hepatic lipid concentration is reduced as the result of the glucogen deposition. During the period of oral feeding, the intravenous use of glucose is of value only for the effect it has in sparing protein stores, because the total calories available from 3,000 c.c. of a five per cent glucose solution are only 600, which is about one-third of the basal caloric requirements.

As the result of anorexia or obstruction adequate oral feeding is often not possible. If the nutritional state of the patient is such that a major operation is extremely hazardous, it is at times wise to perform a jejunostomy to feed the patient. However, the drainage of the stomach for several days by the method of Wangensteen frequently results in the disappearance of some of the edema associated with the obstruction so that a Levin tube will pass into the jejunum. If this can be brought about intensive orojejunal feeding can be begun.

Where feeding is carried out after a gastric resection or simple gastroenterostomy, the special Abbott gastrojejunal tube is passed into the distal loop of jejunum before closing the abdomen. The Abbott tube permits of suction from the stomach through one lumen and feeding into the jujunum through the other.

Either before or after operation, as the case may be, a feeding mixture can be administered through the tube. The feeding mixture used by the authors is a peptone hydrolysate supplied by Merck and Company. The ratio of amino nitrogen to total nitrogen of this preparation is 1 to 1.87. This peptone is put in solution in boiling water and varying amounts of glucose are added, depending upon the concentration of protein and carbohydrate desired in the final feeding mixture. In addition they daily add sufficient sodium choloride to maintain a normal plasma chloride concentration. With this method intravenous fluid and salt administration is not required and the patient can be supplied sufficient calories for energy requirements and for maintaining or replenishing a protein deficiency.

It has been the author's experience that the early introduction of a feeding mixture into the distal jejunum results in the earlier return of peristaltic activity after the operation. They have been impressed by the smoothness of the convalescence and by the fact that the patients did not request food even though oral jejunal feeding in some instances has been continued for as long as 14 days after operation and the caloric intake has not been high. During this period of time, fluid and electrolyte balance, as a rule, can be maintained without resort to intravenous administration. This is of some importance for it has been their experience that phlebitis frequently occurred where prolonged intravenous therapy, especially glucose, is maintained. The injudicious intravenous use of large amounts of sodium chloride in the postoperative period frequently precipitates edema in a patient who would not have developed this complication had nutrition been maintained and had not the water and salt intake been excessive. Ravdin believes that too much emphasis has been placed on the fluid and salt requirements of these patients and too little on associated factors which play in important part in keeping fluids in the blood vessels.

The method need not be used in all cases for not all patients have suffered prolonged nutritional deficits. It can be used, however, in every patient subjected to a gastroenteric anastomosis where suction drainage is to be carried out after operation, for in them it simplifies the postoperative management since the nutritional requirements of the patient can be more adequately fulfilled.

Warren Poole.

Cysts of the Thyroid—Observations—Commentaries (Kystes Thyroidiens — Observations — Commentaires. By Real Dore. L'Union Medicale du Canada, Volume 68, No. 10, October, 1939.

A married woman, 38 years of age, presented herself for examination March 22, 1939. She complained of excessive fatigue, anorexia, nervousness, palpitation of the heart, constipation and insomnia. All these symptoms had begun about three years before, and had gradually increased in intensity.

There was also complaint of a swelling in the front part of the cervical region, noticed for about two years before the examination.

There had been but little change in weight, the weight being usually around 125 pounds.

The general aspect of the patient was bad. There was practically entire loss of pigment in skin and mucous membranes (la peau et la muqueuse sont completement decolorees). The thyroid gland was enlarged to twice its normal size. It was rather firm (plutot dure). The anterior part of the left lobe presented a spherical, renitent swelling (in French "renitente," the spelling being the same as in English, with the exception that an e is aded to the French spelling. In either case, referring to a tumor, the adjective indicates "resistence to pressure"). It was about the size of an egg (du volume d'un oeuf).

The lungs were normal. There was no evidence of excessive irritability of the heart (erethisme cardiaque). No abnormality was discovered in the abdomen, in connection with the pelvic organs, or the kidney areas.

There was no evidence in history or examination of any important hereditary or antecedent difficulty. There was no history of familial goiter.

Blood pressure 120/90. Pulse 80. Weight 134 pounds. B.M.R. minus nine per cent.

An electrocardiogram was normal. Both chemical and microscopic examination of the urine normal.

Both non-protein — nitrogen in the blood, and blood sugar within normal limits.

The author asks the question: "To what category of goitrous patients does this patient belong? (A quelle categorie de goitreuses appartient cette patiente?). The comments in answer to the self-propounded question are so exact and logical that they are referred to here in extenso.

It is remarked that in simple goiter there is enlargement of the thyroid gland without any disturbance of the general condition of the patient. This is not true in the case of this particular patient, and the inference is that simple goiter may be excluded from consideration.

Attention is then called to the fact that toxic goiter is always accompanied by the syndrome of hyperthyroidism. That is not true in the case reported, because the elements that make up such a syndrome, such as tachycardia, cardiac irritability in a state of rest, emaciation, nervousness, tremor and a heightened basal metabolism are not present here.

A consideration of malignancy as an explanation for the enlargement of the thyroid is considered, and in that connection it is indicated that malignancy (cancer) usually arises from an old adenoma, and that this transformation from ordinary adenomatous tissue to malignant tissue is characterised by a woody firmness of the tumor. That is not true in the case of the patient.

One must eliminate a cyst of the thyroid containing lemon-colored or yellowish liquid material, remembering at the same time that such cysts may be simple or frankly toxic. A cyst of this character is designated by the author as "un kyste a liquide citrin."

It is remarked that when a cyst of the thyroid cannot be classified in the category of simple or toxic goiters it must be concluded that it is a hemorrhagic cyst of more or less ancient origin, or a cyst associated with an accumulation of cholesterin.

After making an analysis of the data collected it was concluded that the patient had a hemorrhagic cyst.

The author directs attention to the importance of making a differentiation between hemorrhagic cysts or cysts associated with an accumulation of cholesterin, on the one hand, and a cyst containing colored liquid material (kyste a liquide citrin) on the other hand, bearing in mind always the possibility of cancerization of a pre-existing adenoma. When a cyst contains lemon-colored or yellowish liquid material there can be no question but that it is a cystic goiter, simple or toxic (il ne peut etre question que de goitre kystique simple ou toxique). In the case of such a cyst, whether it be simple or toxic, it is the opinion that surgical operation should be done, and it is indicated that surgical operation for the relief of pathology of this character is gratifyingly successful.

But it is not the same in connection with hemorrhagic cysts or cholesterin cysts. If the average patient who has a cyst of this kind (hemorrhagic or associated with deposits of cholesterin) the patient is often—in fact, usually dilapidated, asthenic and anemic. For this reason operation is approached with caution.

In the case of the patient reported here there was a hemoglobin percentage of 52, R.B.C. 2,050,000, W.B.C. 1,875, polynuclear neutrophiles 67 per cent, lymphocytes 30 per cent.

Acting upon the suggestion of a consultant, the patient was given a few intramuscular injections of pentose nucleatide (pentnucleatide). The author does not say so, but, taking into consideration the very low white blood count, the inference is that was the reason for giving the preparation, such preparations having some supposed value in connection with diseases characterized by an unusually low white blood count. After an investigation covering a period of about two months, a bi-lateral sub-total thyroidectomy was done on May 29, 1939. An examination of the removed tissue confirmed the diagnosis of hemorrhagic cyst of the thyroid.

Convalescence was entirely satisfactory. Within a short time the patient expressed herself as feeling well, and the blood picture was soon of a normal character.

Based upon his observation and experience, the author believes that patients who have hemorrhagic cysts of the thyroid or cysts associated with an accumulation of cholesterin should be treated by surgical operation, not withstanding the poor general condition of the patient, because in old hemorrhagic cysts and cysts associated with an abnormal accumulation of cholesterin the dilapidation of the patient is rapid and progressive, and, for that reason, it would appear that proper surgical operation is more urgent, even, than in the average toxic goiter.

The final conclusions of the author are as follows:

"1. A hemorrhagic cyst, or a cyst associated with abnormal accumulation of cholesterin, rapidly and gravely alters the general condition of the patient.

"2. These cysts ought to be differentiated from cysts containing lemon-colored or yellowish liquid material (gyste a liquide citrin).

3. Consigned to his own means of defence, the carrier of the cysts is quickly overcome, and a surgical operation is feared.

4. A thyroidectomy ought to be done without delay.

5. I have no confidence in the efficacy of medical or physical therapy in this clinical form (Je ne crois pas a l'efficacite d'une therapeutique medicale ou physique dans cette forme clinique)."

LeRoy Long.

Endometriosis of the Lungs: John E. Hobbs, M.D., and A. R. Bortnick, M.D., St. Louis, Missouri; Surgery, Gynecology and Obstetrics, November, 1939, Vol. 69, page 577.

This article reports experimental works carried out on rabbits with autotransplantation of the endometrium through the ear vein of the rabbit and a study of the lungs which demonstrated that the endometrial tissue was able to grow in lung tissue.

The authors quote the work of Sampson, Halban, and others who have demonstrated the presence of uterine mucosa in veins and lymphatic vessels.

Since endometrial tissue can be thus transported through lymphatics and veins, and since their autotransplanted uterine mucosa was found to be viable in lung tissue, they conclude that, therefore, endometrial tissue must occasionally reach the lungs and grow.

It is their contention that this is a plausible explanation for vicarious menstruation since it is possible for endometrial tissue to enter the general circulation either through a patent foramen ovale or by propagation through the pulmonary circulation.

They report a woman of 42 years who had an endometrial implant in the groin and who had hemoptysis at the time of menstruation. X-ray studies of the lungs showed a circumscribed shadow in the apex of the right lung. Upon being given a sterilizing dose of X-rays to the ovaries, she has had only occasional slight hemoptysis usually associated with excitement. They felt that she probably had endometrial tissue in the lung with vicarious menstruation.

They also call attention to the cases reported by Navratil and Kramer and by Mankin in which there was endometrium in the brachioradialis muscle and thigh.

These authors also feel that this aberrant endometrial tissue has characteristics which indicate that it has increased potentiality to become malignant.

Comment: This is a most intriguing explanation for some patients with hemoptysis at menstrual time. However, unfortunately, as far as I know there has been no instance of endometrial tissue demonstrated in the lung at autopsy. This may be due to the fact that the postmortem examinations have not been done carefully enough or that the examinor was not particularly observant about this possibility.

Wendell Long.

———————o———————

EYE, EAR, NOSE AND THROAT
Edited by Marvin D. Henley, M.D.
911 Medical Arts Building, Tulsa

Non-Traumatic Ventilation Treatment of the Nose and Sinuses. Sidney N. Parkinson, Oakland, California. The J o u r n a l of Laryngology and Otology, October, 1939.

This is quite an interesting discussion accompanied by illustrations and a bibliography. The method of treatment and the reason for same is outlined, discussed and defended, adequately. The results claimed are good. The procedure is logical. The article is long and has a comprehensive recapitulation which is given below.

For intranasal medication during acute inflammation of the nose and sinuses it is best to use a drug with known useful action and with known freedom from local tissue resection.

A drug for intranasal use should be prepared in a vehicle known to be physiologically compatible with nasal secretion. This will prevent the occurrence of local tissue reaction from the vehicle. The main factors requiring compatibility are tinicity and hydrogen-ion concentration. Damage to the cilia and to the epithelial cell walls result from errors in either factor. A physiological solution of sodium chloride made with tap water, sterilized by boiling, and free from preservatives and antiseptics appears to be a satisfactory vehicle.

In acute infection of the nose and sinuses treatment solutions are best applied by atomizers and by head-low posture. Thus one avoids the physical trauma to nasal and sinus epithelium inherent in the use of tampons, trocars, cannulas, and other mechanical means.

The head-low posture of choice is the lateral head-low position for the following reasons:

1. It is designed in accordance with the anatomy of the living nose. Although asymmetrical with regard to the skull, it is symmetrical with regard to the nasal structure. All the sinus ostia are reached by this posture.

2. It is practicable from infancy to old age.

3. It is comfortable; in fact, it resembles the position of sleep sufficiently to cause no fear in small children.

4. The head is at the same level as the rest of the body with the exception of part of the chest. Hence there is a minimal gravitation into it of venous blood from the trunk and extremities. This is of real importance, especially in elderly persons.

5. The posture is easily effected in the home or in the office and requires no special equipment. A cot and a pillow are all one needs. With infants and small children the posture is best obtained over one's lap.

6. An intelligent mother or nurse is easily taught the technique.

7. None of the therapeutic fluid need reach the pharynx or mouth in this posture at any stage of treatment. This is important. Drugs used in the nose are for local effect only, and their effect when swallowed or aspirated serves no useful purpose.

———————

Sulfanilimide In The Treatment of Mooren's Ulcer. Marvin J. Blaess, M.D., Detroit, Mich. The Eye, Ear, Nose and Throat Monthly, November, 1939.

This is a report of two cases. Case One was a housewife, age 60, whose chief complaint was severe pain, redness and tearing of the left eye. There was present in the upper nasal quadrant a marginal ulcer. This was covered with a grayish exudate, margins were undermined and the edge was gray and overhanging. Various cauterizations and daily one per cent optochin ointment failed to check its progress. The ulcer continued to enlarge and the patient was hospitalized. Intravenous typhoid vaccine was given ineffectually apparently. Sulfanilimide was then started and the patient did not tolerate it well. However, during one week of the regime the ulcer's progress was stopped. The edges of the ulcer were reduced four days later. As the flap gradually withdrew, epithelization of the corneal defect took place nicely and the patient continued with an uneventful recovery with a remaining moderate translucency of the site of the defect. Fortunately the ulcer did not quite reach the center of the cornea so there is no visual impairment.

Case Two was a white male, age 24, with a marginal ulcer involving two-thirds of the circumference of the left corneal margin, it extended from the 3 o'clock to the 11 o'clock position. The deepest portion involved the entire thickness of the epithelial layer of the cornea. Normal saline instillations and one per cent optochin ointment were used. Fifty grams of sulfanilimide was given daily and tolerated well for four days. At this time the ulcer showed definite improvement. Dosage of the sulfanilimide was reduced to 30 grains daily. By the seventh day the conjunctival injection had subsided, the pain was entirely relieved, and the ulcer stained only lightly. By the tenth day the eye was entirely healed. Because of the variety of treatment instituted in each of the above cases it is difficult to draw a conclusion of definite value; however, the turning point for both cases was after sulfanilimide medication was started.

———————

Blood Cultures in Cases of Otitic Sepsis. Joseph L. Goldman, M.D., New York. Archives of Otolaryngology, October, 1939.

The report and article is derived from 104 cases of thrombosis of the lateral sinus, including primary thrombosis of the jugular bulb, observed in a period of 12 years at the Mount Sinai Hospital. The author's summary is as follows:

Bacteremia is the most constant clinical feature in cases of thrombosis of the lateral sinus. Accordingly, recognition of the bacteremia is an important finding for the diagnosis and clinical management of otitic sepsis.

The micro-organism usually isolated from the blood stream in cases of thrombosis of the lateral sinus is Str. haemolyticus. It was recovered from 95.7 per cent of cases of proved bacteremia associated with otitic sepsis. It appears from bacteriologic investigations that thrombosis of the lateral sinus, with rare exceptions, is essentially a disease caused by Str. haemolyticus.

The demonstration of i n v a s i o n of the blood stream is dependent on the methods used in taking and cultivating the blood. In the interpretation of blood cultures special attention should be directed to the consideration of the number of micro-organisms cultured, and importance should be attached to the growth of micro-organisms in fluid mediums alone. Analysis of the preoperative blood cultures in this series showed that Str. haemolyticus was obtained from the fluid medium in 22.7 per cent of the cultures. It is my opinion that finding Str. haemolyticus in a case of suspected otitic sepsis, even in small numbers and in fluid mediums alone, establishes the diagnosis of thrombosis of lateral sinus or primary thrombosis of the jugular bulb after all other clinical possibilities have been excluded. With this concept in mind, blood cultures should contribute greatly to the diagnosis of septicemia when there is a vague otitic history with inconclusive physical evidence.

Proper interpretation of blood culture can be helpful also in the management of proved otitic sepsis and in the differential diagnosis of conditions simulating otitic sepsis. In cases of clinical sepsis associated with infections of the middle ear, sterile blood cultures also give information of great value. In this connection it is important to emphasize that in my experience infections confined to the middle ear and mastoid bone have not been associated with bacteremia.

It seems pertinent in the discussion of invasion of the blood stream that clinically significant bacteremia should be differentiated from clinically insignificant bacteremia and described as such.

---o---

PLASTIC SURGERY
Edited by
GEO. H. KIMBALL, M.D., F.A.C.S.
404 Medical Arts Building, Oklahoma City

The Treatment of the Patient With Severe Burns. Roy D. McClure, M.D., Detroit, Mich. Journal of A.M.A., November 11, 1939.

The author gives a short statisticians discussion of burns at Henry Ford Hospital, 1937. In a paragraph he summarizes the advancement and treatment of burns since Davidson did his revolutionary work in the Henry Ford Hospital 15 years ago. He states three questions for which the answers should be sought:

1. Are there any new facts concerning the systemic effects of the chemical and tissue changes which follow severe burns?

2. What is the effect on the mortality rate of present methods of treatment?

3. In the light of our present knowledge, what is the best therapeutic procedure in burns?

Three theories according to the author have arisen to account for the marked toxicity of the patient with severe burns:

1. Physical theory which deals with the concentration of the circulatory blood and a failing circulation.

2. Bacterial theory of Aldrich.

3. A specific toxin which is formed at the burned area and distributed by the circulating blood.

The author discusses the pathology of burns and deals principally with that in the liver following massive burns. Specific cases are cited, one in which practically the entire liver was necrosed. Further discussion deals with the changes of the blood chemistry which are well known, and mortality statistics. The treatment of burns used at the Henry Ford Hospital is well summarized and will bear quoting. Summary of Treatment of Burns, Henry Ford Hospital Method:

General Supportive Measures

1. Pain and restlessness are combated by adequate and repeated sedation.

2. Oxygen therapy may be indicated in certain severe cases.

3. External heat is applied: hot water bottles and blankets if area is limited; electrically heated cradle tent and superheated room if extensive.

4. Restoration of fluid balance is undertaken to obtain a 24-hour urinary output of 1,500 cc. Fluids by mouth, rectum, interstitially and intravenously. Continuous intravenous method is often indicated and may be imperative in cases of extensive burns involving the extremities. The solutions used are 5 per cent dextrose and physiologic solution of sodium chloride.

5. Blood plasma transfusions are done.

6. Laboratory investigations are made: (a) frequent hemoglobin or h e m a c r i t determinations should be made. (b) The urine should be analyzed frequently with determinations of the specific gravity and albumin content. (c) Serum protein determination should be made immediately on admission. When facilities are available the following procedures should be done: (d) Chloride estimations should be made at intervals so that depleted chlorides may be restored by intravenous administration of saline solution. (e) Blood cultures may be taken. (f) The nonprotein nitrogen should be determined. (g) The icterus index should be ascertained as a means of recognizing toxic hepatitis or liver damage.

Local Treatment

1. Remove all clothing under as sterile conditions as possible and place patient on sterile sheets in a warm room.

2. Take all precautions to avoid infection of the burned area. Treat as any other large wound. Aseptic conditions: masks, gloves, gowns, must be worn by doctors and nurses.

3. Debridement should be minimal and should be limited to opening blisters and cutting away dead skin.

4. Tannic acid in a 5 per cent fresh solution is applied with atomized or power spray. This is a simple and effective way of tanning the burned area. This solution is sprayed on at frequent intervals until the burned area is thoroughly tanned. Ointments containing tannic acid plus antiseptic are useful in small burns and for burns of the face and the perineum. The addition of antiseptics such as resorcinol or silver nitrate to the tannic acid with the idea of preventing infection has been employed with apparent success, but treating the burned area as a surgical open wound by taking steps to prevent the introduction of infecting organisms is an equally, if not more effective measure.

After Care

1. Cut away all dead skin and open collections of fluids under aseptic precautions and then again spray tannic acid on the bared areas.

2. As the heavy tanned crust forms watch carefully for local signs of infection under the crust and liberate collections of pus. Occasionally the first clue to these collections is evidence of systemic reaction.

3. Prevent contracture deformities by the early use of extension apparatus.

4. Employ skin grafting early and freely.

5. Detect and treat secondary anemia early. Blood transfusion is the best method of doing this in the late stages.

Dr. McClure believes that the original theory that a toxin is formed in the burn and is carried by the circulation throughout the body with the production of systemic effects has not yet been settled. He believes that disagreement regarding the proper local treatment should not distract our attention from the more important problem, the treatment of a very sick patient who has a threatening toxemia, alterations in the blood chemistry, a wound very susceptible to infection and pathologic changes in organs remote from the skin.

Comment

This is an excellent article on the care of the burned patient. The article gives a method of local treatment but does not require that it be used in all cases feeling that this is of secondary importance to the treatment of the patient. There is an excellent discussion of pathology occurring in the liver in severe burns together with a review of the changes occurring in the blood.

Personal experience has led to the opinion that local treatment presents a rather wide choice and should be carefully individualized to the circumstances and to the patient. Major burns which will present a large amount of slough in many cases are perhaps best treated by saline packs since this slough must be removed as soon as separation occurs.

In the first two or three weeks after very extensive burns the major attention must be given to the patient as a whole and active treatment directed toward a maintenance of fluid metabolism; replacement of body salts and dilution of hemoglobin concentration together with the replacement of blood proteins either by whole fresh blood, by blood plasma transfusions, the latter being of course preferable in the presence of marked hemoglobin concentration.

Other complications must be watched fairly closely and treated accordingly. Those paramount are acute toxic nephritis, secondary pneumonia and delirium. It must be borne in mind that the burned patient may have other pathology which should not be overlooked such as diabetes, tuberculosis, lues, etc.

We have seen a patient in the past month who had a bleeding peptic ulcer with a toxic etiology who lost 60 per cent hemoglobin in a period of 48 hours. This man required massive blood daily, 500 cc., transfusions to sustain life.

Treatment of Avulsed Skin Flaps. A l f r e d W. Farmer, M.D., Toronto, Canada. Annals of Surgery, November, 1939.

The author reports four cases of severe avulsion of skin occurring in civil practice, three automobile accidents and one a domestic wringer injury. The treatment that he outlines is that of excision of the avulsed skin and complete cleansing and debridement of the traumatized area. Soap and water and saline are used in cleansing the defect, that is the subcutaneous fat and connective tissue are removed, cut well into the dermis, and the skin being accurately sewed back into position. Pressure bandage and immobilizing splints are placed on the dressing and changed in 10 to 14 days unless otherwise indicated. The author reports four cases treated in this manner with fairly good results. He believes that this is the first time that such a procedure has been described as such, although he cites cases in literature which were treated in this manner, probably unintentionally.

In the discussion of the paper by Dr. Sumner L. Koch of Chicago he brought up the question that many of these flaps which have a wide attachment are best left in position and treated as a pedicle although in certain types of injuries where the pedicle is distal to the circulation and very small it is perhaps better to detach the flap.

Comment: In this type of skin defect probably the agent which causes death of the flap is a congestion from the venous circulation rather than ischemia from lack of blood supply. Therefore it would seem logical that a procedure to permit drainage would be multiple stab wounds in the flap with an agent to prevent coagulation of the cerum, such as sodium citrate, would p e r m i t

sufficient drainage. This together with the pedicle to keep the flap viable until it had re-established its circulation turned loose by the injury.

However, in certain injuries where portions of the skin are crushed and devitalized or where the skin is practically completely detached, procedure as described by the author would be applicable and an acceptable surgical technique.

ORTHOPAEDIC SURGERY
Edited by Earl D. McBride, M.D., F.A.C.S.
717 North Robinson Street, Oklahoma City

Arthroplasty of Hip: A New Method, M. N. Smith-Petersen, Journal of Bone and Joint Surgery, April, 1939.

The author points out that arthroplasties in the past have been confined chiefly to reshaping of two joint surfaces that are mechanically suitable for function, and then covering them with a lining which, in the operator's idea tends to prevent reankylosis. Always the blood clot which formed between these two surfaces organized and resulted in a certain amount of fibrous tissue. The author's method, however, consists of a "two stage, mold arthroplasty." This implies the introduction of an inert mold between the joint surfaces so that repair can go on and the mold later removed, leaving a small joint surface. Several types of molds have been used—the chief one being glass viscaloid which is a form of celluloid; pyrex glass, bakelite and finally Vitallium. The hip joint is the chief joint used although it is not confined entirely to the hip. Very excellent results have been obtained with the use of the latter material; there being objections to the earlier materials used.

The author describes a very excellent new approach to the hip. This approach is similar to that for his acetabulo-plasty previously described. An anterior incision is made along the anterior third of the iliac crest and slightly down and medially along the lateral border of the sartorius muscle. Dissection is carried between the sartorius and tensor fascia later by sharp and blunt dissection. The attachment of the direct head of the rectus femoris to the anterior inferior spine is next defined. A detailed discussion follows of the exact approach to the hip, which is essential for anyone to study in detail before attempting the procedure. It is major surgery and requires a very thorough knowledge of the hip region. However, an excellent exposure is obtained and anatomical closure can be secured.

Post-operatively the patient gets along much better than previously described forms of hip arthroplasty. At the end of the second week the patient uses roller skating exercises with the skates strapped to the backs of the heels and adduction and abduction of the hip being accomplished. At the end of four weeks the patient is up in a chair and may begin exercising on a stationary bicycle. With the Vitallium mold it has not always been necessary to remove it. The author has done 29 patients with this procedure, yet hesitates to give any final end-results since they have all been done since 1938. However, he states the success of the early cases has definitely justified the procedure on following cases.

Internal Fixation of Trochanteric Fractures of the Femur, J. Albert Key, Surgery, Vol. 6, No. 1, July, 1939.

The author points out that during the past few years great emphasis has been placed on the intracapsular fractures or fractures of the femoral neck, and the extreme mortality and morbidity of these fractures. Internal fixation has been developed with the neck fractures to the extent that it is a routine procedure in all well grounded orthopedic clinics. However, the trochanteric fracture has still been treated by various and sundry methods of fixation which keep an elderly patient in bed for several weeks to months and according to records of the St. Louis City Hospital the mortality of 214 trochanteric fractures was 38 per cent while 166 intracapsular fractures in the same hospital was 25.9 per cent. Thus the trochanteric fractures are more frequent and the mortality is greater. The fact that trochanteric fractures heal more kindly than fractures of the neck has probably accounted for considerable attention paid to this type. In fractures of the neck there is much less trauma to the patient as a rule than in trochanteric fractures. There is more pain with trochanteric fractures, and it is the author's belief that this is the chief reason for death in old people. The author describes three general types of trochanteric fractures. First, in which there is little or no visible comminution or displacement. Second, in the usual type with considerable separation and comminution, but with the lateral cortex of the shaft of the femur intact to a point beyond the line with the superior surface of the neck of the femur. The third involves the lateral cortex of the femur and in reality is a subtrochanteric fracture and cannot be nailed, but can be fixed with pins or Parham bands, so that the fragments are fairly stable. Primarily the operation consists of a lateral incision and the drilling of the shaft and the neck by a 3/16 inch drill, followed by three planes with a thin osteotome. This is then fixed firmly with a Smith-Petersen nail of three-flange type. The preliminary drilling is done to prevent splitting the cortex. Casts have not been used in the usual case. It is believed this will give less mortality and morbidity than use of the older methods.

The abstractors have been interested in the nailing of trochanteric fractures for several months and have done a few, following somewhat the same technique as Dr. Key. We feel this is a step forward in the treatment of such fractures.

Howard B. Shorbe, M.D.

---o---

CARDIOLOGY
Edited by F. Redding Hood, M.D.
1200 N. Walker St., Oklahoma City

Functional Cardiac Disorders

The term is here taken to include, cardiac neurosis, neuro circulatory asthenia, irritable hearts and functional murmurs. A patient may have any one or a combination of these.

Cardiac Neurosis

Cardiac neurosis are functional disorders of the nervous system consisting essentially of fear and apprehension about the heart, a fear of death with a secondary fear of partial or complete incapacitation. It may manifest itself by disturbances in rate, rhythm or sensation, or by a combination of these. The most common symptoms are d y s p n e a, palpation, tachycardia, weakness, faintness and dizziness. These are symptoms of organic heart disease but are found in a more exaggerated form. Patients appear flushed and perspire freely but their hands and feet are usually clammy. The heart rate is accelerated but has a normal response to exercise. Where precordial distress is found precordial hyperesthesia is the rule. This distress is usually independent of effort. These patients are definitely below normal in both physical and mental stamina. A history of extreme malaise, helplessness, immobility, weighted sensations, coldness, or extreme prostration may be given. Loss of consciousness is rare but when it occurs it is longer than a simple faint and is probably due to the accelerated pulse rate, the shallow and rapid respiratory effort and vasovagal disturbances.

The physical examination will show evidence of the symptoms found but no evidence of any heart disease or they may accompany heart disease. On this basis, cardiac neurosis has been classified as (1) occurring without heart disease, (2) with heart disease which is not producing symptoms and (3) with severe heart disease producing symptoms of failure.

The signs at the examination of these patients will be a rapid heart rate, snapping first sound at the apex, increased pulmonary second sound, a thrill is rarely found but a systolic murmur at the apex is common. The blood pressure may be elevated at the first examination. As a rule there is no arrhythmia but extra systoles may be present. There is no cardiac enlargement and no signs of failure unless it accompanies severe heart disease. There has been reported cardiac enlargement as a result of cardiac neurosis, however, the effect of exercise and excitement on the heart is to increase the rate and force of the heart beat and if extreme systolic murmur may be present and after such exercise and excitement the heart is actually smaller than before. It is now accepted that there will be no enlargement in uncomplicated cardiac neurosis.

The potential framework for a neurosis of some kind is present in all of us but needs the right set of circumstances and events to set it off. The precipitating or exciting factor may originate in childhood, may come from the death from heart disease of a member of the family or some close friend, may come from death notices in the newspapers. I feel that this is certainly true of cardiac neurosis developing in patients who know that they have heart disease. It may come from palpation following a full meal, excessive use of tobacco, alcoholic imbibition, or it may come from a careless word, action or suggestion on the part of a physician during an examination for other conditions.

In considering treatment of the patient it should start with the history taking since a careless history or a superficial examination is worse than none at all in dealing with these patients. It is above all necessary to establish the patient's confidence and to convince him that he is getting a thorough examination. Much time is needed and well spent in going into details as to tests and results, the diagnosis should be made and then stated as confidentially as possible. There should be no doubtful additions added. To tell a patient that you can find nothing wrong and then to

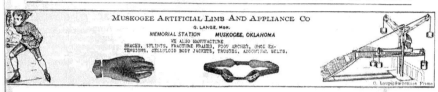

limit his activity or to follow such a statement by administering medication cannot help but arouse in him a suspicion of possibly a more serious heart disease than he may have originally imagined and that you are holding out on him. Should he need a gradation of exercise or medication due to his general physical or nervous condition such procedures should be carried out with ample explanations and it has been suggested that a short time elapse between the examination and the beginning of such medication. A convincing re-assurance is the keynote of success. An exploration with the patient and sometimes a near relative into his fears and doubts will aid in a readjustment. In man, his fears concern himself, his family or his business. Any abnormality such as foci of infection affecting his general systemic well being should be corrected, a budgeting of time as to work, play and rest as needed and general measures as to diet, rest and exercise is important.

Neura Circulatory Asthenia

Neuro circulatory asthenia is to be distinguished from cardiac neurosis in which occurs anxiety, hypochondriasis or hysteria, from irritable hearts due to premature beats or paroxysmal tachycardia, and from ordinary neuroasthenia manifested by lack of energy with mental and physical exhaustion and irritability.

It follows infection, fatigue, salt lack, and hyperventilation. Classification has been made on the basis of etiology, the class depending upon the severity of the predisposing factors which bring about the syndrome. It has also been classified on the basis of the degree of physical activity or excitement which will bring on the symptoms. There is no distinct line between the normal and the abnormal. The symptoms which are brought on in a normal subject by great activity or excitement while in severe cases of neuro circulatory asthenia they may be precipitated by little activity or excitement. It has been said that the syndrome exists, when the symptoms appear in the course of usual efforts of daily life and such activity would not produce them in the patient and when such activity would not produce symptoms in an average subject.

The cardinal symptoms are palpation, respiratory discomfort, precordial aches or pains and exhaustion.

Palpation is the most common symptom complained of. It does not necessarily mean a rapid heart or the presence of irregularities. The patient may feel palpation at a time when the examiner will be finding a normal rate with a regular rhythm. It is more a lowered threshold to heart consciousness.

Respiratory discomfort is not a true dyspnea as found in cardiac failure. There may be a slow respiratory rate with increased inspiratory effort and with periodic sighing type of respiration with actual hyperventilation, yet the patient may insist he has difficulty in getting sufficient air to fill his lungs; one might class this type of dyspnea as a lowered threshold to respiratory consciousness.

Precordial discomfort may quite closely follow the characteristics of that occurring in angina pectoris as to location, radiation and in response to effort.

They differ as to length of time, where in angina pectoris, the time is relatively short, in neuro circulatory asthenia they may last for hours. There is some difference of opinion in literature as to radiation but in reviewing a series of cases, radiation occurred in about 50 per cent, the areas involved corresponding to angina pectoris. The more severe the distress the more likely the radiation. The presence of hyperasthesia of the area and a history of the discomfort occurring without emotional, physical or thermal changes will aid in the diagnosis.

A feeling of physical weakness, exhaustion, dizziness complete the cardinal signs.

The importance of a careful and complete history and examination as stressed under the discussion of cardiac neurosis and the establishment of confidence in the patient for the doctor must not be underestimated. It is necessary to explain his condition, to expell his fears, eliminating complicating cardiac neurosis and then to let him understand fully what his plan of life should be, the limitations that must be met in order to so live that symptoms will not be produced. He must be moderate in work and play, avoiding late hours, excitement, over-indulgence in alcohol and tobacco. In general, to avoid all possible stress and strain, both mental and physical. He should be warned that he should attempt to so live that he does those things that will better his general health and not do those things that will lower his general resistance, and that the period of recovery from other illness will require longer periods than in other individuals. As reassurance is the keynote to success in neuro circulatory asthenia.

Irritable Hearts

An irritable heart may be due to auricular or ventricular premature beats, tachycardias, auricular flutter or fibrilations. They may occur not necessarily due to structural changes in the heart but as a result of disturbance of function. One should be especially careful to ascertain the absence of enlargement of the heart, organic valvular diseases or other forms of cardiac pathology before classifying them as entirely functional. They may occur as part of the clinical picture of cardiac neurosis or neuro circulatory asthenia, or from extra-cardiac conditions such as foci of infections about the tonsils, sinuses, etc., gastro intestinal pathology, may follow infections as pneumonia or influenza, or may be a warning of more serious myocardial condition.

Treatment depends upon the particular type of arrhythmia present, and due to time, cannot be here discussed.

Functional Murmurs

The entire question of functional murmurs has not been decided to our complete satisfaction. A simple classification of the non-organic murmurs would be to divide them into those resulting from disturbances of the heart muscle and those resulting from physical changes.

The functional types resulting from changes in function of the cardiac muscle have been contributed to the asthenia of papillary muscle resulting in a failure of closure of the atrio-ventricular valves with an insufficiency of their action producing systolic m u r m u r s. The other advanced theory of their production is dilatation of the ring about the atrio-ventricular valves which prevents their closure. In either case the disturbance of function of the valve is the same as that from organic valvular disease. One being a temporary condition, the other being more or less permanent.

The physical murmurs may result from a change in the composition of the blood effecting its physical properties as in severe anemias; it may result from a change in velocity, this would occur when the heart is slow, with greater diastolic filling and the murmur would occur when the velocity is increased or during systole. Anatomical changes may bring about abnormal pressure or tortuosity interfering with blood flow and may produce systolic murmurs, such an example would be the systolic murmur over the pulmonary artery in flat chested subjects.

These non-organic murmurs are most frequently heard at the base, but may be heard at any valve area or may be heard all over the precordial area. Although certain types would be expected to be heard only with a slow heart or at least best with a slow heart, we find some that are heard only after exercise, and the area in which they are audible is increased by exercise.

I feel that the important thing about these non-organic murmurs is the possible production of cardiac neurosis by the improper valuation of the murmur by the physician.

Conclusion

In conclusion, I wish to point out the extreme morbidity resulting from functional cardiac disorders; that although many articles have been written on the subject, the standards of today are still expressed in Thomas Lewis treatise on the Soldiers Heart, published in 1919; that establishment of the confidence of the patient in the physician and his reassurance and re-education is the keynote of therapy; that drugs have purposely been left out in this discussion, they are of so little importance in the treatment of cardiac neurosis and neuro circulatory asthenia, and there has been a tendency by some to over-estimate their value; drugs in various cardiac arrhythmias depend upon the type of arrhythmia; and that extreme care should be used not to precipitate cardiac neurosis by miss-evaluation of non-organic murmurs.

---o---

INTERNAL MEDICINE

Edited by Hugh Jeter, M.D., 1200 North Walker,
Oklahoma City

Chronic Leukemia, The Early Phase of Chronic Leukemia, The Results of Treatment and the Effects of Complicating Infections; A Study of Eighty-six Adults. Maxwell M. Wintrobe, M.D., and L. Lee Hasenbush, M.D., Baltimore. (Archives of Internal Medicine, Vol. 64, No. 4, October, 1939.)

This is a very comprehensive report on the study of 86 adult cases of chronic leukemia including both the myelogenous and lymphatic types. Results are given on therapeutics, duration of life, incidence of infection, affects of infection, etc.

It is concluded that there is little evidence to support the theory that a remission of leukemic signs occurs in association with an intercurrent infection. Eighty-six patients with chronic leukemia, 39 of myelogenous and 47 of leukemia showed a predominance (61.5 per cent in males with the myelogenous form and 83 per cent in males with the lymphogenous).

"In 72 per cent of the cases of myelogenous leukemia the age onset was 30 to 59 years, while in 61.7 per cent of the cases of lymphogenous leukemia, symptoms began between 50 and 69 years.

"The early phase of chronic leukemia, as determined by the histories of five patients with myelogenous leukemia and 16 with lymphogenous leukemia, is described.

"These observations indicate that unexplained leukocytosis may be the first and even the only sign of chronic myelogenous leukemia. In these cases mature cells of the myeloid series rather than myelocytes made up the majority of the leukocytes.

"In chronic lymphogenous leukemia, unexplained leukocytosis was the initial sign in only about a third of the cases. Slight glandular enlargement was a frequent early sign. In one case splenomegaly was so pronounced and other signs were so minimal that an erroneous diagnosis of Banti's syndrome had been made.

"Distinct lymphocytosis was found in a number of cases of early lymphogenous leukemia even when the leukocyte count was relatively low.

"Slight anemia was found more often in the early stages of lymphogenous leukemia than in those of myelogenous leukemia.

"It is estimated that the time elapsing from the onset of chronic myelogenous leukemia until symptoms of the disease commonly cause the patient to seek medical attention is about two to five years, whereas this period in cases of lymphogenous leukemia may be only about 1.5 to 2.5 years.

"Treatment with solution of potassium arsenite U.S.P. was found to be of less value that irradiation in myelogenous leukemia. The response to irradiation was slightly better in myelogenous leukemia.

"Statistics concerning the duration of life in cases of chronic leukemia are recorded. It is pointed out that extreme variation occurs in the natural course of the disease in different cases.

"Infections were more c o m m o n in cases of lymphogenous leukemia than in those of myelogenous leukemia.

"Contrary to the opinion frequently expressed, infections in the great majority of the cases did not produce a remission in the physical signs or in the blood picture. In only one instance did a slight change of this nature occur, and in four cases there was an actual increase in the leukocyte count in association with infection."

The One-Hour Two-Dose Dextrose Tolerance Test (Exton-Rose Procedure); Diagnostic Significance. Morgan W. Matthews, M.D., Fellow in Medicine, the Mayo Foundation; Thomas B. Magath, M.D., and Joseph Berkson, M.D. With the Assistance of Robert P. Gage. Rochester, Minn. (J.A.M.A., Vol. 113, No. 17, October 21, 1939.)

In this article the authors have given the results of part of a survey of the dextrose tolerance test used in the Mayo Clinic over about a three-year period and an analysis of the results obtained with the one-hour two-dose test introduced in 1931 by Exton and Rose. Criteria for the interpretation of the test are presented. Several interesting charts are given. Advancing age produced a progressive elevation of the blood sugar level at every phase of the blood sugar curve.

A fasting blood sugar exceeding 120 mg. per 100 cc. of blood is considered to be diagnostic of diabetes.

The most valuable criterion for the diagnosis of diabetes was considered to be the one hour value of the blood sugar. If above 158 mg. per 100 cc. of blood (the so-called critical level) patients are considered to be diabetic, and if below that level non-diabetic. A total of 247 patients were studied and this criterion of laboratory diagnosis of diabetes gave less doubtful results than in any other dextrose test where oral administration was used.

Comment: These results are very interesting inasmuch as the test used is practical, more economical and more convenient than many of the older glucose tolerance tests, the fasting one-half hour and the one-hour blood sugars being the only requirements.

--------o--------

UROLOGY

Edited by D. W. Branham, M.D.
514 Medical Arts Building, Oklahoma City

Affections and Lesions of the Prostatic Urethra. Edgar G. Ballenger, Journal of Urology, October, 1939.

No more neglected anatomical region exists than the prostatic urethra, so far as remediable disease is concerned.

Dr. Ballenger states that for years in his own work, many disorders referable to this region were not recognized because so often he was looking for gross physical factors, such as pus or blood, rather than more intangible evidence of disease.

With the advent of newer types of cystoscopes whereby he can study the posterior urethra more thoroughly, he has been able to recognize etiologic factors responsible for the symptoms. The specific affections of the posterior urethra as viewed by the McCarthy panendoscope are: papillomata, varicose veins, cysts, bullous edema, false passages, diverticula, utriculitis, median bars, valves, fibrous contractions and distortions produced by hypertrophy of the prostate.

A mistake commonly made is to give prolonged courses of prostatic massage merely because pus is present in the secretion. In such cases which do not respond within a reasonable length of time, search should be made to find the cause for the persistence of pus.

The agencies used in the treatment of lesions in the posterior urethra are: dilatation, phenol, nitrate of silver, the cautery current and the fulgurating current. For those familiar with the technic of cystoscopic procedure the correction of the majority of lesions in the posterior urethra is easy; the trouble lies more in the failure to recognize them.

Comment: It is true there are many conditions in the posterior urethra amenable to proper treatment and often neglected to the chagrin of the physician in charge. However, one should use judgement and not be over enthusiastic to use such drastic treatments as much harm is done to those patients who tend to be on the neurotic side so far as their sexual organs are concerned. Before submitting an individual to such strenous procedures it is well to determine definitely by careful examination whether true pathology is actually present.

The Present Day Treatment of Hydrocele. J. Ullman Reaves, M.D. Southern Medical Journal, September, 1939.

The author discusses the modern treatment of hydrocele and finds in his own experience that the injection method is the most convenient and satisfactory. Contraindications to the procedure are: (1) The presence of certain types of hernia; (2) the presence of co-existing disease necessitating surgery; (3) abdomino scrotal hydrocele: (4) the presence of blood or pus in the sac.

His technic for the injection is performed as follows: After careful aspiration of the hydrocele fluid by tunneling under the skin of the scrotum into the sac with an 18 gauge needle, 2 to 4 cc. of quinine urethrane solution is injected into the empty sac and massaged gently to spread it evenly about. A well fitting scrotal support is applied and the patient goes about his duties to return in one week for another injection if it is found necessary. Usually two injections suffice for cure, but often as many as four are given.

--------o--------

Council Seals Speak For Themselves

If they could talk, Council Seals would say: "When you see one of us on a package of medicine or food, it means first of all that the manufacturer thought enough of the product to be willing to have it and his claims carefully examined by a board of critical, unbiased experts. . . . We're glad to tell you that this product was examined, that the manufacturer was willing to listen to criticisms and suggestions the Council made, that he signified his willingness to restrict his advertising claims to proved ones, and that he will keep the Council informed of any intended changes in product or claims. . . . There may be other similar products as good as this one, but when you see us on a package, you know. Why guess, or why take someone's self-interested word? If the product is everything the manufacturer claims, why should he hesitate to submit it to the Council, for acceptance?"

--------o--------

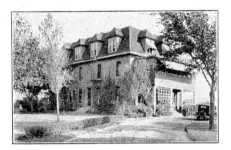
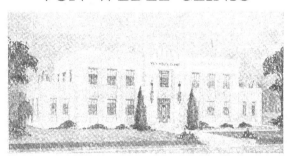

If they could talk,
Council Seals
would say:

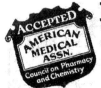

"When you see one of us on a package of medicine
or food, it means first of all that the manufacturer
thought enough of the product to be willing to have
it and his claims carefully examined by a board of
critical, unbiased experts . . . We're glad to tell you
that this product was examined, that the manufacturer
was willing to listen to criticisms and suggestions the
Council made, that he signified his willingness to restrict his advertising claims to <u>proved</u> ones, and that
he will keep the Council informed of any intended
changes in product or claims . . . There may be other
similar products as good as this one, but when you
see us on a package, <u>you know</u>. Why guess, or why
take someone's self-interested word? If the product
is everything the manufacturer claims, why should he
hesitate to submit it to the Council, for acceptance?"

THE FOLLOWING MEAD PRODUCTS ARE COUNCIL-ACCEPTED: Oleum Percomorphum (liquid and capsules);
Mead's Cod Liver Oil Fortified With Percomorph Liver Oil; Mead's Compound Syrup Oleum Percomorphum; Mead's
Viosterol in Halibut Liver Oil (liquid and capsules); Mead's Cod Liver Oil With Viosterol; Mead's Viosterol in Oil;
Mead's Standardized Cod Liver Oil; Mead's Halibut Liver Oil; Dextri-Maltose Nos. 1, 2, and 3; Dextri-Maltose With
Vitamin B; Pablum; Mead's Cereal: Mead's Mineral Oil With Malt Syrup; Mead's Brewers Yeast (powder and tablets);
Mead's Thiamin Chloride Tablets; Mead's Cevitamic Acid Tablets; Mead's Powdered Protein Milk; Mead's Powdered
Whole Milk; Mead's Powdered Lactic Acid Milk Nos. 1 and 2; Alacta; Casec; Sobee; Cemac; Olac.

THE FOLLOWING NEW PRODUCT IS BEFORE THE COUNCIL ON PHARMACY FOR ACCEPTANCE:
Mead's Nicotinic Acid Tablets.

THE JOURNAL
OF THE
OKLAHOMA STATE MEDICAL ASSOCIATION

VOLUME XXXII   McALESTER, OKLAHOMA, DECEMBER, 1939   Number 12

Published Monthly at McAlester, Oklahoma, under direction of the Council.

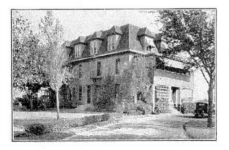
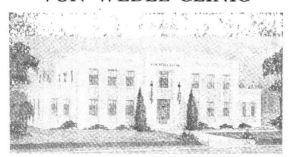

HOW MUCH SUN

Does the Baby Really Get?

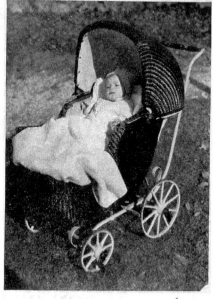

THIS BABY has been placed in the sunlight. (1) The mother discovers the baby is blinking, so she promptly shields its eyes and much of its face from the light. (2) Since the baby's body is covered, the child will then be getting only reflected light or "sky-shine" which is only 50% as effective as direct sunlight as an antiricketic agent (Tisdall). (3) Even if the baby were exposed nude, it has never been determined how much of the ergosterol of the skin is synthesized by the sun's rays (Hess). (4) Time of day also will affect the amount of sunshine or sky-shine reaching this baby's face. At 8:30 A. M., average loss of sunlight, regardless of season is over 31% and at 3:30 P. M. is over 21%. (5) Direct sunlight, moreover, is not always 100% efficient. U. S. Weather Bureau maps show that percentage of possible sunshine varies in different localities, due to differences in meteorological conditions. (6) In cities, smoke and dust, even in summer, are other factors reducing the amount of ultraviolet light.

While Oleum Percomorphum cannot replace the sun, it is a valuable supplement. Unlike the sun, it offers measurable potency in controlled dosage and does not vary from day to day or hour to hour. It is available at any hour, regardless of smoke, season, geography or clothing. A rich source of vitamins A and D, Oleum Percomorphum can be administered in drops, which makes it an ideal year-round antiricketic. Use the sun, too.

●

FOR GREATER ECONOMY, the 50 cc. size of Oleum Percomorphum is now supplied with Mead's patented Vacap-Dropper. It keeps out dust and light, is spill-proof, unbreakable, and delivers a uniform drop. The 10 cc. size of Oleum Percomorphum is still offered with the regulation type dropper.

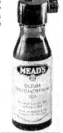

OLEUM PERCOMORPHUM
Ethically Marketed — Not Advertised to the Public

MEAD JOHNSON & COMPANY, EVANSVILLE, INDIANA, U. S. A.

Please enclose professional card when requesting samples of Mead Johnson products to cooperate in preventing their reaching unauthorized persons.

CPB

www.ingramcontent.com/pod-product-compliance
Lightning Source LLC
Chambersburg PA
CBHW071355050326
40689CB00010B/1651